Physics and Engineering of Medical Imaging

NATO ASI Series
Advanced Science Institutes Series

A Series presenting the results of activities sponsored by the NATO Science Committee, which aims at the dissemination of advanced scientific and technological knowledge, with a view to strengthening links between scientific communities.

The Series is published by an international board of publishers in conjunction with the NATO Scientific Affairs Division

A	Life Sciences	Plenum Publishing Corporation
B	Physics	London and New York
C	Mathematical and Physical Sciences	D. Reidel Publishing Company Dordrecht, Boston, Lancaster and Tokyo
D	Behavioural and Social Sciences	Martinus Nijhoff Publishers Boston, Dordrecht and Lancaster
E	Applied Sciences	
F	Computer and Systems Sciences	Springer-Verlag Berlin, Heidelberg, New York
G	Ecological Sciences	London, Paris, Tokyo
H	Cell Biology	

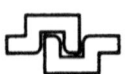

Series E: Applied Sciences – No. 119

Physics and Engineering of Medical Imaging

edited by
Riccardo Guzzardi
Head, Nuclear Imaging Division
C.N.R., Institute of Clinical Physiology
Via P. Savi, 8, 56100 Pisa
Italy

1987 **Martinus Nijhoff Publishers**
Dordrecht / Boston / Lancaster
Published in cooperation with NATO Scientific Affairs Division

Proceedings of the NATO Advanced Study Institute on "Physics and Engineering of Medical Imaging", Maratea, Italy, 23 September-5 October, 1984

```
NATO Advanced Study Institute on "Physics and
   Engineering of Medical Imaging" (1984 : Maratea,
   Italy.
   Physics and engineering of medical imaging.

   (NATO ASI series. Series E, Applied sciences :
no. 119)
   Proceedings of the NATO Advanced Study Institute on
"Physics and Engineering of Medical Imaging," Maratea,
Italy, 23 September-5 October, 1984"--T.p. verso.
   "Published in cooperation with NATO Scientific
Affairs Division."
   Includes index.
   1. Diagnostic imaging--Congresses. 2. Medical
physics--Congresses. 3. Biomedical engineering--
Congresses. I. Guzzardi, Riccardo. II. North Atlantic
Treaty Organization. Scientific Affairs Division.
III. Title. IV. Series. [DNLM: 1. Health Physics.
2. Nuclear Magnetic Resonance--congresses. 3. Nuclear
Medicine--congresses. 4. Radiography--congresses.
5. Radionuclide Imaging--congresses. 6. Technology,
Radiologic--congresses. 7. Ultrasonics--congresses.
WN 160 N2797p 1984]
RC78.7.D53N38 1984      616.07'57      86-28501
ISBN-13: 978-94-010-8081-1
```

ISBN-13: 978-94-010-8081-1   e-ISBN-13: 978-94-009-3537-2
DOI: 10.1007/978-94-009-3537-2
ISBN 90-247-2689-1 (series)

Distributors for the United States and Canada: Kluwer Academic Publishers, P.O. Box 358, Accord-Station, Hingham, MA 02018-0358, USA

Distributors for the UK and Ireland: Kluwer Academic Publishers, MTP Press Ltd, Falcon House, Queen Square, Lancaster LA1 1RN, UK

Distributors for all other countries: Kluwer Academic Publishers Group, Distribution Center, P.O. Box 322, 3300 AH Dordrecht, The Netherlands

All rights reserved. No part of this publication may be reproduced, stored in a retrieval system, or transmitted, in any form or by any means, mechanical, photocopying, recording, or otherwise, without the prior written permission of the publishers,
Martinus Nijhoff Publishers, P.O. Box 163, 3300 AD Dordrecht, The Netherlands
Softcover reprint of the hardcover 1st edition 1987
Copyright © 1987 by Martinus Nijhoff Publishers, Dordrecht

PREFACE & INTRODUCTION

PREFACE

The NATO Advanced Study Institute (ASI) on Physics and Engineering of Medical Imaging has addressed a subject which in the wide area of biomedical technology is one of those which are showing greater impact in the practice of medicine for the ability to picture both Anatomy and Physiology.

The information and accuracy obtained by whatever imaging methodology is a complex result of a multidisciplinary effort of several sciences such as Physics, Engineering, Electronics, Chemistry, Medicine, etc... Development has occurred through work performed in different environments such as basic and applied research laboratories, industries and clinical centers, with the aim of achieving an efficient transfer of know-how and technology for the improvement of both investigation possibilities and health care. On one hand, such an effort requires an ever-increasing committment of human and financial resources at research and industrial level, and, on the other, it meets serious difficulties in recruiting the necessary human expertise oriented to this technology which breaks with the traditional academic borders of the single disciplines.

Furthermore, the scientific community is continually dealing with the problem of increasing the performance and, at the same time, complexity and costs of instruments, applying more and more sophisticated technology in an effort to meet the demand for more complete and accurate clinical information. The scientific program of this ASI and the qualification of the authors reveals the intrinsic complexity of the development process of the Imaging methodologies.

In general, for the various Imaging modalities, the papers in the book provide: a) the introduction on the basic principles, technology and medical criteria, applied in the design of a selected imaging system;b) the description of the state-of-the-art instrumentation at research and industrial level; c) the critical evaluation of the clinical applications together with the indication of limits and future needs; d) the presentation of new concepts or prototype systems.

Special attention has been devoted to individuate those aspects common to the various modalities, e.g. Mathematics for Image Reconstruction, Hard-Copy, 3-D Display, Image Management Systems, as well as the clinical and technological correlation between the different techniques.

Specifically, Digital Radiology, besides the evaluation of its technological content and its future evolution, is examined in correlation with Nuclear Medicine techniques, in order to assess their relative role and merit as far as their applications to cardiac and vascular imaging are concerned. Another important issue is the induced cross-fertilization, which has materialized as a result of the satisfactory achievements of Nuclear Imaging in quantitative analysis of dynamic functions.

Always keeping the X-rays as the source of radiation, a specific section of the book examines how Computed Tomography will evolve in the NMR era, after its significant technological development and diffusion achieved in the past, and towards which objectives time resolution and volumetric imaging will evolve.

In the area of Ultrasound Imaging, which is perhaps the cheapest of the increasingly complex and expensive techniques, the following two apparently different problems are evaluated. On the one hand, how much will ultrasonic instruments be simplified and made compact in order for them to be used with the same simplicity as, for example, the electrocardiograph and, on the other, in order to extract quantitative information about tissues and flow, which new results can be obtained by the integration of the basic devices with the computer techniques.

The variability and the intrinsic technological complexity of Nuclear Magnetic Resonance Imaging is reviewed, including the evaluation of its clinical applications, analyzed in correlation with other imaging methods. Problems concerning the use of MRI for Imaging and Spectroscopy as well as economical and technological implications are evaluated.

The last important field to which this ASI has devoted much attention is Nuclear Medicine, which is divided into two sectors:

the widespread methodology of Single Photon Imaging and that of Positron Emission Tomography using short-lived radionuclides.

Since the beginning, the future of this field has never been accurately predicted and once again, an attempt has been made to analyze the major trends. This has been done in order to explore which new radiopharmaceuticals, using Single Photon Emitters, could strengthen the role of Nuclear Medicine, as a Physiological Imaging Modality, and whether Single Photon Tomography will become a reliable and efficient tool for dynamic studies in the future.

The technology applied to PET is far more complex than SPECT and despite some criticism about the gathered metabolic information, this modality presently offers a unique tool, worthy of being developed today.

Several aspects are carefully examined in order to evaluate whether Radiopharmaceutical Chemistry will be able to become reliable and simple enough to be applied routinely and in which clinical applications the results of PET will have the most significant impact, justifying the presently complex technological developments and the high cost.

The final section of the book is dedicated to the overall assessment of the imaging modalities and to the important problem of the transfer of the technology which is, after all, the actual key to the process and is allowing the evolution in this field.

The qualification of the ASI authors and participants and the time allotted for the topics allowed a deep evaluation of the subjects that I have recalled and many others. The main issues of the discussion for each session have been reported at the end of each specific chapter.

It is my hope that the information contained in this book could contribute to enhancing the development and to improving the application of Medical Imaging technologies.

Pisa, May 1985   Riccardo Guzzardi

Acknowledgments

The Editor wishes to express his appreciation to the following members of the Advisory Committee for the support and the cooperation in the preparation of the Scientific Program of the ASI:

Thomas F. Budinger
Lawrence Berkeley Laboratory, Berkeley, U.S.A.

Luigi Donato
C.N.R., Institute of Clinical Physiology, Pisa, Italy

Roger Gariod
L.E.T.I., Grenoble, France

Roger Griffoul
Thomson CGR, Issy Les Moulineax, France

Richard C. Reba
George Washington University Medical Center, Washington, U.S.A.

Peter N.T. Wells
Bristol General Hospital, U.K.

The Editor is particularly grateful to **Dr. Mario Di Lullo** and **Dr. Craig Sinclair** of the NATO Scientific Affairs Division for their fundamental support and encouragement. Also the organizative suggestions given by **DR. Harold Davidson** (U.S. Army Research) were highly appreciated. The ASI was co-sponsored by the **C.N.R. Special Project of Biomedical and Health Engineering** and it was also supported by:

Azienda Autonoma di Soggiorno e Turismo di Maratea (Italy)
Banca di Lucania (Italy)
Computer Technology @ Imaging (U.S.A.)
EG @ G ORTEC (Italy)

Elscint (Italy)
Face Teleinformatica (Italy)
Hewlett Packard (U.S.A.)
IBM (Italy)
Medimatic A/S (Denmark)
Photon Diagnostic Inc. (U.S.A.)
Regione Lucania (Italy)
Siemens Gammasonics (Italy)
Sorin Biomedica (Italy)
Thomson CGR (Italy)
U.S. Army Research, Development and Standardization Group (U.K.)

The Editor wishes to express a special thank to Miss Laura Bulleri for her indefatigable and enthusiastically performed activity both in the organization of the ASI and, with the essential help of **Miss Judith Brothwell** and **Miss Silvia Pardini**, in the revision and preparation of the manuscripts which are published in this book.

TABLE OF CONTENTS

Preface & Introduction

R. Guzzardi
Preface... VII

T.E. Malone
Research: A Sound Investment in Effective Health Care............ 1

PART I   BASIC ASPECTS OF MEDICAL IMAGING

R.A. Taube, S.J. Adelstein
A Short History of Modern Medical Imaging....................... 9

A. Rescigno
Image Analysis and the Method of Moments....................... 41

P. Garderet
Strategies of Reconstruction Algorithms for Computerized
Tomography... 73

Discussion Summary... 93

PART II   DIGITAL RADIOLOGY: PRINCIPLES, TECHNOLOGY AND
          CORRELATIVE ASPECTS WITH NUCLEAR MEDICINE

R.A. Kruger
Current Status of Digital Radiography.......................... 97

P. Heintzen
Cardiovascular Imaging by Roentgen Television Computer Techniques
.... 110

K.H. Höhne, U. Obermöller, M. Riemer, G. Witte
Advanced Techniques for Digital Angiography of the Heart........ 153

P. Marzullo, O. Parodi, C.R. Bellina, C. Marcassa, D. Neglia, A.
Benassi, A. Riva, A. L'Abbate
Cardiovascular Nuclear Medicine and Functional Imaging.......... 171

C.L. Partain, M.V. Kulkarni, R.R. Price, M.P. Sandler, J.A.
Patton, D.R. Pickens, J.J. Erickson, A.E. James
Digital Radiography and Nuclear Medicine: Correlative Aspects and
Technological Cross-Fertilization............................... 183

Discussion Summary.. 193

R. Bellazzini, A. Brez, A. Del Guerra, M.M. Massai, M.R. Torquati
Digital Radiography Using the Individual Photon Counting
Technique 197

PART III   X-RAY COMPUTED TOMOGRAPHY

R. Allemand
Basic Technological Aspects and Optimization Problems in X-Ray
Computed Tomography (C.T.)... 207

L. Di Guglielmo, A. Villa, L. Biazzi
Clinical Application of X-Ray CT: Results, Limitations and Future
Needs... 218

D.P. Boyd, K.R. Peschmann, R.E. Rand, J.L. Couch, S.A. Napel, R.
Gould, D.W. Farmer, M.J. Lipton, C.B. Higgins
Cine CT: a New Technology for Cardiac Computed Tomography......... 231

Discussion Summary 248

D.J. Hawkes, A.C.F. Colchester, C.R. Mol
The Accurate 3-D Reconstruction of the Geometric Configuration of
Vascular Trees from X-Ray Recordings 250

A. Kettschau, J. Goebbels
Application of Computer-Tomography in Industrial Problems......... 257

PART IV   ULTRASOUND IMAGING: CURRENT TRENDS AND CLINICAL
           APPLICATIONS

L. Masotti
Basic Principles and Advanced Technological Aspects of Ultrasound
Imaging... 263

H.E. Karrer
Phased Array Acoustic Imaging Systems............................. 318

A. Distante, E. Picano, E. Moscarelli
Ultrasounds in Cardiology: Recent Results, Limitations and Future
Needs... 340

L. Angelini
Advanced Applications of Ultrasound Imaging in Internal Medicine:
Results, Limitations and Future Needs............................. 357

P.N.T. Wells
Future Directions in Ultrasound Imaging: a Critical Evaluation... 361

Discussion Summary.. 376

P.A. Payne
High Resolution Medical Ultrasound: Applications in Rheumatology
and Dermatology... 378

PART V   GENERAL PROBLEMS I

D. Kaplan
Digital Archiving of Medical Images................................. 385

PART VI   GENERAL PROBLEMS II

A. Todd-Pokropek
3-D Display... 393

C.L. Partain, J.J. Erickson, J.A. Patton, R.R. Price, D.R. Pickens, A.E. James
Quality Assurance in Medical Imaging................................ 412

V. Cappellini
Medical and Non-Medical Imaging: Cross-Fertilization................ 417

Discussion Summary.. 436

PART VII   OTHER IMAGING MODALITIES

C. Corsi
Current State, Limitations and New Perspectives in Functional Patterns Obtained by Infrared and Microwave Radiometry............ 439

G.L. Romani, R. Leoni
Biomagnetism: a Non-Invasive New Approach for Imaging of Bioelectrical Sources in the Human Body...................................... 455

P.N.T. Wells
Possible Directions of Alternative Imaging Modalities: a Critical Overview.. 474

Discussion Summary.. 484

PART VIII PRINCIPLES AND APPLICATIONS OF NUCLEAR MAGNETIC RESONANCE IMAGING

R. Campanella, C. Casieri, F. De Luca, B.C. De Simone, B. Maraviglia
Basic Principles of NMR Imaging.. 489

P. Mansfield
Comparative Evaluation of NMR Imaging Techniques.................. 500

C.L. Partain, M.V. Kulkarni, M.R. Mitchell, J.A. Patton, M.P. Sandler, A.E. James
Clinical Nuclear Magnetic Resonance Imaging..................... 511

Discussion Summary 546

PART IX APPLICATIVE PROBLEMS AND FUTURE DIRECTIONS OF NMR FOR IN VIVO STUDIES

J.D. Weissman
State of the Art Magnetic Resonance Imaging....................... 551

Discussion Summary.. 561

PART X NUCLEAR MEDICINE AGENTS AND INSTRUMENTATION

P.H. Cox
Radiopharmaceuticals for In Vivo Diagnosis - Current Topics and Future Prospects... 569

A. Todd-Pokropek
Single Photon Imaging: State of the Art, Limitations and Future Needs... 575

J. Salomon
Digital Imaging in Nuclear Medicine.............................. 595

Discussion Summary.. 606

S. Ghione, E. Fommei, C.R. Bellina, C. Palombo, P. Meconi, L.S. Palla, C. Rosa
Transient Changes in Renal Uptake Rate of 99mTc DMSA as Possible Indicators of Changes of Renal Function During Stress............. 611

D. Neglia, C. Marcassa, O. Parodi, C.R. Bellina, P. Marzullo, C. Michelassi, S. Berti, C. Contini, A. L'Abbate
Optimization of Right Ventricular Ejection Fraction Measurements from First Pass and Gated Blood Pool Scintigraphy 615

PART XI STATE-OF-THE-ART AND FUTURE TRENDS IN SINGLE PHOTON TOMOGRAPHY

G. van Oortmarssen
Emission Tomography Using Rotating Cameras........................ 623

P. Rommer, J.R. Olsson, N.A. Lassen
High Efficiency Multislice Approach for Single Photon Tomography
of the Brain... 646

H.F. Stoddart
Design and Performance of the Cleon Two-Dimensional Focused-Ray
Geometry Scanner for Single Photon Tomography..................... 674

T.C. Hill, B.L. Holman, S. Moore, P. Kasulis, M.E. Clouse
Clinical Comparison between Multi-Ring Detector and Rotating Gamma
Camera for Single Photon Tomography 682

Discussion Summary... 691

U. Biader Ceipidor, F. Fusco, E. Muciaccia, M.A. Macrì
Evaluation of the Computer Artifacts Generated in SPECT
Reconstruction... 694

K. Knesaurek
Limited Angle Sampling in SPECT................................... 699

G. Perri, B. Fedeli, F. Zito, M. Mey, R. Guzzardi, V. Giordano
X-Ray Tomography vs Compton Scattering in the Diagnosis of
Pulmonary Diseases... 704

M.A. Viergever, J.W. van Giessen
Seven Pinhole Tomography of the Heart............................. 708

L.P. Clarke, A. Gentili, C.B. Saw, P.Kenny, A.N. Serafini
SPECT Collimation for Medium-High Energy: Influence of Spatial
Resolution and Image Contrast Within Transverse Plane............. 714

PART XII POSITRON EMITTERS RADIONUCLIDES, RADIOCHEMISTRY AND BIOTRACERS

A.P. Wolf, J.S. Fowler
Cyclotrons and Positron Emitting Radiopharmaceuticals............. 721

C. Crouzel
Radiopharmaceuticals for Positron Tomography...................... 750

J.A.G. Russell, D.L. Alexoff, A.P. Wolf
Distributed Microprocessor Automation Network for Synthesizing
Radiotracers used in Positron Emission Tomography.................. 765

P.A. Salvadori
Design Aspects of Installation for PET Radiochemistry............. 782

E.M. Ferdeghini, P.A. Salvadori, R. Guzzardi, A. Benassi
An Automatic Line for the Production of Radiopharmaceuticals...... 792

PART XIII   PHYSIOLOGICAL MEASUREMENTS BY POSITRON EMISSION TOMOGRAPHY

T. Jones
In Vivo Biochemistry, Physiology and Pharmacology Studies using
Positron Emitting Radionuclides................................... 797

E.J. Hoffman
Evaluation of Performance and Accuracy in PET..................... 802

O. Parodi, P. Camici
Advanced Cardiological Application of PET......................... 813

G.L. Lenzi, C. Fieschi
PET in Neurology: an Outline of Problems, Recent Acquisitions and
Future Perspectives... 829

A. Rescigno, R.M. Lambrecht, C.C. Duncan, C.Y. Shiue, L.R. Ment
Simultaneous Determination of Cerebral Blood Flow and Partition
Coefficient with a Freely Diffusable Tracer....................... 836

Discussion Summary 845

C. Paoli, R. Porinelli, M.G. Trivella, R. Bellazzini, M. Massai,
M. Dalle Vacche, G. Pelosi, A. L'Abbate
Computerized Millimetric Mapping of Myocardial Blood Flow and
Metabolism.. 846

PART XIV   STATE-OF-THE-ART AND FUTURE TRENDS IN PET INSTRUMENTATION

S.E. Derenzo, T.F. Budinger
Advanced Instrumentation for Positron Emission Tomography......... 855

E.J. Hoffman
Signal to Noise Improvement in PET Using BGO...................... 874

R. Nutt, M. Crabtree
The ECAT: A Recent Solution to High Efficiency, High Resolution
Tomography... 882

R. Allemand
Time-of-Flight Positron Emission Tomography (T.O.F. P.E.T.)....... 902

S. E. Derenzo
Potential Improvements in Instrumentation for PET................. 913

Discussion Summary 926

A.R. Ricci, M. Dahlbom, E.J. Hoffman
Comparison of Resolution and Crosstalk among Detectors Used in
Positron Emission Tomography...................................... 928

PART XV   GENERAL REMARKS

S.J. Adelstein
Comparative Assessment of Imaging................................. 937

R. Gariod
Perspective of Diffusion of Imaging Technologies.................. 948

Subject Index... 971

List of Participants.. 979

Colour Section 997

RESEARCH: A SOUND INVESTMENT IN EFFECTIVE HEALTH CARE

Thomas E. Malone

National Institutes of Health, Bethesda, Maryland, U.S.A.

A virtual revolution has occurred in the practice of medicine over the past 50 years, but in the very recent past, we have seen the development of powerful new technologies for the diagnosis and treatment of disease. Among the most spectacular advances are those accociated with imaging techniques made possible by the almost incredible leaps of understanding that have taken place in electronics, computer science, physics, molecular biology and physiology. Within the biomedical scientific enterprise itself during recent years there has been a convergence having profound implications. Nobel laureate Arthur Kornberg recently called attention to the 'confluence of many discrete and previously unrelated medical subjects into a single unified discipline'. He observed that 'anatomy, physiology, biochemistry, microbiology, immunology and genetics have now been merged and are expressed in a common language of chemistry'.

In writing about the exciting time in medical history when antibiotics were discovered, Lewis Thomas stated that 'It needs emphasizing that it took about 50 years of concentrated effort in basic research to reach this level' and 'if this research had not been done, we could not have guessed that streptococci and pneumococci exist and the search for antibiotics would have made no sense at all'.

The distinguished British physician and scientist, Sir Harold Himsworth expressed the same thought in somewhat different words. He said that 'When future historians look back at the period in which we are living, they are likely to see it as that time in which scientific knowledge emerged from its adolescence to become a major factor in the affairs of human societies'.

Indeed I can think of no clearer example of the emergence of mature science as a factor in society than the technologies that are discussed in this book.

The progress in the last two generations in the application of science to health has stimulated expectations. People today are being taught to expect good health care. In the past, throughout history man has tended to accept illness, plagues and personal injury as 'normal'. This is no longer the case, the newfound ability of medicine to control or even to eradicate disease - a direct legacy of research - has brought into being new human expectations and even demands. Inevitably, such a development has major economic implications.

The complex calculus of cost-benefit analysis of medical progress is illustrated in an example cited 20 years ago by Dr. Lowell Coggeshall, then Vice President for Medical Affairs of the University of Chicago. Writing in a report on medical education, he compared costs of the old and new medicine. 'Once', he said 'it took only one doctor to resign himself and the child's parents to the inevitable death of a blue baby; it now takes a team of medical specialists and auxiliary personel to correct the congenital abnormality of a baby's heart to ensure the child a normal lifespan. More than 100 medical specialists, nurses and skilled technicians are involved in preparations for and performance of the operation as well as in the postsurgical care of the patient. This example points to the fallacy inherent in using dollars or lira or pounds or francs to measure the costs versus benefits of medical research and innovations. Basically, the costs of research and the health benefits it makes possible are incommensurable. However, in the course of seeking funds for research enterprise, persons in positions like mine are constantly being called upon to justify the purpose of the substantial investment required. To justify to the Congress and the Administration our request for funds at the NIH, my colleagues and I have emphasized the intangible and incalculable human benefits - the improvements in the quality of life - that have come from research and frankly, I cannot suggest a better reason for the current national investment in biomedical research and development. But there is another effect of biomedical research, a benefit that is perhaps more evident to economists than to bioscientists.

We are not accustomed to viewing biomedical research as a financier might scrutinize the cost-benefit track record of an industry. A five-year study attempting to quantify the worth of biomedical research was conducted in the United States in the late seventies.

The results were published in 1979 in a book by Selma J. Mushkin titled 'Biomedical Research: Costs and Benefits'. The study addressed the question, 'Is the public getting an appropriate return for the multibillion dollar yearly expenditure on health research? The answer was an emphatic 'yes' when the measures used included actuarial estimates of the dollar value of the productivity of the lives saved and the years of sickness averted. For the 75-year period beginning in 1900, the ratio of total cumulative benefits to total research and development costs was about 13 to 1. In more recent years since 1930, the ratio was 5 to 1. The recent somewhat lower but still spectacular return includes the high level of basic research during the past 40 years, whose pay-offs are certain to affect strongly and favourably the future ratios of benefits to costs.

Recent events have highlighted other beneficial and tangible effects of the national investment in biomedical research. For example, in the past 7 or 8 years, a totally new industry has emerged from the utilization of recombinant DNA, cell fusion and related technologies that were developed with public funds. In just one year - 1983 - a billion dollars was invested in the United States by the private sector for the commercialization of the products of these new discoveries. Similar and perhaps even more spectacular findings would result from economic case studies of the impact of the various technologies for imaging. I read a recent report that although NMR diagnostic imaging systems are barely past the research stage, this equipment will emerge in 1984 as a significant and high-growth commercial activity. Worldwide sales are forecast to reach over 150 million USD in 1984 and 700 million USD by 1988.

In the context of these economic benefits, we encounter a paradox: namely, that a substantial number of medicine's discoveries in recent years have increased rather than decreased the costs of medical care. This is an aspect of the economics of research about which there has been considerable public discussion of late. Writing in the Washington Post last June, staff writer Spencer Rich summarized the predictions of a number of experts in health care and research as follows: 'Costly medical innovations such as heart and liver transplant and expensive futuristic diagnostic techniques could plunge the Nation into vast additional expenditures over the next generation and confound efforts to rein in health outlays'. When considering this question, however, we must not forget that each of these innovations represents for the patients involved supremely important progress, hope and benefits that cannot be measured.

In speaking of the human side of the use of modern technology and the practice of medicine, I am aware that there are those who say with some validity that as the technology and complexity of medicine have increased, medical care has become more institutionalized and its delivery depersonalized. A widely held view, particularly among nonphysicians, is that the science and technology of medicine are responsible for the perceived decline of compassion in medicine as though there were something inherently contradictory between science and humanity - between technology and compassion. There is, of course, no evidence for such an inherent contradiction. Science and technology underlie most of the advances of medicine that enable contemporary physicians to render more effective medical care than their professional forebears were able to offer. From this perspective computed tomography, for example, can be viewed as a technological advance of extraordinary compassion. Its use has spared patients many difficult, painful and dangerous procedures and has permitted definitive diagnoses to be made earlier. With recent advances in tomography and ultrasound, exploratory surgery, for example, has become almost a thing of the past. Good science and complex technology applied for the patient constitutes the prime example of human medicine. Physicians cannot be made more compassionate by downgrading science. On the other hand, their efforts can be made infinitely more effective through the application of the fruits of basic science. The CAT scanner, for example, has altered forever the practice of neurology and neurosurgery. It has become the single most valuable tool for prying open the armor encasing the brain and spinal cord and for detecting and pinpointing nervous system disorders. Just as the tremendous advances in imaging involved multiple stages of development - so the optimal uses of such promising devices must be evolved. A kind of Newton's third law operates with respect to the powerful means that have been developed in the past few generations for diagnosis, treatment or prevention of disease. The same capabilities that make such measures tremendously useful can also make them capable of serious abuse. Let me mention a few examples of well-intentioned but potentially dangerous misuse of medical devices. Most of us well remember mass X-ray screening for tuberculosis. It was less than 10 years ago when our agency, the NIH, decided to terminate its support for breast cancer. Perhaps a few of you are old enough to remember when typical large shoe stores used the fluoroscope for assuring that new shoes fit properly.

While the newer techniques for imaging have largely eliminated the hazardous aspects of the former methods, there has been some tendency to employ these complex and expensive devices for less than optimal if not trivial purposes. In the United States, there is a great deal of concern about the rising costs of medical care and, in this context, the new techniques for imaging, properly employed, offer the potential for savings in the costs of medical care by assisting in early diagnosis and minimizing the need for exploratory surgery. The part of the department where I am employed, the National Institutes of Health, centers its concerns on the medical and scientific issues concerning the use of the new methods of imaging.

In November 1981 the National Institutes of Health sponsored a conference at which the scientific evidence related to computed tomographic scanning of the brain was reviewed. The session was one of a series we call Consensus Development Conferences where we bring together investigators in the biomedical sciences, clinical investigators, physicians and consumer and special interest groups to make a scientific assessment of technologies and to seek agreement on their safety and effectiveness. Presentation by experts from a variety of fields indicated that the CT is a safe, accurate and powerful tool in the primary diagnosis of, among other conditions, brain tumors, brain hemorrhages, effects of major head injury, certain infections of the brain. Given its speed, accuracy and low dosage, CT has displaced a number of other radiological diagnostic procedures, many of which in comparison are more uncomfortable, more dangerous and more costly to the patients. In addition, the panel considered the geographic distribution of CT scanners and the current patterns of diagnostic usage. Two important considerations emerged. It appeared to the panel that in the United States, CT may not be sufficiently available for the public to derive the full benefit of this diagnostic tool. Evidence pointed to an insufficient number of instruments in several large metropolitan areas in medically underserved areas and in some sparsely populated regions where the prevalence of head trauma is high. In some instances, however, the indiscriminate use of CT occurred in patients unlikely to have structural disease and this resulted in the displacement of patients for whom the technology is critical. Accordingly, the consensus report suggested appropriate criteria for the use of CT in current medical practice. My colleagues at NIH tell me that magnetic resonance imaging is at the moment the most exciting new diagnostic imaging modality. In March of this year, the chief of the diagnostic radiology department of the Clinical Center of the National Institutes of Health began a two-year study in an attempt to evaluate the role of NMR imaging with respect to its ability to provide useful and unique diagnostic information on a variety of diseases. We plan to study a wide range of diseases during the initial year of imaging involving perhaps as many as a thousand patients. The study will utilize Whole Body NMR Imaging. Among the tentatively proposed protocols, the National Institute of Neurological and Communicative Disorders and Stroke will conduct studies on post-trauma paraplegia patients on cerebellopontine angle tumors, acoustic neuromas and multiple sclerosis. For the National Institute of Mental Health, the studies will include pediatric and adult development dyslexias. For the National Heart, Lung and Blood Institute, iron storage overload studies in the heart, pituitary and pancreas. In addition, studies will be made of septal asymmetry and cardiac outflow. For the Cancer Institute, presurgical NMR imaging for lung cancer, for ovarian carcinoma or pediatric sarcomas of the extremities. For such studies, we hope to add to the general information about the optimal uses of this important new technique as compared with computerized tomography, ultrasound and positron emission tomography. Earlier in my remarks, I talked of the confluence of disciplines within the biomedical field and - of the example provided by imaging devices - of the convergence of mathematics, physics, physiology and molecular biology. This conference itself exemplifies convergence in a different realm, the exciting developments discussed during the meeting represent the joint and complementary efforts of scientists and engineers based in academic institutions, in industrial organizations and in governmental agencies.

PART I BASIC ASPECTS OF MEDICAL IMAGING

Chairman: Andrew Todd Pokropek (U.K.)

A Short History of Modern Medical Imaging

R.A. Taube and S.J. Adelstein

Department of Radiology
Harvard Medical School
Boston, Ma, U.S.A.

INTRODUCTION

Roentgen's discovery of x-rays revolutionized diagnostic medicine. For the first time, physicians could visualize internal organs and determine with precision whether bones were broken, hearts enlarged, or lungs opacified. Cannon's introduction of heavy element contrast material to study the physiology of the gastrointestinal system opened up another dimension and increased the utility of radiological procedures. Heavy element contrast material was used, albeit briefly, to visualize the liver and spleen with thorotrast and, more lastingly, as iodinated material to display the kidneys, vascular system and spinal canal. Obversely, air has been used as a contrast agent in the nervous system and bowel as well. With these important but relatively primitive tools, a vast experience with two-dimensional radiology was developed along with procedures that by the early 1960s were providing some 60% of all medical diagnoses.

In the past two decades, there has been a second revolution in medical imaging, one that has greatly extended our ability to define disease in terms of anatomic and physiological detail. This revolution was born from the confluence of several factors: an explosion in instrumental technology stemming from advances in electronics, nuclear and information sciences; progress in the life sciences leading to a deeper understanding of disease processes; and a marked increase in the range of human disorders amenable to treatment, if not to cure. The chemical and physical nuclear sciences produced the first practical breakthrough in nuclear medicine, followed rapidly by the medical application of acoustical science to ultrasound. With some lag, advances in tomography and data processing requiring substantial computer power led to developments in transmission and emission computed tomography and digital angiography. Last to be introduced was a modality (nuclear magnetic resonance) that reflects progress in magnet, microwave, and computer-based technology.

It should be recognized that in each of the new modalities positional signals, whether they be gamma or x-ray photons, sound waves or radio waves are rendered into visual images. We have transformed the invisible electromagnetic and acoustic spectra into charts of optical frequencies that contain the positional (and textural) information best processed by the human brain.

In this essay, we will try to follow the several threads which have led to this second revolution in medical imaging. We will not attempt to present the basic antecedents in the general sciences which have made the new methods possible or to trace the historical development of each of these modalities. Instead we shall focus on a few particular situations in which the potential application to medical diagnosis became apparent. Without doubt, we are much too close to these events and a still evolving technology to have a true perspective.

ULTRASOUND IMAGING

In the nineteenth century as methods evolved for the generation and detection of ultrasound, scientists began to explore its characteristics. Pierre and Jacques Curie in 1880 discovered the phenomenon of piezoelectricity, and it was in France that the approaches and methodology for producing directed ultrasonic waves were developed. In the years before and during World War One attempts were made to use ultrasound for locating submarines, mapping the ocean bottom, and communicating underwater. With the development of vacuum tube technology and the increased availability of sources based on piezoelectricity or magnetostriction in the 1920s, considerable progress was made in applying ultrasonic energy to maritime use as described by Langevin in 1928 (1). By March of that year there was an experimental apparatus mounted on the ocean liner Ile de France for mapping the sea floor. Undersea communication between ships and also between a fixed transmitting station and ships had reached a fair degree of precision.

Dussik was the first to research the use of ultrasound for medical diagnosis. Beginning in 1937, he developed a "through transmission" technique to detect intracranial tumors, sending the ultrasonic energy through transmitting and receiving transducers placed on opposite sides of the head and mapping changes in attenuation (2). The data obtained were of questionable value, but this work later stimulated other investigators who had much improved instrumentation based on pulsed echo detection techniques developed during World War Two for SONAR (sound navigation and ranging) and metal flaw detection.

In the late 1940s three independent investigators in the United States demonstrated that as ultrasound waves were sent into the body echoes would return to the same transducer by reflection from tissue interfaces of different density. Ludwig working with Struthers at the Naval Medical Research Institute implanted gallstones into the back muscles of dogs. Following wound healing, the calculi were localized by ultrasound (3). He soon recognized the difficulties inherent in the clinical use of the technique, particularly those associated with marked attenuation of sound produced by gas filled intestines. One of his most significant contributions consisted in measuring the velocity of sound transmission through a variety of soft tissues (4).

Wild at the University of Minnesota was able to measure bowel wall thickness in vitro utilizing elements from a U.S. Navy Ultrasonic Trainer device 15-Z-1. The calculation of wall thickness was based on the rate of sound transmission and the ultrasonically measured distance between anterior and posterior wall echoes. He also recognized that the echo pattern from normal stomach tissue differed significantly from that of cancerous stomach tissue, and demonstrated three different echoes from the intestine wall which he assumed represented the three layers of the intestine. His work firmly established the pulse-echo technique in ultrasound diagnosis. The first two-dimensional echograms were obtained in 1952 from an apparatus designed by Wild and Reid whose major clinical interests lay in the diagnosis of breast lesions. This technique is now known as brightness mode (B-mode) display (5). Wild was the first to conceive of ultrasound as a method for tissue characterization rather than an anatomical imaging technique.

Howry working in his basement with two engineers, Bliss and then Posakony, demonstrated that an ultrasonic echo interface existed between fat and muscle and that the return echoes could be recorded on a scope (6). He developed a water path scanner in which the subject's extremity was submerged in water in a cattle tank and the transducer carriage moved along a wooden rail at the side of the tank. The echo picture obtained lacked a two-dimensional appearance. In the 1950s, in collaboration with Holmes at the University of Colorado, he developed compound scanning which eliminated most artifacts and permitted the recording of curved or angular tissue interfaces thus producing an accurate anatomical picture in the B mode (7). Good scans of the liver (abscesses and cysts), spleen, kidney, bladder and breast were obtained.

Donald of Glasgow, Scotland, also initiated studies of diagnostic soft-tissue ultrasound in 1954, taking pathological specimens to an atomic boiler plant to examine them with a metal flaw detector. After he borrowed A-mode equipment from Mayneord at the Royal Marsden Hospital in England, he was able to substantiate his conviction that tumor tissue had a different echo pattern from normal tissue and to detect ovarian cysts, ascites, and hydramnios (8). Working with Brown, an engineer at Kelvin Hughes, Donald helped to design a contact-compound scanner which was mounted on a bedside table and suspended over the patient. The transducer was manipulated by hand underneath the table. The B-mode pictures obtained were crude, but marked the beginning of the use of this mode in obstetrics, a field which has benefited enormously from further developments. Among those exploring its use in obstetrical diagnosis were Kossoff and Garrett in Australia who constructed a contact-compound water path scanner and performed many of the early studies (9).

Echocardiography had its beginnings in Sweden in 1954 when Edler and Hertz, borrowing a flaw detector from the Malmo Ship Yards, used intensity modulation and motion displays as wave patterns to demonstrate intracardiac structures. The work laid the foundations of one-dimensional time-motion display or M-mode sonography (10). After the two investigators obtained a more sensitive Siemens flaw detector, they were more successful, and when Edler established the characteristic motion pattern for the anterior leaflet of the mitral valve, the diagnostic potential of echocardiography was established (11). Hertz spent a year at Siemens constructing additional equipment, one unit of which was given to Effert who placed the transducer directly on the heart and verified previous identifications of the intracardiac motion patterns (12).

Work continued in the fields of echocardiography (13,14) and echoencephalography (15-18) and ophthalmic techniques were developed (19,20). By the early 1960s ultrasound had become a promising diagnostic modality for soft tissue imaging. The field has progressed along two parallel pathways with technical efforts producing more sophisticated instrumentation and empirical studies leading to new clinical procedures.

TRANSMISSION COMPUTED TOMOGRAPHY

The practical history of x-ray transmission computed tomography is relatively brief, but the impact of this modality has already been enormous. In addition to revolutionizing roentgenology, it has fostered major advances in nuclear magnetic resonance and radionuclide imaging and promising developments in ultrasound.

The principles of computed tomography were based on the work of Radon, an Austrian mathematician interested in gravitational fields, who proved in 1917 that a three-dimensional object could be reconstructed from the infinite set of all its projections. The evolution of reconstruction techniques as an imaging tool occurred in several disciplines: solar astronomy where they were used to produce a map of the emission of microwave radiation from the sun (21,22); electron micrography where the structure of complex molecules could be reconstructed from electron transmission images obtained as the specimen was rotated in an electron beam (23,24); and the interpretation of optical problems (25,26). The components necessary for building the CT scanner were also in place: that x-rays cause crystals to scintillate was observed shortly after Roentgen's discovery, followed over the next half century by the development of electronics and computer technology.

In 1956, Cormack, as attending nuclear physicist at the Groote Schuur Hospital in Capetown, South Africa, had occasion to observe the planning of radiotherapy treatment. Realizing that the isodose charts used by hospital physicists were for homogeneous materials and that the human body is inhomogeneous, it occurred to him that the accuracy of treatment planning could be improved if the distribution of the attenuation coefficient of tissues in the body could be determined. Shortly thereafter, he realized that this distribution, found by measurements made external to the body, would also be useful for diagnostic purposes. The exponential attenuation of x- and gamma-rays had been known and used for over 60 years in terms of parallel-sided homogeneous slabs of material. Cormack assumed the generalization had been extended to inhomogeneous materials, but his search through the literature did not turn up the information, and it was not until 14 years later that he learned Radon had previously solved the problem (27).

In 1957, Cormack moved to Tufts University in Medford, Massachusetts, where he worked intermittently on reconstruction tomography. By 1963, he had dealt with many of the mathematical problems involved and was ready to experiment using a nonsymmetrical phantom consisting of an outer ring of aluminum, representing the skull, an inner core of lucite representing soft tissue and two aluminum disks representing tumors. A computer was used for processing the transmission data obtained at 7-1/2 degree angular increments. The computed tomography scanner was assembled at a cost of approximately $100. The results obtained and those from the early studies begun in 1956 were published in 1963-64 (28,29) and received virtually no response. It is this work on which was based Cormack's 1979 Nobel Prize in physiology and medicine which he shared with Hounsfield.

During the decade of the 60s, there were other investigators exploring various approaches to reconstruction tomography as potential imaging techniques including its use as a possible aid to planning radiation therapy - Oldendorf (30), Kuhl and Edwards (31), Tretiak, Eden and Simon (32), Gordon, Bender and Herman (24), Bates and Peters (33). The final breakthrough to a practical photon x-ray scanner was made by Hounsfield, an electronics engineer at Electro Musical Industries in England, who was involved in research into pattern recognition using computers. He had investigated the possibility that a computer might be able to reconstruct an object from sets of very accurate x-ray measurements taken through the body at many different angles.

Hounsfield decided the most convenient form of presenting the data would be a series of slices from which a three-dimensional representation of the object could be built up. Therefore, the transmission readings taken through the object could be limited to a single plane. All measurements would be contained within the slice so that a closed solution of the contents would be possible. Many hundreds of thousands of measurements would have to be taken and it was thought at the time an equal number of simultaneous equations would have to be solved, so the task seemed a tremendous undertaking. However, upon calculation it appeared that this kind of a system could handle data very efficiently and might be two orders of magnitude more sensitive than conventional x-rays. Although Hounsfield could find no references in the literature which suggested that x-ray absorption differences existed among the various tissues, he hoped that the technique would be able to distinguish between the tissues of the body (34).

Hounsfield constructed a prototype CT scanner in order to obtain data for confirming his computer calculations. The machine consisted of a collimated americium-241 gamma source and a sodium iodide detector positioned on opposite sides of a motorized lathe bed that could undergo both rotational and translational motion. The original objects scanned were perspex models. Because of the low intensity gamma source, each scan took 9 days. Processing the data on the computer consumed 2-1/2 hours. The results were obtained on punched paper tape which was then fed through a paper tape recorder - a 2 hour procedure - connected to a modified oscilloscope that displayed the readings as a trace on its screen. In order to obtain a more intense source of radiation, the gamma source was soon replaced by an x-ray tube, and the time needed to collect the data was reduced to 9 hours.

Thinking that the method, if speeded up, might have clinical application, Hounsfield visited radiologists at a number of hospitals and then approached the Department of Health in London. He told them that he had a technique for resolving differences in absorption coefficients to 1 in 1000, and he demonstrated this by showing them a computer print-out and a polaroid picture of three synthetic materials in a bowl of water. A preserved brain specimen was obtained from a hospital museum and gave very encouraging pictures distinguishing gray and white matter, although some of the differences were later determined to be artifactual.

The first computed tomographic scanner for clinical use was installed at Atkinson Morley's Hospital in Wimbledon and was ready for use by October 1, 1971. The time from design to working model was just over a year. The scanner employed synchronous translation of the x-ray source and the sodium iodide detector with each translation occurring in a separate angular increment of one degree over a 180 degree arc. A water bag placed around the patient's skull functioned to make the x-ray transmission path equal in all directions. A total of 28,800 measurements recorded on magnetic tape was made in 4-1/2 minutes; the picture processing could be completed in 20 minutes. The original specifications stipulated that the picture should be produced on a 160 x 160 matrix, but using the available computer program would have required 80 minutes for processing the data. The first diagnostic scan demonstrated a left frontal lobe tumor. The positive results were obtained two days after the data were collected at the hospital, as the magnetic tape had to be taken to the Electro Musical Industries factory for computer processing. In April 1972, the clinical CT data obtained on this scanner were presented at the annual meeting of the British Institute of Radiology and later in the same year similar material was presented at the International Congress of Radiology and the Radiological Society of North America. Clinical papers were first published in 1973 (35,36).

EMISSION COMPUTED TOMOGRAPHY

Emission computed tomography (ECT) uses the principles of computed tomography to reconstruct the distribution of a radioactive nuclide in the body. It shares with x-ray computed tomography its early history, and advances in the latter modality have stimulated investigators in this area. While transmission computed tomography generates structural and morphological data, emission computed tomography tends to provide information on the physiological and biochemical state of an organ or tissue (37).

Although the clinical potential of emission computed tomography was initially explored well in advance of that of transmission computed tomography, the field has not evolved so rapidly. The reconstruction process is more difficult when the radiation is emitted from a radionuclide in a patient, because corrections are required for attenuation of the radiation through different thicknesses of tissue and for variations in distance between the detector and the radionuclide. These problems can be solved in part by using positron-emitting radionuclides, but these present other complications including the need for a convenient source of short-lived cyclotron-produced nuclides, and the development of appropriate radiopharmaceuticals and instruments for high resolution imaging.

Depending on the kind of radiation released from the administered radiopharmaceutical, ECT can be divided into two separate branches: single photon emission computed tomography (SPECT) in which conventional scintillation cameras or specifically designed detector arrays process the gamma emissions from readily available radionuclides such as technetium-99m, thallium-201, and iodine-131, and positron emission tomography (PET) in which specially designed instruments of two types assay the annihilation radiation emitted from the decay of positron emitters such as fluorine-18, oxygen-15, nitrogen-13, and carbon-11 (38).

The history of SPECT begins with the work of Kuhl, Edwards and coworkers at the University of Pennsylvania. As early as 1959, Kuhl began to apply tomographic principles developed in diagnostic radiology to radionuclide scanning in order to separate images. He was also interested in exploring the possibility that scans could be used as autoradiographs for the analysis of the distribution of radioactivity in the body. He proposed that discrimination of an image from its background could be improved by separation of the images according to their depth in the body. Focal-plane tomography, section scanning and stereoscopic methods were explored using phantoms (31). Kuhl and Edwards constructed a scanning instrument consisting of a dual detection system, perforated paper tape data storage, and time compression read-out of the image (Mark II). With this instrument, transverse section scanning of the liver and brain was initiated (39). The investigators were hampered by the lack of sophisticated computer software. Technetium-99m labeled radiopharmaceuticals were also in their infancy (40), and the reconstructions were quite photon limited. The early scans did not have good resolution, but they seemed to provide more effective localization of lesions in these organs. This group continued to focus on transverse section imaging of the brain, and with the evolution of computer technology, their Mark III scanner was completely computerized (41). The next improvement was the development of the orthogonal tangent correction, an iterative technique in which the profile from a detector was corrected using the count rate profile from an orthogonal detector. The final matrix formed was a high contrast image of the cross-section, and there was a linear relationship between matrix counts and radioactivity in the scanned object (42). This approach to SPECT provides images perpendicular to the detector surfaces and is called transaxial tomography. There have been other multidetector tomographic scanners marketed commercially - the first of which was the Cleon 710 Brain Imager (43), followed by the Tomogscanner, and the Tomomatic 64. All of these multiple crystal instruments require considerable time for image formation which limits their clinical utility.

Transaxial tomography can also be performed using either a single-crystal scintillation camera with parallel hole collimators which rotates around the patient, or the reverse, a stationary camera and a rotating patient. Early efforts to develop a rotating camera system include those of Freedman from Yale University (44), Budinger, Gullberg, McRae and Anger at the University of California, Berkeley (45), Keyes and his group at the University of Michigan Medical Center (46), Jaszczak, Huard, Murphy and their associates at Baylor College of Medicine in Houston (47). Advantages of the scintillation camera include the ability to record images simultaneously from multiple planes and the capability of employing the system for routine frontal plane imaging. The disadvantages are the loss of spatial resolution and sensitivity with depth. There have been some commercial instruments; the earliest was that produced by SELO Corporation of Milan. Siemens Gammasonics and Picker International have also marketed units. The General Electric 400 T is mounted in a gantry so that the detector assembly can be rotated at any desired radius around the patient. Variations on the basic systems continue to be advanced and to be evaluated with respect to resolution, sensitivity and imaging times (48-51).

The second approach to SPECT, longitudinal or limited angle tomography, in which images are formed in planes parallel to the surfaces of detectors will not be discussed in detail. The general idea was applied to radioisotope imaging in 1965 by Anger, and by 1967 he had built the multiplane tomographic scanner (52). Several modes have been developed for use with conventional scintillation cameras including pinhole arrays (53,54), stochastic coded apertures (55-57), and Fresnel coding (58). Attempts have also been made to solve mathematically with iterative techniques some of the problems inherent in this approach (59).

Interest has existed for many years in the formation of radionuclide images by detection of annihilation radiation released during positron decay of internally deposited radionuclides. Wrenn (60) and Brownell (reported by Sweet, 61) in 1951 independently suggested the possibility of imaging brain tumors with this method. The first practical positron imaging device was created by Brownell and Sweet and consisted of a pair of sodium iodide detectors which scanned mechanically over the head to record the number of annihilation photons detected in coincidence. This system was used for evaluating the localization of arsenic-74 in brain tumors (75 percent accuracy) and abscesses (83 percent accuracy). Subsequently other organs such as the liver, pancreas, kidney and lung were scanned with copper-64 and zinc-65 (62). Based on this experience the group at the Massachusetts General Hospital developed a more sophisticated single pair scanning system (63); from 1956 to the present, this device and its successors have been in continuous routine clinical and research use.

In addition to the group at the Massachusetts General Hospital, there were other workers involved in positron imaging. Anger in 1966 demonstrated that two static scintillation cameras could produce images without the use of a conventional collimator (64). The system produced excellent high resolution images in a variety of biological applications and demonstrated the tomographic properties inherent in any device using nonparaxial rays. Similar focusing techniques have been used in later instrumentation. Limitations in count rate were a major drawback to the system. The possibility of transverse section imaging with positron-emitting radioisotopes had also been realized for some time. Rankowitz, Robertson, Bozzo, Marr and their associates at Brookhaven National Laboratory had developed a ring system with discrete detectors for quantitating annihilation radiation (65-67). Reconstruction algorithms had not yet been realized, so there was no way to process the data for image formation. The device did demonstrate the concept of transverse section imaging, and was later refined further (68,69).

Three approaches to detector geometry have evolved. The detector assemblies can be classified as parallel-opposed multicrystal arrays, hexagonal arrays, and circular tomographic units. Different techniques have been developed to provide multisection capability and adequate linear and angular sampling of emitted radiation.

Brownell and his group have developed a series of instruments using parallel-opposed multicrystal arrays that extends from the Hybrid Positron Scanner of 1970 to the PC 4200, a commercial instrument marketed for a time by the Cyclotron Corporation (70). This Hybrid Positron Scanner used two rows of nine detectors each to yield higher sensitivity than the single pair systems (71). The resultant images could be focused on planes lying between the two detector banks. This device led to the development of the first positron camera, the PC-I, which had two banks of 127 NaI(Tl) detectors coded to 72 photomultipliers (72). Each detector in one bank was in coincidence with 25 in the opposite bank yielding 2549 coincidence pairs or data channels. Images were prepared by focusing the data channels on planes lying between and parallel to the detector banks. The use of discrete detectors permitted high single photon count rates and high coincidence count rates. Since the detectors were separated by 2.8 centimeters, the device incorporated a small translational motion to permit higher sampling frequency and eliminate off-focal plane patterning (73). Dynamic images containing 2000 to 5000 events could be obtained in 0.1 second. Static images using interpolative motion took 10 to 100 seconds (74). Transverse section images of phantoms and animals could be obtained by rotation of the object. A transverse section version of the camera, the PC-II, has been developed for both transverse section and conventional imaging. Transverse section images are produced by rotation and translation of the two camera heads around the object to be imaged. Multiple transmission and emission images can be constructed from one set of transmission and one set of emission data. In the commercial instrument, the PC 4200, the detector assembly consisted of opposing banks of 140 crystals arranged as 12 x 12 arrays (less the corner crystals) with each crystal in one array operated in coincidence with a 5 x 5 matrix of crystals in the opposite array. The detector assembly furnished 2848 possible coincidence pairs. During a single scan, data was collected at 29 angular positions to give images of 23 separate tomographic sections 1 to 4 centimeters apart.

Ter-Pogossian, Phelps, Hoffman, Mullani and their associates at Washington University in St. Louis used the hexagonal-array approach to the design of detector assemblies. Their instrument evolved through four stages from PETT-I (positron-emission transaxial tomography) to PETT-IV. The PETT-III detector system consists of 48 NaI(Tl) scintillation detectors placed in a hexagonal array of six banks each with eight detectors. The electronic circuitry is such that every detector is operated in coincidence with each detector on the opposite bank. Thus there are 192 coincidence lines. The design of the PETT-III was incorporated into the commercial ECAT unit with a hexagonal array of 66 NaI(Tl) detectors, in which each detector in a given bank is operated in coincidence with all 11 detectors in the opposite bank (75). During a scan, each bank of detectors moves linearly about 4 centimeters and then rotates through 5-degree (or multiples thereof) angular increments over a total rotational arc of 60 degrees. The scanning motion, data collection, indexing of the patient bed, data processing and display are all under computer control. The unit has cardiac gating capability by using a buffer memory to partition data collected during different phases of the cardiac cycle. The PETT-IV is a tomographic unit that uses one-dimensional Anger logic to determine the location of a photon interaction in a long NaI(Tl) detector positioned normal to the transverse section plane. Four planes can be reconstructed simultaneously, and if cross-plane coincidences are used, the number may be increased to seven.

Recent trends in positron instrumentation have been in two directions: toward high resolution positron instruments and toward the use of time-of-flight concepts to improve image quality. Positron cameras consisting of one or more rings of scintillation detectors surrounding the patient offer the advantages of increased sensitivity per section and the capability of producing as many as nine tomographic sections simultaneously. Recent versions of the PETT scanner (the PETT-V and VI), the instruments at Brookhaven National Laboratory, the Montreal Neurological Institute (68), the Donner Laboratory at the University of California, Berkeley (76) and other centers (77-80) as well as the commercial systems now available all illustrate this increased sensitivity with better rejection of scattered events.

Developments in the cyclotron production of radionuclides (81-84) and the synthesis of useful positron-emitting compounds (85-87) have proceeded along with progress in instrumentation. Radiopharmaceuticals have been developed for substrate labeling (carbon-11 labeled glucose, 88; oxygen-15 labeled water, 89,90; oxygen-15, 91; nitrogen-13 labeled amino acids, 92,93), substrate analog labeling (fluorine-18 labeled 2-deoxyglucose, 94,95), labeling of drugs involved in normal or pathological biochemical pathways (96), labeling of ligands for receptor site binding (spiroperidol, 97; flunitrazepam, 98), and labeling of antibodies, particles, proteins and cells.

DIGITAL RADIOGRAPHY

The initial impetus for the development of digital radiography was a search for techniques to replace invasive intraarterial angiographic methods and their attendant dangers with a more benign procedure. In 1896, less than a month after the publication of Roentgen's paper introducing the x-ray, Haschek and Lindenthal in Vienna performed postmortem angiography of the hand using as contrast agent calcium oxide and mercuric sulfide suspended in a petroleum vehicle (99). During the next seventy-five years various improvements in contrast medium, injection technique, x-ray and film handling equipment led to the successful visualization of many of the peripheral and systemic arteries. By the late 1930s, Castellanos and coworkers in Cuba (100) and Robb and Steinberg in New York (101) using intravenous injection of contrast media were obtaining adequate pictures of the cardiac chambers. However, with the introduction of the Seldinger technique, direct (intraarterial) arteriography giving improved resolution and contrast and more consistent results became the method of choice.

In recent years, technical developments in television, image intensification, and digital electronics have improved the electronic recording of images and have led to the technique of digital subtraction angiography in which the traditional silver halide film/screen radiation receptor has been replaced by a photoelectronic receptor controlled by a computer. It is hoped that by using digitized video images from an intensifier, it may be possible to return to intravenous arteriography while maintaining the good image contrast and acceptable resolution of intraarterial studies.

Subtraction techniques have been used in radiology for many years. Des Plantes first described a photographic subtraction technique in 1934. Both photographic and electronic methods of subtraction have been used increasingly as an adjunct in contrast procedures to suppress the appearance of bony structures overlying areas of interest. In 1972 Sashin, Goldman and coworkers reported a subtraction technique using video disc storage to produce a guide to help the radiologist during catheterization (102).

After hearing a seminar delivered by Cameron in which he described differences in x-ray transmission attenuation through the lungs that reflected the systolic and diastolic variations of the heart, Mistretta at the University of Wisconsin thought that it might be possible to image pulmonary arteries without using contrast material by subtracting a sum of gated images obtained at systole from a sum of images obtained at diastole. With the help of Ort he devised a scheme for performing image subtraction on an analog storage tube by operating the tube at two separate voltages, one of which resulted in the addition of charge to the target when it was scanned with a video-modulated electron beam and another which resulted in the subtraction of charge.

During 1972 to 1973, the Wisconsin group became aware of Jacobson's work in Sweden on iodine K-edge energy subtraction imaging. By scanning with beam energies centered above and below the K-edge of iodine, Jacobson and associates were able to produce subtraction images in which the iodine was greatly enhanced relative to bone and soft tissue (103). Kelcz using this principle was able to generate iodine and cerium-filtered beams which, when used in conjunction with image-intensified fluoroscopy and the dual storage tube video subtraction apparatus, provided a K-edge subtraction system with a data collection rate 10,000 times faster than anything available at that time (104). In order to separate iodine, soft tissue, and bone, Kelcz extended the technique to include three beams, one with energy just below the K-edge and two with energies just above the K-edge. The technique was so successful in cancelling bone and tissue that a projected iodine concentration of 1 to 2 milligrams/s gm cm could be imaged. The technique did not become clinically useful because the intensity of the filtered x-ray beams was too low, and the storage tube apparatus had too many adjustable parameters and was not reliable.

The next development, which occurred during 1974 to 1975, was the construction, at the University of Wisconsin Physical Laboratory, of a digital version of the three-beam K-edge apparatus which included three 256 x 256-pixel digital memories. The digital approach removed the unreliability of the storage tubes, but the beam intensity limitations kept the technique from becoming clinically practical. Earlier studies had successfully shown enhancement of the visibility of iodine and suppression of bone and tissue shadows in the cerebral cisterns of a monkey (105).

A fortuitous observation of the passage of cholografin through the heart of a dog on its way to the liver changed the focus of the research to cardiac applications. It was discovered that high quality heart images could be obtained using a blurry preinjection mask image integration over a large fraction of a heart beat. This mask was adequate to cancel sufficient anatomical information so that the iodine in the subtraction display could be amplified by a factor of eight (106). However, other sorts of patient motion, such as respiration, produced enormous misregistration signals and needed to be overcome. As a result two new imaging modes were explored to deal with the problem of patient motion in cardiac imaging.

During the time that Mistretta and the Wisconsin group were pursuing various energy and time subtraction studies with their digital video image processor, digital video imaging programs were being developed independently by Brennecke, Heintzen and colleagues in Kiel, (107-109) Höhne and his group in Hamburg (110) and by Capp and Nudelman at the University of Arizona (111,112). Sashin, who had begun investigating analog disc subtraction techniques in the 1960s, had established a digital imaging program at the University of Pittsburgh using a non-video approach similar conceptually to that reported by Brody and associates (113). The techniques utilize a linear scanned projection geometry which provides high detector dynamic range and improved scatter rejection achieved at the expense of temporal resolution and dynamic capabilities. These systems have been used successfully with both time and energy subtraction for intravenous angiography. It is not yet clear what role each system will play in clinical diagnosis.

By February 1980, the first one hundred patients had been studied on the original University of Wisconsin apparatus. In March of the same year, commercial prototypes were installed both at the University of Wisconsin and at the Cleveland Clinic in Ohio where a large scale patient study was begun (114). Clinical activity was also on the increase at the University of Arizona and at the Kiel Kinderklinik. With digital subtraction arteriographic techniques, the major disadvantages of intravenous arteriography (115) have been overcome: percutaneous placement of a small catheter in the vena cava is safe and simple; the volume of contrast is only 40 to 60 percent of that previously used; logarithmic amplification of the iodine signal permits cancellation of the inequality of tissue density; and because of electronic processing, the images can be subtracted in unlimited number and viewed immediately. There are some limitations: contrast levels are 10 to 20-fold lower than those achieved by direct arterial injections, and therefore image quality is not adequate for examinations requiring high spatial resolution; and the problem of superimposed iodine precludes use of intravenous techniques for definitive evaluation of native coronary vessels.

NUCLEAR MAGNETIC RESONANCE IMAGING

Nuclear magnetic resonance imaging, the newest technique for obtaining cross sectional pictures through the human body, offers several unique advantages. It does not require ionizing radiation. The position and direction of the plane to be imaged can be controlled electronically instead of by mechanically moving the instrument around a patient. The potential for discriminating between healthy and diseased soft tissue and for defining organ chemistry and function seems greater. In addition since bone is "transparent" on NMR images, it appears possible to visualize structures hidden by bone which absorbs many of the x-rays required for x-ray computed tomography.

All of the instrumentation necessary for demonstrating nuclear magnetic resonance had been available for the previous 25 years, but it was not until the early 1940s when Bloch at Stanford University and Purcell at Harvard University independently developed the theoretical analyses and designed the appropriate experiments that nuclear magnetic resonance was discovered. They observed that energy is absorbed and subsequently released by selected nuclei at particular frequencies following irradiation with radio waves (116,117), and for this work they shared the Nobel Prize in 1952. Nuclear magnetic resonance spectroscopy has been used for over 30 years by physicists, chemists, biologists, and biochemists to study atomic and molecular structure in pure homogeneous samples. More recently NMR techniques have been used to help characterize the metabolic activity of tissues, and thus alterations in enzyme function, which reflects disease processes and their treatment by drugs (118,119). In vivo analyses of certain changes in the chemistry of internal organs may be possible (120) and also the assessment of cardiovascular and cerebrovascular damage and repair after therapy.

The potential of NMR as a medical imaging modality was first recognized in the early 1970s. Damadian suggested in 1971 that spin echo nuclear magnetic resonance measurements might be used to distinguish between malignant tumors and normal tissue on the basis of differences in their spin-lattice (T_1) and spin-spin (T_2) magnetic relaxation times (121). In 1973 Lauterbur published a technique by which a two-dimensional image could be generated by processing in a computer a series of one-dimensional projections obtained when an object interacts with two magnetic fields, a static one with a superimposed linear magnetic gradient and one alternating at radiofrequencies (122). He made use of an observation published by Gabillard of the Universite de Lille in 1951 (123). The latter noted that partial information can be obtained from NMR signals by using a nonuniform magnetic field. The resonance frequencies of the precessing nuclei depend primarily on their positions along the direction of the magnetic gradient and can be used to generate a one-dimensional projection of the structure of the object. By taking a series of these projections at different gradient orientations, a two- or three-dimensional image of the object can be constructed. Because the object interacts with two magnetic fields, Lauterbur named the procedure zeugmatography from the Greek word meaning "that which joins together."

Four basic methods for characterizing an object in three dimensions by NMR have been developed and within each method several techniques have been elaborated by various research groups. These include sequential point methods (sensitive point - Hinshaw, 124; and focused nuclear resonance - Damadian 125), sequential line methods (selective excitation line scan -Mansfield and his associates, 126; Crooks, 127; sensitive line or multiple sensitive point techniques - Hinshaw, Andrew and co-workers, 128), sequential plane methods (two-dimensional projection-reconstruction - Lauterbur, 129; two-dimensional Fourier imaging - Brunner, Ernst, 130; Kumar, Welti, 131; Edelstein, Hutchison and associates, 132; planar imaging - Mansfield and Maudsley, 133; two-dimensional echo planar imaging, 134; rotating frame imaging, 135), and simultaneous methods (three-dimensional projection-reconstruction, 136; three-dimensional Fourier imaging, 131; multiplanar imaging, 133; three-dimensional echo planar imaging, 134, 137).

The basic technology required for NMR imaging is the same as that used in NMR spectroscopy. Many of the early imaging studies were obtained with modified NMR spectrometers including the work of Hutchison, Mallard and their associates in Aberdeen (138), and that of Hinshaw and his group in Nottingham (139,140). The first whole body human scanner was constructed at the Downstate Medical Center in Brooklyn, New York, from early 1976 to early 1977 under the supervision of Damadian, Goldsmith and Minkoff. The first successful scan on July 3, 1977, yielding an image of the human torso (that of Minkoff), took 4-1/2 hours (141). Early in the following year this group produced a successful FONAR scan of a patient with cancer (142). Other groups made images of various body parts - Hinshaw and his associates a successful scan of the wrist (143), Clow and his group at the EMI laboratory a reconstruction image across the principal investigator's head (144). The Aberdeen group, using a whole body scanner built by Oxford Instruments, produced successful human trunk images early in 1979 (145). Increasing clinical experience, coming from a number of NMR research centers, has suggested that the modality may produce images containing unique chemical and structural information (146).

CONCLUSION

These brief vignettes representing some episodes in the development of the several modalities which are the subject of this advanced study institute hardly do justice to the intellectual and technical efforts that have made them possible. We hope they demonstrate the enormous impact that physics and engineering have had on diagnostic medicine in the past two decades. These developments, of course, have had important consequences - particularly as we have had to learn how to incorporate them into medical practice. First, they have permitted direct direct visualization of anatomic and physiological phenomena only implied by inference in the past (or not at all): e.g., hemorrhage into the brain, fetal abnormalities of soft tissues, regional carbohydrate metabolism. Second, their evolution and diffusion have been so rapid that our ability to absorb the information that is and can be provided often lags behind technological advances. Keep in mind that most physicians today received their training when these modalities were not generally available. Third, the technology is relatively expensive, leaving those who allocate health resources wondering as to the relative costs and benefits. This question is particularly difficult to address as technologies are emerging, and there is considerable overlap between new procedures and older ones still in place.

1. Langevin, M.P. Les ondes ultrasonores. Rev. Gen. Electr. 23 (1928) 626.

2. Dussik, K.T. Uber die mogleckeit hochfrequent mechanische schwingungen als diagnostiches hilfmittel zu verwenden. Ages. Neurol. Psych. 174 (1942) 143.

3. Ludwig, G.D. and F.W. Struthers. Considerations underlying the use of ultrasound to detect gallstones and foreign bodies in tissues. Naval Medical Research Institute Project NM 004 001 4 (1949) 1-23.

4. Ludwig, G.D. The velocity of sound through tissues and the acoustic impedance of tissues. J. Accoust. Soc. Am. 22 (1950) 862.

5. Wild, J.J. and J.M. Reid. Application of echo-ranging techniques to the determination of structure of biological tissues. Science 115 (1952) 226.

6. Howry, D.H. and W.R. Bliss. Ultrasonic visualization of soft tissue structures of the body. J. Lab. Clin. Med. 40 (1952) 579.

7. Holmes, J.H. and D.H. Howry. Ultrasonic visualization of edema. Trans. Am. Clin. Climatol. Assoc. 70 (1958) 225.

8. Donald, I., J. MacVicar and T.G. Brown. Investigation of abdominal masses by pulsed ultrasound. Lancet 1 (1958) 1188.

9. Kossoff, G., D.E. Robinson and W.J. Garrett. Two dimensional ultrasonography in obstetrics. In Diagnostic Ultrasound, ed. C.C. Grossman, J.H. Holmes, C. Joyner and E.W. Purnell. New York, Plenum Press, 1966, pp. 333-347.

10. Edler, I. and C.H. Hertz. The use of ultrasonic reflectoscope for the continuous recording of the movements of heart walls. K. Fysiogr. Saellsk. Lund Foerh. 24 (1954) 40.

11. Edler, I. Ultrasound-cardiogram in mitral valvular diseases. Acta Chir. Scand. 111 (1956) 230.

12. Effert, S., W. Bleifeld, F.J. Deupmann and J. Karitsiotis. Diagnostic value of ultrasonic cardiography. Br. J. Radiol. 37 (1964) 920.

13. Joyner, C.R., J.M. Reid and J.P. Bond. Reflected ultrasound in the assessment of mitral valve disease. Circulation 27 (1963) 503.

14. Feigenbaum, H., J.A. Waldhausen and L.P. Hyde. Ultrasound diagnosis of pericardial effusion. JAMA 191 (1965) 711.

15. Leksell, L. Echo-encephalography. I. Detection of intracranial complications following head injury. Acta Chir. Scand. 110 (1955-1956) 301.

16. Gordon, D. Echo-encephalography, ultrasonic rays in diagnostic radiology. Br. Med. J. 1 (1959) 1500.

17. deVlieger, M. and H.J. Ridder. Use of echoencephalography. Neurology 9 (1959) 216.

18. Ford, R. and J. Ambrose. Echoencephalography: The measurement of the position of mid-line structures in the skull with high frequency pulsed ultrasound. Brain 86 (1963) 189.

19. Oksala, A. Ultrasound equipment in the examination of the eye and its diseases. Nord. Med. 59 (1958) 721.

20. Baum, G. and I. Greenwood. The application of ultrasonic locating techniques to ophthalmology. Arch. Ophthalmol. 60 (1958) 263.

21. Bracewell, R.N. Strip integration in radio astronomy. Aust. J. Phys. 9 (1956) 198.

22. Branson, N.J.B. The emission spectrum of the crab nebula. Observatory 85 (1965) 250.

23. DeRosier, D.J. and A. Klug. Reconstruction of three dimensional structures from electron micrographs. Nature 217 (1968) 130.

24. Gordon, R., R. Bender and G.T. Herman. Algebraic reconstruction techniques (ART) for three-dimensional electron microscopy and x-ray photography. J. Theor. Biol. 29 (1970) 471.

25. Rowley, P.D. Quantitative interpretation of three-dimensional weakly refractive phase objects using holographic interferometry. J. Opt. Soc. Am. 59 (1969) 1496.

26. Berry, M.V. and D.F. Gibbs. The interpretation of optical projections. Proc. R. Soc. London A. 314 (1970) 143.

27. Cormack, A.M. Early two-dimensional reconstruction and recent topics stemming from it. Science 209 (1980) 1482.

28. Cormack, A.M. Representation of a function by its line integrals, with some radiological applications. J. Appl. Phys. 34 (1963) 2722.

29. Cormack, A.M. Representation of a function by its line integrals, with some radiological applications. II. J. Appl. Phys. 35 (1964) 2908.

30. Oldendorf, W.H. Isolated flying spot detection of radiodensity discontinuities displaying the internal structural pattern of a complex object. IRE Trans. Bio-Med. Electron. BME-8 (1961) 68.

31. Kuhl, D.E. and R.Q. Edwards. Image separation radioisotope scanning. Radiology 80 (1963) 653.

32. Tretiak, O.J., M. Eden and W. Simon. Internal structure from x-ray images. In Proceedings of the Eighth International Conference on Medical and Biological Engineering. IEEE, Chicago, 1969.

33. Bates, R.H.T. and T.M. Peters. Towards improvements in tomography. N. Z. J. Sci. 14 (1971) 883.

34. Hounsfield, G.N. Computed medical imaging. Science 210 (1980) 22.

35. Hounsfield, G.N. Computerized transverse axial scanning (tomography): Part 1. Description of system. Br. J. Radiol. 46 (1973) 1016.

36. Ambrose, J. Computerized transverse axial scanning (tomography): Part 2. Clinical application. Br. J. Radiol. 46 (1973) 1023.

37. Brownell, G.L., J.A. Correia and R.G. Zamenhof. Positron instrumentation. In Recent Advances in Nuclear Medicine, Vol. 5, ed. J.H. Lawrence and T.F. Budinger. New York, Grune and Stratton, Inc., 1978, pp. 1-49.

38. Soussaline, F. Emission tomography: Physical aspects. In Computerized Tomography, INSERM Symposium, Bordeaux 1979, ed. J.M. Caillé and G. Salamon. Berlin, Springer-Verlag, 1980, pp. 211-217.

39. Kuhl, D.E. and R.Q. Edwards. Cylindrical and section radioisotope scanning of the liver and brain. Radiology 83 (1964) 926.

40. Harper, P.V., R. Beck, D. Charleston and K.A. Lathrop. Optimization of a scanning method using Tc^{99m}. Nucleonics 22, No. 1 (1964) 50.

41. Kuhl, D.E. and R.Q. Edwards. The Mark III scanner: A compact device for multiple-view and section scanning of the brain. Radiology 96 (1970) 563.

42. Kuhl, D.E., R.Q. Edwards, A.R. Ricci and M. Reivich. Quantitative section scanning using orthogonal tangent correction. J. Nucl. Med. 14 (1973) 196.

43. Stoddart, H.F. and H.A. Stoddart. A new development in single gamma transaxial tomography. Union Carbide focussed collimator scanner. IEEE Trans. Nucl. Sci. NS-26 (1979) 2710.

44. Freedman, G.S. Tomography with a gamma camera. Concise communication. J. Nucl. Med. 11 (1970) 602.

45. Budinger, T.F., G.T. Gullberg, J. McRae and H.O. Anger. Isotope distribution reconstruction from multiple gamma camera views. J. Nucl. Med. 15 (1974) 480 (abst).

46. Keyes, J.W., Jr., N. Orlandea, W.J. Heetderks, P.F. Leonard and W.L. Rogers. The Humongotron - A scintillation-camera transaxial tomograph. J. Nucl. Med. 18 (1977) 381.

47. Jaszczak, R., D. Huard, P. Murphy and J. Burdine. Radionuclide emission computed tomography with a scintillation camera. J. Nucl. Med. 17 (1976) 551 (abst).

48. Hill, T.C., P. Costello, H.F. Gramm, R. Lovett, B.J. McNeil and S. Treves. Early clinical experience with a radionuclide emission computed tomographic brain-imaging system. Radiology 128 (1978) 803.

49. Murphy, P.H., W.L. Thompson, M.L. Moore and J.A. Burdine. Radionuclide computed tomography of the body using routine radiopharmaceuticals. I. System characterization. J. Nucl. Med. 20 (1979) 102.

50. Budinger, T.F. Physical attributes of single-photon tomography. J. Nucl. Med. 21 (1980) 579.

51. Goodwin, P.N. Recent developments in instrumentation for emission computed tomography. Semin. Nucl. Med. X (1980) 322.

52. Anger, H.O. Multiplane tomographic scanner. In Tomographic Imaging in Nuclear Medicine, Proceedings of Symposium, September 1972, ed. G.S. Freedman. New York, The Society of Nuclear Medicine, 1973, pp. 2-18.

53. Mathieu, L. and T.F. Budinger. Pinhole digital tomography. In Recent Advances in Nuclear Medicine, Proceedings of the First World Congress of Nuclear Medicine, Tokyo, 1974, pp. 1264-1266.

54. Vogel, R.A., D. Kirch, M. LeFree and P. Steele. A new method of multiplanar emission tomography using a seven pinhole collimator and an Anger scintillation camera. J. Nucl. Med. 19 (1978) 648.

55. Koral, K.F., W.L. Rogers and G.F. Knoll. Digital tomographic imaging with time-modulated pseudorandom coded aperture and Anger camera. J. Nucl. Med. 16 (1975) 402.

56. Chang, W., S.L. Lin and R.E. Henkin. A rotatable quadrant slant hole collimator for tomography (QSH): A stationary scintillation camera based SPECT system. In Single-Photon Emission Computed Tomography and Other Selected Computer Topics. Proceedings of Symposium on Sharing of Computer Programs and Technology in Nuclear Medicine. New York, The Society of Nuclear Medicine, 1980, pp. 81-94.

57. Williams, J.J and G.F. Knoll. Initial performance of SPRINT: A single photon system for emission tomography. IEEE Trans. Nucl. Sci. NS-26 (1979) 2732.

58. Barrett, H.H. Fresnel zone plate imaging in nuclear medicine. J. Nucl. Med. 13 (1972) 382.

59. Myers, M.J., W.I. Keyes and J.R. Mallard. An analysis of tomographic scanning systems. In Medical Radioisotope Scintigraphy 1972, Vol. I, Proceedings of Symposium, Monte Carlo 1972. Vienna, IAEA, 1973, pp. 331-345.

60. Wrenn, F.R., Jr., M.L. Good and P. Handler. The use of positron-emitting radioisotopes for the localization of brain tumors. Science 113 (1951) 525.

61. Sweet, W.H. The uses of nuclear disintegration in the diagnosis and treatment of brain tumor. N. Engl. J. Med. 245 (1951) 875.

62. Brownell, G.L and W.H. Sweet. Scanning of positron-emitting isotopes in diagnosis of intracranial and other lesions. Acta Radiol. 46 (1956) 425.

63. Aronow, S. and G.L. Brownell. An apparatus for brain tumor localization using positron emitting isotopes. IRE International Convention Record Part 9 (1956) 8-16.

64. Anger, H.O. Sensitivity, resolution and linearity of the scintillation camera. IEEE Trans. Nucl. Sci. NS-13, No. 3 (1966) 380.

65. Rankowitz, S., J.S. Robertson, W.A. Higinbotham and M.J. Rosenblum. Positron scanner for locating brain tumors. IRE International Convention Record Part 9 (1962) 49-56.

66. Robertson, J.S. and S.R. Bozzo. Positron scanner for brain tumors. In Proceedings of VIth IBM Medical Symposium, 1964, pp. 631-645.

67. Robertson, J.S., R.B. Marr, M. Rosenblum, V. Radeka and Y.L. Yamamoto. 32-Crystal positron transverse section detector. In Tomographic Imaging in Nuclear Medicine, Proceedings of Symposium, September 1972, ed. G.S. Freedman. New York, The Society of Nuclear Medicine, 1973, pp. 142-153.

68. Thompson, C.J., Y.L. Yamamoto and E. Meyer. A positron imaging system for the measurement of regional cerebral blood flow. Application of Optical Instrumentation in Medicine V, Proc. Soc. Photo-Opt. Instr. Eng. 96 (1976) 263-268.

69. Yamamoto, Y.L., C.J. Thompson, E. Meyer, J.S. Robertson and W. Feindel. Dynamic positron emission tomography for study of cerebral hemodynamics in a cross section of the head using positron-emitting ^{68}Ga-EDTA and ^{77}Kr. J. Comput. Assist. Tomogr. 1 (1977) 43.

70. Carroll, L.R. Design and performance characteristics of a production model positron imaging system. IEEE Trans. Nucl. Sci. NS-25 (1978) 606.

71. Brownell, G.L., C.A. Burnham, S. Wilensky, S. Aronow, H. Kazemi and D. Streider. New developments in positron scintigraphy and the application of cyclotron-produced positron emitters. In Medical Radioisotope Scintigraphy, Vol. I, Proceedings of Symposium, Salzburg 1968. Vienna, IAEA, 1969, pp. 163-176.

72. Brownell, G.L., C.A. Burnham, B. Hoop and H. Kazemi. Positron scintigraphy with short-lived cyclotron-produced radiopharmaceuticals and a multicrystal positron camera. In Medical Radioisotope Scintigraphy, Proceedings of Symposium. Vienna, IAEA, 1973, p. 313.

73. Brownell, G.L and C.A. Burnham. MGH positron camera. In Tomographic Imaging in Nuclear Medicine, Proceedings of Symposium, September 1972, ed. G.S. Freedman. New York, The Society of Nuclear Medicine, 1973, pp. 154-164.

74. Wilensky, S., A.B. Ashare, S.M. Pizer, B. Hoop and G.L. Brownell. Computer processing and display of positron scintigrams and dynamic function curves. In Medical Radioisotope Scintigraphy, Vol. I, Proceedings of Symposium, Salzburg 1968. Vienna, IAEA, 1969, pp. 815-827.

75. Ter-Pogossian, M.M., M.E. Phelps, E.J. Hoffman and N.A. Mullani. A positron-emission transaxial tomograph for nuclear imaging (PETT). Radiology 114 (1975) 89.

76. Derenzo, S.E., T.F. Budinger, R.H. Huesman, J.L. Cahoon and T. Vuletich. Imaging properties of a positron tomograph with 280 BGO crystals. IEEE Trans. Nucl. Sci. NS-28 (1981) 81.

77. Brooks, R.A., V.J. Sank, G. DiChiro, W.S. Friauf and S.B. Leighton. Design of a high resolution positron emission tomograph. The Neuro-PET. J. Comput. Assist. Tomogr. 4 (1980) 5.

78. Tanaka, E., N. Nohara, M. Yamamoto, T. Tomitani, H. Murayama, K. Ishimatsu and K. Takami. "Positology" - The search for suitable detector arrangements for a positron ECT with continuous rotation. IEEE Trans. Nucl. Sci. NS-26 (1979) 2728.

79. Bohm, Chr., L. Eriksson, M. Bergstrom, J. Litton, R. Sundman and M. Singh. A computer assisted ring-detector positron camera system for reconstruction tomography of the brain. IEEE Trans. Nucl. Sci. NS-25 (1978) 624.

80. Kanno, I., K. Uemura, S. Miura and Y. Miura. HEADTOME: A hybrid emission tomograph for single photon and positron emission imaging of the brain. J. Comput. Assist. Tomogr. 5 (1981) 216.

81. Yano, Y. and H.O. Anger. Visualization of heart and kidneys in animals with ultrashort-lived ^{82}Rb and the positron scintillation camera. J. Nucl. Med. 9 (1968) 412.

82. Myers, W.G. ^{11}C-Acetylene. J. Nucl. Med. 13 (1972) 699.

83. Grant, P.M., B.R. Erdal and H.A. O'Brien, Jr. A ^{82}Sr-^{82}Rb isotope generator for use in nuclear medicine. J. Nucl. Med. 16 (1975) 300.

84. Budinger, T.F., Y. Yano and B. Hoop. A comparison of ^{82}Rb$^+$ and ^{13}NH$_3$ for myocardial positron scintigraphy. J. Nucl. Med. 16 (1975) 429.

85. Clark, J.C. and P.D. Buckingham. The preparation and storage of carbon-11 labelled gases for clinical use. Int. J. Appl. Radiat. Isot. 22 (1971) 639.

86. Wolf, A.P. and C.S. Redvanly. Carbon-11 and radiopharmaceuticals. Int. J. Appl. Radiat. Isot. 28 (1977) 29.

87. Welch, M.J. and S. Wagner. Preparation of positron-emitting radiopharmaceuticals. In Recent Advances in Nuclear Medicine, Vol. 5, ed. J.H. Lawrence and T.F. Budinger. New York, Grune and Stratton, Inc., 1978, pp. 51-69.

88. Lifton, J.F. and M.J. Welch. Preparation of glucose labeled with 20-minute half-lived carbon-11. Radiat. Res. 45 (1971) 35.

89. Ter-Pogossian, M.M., J.O. Eichling, D.O. Davis and M.J. Welch. The measure in vivo of regional cerebral oxygen utilization by means of oxyhemoglobin labeled with radioactive oxygen-15. J. Clin. Invest. 49 (1970) 381.

90. Ter-Pogossian, M.M., J.O. Eichling, D.O. Davis, M.J. Welch and J.M. Metzger. The determination of regional cerebral blood flow by means of water labeled with radioactive oxygen-15. Radiology 93 (1969) 31.

91. Subramanyam, R., N.M. Alpert, B. Hoop, Jr., G.L. Brownell and J.M. Taveras. A model for regional cerebral oxygen distribution during continuous inhalation of $^{15}O_2$, $C^{15}O$, and $C^{15}O_2$. J. Nucl. Med. 19 (1978) 48.

92. Gelbard, A.S., L.P. Clarke and J.S. Laughlin. Enzymatic synthesis and use of ^{13}N-labeled L-asparagine for myocardial imaging. J. Nucl. Med. 15 (1974) 1223.

93. Gelbard, A.S., L.P. Clarke, J.M. McDonald, W.G. Monahan, R.S. Tilbury, T.Y.T. Kuo and J.S. Laughlin. Enzymatic synthesis and organ distribution studies with ^{13}N-labeled L-glutamine and L-glutamic acid. Radiology 116 (1975) 127.

94. Ido, T., C.-N. Wan, J.S. Fowler and A.P. Wolf. Fluorination with F_2. A convenient synthesis of 2-deoxy-2-fluoro-D-glucose. J. Org. Chem. 42 (1977) 2341.

95. Gallagher, B.M., A. Ansari, H. Atkins, V. Casella, D.R. Christman, J.S. Fowler, T. Ido, R.R. MacGregor, P. Som, C.N. Wan, A.P. Wolf, D.E. Kuhl and M. Reivich. Radiopharmaceuticals XXVII. ^{18}F-labeled 2-deoxy-2-fluoro-D-glucose as a radiopharmaceutical for measuring regional myocardial glucose metabolism in vivo: Tissue distribution and imaging studies in animals. J. Nucl. Med. 18 (1977) 990.

96. Receptor-Binding Radiotracers Vol. 1 and 2, ed. W.C. Eckelman. Boca Raton, CRC Press, 1982.

97. Comar, D., M. Maziere and C. Crouzel. Synthesis and metabolism of ^{11}C-chlorpromazine methiodide. In Radiopharmaceuticals and Labelled Compounds, Vol. 1, Proceedings of Symposium, Copenhagen 1973. Vienna, IAEA, 1973, pp. 461-469.

98. Comar, D., M. Maziere, J.M. Godet, G. Berger and F. Soussaline. Visualization of ^{11}C-flunitrazepam displacement in the brain of the live baboon. Nature (London) 280 (1979) 329.

99. Haschek, E. and O.T. Lindenthal. A contribution to the practical use of the photography according to Röntgen. Wien. Klin. Wschr. 9 (1896) 63.

100. Castellanos, A., R. Pereiras and A. Garcia. La angiocardiografia radioopaca. Arch. Soc. Estud. Clin. (Habana) 31 (1937) 523.

101. Robb, G.P. and I. Steinberg. Visualization of the chambers of the heart, the pulmonary circulation, and the great blood vessels in man. AJR 41 (1939) 1.

102. Sashin, D., R.L. Goldman, P. Zanetti and E.R. Heinz. Electronic radiography in stereotaxic thrombosis of intracranial aneurysms and catheter embolization of cerebral arteriovenous malformations. Radiology 105 (1972) 359.

103. Jacobson, B. and R.S. Mackay. Radiological contrast enhancing methods. Adv. Biol. Med. Phys. 6 (1958) 201.

104. Kelcz, F. and C.A. Mistretta. Absorption-edge fluoroscopy using a three-spectrum technique. Med. Phys. 3 (1976) 159.

105. Houk, T.L., R.A. Kruger, C.A. Mistretta, S.J. Riederer, C.-G. Shaw, J.C. Lancaster and D.C. Flemming. Real time digital K-edge subtraction fluoroscopy. Invest. Radiol. 14 (1979) 270.

106. Kruger, R.A., C.A. Mistretta, T.L. Houk, S.J. Riederer, C.G. Shaw, M.M. Goodsitt, A.B. Crummy, W. Zwiebel, J.C. Lancaster, G.G. Rowe and D. Flemming. Computerized fluoroscopy in real time for noninvasive imaging of the cardiovascular system. Preliminary studies. Radiology 130 (1979) 49.

107. Heintzen, P.H., R. Brennecke, J.H. Bürsch, P. Lange, V. Malerezyk, K. Moldenhauer and D. Onnasch. Automated video-angiocardiographic image analysis. In Computers in Cardiology, Proceedings of Conference, October 1974. Long Beach, IEEE Inc., 1974, pp. 67-75.

108. Brennecke, R., T.K. Brown, J.H. Bürsch and P.H. Heintzen. Digital processing of video-angiocardiographic image series using a minicomputer. In Computers in Cardiology, Proceedings of Conference, October 1976. Long Beach, IEEE Inc., 1976, pp. 255-260.

109. Brennecke, R., T.K. Brown, J.H. Bürsch and P.H. Heintzen. Computerized video-image preprocessing with application to cardioangiographic roentgen image series. In Digital Image Processing, ed. H.H. Nagel. New York, Springer-Verlag, 1977, pp. 244-262.

110. Höhne, K.H., G. Nicolae, G. Pfeiffer, W.-R. Dix, W. Ebenritter, D. Novak, M. Böhm, B. Sonne and E. Bücheler. An interactive system for clinical application of angiodensitometry. Informatik Fachb. 8, Digitale Bildverarbeitung. Berlin, Springer-Verlag, 1977, pp. 234-243.

111. Nudelman, S., M.P. Capp, H.D. Fisher, M.M. Frost and H. Roehrig. Photoelectronic imaging for diagnostic radiology and the digital computer. 4th European Electro-optics Conference, Proc. Soc. Photo-Opt. Instr. Eng. 164 (1978) 138.

112. Ovitt, T.W., M.P. Capp, H.D. Fisher, M.M. Frost, J.L. Lebel, S. Nudelman and H. Roehrig. The development of a digital video subtraction system for intravenous angiography. In Noninvasive Cardiovascular Measurements. Bellingham, Society of Photo-Optical Instrumentation Engineers, 1978, pp. 61-65.

113. Brody, W.R., A. Macovski, L. Lehmann, F.A. DiBianca, D. Volz and L.S. Edelheit. Intravenous angiography using scanned projection radiography: Preliminary investigation of a new method. Invest. Radiol. 15 (1980) 220.

114. Meaney, T.F., M.A. Weinstein, P. Buonocore, W. Pavlicek, G.P. Borkowski, J.H. Gallagher, B. Sufka and W.J. MacIntyre. Digital subtraction angiography of the human cardiovascular system. Application of Optical Instrumentation in Medicine VIII, Proc. Soc. Photo-Opt. Instr. Eng. 233 (1980) 272-278.

115. Mistretta, C.A., A.B. Crummy and C.M. Strother. Digital angiography: A perspective. Radiology 139 (1981) 273.

116. Bloch, F. The principle of nuclear induction. Science 118 (1953) 425.

117. Purcell, E.M. Research in nuclear magnetism. Science 118 (1953) 431.

118. Burt, C.T., T. Glonek and M. Barany. Analysis of living tissue by phosphorus-31 magnetic resonance. Science 195 (1977) 145.

119. Marx, J.L. NMR research: Analysis of living cells and organs. Science 202 (1978) 958.

120. Ross, B.D., G.K. Radda, D.G. Gadian, G. Rocker, M. Esiri and J. Falconer-Smith. Examination of a case of suspected McArdle's syndrome by ^{31}P nuclear magnetic resonance. N. Engl. J. Med. 304 (1981) 1338.

121. Damadian, R. Tumor detection by nuclear magnetic resonance. Science 171 (1971) 1151.

122. Lauterbur, P.C. Image formation by induced local interactions: Examples employing nuclear magnetic resonance. Nature 242 (1973) 190.

123. Gabillard, R. Measurement of relaxation time T_2 in the presence of an inhomogeneous magnetic field. C.R. Acad. Sci. Paris 232 (1951) 1551.

124. Hinshaw, W.S. Spin mapping: The application of moving gradients to NMR. Phys. Lett. 48A (1974) 87.

125. Damadian, R., L. Minkoff, M. Goldsmith, M. Stanford and J. Koutcher. Tumor imaging in a live animal by field focusing NMR (FONAR). Physiol. Chem. Phys. 8 (1976) 61.

126. Garroway, A.N., P.K. Grannell and P. Mansfield. Image formation in NMR by a selective irradiative process. J. Phys. C: Solid State Phys. 7 (1974) L457.

127. Crooks, L.E. Selective irradiation line scan techniques for NMR imaging. IEEE Trans. Nucl. Sci. NS-27 (1980) 1239.

128. Andrew, E.R., P.A. Bottomley, W.S. Hinshaw, G.N. Holland, W.S. Moore and C. Simaroj. NMR images by the multiple sensitive point method: Application to larger biological systems. Phys. Med. Biol. 22 (1977) 971.

129. Lauterbur, P.C., C.S. Dulcey, C.M. Lai, M.A. Feiler, W.V. House, D.M. Kramer, C.N. Chen and R. Dias. Magnetic resonance zeugmatography. In Proceedings of XVIII Ampere Congress, Nottingham, ed. P.S. Allen, E.R. Andrew and C.A. Bates. Amsterdam, North-Holland, 1974, pp. 27-29.

130. Brunner, P. and R.R. Ernst. Sensitivity and performance time in NMR imaging. J. Magn. Reson. 33 (1979) 83.

131. Kumar, A., D. Welti and R.R. Ernst. NMR Fourier zeugmatography. J. Magn. Reson. 18 (1975) 69.

132. Edelstein, W.A., J.M.S. Hutchison, G. Johnson and T. Redpath. Spin warp NMR imaging and applications to human whole-body imaging. Phys. Med. Biol. 25 (1980) 751.

133. Mansfield, P. and A.A. Maudsley. Planar spin imaging by NMR. J. Phys. C: Solid State Phys. 9 (1976) L409.

134. Mansfield, P. Multi-planar image formation using NMR spin echoes. J. Phys. C: Solid State Phys. 10 (1977) L55.

135. Hoult, D.I. Rotating frame zeugmatography. J. Magn. Reson. 33 (1979) 183.

136. Lai, C.-M. and P.C. Lauterbur. A gradient control device for complete three-dimensional nuclear magnetic resonance zeugmatographic imaging. J. Phys. E: Sci. Instrum. 13 (1980) 747.

137. Ordidge, R.J., P. Mansfield and R.E. Coupland. Rapid biomedical imaging by NMR. Br. J. Radiol. 54 (1981) 850.

138. Hutchison, J.M.S., J.R. Mallard and C.C. Goll. In vivo imaging of body structures using proton resonance, Nottingham. In Proceedings of XVIII Ampere Congress, Nottingham, ed. P.S. Allen, E.R. Andrew, and C.A. Bates. Amsterdam, North-Holland, 1974, pp. 283-284.

139. Hinshaw, W.S. Image formation by nuclear magnetic resonance: The sensitive-point method. J. Appl. Phys. 47 (1976) 3709.

140. Hinshaw, W.S., E.R. Andrew, P.A. Bottomley, G.N. Holland, W.S. Moore and B.S. Worthington. Display of cross sectional anatomy by nuclear magnetic resonance imaging. Br. J. Radiol. 51 (1978) 273.

141. Damadian, R., M. Goldsmith and L. Minkoff. NMR in cancer: XVI. FONAR image of the live human body. Physiol. Chem. Phys. 9 (1977) 97.

142. Damadian, R., M. Goldsmith and L. Minkoff. NMR in cancer: XX. FONAR scans of patients with cancer. Physiol. Chem. Phys. 10 (1978) 285.

143. Hinshaw, W.S., P.A. Bottomley and G.N. Holland. Radiographic thin-section image of the human wrist by nuclear magnetic resonance. Nature 270 (1977) 722.

144. Reported in New Scientist 80 (1978) 588.

145. Mallard, J., J.M.S. Hutchison, W.A. Edelstein, C.R. Ling, M.A. Foster and G. Johnson. In vivo NMR imaging in medicine: The Aberdeen approach, both physical and biological. Philos. Trans. R. Soc. London. B. 289 (1980) 519.

146. Brownell, G.L., T.F. Budinger, P.C. Lauterbur and P.L. McGeer. Positron tomography and nuclear magnetic resonance imaging. Science 215 (1982) 619.

The material in this lecture note was drawn in part from the following:

Holmes, J.H. Diagnostic ultrasound during the early years of A.I.U.M. J. Clin. Ultrasound 8 (1980) 299.

Hendee, W.R. The Physical Principles of Computed Tomography. Boston, Little, Brown and Company, 1983.

Digital Subtraction Arteriography: An Application of Computerized Fluoroscopy, ed. C.A. Mistretta, A.B. Crummy, C.M. Strother, J.F. Sackett. Chicago, Year Book Publishers, 1982.

Imaging for Medicine, Vol. 1, Nuclear Medicine, Ultrasonics, and Thermography, ed. S. Nudelman, D.D. Patton. New York, Plenum Press, 1980.

IMAGE ANALYSIS AND THE METHOD OF MOMENTS

Aldo Rescigno

Section of Neurological Surgery,
Yale University School of Medicine,
New Haven, CT, U.S.A.

0. INTRODUCTION

I would like to start this chapter by stressing an important distinction between **pattern recognition** and **image analysis**. As their etymologies show, recognition means "perception of identity as already known", while analysis means "resolution of components parts"; therefore by pattern recognition I mean the identification of an observed pattern with a preestablished pattern, while by image analysis I mean the discovery on unknown patterns; of course the two problems have a number of features in common, and some of the methods employed are similar, but their philosophies are quite different. In the following pages I shall try to emphasize this distinction.

The problem of image analysis, in simple words, consists in discovering specific features of the external world. This is done sequentially by:
a) collecting data with an appropriate detector,
b) encoding the data in a suitable form,
c) storing the data in a memory,
d) elaborating the stored data,
e) decoding the data to reveal their specific features.

Each of the above steps presents its own problems, but they are all strictly connected. For instance step $\underline{c}$ is limited by the available storage space; a three-dimensional image of 1 dm^3 with a resolution of 1 mm includes 10^6 voxels; if the image is to be followed kinetically at a rate of 50 sec^{-1}, a one-minute observation requires the storage of the content of 3×10^9 voxels; a discrimination of 256 levels for the content of each voxel requires then the storage of 2.4×10^{10} bits/min or more than 10^6 Megabyte/hour. Obviously most of this information is useless, as it represents unneeded redundancy for contiguous voxels; a convenient encoding of the information collected could considerably reduce the redundancy without reducing the reliability of the data.

Similarly step b needs not be separate from step a; as we shall see below, the data can be collected by the detector in a form suitable for immediate coding.

More specifically our problem consists in observing two-dimensional or three-dimensional pictures of time varying objects, then compute some parameters that express in mathematical form the underlying physical phenomenon. For instance from sequential autoradiographies of the brain we want to know the local rate of utilization of a particular drug.

How to condense a very large number of data in a few, meaningful parameters is a common problem of statistical analysis; analysis of moments is a natural answer to this problem. Such parameters as Expected Value, Variance, Skewness, Kurtosis,etc.describe some very important properties of a collection of data, and very frequently can be given a meaningful physical interpretation. Image analysis faces an analogous problem, namely from all visual information available one should retain only that part revealing any deviation of the observed image from the most probable pattern as determined by that part of the observed image bordering the part under analysis. For the study of sequential images the problem is substantially the same, but in one more dimension.

All these problems have one thing in common, i.e. the total _amount of information_ available is reduced, but the _value of the information_ is not, and sometimes it is increased. I have used here the term "value of information" in a rather loose sense; a mathematical theory dealing with the relations between information and observer, thus treating the value as well as the quantity of information, has not yet been developed. Therefore rather than giving here a rigid definition of "value of information", I shall proceed and use this undefined term; its meaning will become clear through its use.

1. CHOICE OF A MODEL

Most experimental workers first define a qualitative model, then use experimental data to compute the parameters of that model. For instance the model appropriate to dilution phenomena is a set of ordinary differential equations with constant coefficients, while for diffusion phenomena partial differential equations are to be used, for delay phenomena finite difference equations, etc. Of course the gnoseological value of the parameters computed in this way depends on the chosen model.

For instance the compartment model, so often used in Nuclear Medicine and in Pharmacokinetics (1), is formed by a set of linear differential equations of order one with constant coefficients; its validity depends upon the hypotheses that the system described contain a finite number of components, and that each component be homogeneous. These hypotheses exclude the presence of diffusion and of age-dependent processes, or in general of transport of a non-Markovian nature. The fact that frequently the experimental data agree with this model does not necessarily prove the model is appropriate, but only that it is flexible (2).

In fact many classes of functions and an infinity of specific functions in each class can fit any contiguous single-valued correspondence with time to any arbitrary closeness. Among the best known demonstrations are those for polynomials (3) and for trigonometric functions (4).

In the specific case of n compartments, the model is a set of n first order, constant coefficient, linear differential equations in n state variables; they contain n^2 parameters. With n large enough, this model can be made consistent with many experimental data, but at the price of a considerable complexity of the model itself. Frequently this model is considerably simplified by making many coefficients of the differential equations equal to zero; but the price paid for this simplification is a reduced flexibility of the model.

In addition to the consistency with the experimental data, an obvious conceptual requirement of the model is that its parameters could be interpreted in terms of perceivable physical properties.

All this considered, a model is useful only if it allows us to determine a number of parameters (quantitative or qualitative), and if these parameters have a physical interpretation independent of the model itself; in fact no knowledge is acquired if the parameters obtained by elaboration of the experimental data through a model do not have a justifiable existence outside of the model.

Going back to the compartment model, its validity (when it is valid!) is based on the fact that at least some of the coefficients of the differential equations of the compartments can be measured directly or computed from different physical setups. The ideal situation of course is to compute parameters not dependent upon any model; this is rarely attainable, but we can at least try to examine the experimental data in terms of a model implying a minimum number of assumptions, and elaborate therefrom "robust" parameters, i.e. parameters as independent as possible from the model, giving them the best physical interpretation.

In the next few section I shall try to show how some robust parameters of pharmacokinetic interest can be defined and measured, and later how the same methods can be extended to image analysis.

2. STOCHASTIC TRANSPORT

Consider the transport of a particle through a living system as a stochastic process, i.e. as a random phenomenon that arises through a process controlled by probabilistic rather than deterministic laws. The only hypothesis required here is that the particle itself behaves in a way that depends on its present location and chemical association, but not on its past history.

Many papers have been published on stochastic compartments (5, 6, 7), where the time-dependent random variable is equal to the number of particles present in a compartment; those models require the same general assumptions made with the ordinary compartments, and in most cases lead to distributions with very small relative variances (8).

Alternatively, consider as random variable the time when a given particle reaches a certain state in the system, or the interval of time it takes to move from one state to another (9); the distribution of this random variable can be analyzed and compared with the available experimental data.

Under the present hypotheses, call A(t) the probability density function of the time when a given particle is present in a certain state, B(t) the probability density function of the interval of time for the transition from that state to another specified state, and finally C(t) the probability density function of the time when the same particle is present in this last state. More precisely,

A(t)dt = probability that a given particle is in the first state during the interval of time from t to t+dt,

B(t)dt = probability that a given particle takes a length of time from t to t+dt to move from the first to the second state,

C(t)dt = probability that a given particle is in the second state during the interval of time from t to t+dt.

Then, ignoring infinitesimals of higher order, A(u)duB(t−u)dt is the probability that a given particle that was in the first state during the interval u, u+du will be in the second state during the interval t,t+dt. Integrating the expression above for all values of u from 0 to t, one gets the probability that that particle is in the second state at a time between t and t+dt if it was in the first state at any time from 0 to t,

$$(1) \qquad \int_0^t A(u)B(t-u)du = C(t).$$

This is the well known convolution integral representing a linear, invariant system, without invoking the properties of homogeneous, well-mixed compartments.

3. DEFINITION OF THE MOMENTS

Many properties of the convolution integral in equation 1 can be analyzed by first defining the moments of the functions in it.

Given a generic function $F(t)$ defined for all values of t from 0 to $+\infty$, define the **moments**,

(2) $$F_i = \int_0^\infty t^i/i!\, F(t)dt, \quad i=0,1,2,\ldots$$

the **relative moments**,

(3) $$f_i = F_i/F_0,$$

and the **central moments**,

(4) $$\varphi_i = \int_0^\infty (t-f_1)^i/i!\, F(t)dt/F_0, \quad i=2,3,4,\ldots$$

provided that the integrals above converge.

A few comments are necessary here. First, the definition of moment in equation 2 differs from the most common definition by a factor $i!$; I have introduced this factor because it considerably simplifies many expressions we shall find later on. I shall not discuss the obvious, general conditions necessary for the convergence of the integrals in definitions 2 and 4, but section 8 shows what can be done when one of those integrals does not converge. Finally, definition 4 applies only to values of i larger than one; for convenience we complete that definition with

(5) $$\varphi_1 = f_1,$$

so that in the following pages we shall use central moments for any positive integer i.

To express a central moment in terms of the relative moments, expand the binomial in definition 4,

$$\varphi_i = \int_0^\infty \sum_{j=0}^{i} (-1)^j f_1^j/j!\cdot t^{i-j}/(i-j)!\cdot F(t)dt/F_0$$

$$\varphi_i = \sum_{j=0}^{i-2}(-1)^j f_1^j/j!\cdot f_{i-j} +$$
$$\quad + (-1)^{i-1}f_1^{i-1}/(i-1)!\cdot f_1 + (-1)^i f_1^i/i!$$

(6) $$\varphi_i = \sum_{j=0}^{i-2}(-1)^j f_1^j f_{i-j}/j! + (-1)^{i-1}(i-1)f_1^i/i!.$$

In particular we can write

$$\varphi_1 = f_1$$
$$\varphi_2 = f_2 - f_1^2/2$$
$$\varphi_3 = f_3 - f_1 f_2 + 2f_1^3/3!$$

$$\varphi_4 = f_4 - f_1 f_3 + f_1^2 f_2/2! - 3 f_1^4/4!$$

and so on.

4. PROPERTIES OF THE CONVOLUTION

Multiply both sides of equation 1 by $t^i/i!$ and integrate from 0 to $+\infty$,

$$\int_0^\infty t^i/i! \int_0^t A(u) B(t-u) du \, dt = \int_0^\infty t^i/i! \, C(t) dt,$$

where i is any non-negative integer; change the order of integration,

$$\int_0^\infty A(u) \, t^i/i! \int_u^\infty B(t-u) dt \, du = C_i;$$

change the variable of the inner integral,

$$\int_0^\infty A(u) \int_0^\infty (t+u)^i/i! \, B(t) dt \, du = C_i,$$

expand the binomial to obtain finally,

(7) $$\sum_{j=0}^{i} A_{i-j} \cdot B_j = C_i; \quad i=0,1,2,\ldots$$

in particular,

$$A_0 B_0 = C_0$$

$$A_1 B_0 + A_0 B_1 = C_1$$

$$A_2 B_0 + A_1 B_1 + A_0 B_2 = C_2$$

$$A_3 B_0 + A_2 B_1 + A_1 B_2 + A_0 B_3 = C_3.$$

Dividing both sides of equation 7 by $A_0 B_0$ we get

(8) $$\sum_{j=0}^{i} a_{i-j} b_j = c_i. \quad i=1,2,3,\ldots$$

Now call α_i, β_i, and γ_i the central moments of $A(t)$, $B(t)$, and $C(t)$. From equation 1 again we get

$$\int_0^\infty (t-c_1)^i/i! \int_0^t A(u) B(t-u) du \, dt = \int_0^\infty (t-c_1)^i/i! \, C(t) dt,$$

where i is any integer larger than one; invert the order of integration and observe that

$$A_0 \cdot B_0 = C_0,$$

$$a_1 + b_1 = c_1;$$

then
$$\int_0^\infty A(u)/A_0 \int_u^\infty (t-a_1-b_1)^i/i! \cdot B(t-u)/B_0 \cdot dt \cdot du = \gamma_i$$
or
$$\int_0^\infty A(u)/A_0 \int_0^\infty (t+u-a_1-b_1)^i/i! \cdot B(t)/B_0 \cdot dt \cdot du = \gamma_i;$$

with a binomial expansion we get

$$\sum_{j=0}^{i} \int_0^\infty (u-a_1)^{i-j}/(i-j)! \cdot A(u)/A_0 \int_0^\infty (t-b_1)^j/j! \cdot B(t)/B_0 \cdot dt \cdot du = \gamma_i$$

and observing that

$$\int_0^\infty (t-a_1)A(t)dt = \int_0^\infty (t-b_1)B(t)dt = 0$$

we get finally

(9) $\qquad \alpha_i + \sum_{j=2}^{i-2} \alpha_{i-j}\beta_j + \beta_i = \gamma_i,$

and in particular from definition 5 and from equation 9,

$$\alpha_1 + \beta_1 = \gamma_1$$
$$\alpha_2 + \beta_2 = \gamma_2$$
$$\alpha_3 + \beta_3 = \gamma_3$$
$$\alpha_4 + \alpha_2\beta_2 + \beta_4 = \gamma_4$$
$$\alpha_5 + \alpha_3\beta_2 + \alpha_2\beta_3 + \beta_5 = \gamma_5$$

and so on.

In general the number of particles in a given state is very large, and if it can be observed as a function of time it is a very good approximation of the probability density function defined in section 2. This means that the functions A(t) and C(t) corresponding to two given states can be measured, their moments computed, and finally the moments of the unknown function B(t) obtained using equations 7, 8, or 9.

These last moments can be given a clear physical meaning; for instance B_0 is the fraction of particles leaving the first state that actually reach the second state (a quantity analogous to the Bioavailability as defined in Pharmacokinetics), b_1 is the expected interval of time for a particle to move from the first to the second state, β_2 is twice the variance of the above time, etc. (10).

5. A SIMPLE COMPARTMENT

It may be interesting to compare the actual values of the moments of a specific system. Take for instance a single compartment, i.e. a well mixed pool of homogeneous particles, all with the same probability $m\,dt$ of leaving in the interval from t to $t+dt$, where m is a constant; in other words the probability of leaving the compartment does not depend on the absolute time or on the time when a particle entered it. If $A(t)$ is the probability density function characteristic of the compartment, i.e., the probability that a particle is in the compartment at time t, then

$$A(t+dt) = A(t).(1-m\,dt)$$

is the probability that a given particle present in the compartment at time t is still there at time $t+dt$; rearranging this equation,

$$dA/dt = -mA(t),$$

and integrating,

$$A(t) = A(0).e^{-mt},$$

where the constant of integration $A(0)$ is the probability that a given particle is present in the compartment at the initial time. Using definitions 2, 3, and 4 we get for a simple compartment,

$$A_i = A(0)/m^{i+1}, \quad i=0,1,2,\ldots$$

$$a_i = 1/m^i, \quad i=1,2,3,\ldots$$

$$\alpha_1 = 1/m$$

$$\alpha_2 = 1/2m^2$$

$$\alpha_3 = 1/3m^3$$

$$\alpha_4 = 3/8m^4$$

and so forth.

6. SYNTHESIS

Consider two systems in series, that is two systems such that all particles entering the second of them are originating from the first; the first system is called the _unique precursor_ of the second (11). If

$A(t)dt$ = probability that a particle entering the first system at time 0 leaves it during the interval $t, t+dt$,

$B(t)dt$ = probability that a particle entering the second system at time 0 leaves it during the interval $t, t+dt$,

then, ignoring infinitesimals of order higher than dt, the probability that a particle entering the first system at time 0 moves to the second in the interval $u, u+du$ and leaves this one in the interval $t, t+dt$ is $A(u)du \cdot B(t-u)dt$. Taking the integral of the expression above for all values of u from 0 to t, one gets the probability that a particle that entered the first system at time 0 leaves the second at a time between t and $t+dt$, no matter when it moved from the first to the second, i.e. the convolution

$$\int_0^t A(u)B(t-u)du$$

is the probability density function characteristic of the system formed by two systems in series.

Obviously the properties of the convolution described in section 4 apply in this case also.

If two systems are in parallel, i.e. a particle can enter either system and be detected when it leaves either of them, then calling $A(t)$ and $B(t)$ the probability density functions of the two separate systems, the probability density function of the two systems taken globally is $A(t)+B(t)$. Obviously in this case the moments of the resulting system are

$$A_0 + B_0$$

$$A_1 + B_1$$

$$A_2 + B_2$$

$$\cdots\cdots\cdots$$

For the relative moments we have

(10) $$\frac{A_i+B_i}{A_0+B_0} = \frac{A_i}{A_0} \frac{A_0}{A_0+B_0} + \frac{B_i}{B_0} \frac{B_0}{A_0+B_0}$$

$$= a_i w_a + b_i w_b,$$

where i is any positive integer and

$$w_a = A_0/(A_0+B_0), \quad w_b = B_0/(A_0+B_0),$$

called the _weights_ of the two systems (12), are factors representing the probability that a particle goes through one rather than the other system.

If a system forms a loop, i.e. a particle can reenter it after leaving it, put

$A(t)dt$ = probability that a particle that entered the system at time 0 leaves it for the first time in the interval t, $t+dt$,

$M(t)dt$ = probability that a particle that entered the system at time 0 leaves it in the interval $t, t+dt$ irrespective of the number of passages through it.

The convolution

$$\int_0^t M(u)A(t-u)du$$

is the probability density function corresponding to a particle going through that system two or more times; by adding to it the probability density function corresponding to just one passage, we should get again the function $M(t)$, i.e.,

$$M(t) = \int_0^t M(u)A(t-u)du + A(t);$$

taking the moments of the functions above, using equation 7,

$$M_0 = M_0 A_0 + A_0$$

$$M_1 = M_0 A_1 + M_1 A_0 + A_1$$

$$M_2 = M_0 A_2 + M_1 A_1 + M_2 A_0 + A_2$$

$$\cdots\cdots\cdots$$

hence

(11)
$$M_0 = A_0/(1-A_0)$$

$$M_1 = A_1(M_0+1)/(1-A_0)$$

$$M_2 = [A_2(M_0+1)+A_1 M_1]/(1-A_0)$$

$$\cdots\cdots\cdots$$

and

$$m_1 = a_1(M_0+1)$$

$$m_2 = a_2(M_0+1) + a_1 M_1$$

$$\cdots\cdots\cdots$$

(12)
$$m_i = a_i(M_0+1) + \sum_{j=1}^{i-1} a_j M_{i-j}.$$

7. ANALYSIS

The formulas of the previous section can be inverted to compute the moments of separate subsystems from the moments of the global system, if enough data are available. At this point it is convenient to introduce a new notation. Call $F_n{}^{ij}$ the n-moment of the transport of a particle from state i to state j, and $F_n{}^{ii}$ the n-moment of the transport through a cycle beginning and ending in state i. Also call $F_n{}^{ii*}$ the n-moment of the onetime transport through the cycle around i, and $F_n{}^{ij}(l,m,...)$ the n-moment of the transport from i to j excluding the particles that are going through the states $l,m,...$, indicated in parenthesis. Furthermore, if j is one of the superscripts in parenthesis, then from that moment the transport along a cycle through j is excluded. Lower case letters represent the corresponding relative moments.

With this notation equation 11 for instance becomes

(13) $$F_0{}^{jj} = F_0{}^{jj*}/(1-F_0{}^{jj*})$$

and equation 12

(14) $$f_n{}^{jj} = f_n{}^{jj*}(F_0{}^{jj}+1) + \sum_{\ell=1}^{n-1} f_1{}^{jj*} F_{n-1}{}^{jj};$$

by inversion,

$$F_0{}^{jj*} = F_0{}^{jj}/(1+F_0{}^{jj}),$$

$$f_n{}^{jj*} = 1/(F_0{}^{jj}+1) \cdot (f_n{}^{jj} - \sum_{\ell=1}^{n-1} f_1{}^{jj*} F_{n-1}{}^{jj}).$$

Suppose now that two states, say i and j, have been observed, and from the experimental data the moments $F_n{}^{ij}$ have been computed for a sufficient number of values of n. From section 6, remembering equation 7,

$$F_0{}^{ij} = F_0{}^{ij}(j) F_0{}^{jj}$$

and remembering equation 8,

$$f_n{}^{ij} = \sum_{\ell=0}^{n} f_{n-1}{}^{ij}(j) f_1{}^{jj}, \quad n=1,2,...$$

because the direct transfer of a particle from state i to state j is followed by an indeterminate number of recyclings of that particle around state j. If in the two equations above we substitute the values of $F_0{}^{jj}$ and $f_n{}^{jj}$ given by equations 13 and 14, we have a number of equations showing the relationships between, on one side the moments $F_0{}^{ij}$, $f_n{}^{ij}$ of the global transfer from i to j, as observed experimentally, and on the other side the unknown moments $F_0{}^{ij}(j)$, $f_n{}^{ij}(j)$ of the direct transfer from i to j, and $F_0{}^{jj*}$, $f_n{}^{jj*}$ of a single recycling around j. By inversion of those equations, the moments of the subsystems can be computed; they describe the behavior of a particle during transfers not directly observable.

8. NON-CONVERGING MOMENTS

The definitions given in section 3 require the convergence of certain integrals, in particular of

(15) $$\int_0^\infty t^i/i! \, F(t) dt;$$

this requires that function F(t) decreases fast enough when t approaches infinity. It is a known fact (12) that most functions of biological interest are of exponential order, i.e. they have the property that a constant a>0 exists such that the product $e^{-at}F(t)$ is bounded for all values of t larger than some finite value; for a function of exponential order the integral above always converges, no matter how large i is. A notable exception is given by a closed system, i.e. a system from where not all particles are eventually lost; in this case

$$\lim_{t\to\infty} F(t) \neq 0,$$

and integral 15 does not converge for any non-negative value of i. Obviously the expected time spent by a particle in such a system is infinite. We shall not consider this case, but the more interesting case when function B(t), as defined in section 2, is of exponential order, while function A(t) is bounded but does not approach zero as t approaches infinity. This corresponds to feeding a "regular" system with an endless stream of particles. Equation 1 shows that function C(t) also will have a non-zero limit, therefore neither the moments of A(t) or C(t) are defined, while B(t) has defined, but unknown moments.

From the hypothesis that A(t) is bounded, it follows that $e^{-gt}A(t)$ is of exponential order for any g>0; the convolution integral in 1 can be rewritten as

$$\int_0^t e^{-gu}A(u) \cdot e^{-g(t-u)}B(t-u) du = e^{-gt}C(t),$$

showing that multiplying both A(t) and C(t) by e^{gt} is equivalent to multiplying B(t) by the same exponential function. The new functions $e^{-gt}A(t)$ and $e^{-gt}C(t)$ have finite moments, and using equations 7, 8, 9 we can compute the moments of $e^{-gt}B(t)$; calling B_i^* the moments of this last function, then

$$B_i^* = \int_0^\infty t^i/i! \cdot e^{-gt}B(t)dt$$

$$= \int_0^\infty \sum_{j=0}^\infty (-gt)^j/j! \cdot t^i/i! \cdot B(t)dt$$

$$= \sum_{j=0}^\infty (-1)^j g^j (i+j)!/i!j! \cdot B_{i+j}, \qquad i=0,1,2,\ldots$$

and by inversion

(16) $$B_i = \sum_{j=0}^{\infty} g^j (i+j)!/i!j! \cdot B_{i+j}^*, \qquad i=0,1,2,\ldots$$

In the special case when functions A(t) and C(t) are evaluated by measuring the activity of a radioactive tracer in two states of the system, then the "true" probability density functions are multiplied by the exponential function e^{-gt}, where g is the decay constant of the nuclide used. If the true functions A(t) and C(t) are not corrected for the radioactive decay, then the moments B_i^* should be corrected using equations 16; these last corrections are frequently easy because in general the infinite series in equation 16 converges very rapidly. More important is the fact that the direct correction of A(t) and C(t) for the disintegration rate of the nuclide involves a non-negligible error when that rate is very high, as shown in the next section.

9. RECORDING THE MOMENTS

In section 4 we saw that functions A(t) and C(t) can be measured, for instance, by counting the number of particles present in a state at a given time t, and then their moments computed. Several observations are needed at this point.

First, very rarely a direct count of particles is possible; more often than not what can be counted are not the particles themselves, but a _tracer_ thereof, i.e. a subset of the _tracee_, sharing all or most of its properties but having some additional property that can be easily measured by an appropriate detector. This implies the introduction of a factor representing the trueness of the tracer to the tracee; this factor can be determined by calibration, but it may also contain some non-deterministic components. For instance when using an isotopic tracer one must consider the random nature of the mixing tracer-tracee, and if the isotope is a radioactive one also the randomness of the disintegration events.

Second, any detector has a finite resolution time, therefore it does not measure the exact number of particles present at time t, but the average number of particles present in a certain interval of time; this implies an error when the number of particles changes fast enough compared to the resolution time of the detector (13, 14).

Third, the obvious method of computing the moments of A(t) and C(t) is by a number of integrations; they introduce some computational errors that are added to the measuring errors intrinsic to the counter.

The method described here tries to reduces to their theoretical minimum all errors due to computations, and at the same time allows a direct evaluation of the errors due to the random nature of the phenomenon to be detected.

Consider X(t) to be the number of particles to be counted in a particular voxel, or alternatively the number of photons transmitted through a particular pixel; then kX(t) is the probability that an event will be detected in the interval from t to t+dt, where k is a constant depending upon the efficiency of the detector and, if the case, upon the disintegration rate of the radiotracer used; the probability of a double event in the infinitesimal time interval dt is an infinitesimal of order higher than dt and can be neglected. The constant k can be determined by counting for a sufficiently long interval of time the particles present in, or the photons emitted by, a calibrated phantom.

Also define the random variable N(t) equal to the number of events (for instance photons) recorded in the interval of time from 0 to t, with distribution

$$p(r,t) = \text{Prob}\{N(t)=r\}.$$

Each time an event is recorded, the value of the random variable N(t) increases by one unit; it stays constant if no events are recorded. Therefore

$$p(0,t+dt) = [1-kX(t)dt] \cdot p(0,t)$$

$$p(r,t+dt) = kX(t)dt \cdot p(r-1,t) + [1-kX(t)dt] \cdot p(r,t), \quad r>0$$

and of course
$$p(0,0) = 1$$

because the counter is set to zero at the beginning of the experiment.

Rearranging,

$$\partial p(0,t)/\partial t = -kX(t) \cdot p(0,t),$$

$$\partial p(r,t)/\partial t = -kX(t) \cdot [p(r,t)-p(r-1,t)]. \quad r>0$$

Integrating,

$$p(r,t) = 1/r! \cdot [\int_0^t kX(u)du]^r \cdot \exp[-\int_0^t kX(u)du], \quad r=0,1,2,\ldots$$

i.e. N(t) is a Poisson random variable with intensity f(t) given by
$$f(t) = \int_0^t kX(u)du.$$

It follows that its expected value, variance, and third moment around the mean are

$$E[N(t)] = \text{Var}[N(t)] = M_3[N(t)] = f(t).$$

10. HIGHER MOMENTS

We introduce now the random variable $N_i(t)$ equal to the sum of the i-th power of the times of recording an event in the interval from 0 to t, divided by $i!$, ($i=1,2,3,\ldots$); in other words, if $t_1, t_2, \ldots$ are the times when the first, second, ... event are recorded, with

$$0 < t_1 < t_2 < \ldots < t_n < t,$$

where n is the number of pulses recorded in the interval from 0 to t, then

$$N_i(t) = (t_1^i + t_2^i + \ldots + t_n^i)/i!, \quad i=1,2,\ldots$$

$$p_i(r,t) = \text{Prob}\{r < N_i(t) < r+dr\};$$

we can also define

$$N_0(t) = n,$$

a random variable identical to N(t) as defined in section 9.

If several registers are used, each time an event is detected, its instant of occurrence is read on a clock, this value is raised to the power i, divided by $i!$, and this number is added to its corresponding register. When time t is reached, the different registers will show a particular realization of the random variables $N_0(t), N_1(t), N_2(t), \ldots$

If an event is recorded in the interval from t to t+dt, the value of the random variable $N_i(t)$ increases by an amount $t^i/i!$, while it does not change if no events are recorded, therefore

$$p_i(r,t+dt)dr = [1-kX(t)dt].p_i(r,t)dr, \quad r < t^i/i!$$

$$= kX(t)dt.p_i(r-t^i/i!,t)dr +$$
$$+ [1-kX(t)dt].p_i(r,t)dr, \quad r \geq t^i/i!$$

for any positive integer i. Rearranging,

(17) $\quad \partial p_i/\partial t.dr = -kX(t).p_i(r,t)dr, \quad r < t^i/i!$

(18) $\quad \partial p_i/\partial t.dr = -kX(t).[p_i(r,t)dr - p_i(r-t^i/i!,t)dr].$
$$r \geq t^i/i!$$

Define the moment generating function

$$F_i(s,t) = \int_0^\infty e^{rs} p_i(r,t) dr;$$

multiply both equations 17 and 18 by e^{rs}, then integrate the first from 0 to $t^i/i!$ and the second from $t^i/i!$ to ∞; add them together,

$$\partial F_i/\partial t = -kX(t)[1-\exp(st^i/i!)]F_i(s,t);$$

at time 0 no pulses are recorded and by hypothesis all registers read zero, therefore

$$F_i(s,0) = 1;$$

by integration we get

$$F_i(s,t) = \exp[-\int_0^t (1-\exp[su^i/i!])kX(u)du]. \quad i=0,1,2,\ldots$$

By taking successive derivatives with respect to s,

$$\partial F_i/\partial s = \int_0^t u^i/i!\cdot\exp(su^i/i!)\cdot kX(u)du\cdot F_i$$

$$\partial^2 F_i/\partial s^2 = \int_0^t (u^i/i!)^2\cdot\exp(su^i/i!)\cdot kX(u)du\cdot F_i +$$
$$+ \int_0^t u^i/i!\cdot\exp(su^i/i!)\cdot kX(u)du\cdot \partial F_i/\partial s$$

$$\partial^3 F_i/\partial s^3 = \int_0^t (u^i/i!)^3\cdot\exp(su^i/i!)\cdot kX(u)du\cdot F_i +$$
$$+ 2\int_0^t (u^i/i!)^2\cdot\exp(su^i/i!)\cdot kX(u)du\cdot \partial F_i/\partial s +$$
$$+ \int_0^t u^i/i!\cdot\exp(su^i/i!)\cdot kX(u)du\cdot \partial^2 F_i/\partial s^2,$$

and making s=0 we get the first three moments of $N_i(t)$ around the origin,

(19) $E[N_i(t)] = \int_0^t u^i/i!\cdot kX(u)du$

$E[N_i(t)^2] = \int_0^t (u^i/i!)^2\cdot kX(u)du + [\int_0^t u^i/i!\cdot kX(u)du]^2$

$E[N_i(t)^3] = \int_0^t (u^i/i!)^3\cdot kX(u)du +$
$$+ 3\int_0^t (u^i/i!)^2\cdot kX(u)du\cdot \int_0^t u^i/i!\cdot kX(u)du +$$
$$+ [\int_0^t u^i/i!\cdot kX(u)du]^3$$

and from these the variance and the third central moment,

(20) $\text{Var}[N_i(t)] = \int_0^t (u^i/i!)^2\cdot kX(u)du =$

$$= (2i)!/(i!)^2\cdot E[N_{2i}(t)]$$

$M_3[N_i(t)] = \int_0^t (u^i/i!)^3\cdot kX(u)du =$

$$= (3i)!/(i!)^3\cdot E[N_{3i}(t)].$$

Observe that while equations 17 and 18 were written only for positive integer values of i, the moments computed here are valid for any non-negative integer i, because for i=0 they coincide with the results of the previous section.

The value given by register i is the best estimator of the i-moment of kX(t), while from register 2i we compute the best estimator of its variance, and so forth. Of course k can be determined for a particular experimental set-up by measuring N_0 with a calibrated phantom.

In short, by this method the successive moments of the function kX(t) are accumulated in separate registers; because no analog transformations are required as with ordinary ratemeters, the only errors involved are due to the random fluctuations of the photon production and transmission, and these are estimated by higher moments.

11. SCALING THE COUNTING RATE

If the counting rate is too fast, it may be necessary to scale the events before recording their time. Suppose that only every m-th event is recorded; define, for i=1,2,...,

$N_i(m)$ = sum of the i-th power of the time of recording every m-th event in the interval 0, t;

$p_i(m)(r,a,t)dr = \text{Prob}\{r<N_i(m)(t)<r+dr. N(t) \equiv a \pmod{m}\}$;

$0 \leq a < m$

proceeding as in section 10,

$p_i(m)(r,0,t+dt)dr = [1-kX(t)dt] \cdot p_i(m)(r,0,t)dr,$

$r < t^i/i!$

$= kX(t)dt \cdot p_i(m)(r-t^i/i!, m-1, t)dr +$

$+ [1-kX(t)dt] \cdot p_i(m)(r,0,t)dr. \quad r \geq t^i/i!$

$p_i(m)(r,a,t+dt)dr = kX(t)dt \cdot p_i(m)(r,a-1,t)dr +$

$+ [1-kX(t)dt] \cdot p_i(m)(r,a,t)dr,$

$a=1,2,...,m-1$

Rearranging,

$\partial p_i(m)(r,0,t)/\partial t \cdot dr = -kX(t) \cdot p_i(m)(r,0,t)dr, \quad r<t^i/i!$

$= -kX(t)[p_i(m)(r,0,t)dr -$

$- p_i(m)(r-t^i/i!, m-1, t)dr], \quad r \geq t^i/i!$

$\partial p_i(m)(r,a,t)/\partial t \cdot dr = -kX(t)[p_i(m)(r,a,t)dr -$

$- p_i(m)(r,a-1,t)dr]. \quad a=1,2,...,m-1$

Adding these equations together,

(21) $\partial P_i^{(m)}/\partial t \cdot dr = -kX(t) \cdot p_i^{(m)}(r,m-1,t)dr,$ $r < t^i$

(22) $\partial P_i^{(m)}/\partial t \cdot dr = -kX(t)[p_i^{(m)}(r,m-1,t)dr -$
$- p_i^{(m)}(r-t^i/i!,m-1,t)dr],$ $r \geq t^i$

where

$$P_i^{(m)}(r,t)dr = \sum_{a=0}^{m-1} p_i^{(m)}(r,a,t)dr$$
$$= \text{Prob}\{r < N_i^{(m)}(t) < r+dr\}.$$

Define now the moment generating functions

$$F_i^{(m)}(s,t) = \int_0^\infty e^{rs} P_i^{(m)}(r,t)dr,$$
$$f_i^{(m)}(s,t) = \int_0^\infty e^{rs} p_i^{(m)}(r,m-1,t)dr;$$

multiply equations 21 and 22 by e^{rs}, then integrate the first from 0 to $t^i/i!$, the second from $t^i/i!$ to ∞, and add them together,

$$\partial F_i^{(m)}/\partial t = -kX(t)[1-\exp(st^i/i!)]f_i^{(m)}(s,t).$$

From this equation, by differentiation, we get

$$\partial^2 F_i^{(m)}/\partial s \partial t = kX(t)[t^i/i! \cdot \exp(st^i/i!)f_i^{(m)}(s,t) -$$
$$- (1-\exp(st^i/i!))\partial f_i^{(m)}/\partial s]$$

$$\partial^3 F_i^{(m)}/\partial s^2 \partial t =$$
$$= kX(t)[(t^i/i!)^2 \exp(st^i/i!)f_i^{(m)}(s,t)$$
$$+ 2t^i/i! \cdot \exp(st^i/i!)\partial f_i^{(m)}/\partial s -$$
$$- (1-\exp(st^i/i!))\partial^2 f_i^{(m)}/\partial s^2];$$

for $s = 0$ these two equations become

$$dE[N_i^{(m)}(t)]/dt = kX(t) \cdot t^i/i! \cdot f_i^{(m)}(0,t),$$
$$dE[N_i^{(m)}(t)^2]/dt = kX(t) \cdot t^i/i![t^i/i! \cdot f_i^{(m)}(0,t) +$$
$$+ 2\partial f_i^{(m)}(0,t)/\partial s].$$

Observe that, by definition,

$$f_i^{(m)}(0,t) = \int_0^\infty p_i^{(m)}(r,m-1,t)dr$$
$$= \text{Prob}\{N(t) \equiv m-1 \pmod{m}\}$$

and, as a consequence,

$$\partial f_i{}^{(m)}(0,t)/\partial s = \int_0^\infty r p_i{}^{(m)}(r,m-1,t)dr$$

$$= E[N_i{}^{(m)}(t) | N(t) \equiv m-1 (\bmod\ m)] \cdot \text{Prob}\{N(t) \equiv m-1 (\bmod\ m)\} ;$$

from section 9 we have

$$\text{Prob}\{N(t) \equiv m-1 (\bmod\ m)\} = \sum_{j=1}^\infty p(jm-1,t)$$

$$= \sum_{j=1}^\infty 1/(jm-1)! \left([\int_0^t kX(u)du]^{jm-1} \cdot \exp[-\int_0^t kX(u)du] \right) ;$$

therefore,

(23) $dE[N_i{}^{(m)}(t)]/dt =$

$$= kX(t) \cdot t^i/i! \cdot \exp[-\int_0^t kX(u)du] \cdot \sum_{j=1}^\infty [\int_0^t kX(u)du]^{jm-1}/(jm-1)!$$

$dE[N_i{}^{(m)}(t)^2]/dt =$

$$= dE[N_i{}^{(m)}(t)]/dt \cdot$$

$$\cdot \left(t^i/i! + 2E[N_i{}^{(m)}(t) | N(t) \equiv m-1 (\bmod\ m)] \right),$$

thence

$$dVar[N_i{}^{(m)}(t)]/dt = dE[N_i{}^{(m)}(t)^2]/dt -$$

$$- 2E[N_i{}^{(m)}(t)] \cdot dE[N_i{}^{(m)}(t)]/dt$$

(24) $dVar[N_i{}^{(m)}(t)]/dt = dE[N_i{}^{(m)}(t)]/dt \cdot$

$$\cdot \left(t^i/i! + 2E[N_i{}^{(m)}(t) | N(t) \equiv m-1 (\bmod\ m)] - 2E[N_i{}^{(m)}(t)] \right).$$

12. AN APPROXIMATE SOLUTION

The two differential equations 23 and 24 must be solved to evaluate the expected value and the variance of the random variable $N_i{}^{(m)}(t)$.

Equation 23 can be written

(25) $\quad dE[N_i{}^{(m)}(t)]/dt = 1/m \cdot t^i/i! \cdot kX(t) \cdot Y(w) \cdot \exp(-w),$

where

(26) $\quad Y(w) = m \cdot \sum_{j=1}^\infty w^{jm-1}/(jm-1)!,$

$$w(t) = \int_0^t kX(u)du.$$

Observe that $w(t)$ is the expected value of the random variable $N(t)$, as found in section 9. For $m=1$,

$$Y(w) = \exp(w)$$

and this case reverts to the case of no scaling; for m=2,

$$Y(w) = 2.\sinh(w);$$

for any values of m>1 we have

$$Y(0) = Y'(0) = Y''(0) = \ldots = Y^{(m-2)}(0) = 0,$$

$$Y^{(m-1)}(0) = 1,$$

$$Y(w) = Y^{(m)}(w),$$

therefore, in operational notation (15),

(27) $\{Y(w).\exp(-w)\} = m/[(s+1)^m - 1]$.

The most logical scaling factors are the powers of two; equation 27 for n = 2, 4, 8 becomes

n = 2: $Y(w).\exp(-w) = 1 - \exp(-2w)$
n = 4: $Y(w).\exp(-w) = 1 - \exp(-2w) - 2.\exp(-w).\sin(w)$
n = 8: $Y(w).\exp(-w) = 1 - \exp(-2w) - 2.\exp(-w).\sin(w) -$
            $- 2.\exp[-(1+\sqrt{2}/2)w].\cos(\sqrt{2}/2.w - \pi/4) -$
            $- 2.\exp[-(1-\sqrt{2}/2)w].\sin(\sqrt{2}/2.w - \pi/4).$

It is clear from these examples that the product Y(w) approaches one very rapidly when w increases. As a first approximation we can take

$$Y(w).\exp(-w) = 1$$

and from equation 25,

(28) $E[N_i(t)] = m.E[N_i^{(m)}(t)].$

Thus the moments on $N_i^{(m)}(t)$ multiplied by m are an approximation of the corresponding moments of $N_i(t)$; the goodness of this approximation depends of course on how fast w increases with t and how fast $Y(w).\exp(-w)$ approaches one. This of course depends on the particular function kX(t) one is trying to evaluate.

As an example consider the function

$$kX(t) = 1 - \exp(-at);$$

tables I, II, III show the correct expected values of $N_0(t)$, $N_1(t)$, $N_2(t)$ for some selected values of a.t, together with the relative errors of the approximations given by equation 28.

TABLE I

Evaluation of $E[N_0(t)]$ from $E[N_0^{(m)}(t)]$

a.t	Correct value	Error for m=2	Error for m=4	Error for m=8
5	4.007	.125	.381	.897
10	9.000	5.6×10^{-2}	.167	.379
20	19.000	2.6×10^{-2}	7.9×10^{-2}	.184
50	49.000	1.0×10^{-2}	3.1×10^{-2}	7.1×10^{-2}
100	99.000	5.1×10^{-3}	1.5×10^{-2}	3.5×10^{-2}
200	199.000	2.5×10^{-3}	7.5×10^{-3}	1.8×10^{-2}

TABLE II

Evaluation of $E[N_1(t)]$ from $E[N_1^{(m)}(t)]$

a.t	Correct value	Error for m=2	Error for m=4	Error for m=8
5	11.541	4.7×10^{-2}	.216	.845
10	49.001	1.1×10^{-2}	4.8×10^{-2}	.146
20	199.00	2.8×10^{-3}	1.2×10^{-2}	4.1×10^{-2}
50	1249.00	4.4×10^{-4}	1.9×10^{-3}	6.6×10^{-3}
100	4999.00	1.1×10^{-4}	4.8×10^{-4}	1.6×10^{-3}
200	19999.00	2.8×10^{-5}	1.2×10^{-4}	4.1×10^{-4}

TABLE III

Evaluation of $E[N_2(t)]$ from $E[N_2^{(m)}(t)]$

a.t	Correct value	Error for m=2	Error for m=4	Error for m=8
5	19.958	2.1×10^{-2}	.125	.803
10	165.671	2.5×10^{-3}	1.3×10^{-2}	1.2×10^{-2}
20	1332.33	3.1×10^{-4}	1.6×10^{-3}	5.1×10^{-3}
50	20832.33	2.0×10^{-5}	1.0×10^{-4}	4.2×10^{-4}
100	166665.7	5.4×10^{-6}	1.2×10^{-5}	5.2×10^{-5}
200	333332.0	1.5×10^{-6}	3.9×10^{-6}	5.2×10^{-6}

As for equation 24, using the approximation given by equation 26 we get

(29) $d\text{Var}[N_i^{(m)}(t)]/dt = 1/m \cdot dE[N_i(t)]/dt \cdot (t^i/i! + 2\varepsilon)$,

where the quantity

$$\varepsilon = E[N_i^{(m)}(t) \mid N(t) \geq m-1 \pmod{m}] - E[N_i^{(m)}(t)]$$

become negligible when $N(t)$ increases. Again a general solution of equation 29 is impossible because ε depends on the particular function $kX(t)$, but as long as ε can be ignored, we can write, using equation 19,

$$dVar[N_i^{(m)}(t)] = 1/m \cdot (t^i/i!)^2 \cdot kX(t)$$

thence, using equation 20,

$$Var[N_i(t)] \cong m \cdot Var[N_i^{(m)}(t)],$$

13. TRUNCATED MOMENTS

The measurement of the moments with a minimum error requires that the integral in definition 2 converges rapidly enough during the time interval of the experiment; this is not always the case, and the problem of incomplete measurements have been studied by many authors in various contexts (see for instance 16).

A method of correcting this error is sketched here.

Because the moments F_i cannot be measured exactly, a reconstruction of the unknown function $f(t)$ is possible only by making some additional assumptions. Let us assume that

(30) $$f(t) = \sum_{i=1}^{n} b_i \exp(-a_i t),$$

where the b_i's, the a_i's and n are unspecified constants, with the only restriction that $a_i \geq 0$; this is the case when the system under observation is formed by a finite number of perfect compartments with different turnover times and is fed by an instantaneous injection or by a constant function; in other cases this provides a good approximation if the system is sufficiently "regular" and n is large enough.

There is no loss of generality if we suppose that all a_i's are different; in some special cases it may be necessary to consider some of the b_i's not constants but polynomials in t, and some of the a_i's complex; these cases will be discussed in the next section.

According to the results of section 5 the moments of $f(t)$ are

$$F_j = \sum_{i=1}^{n} b_i/a_i^{j+1}; \quad j=0,1,2,\ldots$$

With these moments we form the persymmetric matrix (17)

$$P\{F\} = \begin{bmatrix} f(0) & F_0 & F_1 & \cdots & F_{j-1} \\ F_0 & F_1 & F_2 & \cdots & F_j \\ F_1 & F_2 & F_3 & \cdots & F_{j+1} \\ \cdots & \cdots & \cdots & \cdots & \cdots \\ F_{j-1} & F_j & F_{j+1} & \cdots & F_{2j-1} \end{bmatrix}$$

where j is an arbitrary integer not smaller than n-1.
With the coefficients a_i we form the matrix

$$A = \begin{bmatrix} 1 & 1/a_1 & 1/a_1^2 & 1/a_1^3 & \ldots & 1/a_1^j \\ 1 & 1/a_2 & 1/a_2^2 & 1/a_2^3 & \ldots & 1/a_2^j \\ 1 & 1/a_3 & 1/a_3^2 & 1/a_3^3 & \ldots & 1/a_3^j \\ \multicolumn{6}{c}{\dotfill} \\ 1 & 1/a_n & 1/a_n^2 & 1/a_n^3 & \ldots & 1/a_n^j \end{bmatrix};$$

the rank of A is n; in fact the determinant formed by the first n columns of A is a Vandermonde determinant (18, 19) and is equal to the product of the differences, two by two, of the a_i coefficients, all different by hypothesis. Also observe that the <u>kernel</u> of A is the vector C formed by the coefficients c_0, c_1, c_2, ..., c_n of the polynomial

(31) $c_0 + c_1 x + c_2 x^2 + \ldots + c_n x^n = (x - 1/a_1) \ldots (x - 1/a_n)$;

in fact the product of the matrix formed by any n+1 consecutive columns of A by vector C is identically zero.

Define also the diagonal matrix

$$B = [b_1 \quad b_2 \quad b_3 \quad \ldots \quad b_n]$$

formed by the b_i coefficients. It is easy to check that

(32) $P\{F\} = A^{tr} \cdot B \cdot A,$

where A^{tr} is the transpose of A, and that vector C is also the kernel of $P\{F\}$,

$$P\{F\} \cdot C = 0,$$

and of any of its principal minors of order not less than n.

If the moments of f(t) were known, from vector C we could compute the coefficients a_i. In this case the moments F_0, F_1, F_2, ... are unknown, but the <u>truncated moments</u>

$$G_i = \int_0^T t^i/i! \cdot f(t) dt, \quad i=0,1,2,\ldots$$

have been measured in their stead, where T is a finite value of t such that f(T) is different from zero. The differences

$$F_i - G_i = H_i$$

are the moments of the unknown <u>tail</u> of function f(t), i.e.

$$H_i = \int_T^\infty t^i/i! \cdot f(t) dt.$$

If the tail of f(t) is shifted toward the origin, the moments of this new function are

$$H_i^* = \int_0^\infty t^i/i! \cdot f(t+T) dt;$$

from the previous equation, with a change of variable,

$$H_i = \int_0^\infty (t+T)^i/i! \cdot f(t+T) dt$$
$$= \sum_{j=0}^{i} T^j/j! \int_0^\infty t^{i-j}/(i-j)! \cdot f(t+T) dt$$
$$= H_i^* + T \cdot H_{i-1}^* + T^2/2! \cdot H_{i-2}^* + T^i/i! \cdot H_0^*.$$
$$i=0,1,2,\ldots$$

According to assumptions 30, the moments of H_i^* are the moments of

$$\sum_{i=1}^{n} b_i \exp[-a_i(t+T)] = \sum_{i=1}^{n} b_i \exp(-a_i T) \exp(-a_i t),$$

therefore

$$P\{H^*\} = \underline{A}^{tr} \cdot \underline{B}^* \cdot \underline{A},$$

where $\underline{B}^*$ is the diagonal matrix formed by the coefficients $b_1 \exp(-a_1 T)$, $b_2 \exp(-a_2 T)$, and so forth. It follows that the kernel of $P\{H^*\}$ is the same as the kernel of $P\{F\}$.

Observe that the kernel of a matrix does not change if that matrix is multiplied by a non-singular matrix, and that if two matrices have the same kernel, their difference also has the same kernel; therefore if

$$\underline{T} = \begin{bmatrix} 1 & 0 & 0 & 0 & 0 & \ldots \\ T & 1 & 0 & 0 & 0 & \ldots \\ T^2/2! & T & 1 & 0 & 0 & \ldots \\ T^3/3! & T^2/2! & T & 1 & 0 & \ldots \\ \ldots\ldots\ldots\ldots\ldots\ldots\ldots\ldots\ldots\ldots \end{bmatrix}$$

then the kernel of

$$P\{F\} - \underline{T} \cdot P\{H^*\}$$

is still $\underline{C}$. This last matrix can be written

$$P\{G+H\} - \underline{T} \cdot P\{H^*\} = [G_{i+j} + \sum_{\ell=0}^{i+j} H_{i+j-1}^* T^\ell/\ell!] -$$
$$- \underline{T} \cdot [H_{i+j}^*]$$
$$= [G_{i+j} + \sum_{\ell=i+1}^{i+j} H_{i+j-1}^* T^\ell/\ell!] \quad i,j=0,1,2,\ldots$$

where i indicates the row and j the column.

Observe also that the kernel of a matrix does not change if from each element of a row we subtract the corresponding elements of another row multiplied by the same quantity; now from row i (i=1,2,...) subtract the previous row multipled by $T/(i+1)$; from row i of the new matrix subtract the previous row multiplied by $iT/(i+1)(i+2)$; from row i of the this new matrix subtract the previous row multiplied by $iT/(i+2)(i+3)$; and so forth. After each such transformation one of the unknown moments disappears; it is easy to prove by induction that after m such transformations the element of row i (i>m) and column j (j=0,1,2,...) is

$$\sum_{l=0}^{i+j}(-1)^l\binom{m}{l}\Big/\binom{i+m}{l}\cdot T^l/l!\ G_{i+j-l} + \text{terms with } H_0, H_1, \ldots, H_{j-m}.$$

By making m=n, the rows from the n-th down contain only the truncated moments of $f(t)$, which are known.

If enough truncated moments G_j have been measured, the transformations above can be repeated for increasing values of n until one finds a singular matrix, or a determinant sufficiently small to consider its matrix singular within the bounds of the expected experimental errors. The kernel of that matrix is the vector $\underline{C}$, and from it the a_i coefficients can be computed. Using again assumption 30, the truncated moments of $f(t)$ are given by

$$G_j = \sum_{i=1}^{n} b_i/a_i [1/a_i{}^j - (1/a_i{}^j + 1/a_i{}^{j-1}\cdot T + 1/a_i{}^{j-2}\cdot T^2/2! + \ldots + T^j/j!)\exp(-T/a_i)]; \quad j=0,1,2,\ldots$$

these are linear expressions in the b_i's; if the G_j's are measured and the a_i's are computed, the b_i's can be determined from n of those equations.

14. SPECIAL CASES

Polynomial 31 may have multiple or complex conjugate zeros.
Suppose $1/a_i$ is a zero of multiplicity p; then in matrix $\underline{A}$ the row with the powers of that zero, i.e.

$$1 \quad 1/a_i \quad 1/a_i{}^2 \quad 1/a_i{}^3 \quad \ldots$$

will be followed by p-1 rows with the successive derivatives of that row with respect to a_i, thus

$$1 \quad -1/a_i{}^2 \quad -2/a_i{}^3 \quad -3/a_i{}^4 \quad \ldots$$

$$1 \quad 2/a_i{}^3 \quad 6/a_i{}^4 \quad 12/a_i{}^5 \quad \ldots$$

$$\cdots\cdots\cdots\cdots\cdots\cdots\cdots\cdots\cdots\cdots\cdots\cdots$$

In function $f(t)$ the coefficient of $\exp(-a_i t)$ will be a polynomial in t of degree p-1; matrix $\underline{B}$ from equation 32 will not be diagonal anymore, but still independent on the a_i coefficients.

If polynomial 31 contains complex conjugate zeros, then matrix **A** has two rows for each pair of zeros, formed respectively by the real and the imaginary parts of the successive powers of their inverses; for instance from the successive powers of $p \pm iq$,

$$1, (p+iq)/Q, (p^2+2ipq-q^2)/Q^2, (p^3+3ip^2q-3pq^2-iq^3)/Q^3,$$

the two rows are formed,

$$1, \quad p/Q, \quad (p^2-q^2)/Q^2, \quad (p^3-3pq^2)/Q^3, \quad \ldots$$

$$0, \quad q/Q, \quad 2pq/Q^2, \quad (3p^2q-q^3)/Q^3, \quad \ldots$$

where

$$Q = p^2 + q^2.$$

Function $f(t)$ in this case contains the terms

$$[b.\cos(qt) + c.\sin(qt)]\exp(-pt),$$

and the coefficients b and c can be determined from matrix **B** in equation 32.

15. MULTIDIMENSIONAL MOMENTS

Using the algorithm sketched in section 7 the moments derived from each particular pixel can be analyzed to provide information about the subsystems thereof.

The next logical step is the extension of this algorithm to a larger number of dimensions so that the information content of all pixels is treated as a whole and then analyzed in an analogous way (20).

Let function $f(t,x,y,z)$ represent a state variable at time t at a point of coordinates x,y,z; as usual $f(t,x,y,z)$ may be an intensive quantity (concentration of a drug, activity of a tracer, intensity of a light source, etc. at time t and point of coordinates x,y,z) of unspecified dimensions. Define the moments

$$F_{ijkl} = \iiiint t^i/i!\ x^j/j!\ y^k/k!\ z^l/l!\ f(t,x,y,z)\,dt\,dx\,dy\,dz$$

$$i,j,k,l = 0,1,2,\ldots$$

and the relative moments

$$f_{ijkl} = F_{ijkl}/F_{0000},$$

with the quadruple integral above extended to the whole domain where the function has positive values; obviously the set $F_{0000}, F_{1000}, F_{2000}, \ldots$ coincides with the moments defined for a function of one variable t. The four-dimensional moments F_{ijkl} can be recorded using separate registers that accumulate the instantaneous values of $f(t,x,y,z)$ multiplied by the appropriate powers of the coordinates (both spatial and temporal) of the point under observation, divided by the corresponding factorial; the reconstruction of $f(t,x,y,z)$ from these moments can be made with a method analogous with the one described for fewer dimensions (21).

It is interesting to enumerate the different moments of a function in any number of dimensions.

Each moment of order k of a function of n variables is represented by a string $i_1, i_2, \ldots, i_n$ of subscripts, this string being formed by n non-negative integers whose sum is k; the number of such different strings is equal to the number of combinations with repetition of k objects chosen among n objects, i.e.

$$C_k^n = \binom{n+k-1}{k};$$

to enumerate the moments of order up to i, to the string above add the number

$$i - (i_1 - i_2 - \ldots - i_n)$$

representing the difference between the maximum order i and the actual order k; the number of these augmented strings is equal to the number of combinations with repetition of i objects chosen among n+1 objects, i.e.

$$C_i^{n+1} = \binom{n+i}{i};$$

The following table shows the values of this coefficient for some selected values of n and i.

i	n = 1	2	3	4
0	1	1	1	1
1	2	3	4	5
2	3	6	10	15
3	4	10	20	35
4	5	15	35	70
5	6	21	56	126
6	7	28	84	210
7	8	36	120	330
8	9	45	165	495
9	10	55	220	715
10	11	66	286	1001

16. RECONSTRUCTION OF $f(t,x,y,z)$

It is a well known fact that, in general, a function is uniquely determined by its moments (22); therefore if the moments of a function are recorded with the method outlined in section 10, the original function can be reconstructed with a precision depending upon the number of moments available. Even if only few of its moments are known, a function can be reconstructed with some accuracy using Chebyshev's inequality and its generalizations.

Nevertheless in most instances the investigator does not need to know the original function itself, but some of its characteristics, as illustrated in section 6 for the one-dimensional case, where the moments are observed in each single pixel. Parameters like transit time, residence time, transfer time, fraction recirculated (23), and so forth, are much more valuable to the investigator than the mere shape of a distribution curve, even though the amount of information they contain is no greater than the information content of the full curve.

As a first elementary example consider the case when function $f(t,x,y,z)$ is a simple "box", i.e.

$$f(t,x,y,z) = g(t) \text{ for } x_1<x<x_2,\ y_1<y<y_2,\ z_1<z<z_2,$$

$$= 0 \quad \text{everywhere else};$$

then the moment F_{ijkl} is given by

$$\frac{x_2^{j+1}-x_1^{j+1}}{(j+1)!} \cdot \frac{y_2^{k+1}-y_1^{k+1}}{(k+1)!} \cdot \frac{z_2^{l+1}-z_1^{l+1}}{(l+1)!} \cdot G_i,$$

and the relative moment f_{ijkl} by

$$\frac{\sum_{p=0}^{j} x_1^p x_2^{j-p}}{(j+1)!} \cdot \frac{\sum_{p=0}^{k} y_1^p y_2^{k-p}}{(k+1)!} \cdot \frac{\sum_{p=0}^{l} z_1^p z_2^{l-p}}{(l+1)!} \cdot g_i,$$

where G_i and g_i are the one-dimensional moments and relative moments, respectively, of the one-variable function $g(t)$. In particular we can write

$$F_{0000} = (x_2-x_1)(y_2-y_1)(z_2-z_1)G_0,$$

$$f_{1000} = g_1,$$

$$f_{0100} = (x_1+x_2)/2,$$

$$f_{0010} = (y_1+y_2)/2,$$

$$f_{0001} = (z_1+z_2)/2.$$

It is clear that f_{0100}, f_{0010}, f_{0001} are the coordinates of the center of the box; the other first-order relative moment f_{1000} can be seen as a "temporal" coordinate of the box, this one measuring the average time of presence of the particles observed in the box.

From the relative moments

$$f_{i000} = g_i, \quad i=1,2,\ldots$$

the original function $g(t)$ can be reconstructed, but even better its important parameters can be obtained, as seen in the previous sections.

From the second-order relative moments

$$f_{0200} = (x_1^2 + x_1 x_2 + x_2^2)/3!,$$

$$f_{0020} = (y_1^2 + y_1 y_2 + y_2^2)/3!,$$

$$f_{0002} = (z_1^2 + z_1 z_2 + z_2^2)/3!,$$

the coordinates of the box can be computed; in fact

$$4(f_{0100})^2 - 6f_{0200} = x_1 x_2,$$

$$2f_{0100} = x_1 + x_2;$$

similarly for the other coordinates.

From the other higher moments like

$$f_{i200} = (x_1^2 + x_1 x_2 + x_2^2)/3! \cdot g_i,$$

$$f_{i110} = (x_1 + x_2)/2! \cdot (y_1 + y_2)/2! \cdot g_i,$$

and so on, no additional information can be acquired, but they can be used to verify the correctness of the hypotheses made on the system under observation.

Consider now the case when function $f(t,x,y,z)$ is formed by b different boxes. The unknown quantities are $2 \cdot b$ spacial coordinates for each dimension, plus $b \cdot (i+1)$ moments of the state functions of all separate boxes, where i is the order of the highest moment to be considered. Therefore the problem can be solved when

$$\binom{n+i}{i} \geq b \cdot (i+1) + 2 \cdot b \cdot n.$$

The following table shows the number of boxes that can be identified for different dimensions n and moments up to order i.

i	n = 2	3	4
1	<1	<1	<1
2	<1	1+	1+
3	1+	2	2+
4	1+	3+	5+
5	2+	4+	9
6	2+	6+	14
7	3	8+	20+
8	3+	11	29+
9	3+	13+	39+
10	4+	16+	52+

Once the coordinates of the boxes have been determined, the relative moments of order i of the b unknown one-variable functions of the different boxes can be computed using different relative moments f_{ijkl}, where i is fixed and $j,k,l=0,1,2,\ldots$, up to the value needed to form b equations.

These equations are all of the form

$$\sum \frac{\sum_{p=0}^{j} x_1^p x_2^{j-p}}{(j+1)!} \cdot \frac{\sum_{p=0}^{k} y_1^p y_2^{k-p}}{(k+1)!} \cdot \frac{\sum_{p=0}^{l} z_1^p z_2^{l-p}}{(l+1)!} \cdot g_i = f_{ijkl},$$

where the big sum includes b terms, each of them corresponding to a separate box; the above equations are linear in the unknown functions g_i of the different boxes, therefore they always have a unique solution.

Consider now the more complex case when the substance observed diffuses following Fick's law; then

$$\partial^2 f/\partial x^2 + \partial^2 f/\partial y^2 + \partial^2 f/\partial z^2 = D \, \partial f/\partial t,$$

where D is the diffusion coefficient; this equation of course must be completed by appropriare boundary condition that describe the effective physical situation.

With the usual hypothesis that the system is open, therefore the state variable and its derivatives have a limit of zero for t going to infinity, it is easy to verify that the functions in the following table have the moments indicated.

Function	i,j,k,l moment
$\partial f/\partial t$	$-F_{i-1,j,k,l}$ (i>0)
$\partial^2 f/\partial x^2$	$F_{i,j-2,k,l}$ (j>1)
$\partial^2 f/\partial y^2$	$F_{i,j,k-2,l}$ (k>1)
$\partial^2 f/\partial z^2$	$F_{i,j,k,l-2}$ (l>1)

For $i = 0$, the $0,j,k,l$ moment of $\partial f/\partial t$ is the j,k,l moment of the three-variable function $-f(0,x,y,z)$; for $j = 0$, the $i,0,k,l$ moment of $\partial^2 f/\partial x^2$ is equal to the i,k,l moment of the three variable function $-\partial f(t,o,y,z)/\partial x$; for $j = 1$, the $i,1,k,l$ moment of $\partial^2 f/\partial x^2$ is equal to the i,k,l moment of the three variable function $f(t,o,y,z)$. Similar relationships are valid for k and l equal to zero or one.

17. REFERENCES

1. A.Rescigno and G.Segre. Drug and Tracer Kinetics (Blaisdell, Waltham, Mass., 1964).
2. J.S.Beck and A.Rescigno. Calcium Kinetics: The Philosophy and Practice of Science. Phys.Med.Biol. 15(1970)566-567.
3. K.Weierstrasse. Sitzungberichte Akademie Berlin (1885), pages 633 and 789.
4. J.B.Fourier. Théorie Analytique de la Chaleur. (Paris, 1822), page 212.
5. J.H.Matis and H.O.Hartley. Stochastic Compartmental Analysis: Model and Least Square Estimation from Time Series Data. Biometrics 27(1971)77-102.
6. A.K.Thakur, A.Rescigno and D.A.Schafer. On the Stochastic Theory of Compartments: I. A Single-Compartment System. Bull.Math. Biol. 34(1972)53-63.
7. P.Purdue. Stochastic Theory of Compartments. Bull.Math.Biol. 36(1974)305-309.
8. A.Rescigno and J.H.Matis. On the Relevance of Stochastic Compartmental Models to Pharmacokinetic Systems. Bull.Math.Biol. 43(1981)245-247.
9. A.Rescigno. Multiple Compartmental Localization by Diffusion; in Principles of Radiopharmacology (L.Colombetti editor), Vol.3 (CRC Press, Boca Raton, Florida, 1978).
10. A.Rescigno and L.D.Michels. Compartment Modeling from Tracer Experiments. Bull.Math.Biol. 35(1973)245-257.
11. A.Rescigno and G.Segre. The Precursor-Product Relationship. J.Theor.Biol. 1(1961)498-513.
12. A.Rescigno. On Transfer Times in Tracer Experiments. J.Theor.Biol. 39(1973)9-27.
13. C.C.Duncan, R.M.Lambrecht, A.Rescigno, C.Y.Shiue, C.W.Bennett, L.R.Ment. The Ramp Injection of Radiotracers for Blood Flow Measurement by Emission Tomograpgy. Phys.Med.Biol. 8(1983)963-972.
14. A.Rescigno and R.M.Lambrecht. An Algorithm for Reconstruction of Count Rate Curves from Total Counts. Mathematics in Biology and Medicine (Paveri-Fontana and Capasso editors). (Springer-Verlag, Berlin, in press).
15. J.Mikusinski. Operational Calculus. (Pergamon Press, London, 1959).

16. I.Isenberg, R.D.Dyson, and R.Hanson. Studies on the Analysis of Fluorescence Decay Data by the Method of Moments. *Biophys. J.* 13(1973)1090.
17. J.J.Sylvester. *The Philosophical Transactions of the Royal Society of London* 143(1853)424 and 546.
18. A.T.Vandermonde. *Histoire de l'Académie Royale des Sciences de Paris*. (Paris, 1771), page 369.
19. A.L.Cauchy. *Exercices d'Analyse et de Physique Mathématique*. (Paris, 1841), page 151.
20. A.Rescigno. The Two-Variable Operational Calculus in the Construction of Compartmental Ecological Models; in *Compartmental Analysis of Ecosystem Models* (Matis, Patten, White, editors).(Int.Coop.Publ.House, Burtonsville, MD.,1979)
21. A.Rescigno. Multidimensional Operators for the Construction of Mathematical Models; in *Modeling and Analysis in Biomedicine* (C. Nicolini editor). (World Scientific Publ.Co., Singapore, in press).
22. A.Wald. Limits of a Distribution Function Determined by Absolute Moments and Inequalities Satisfied by Absolute Moments. *Trans. Amer. Math. Soc.* 46(1939)280-306.
23. A.Rescigno and E.Gùrpide. Estimation of Average Times of Residence, Recycle and Interconversion of Blood-borne Compounds Using Tracer Methods. *J. Clin. Endocrin. Metab.* 36(1973)263-276.

STRATEGIES OF RECONSTRUCTION ALGORITHMS
FOR COMPUTERIZED TOMOGRAPHY

Ph. GARDERET

CEA - CENG LETI/MCTE - 85 X 38041 GRENOBLE CEDEX FRANCE

SUMMARY

Image reconstruction from projections has progressively spread out over all fields of medical imaging.

As the mathematical aspects of the problem become more and more comprehensively explored a great variety of numerical solutions have been developed best suited to certain medical imaging application and taking into account the physical phenomena related to data collection (a priori properties for signal and noise).

The purpose of that survey is to present the general mathematical frame and the fundamental assumptions of various strategies; Fourier methods approximate an explicit deterministic inversion formula for the Radon transform. Algebraic reconstruction techniques set up an a priori discrete model through a series expansion approach to the solution. The numerical system to be solved is huge when a fine grid of pixels is to be reconstructed ; iterative solutions may then be found. Recently some least square procedures have been shown to be tractable which avoid the use of iterative methods. Finally the maximum likelihood approach incorporates accurately the Poisson nature of photon noise and is well adapted to emission computed tomography.

The various strategies will be analyzed from the aspects of both theoretical assumptions needed for suitable use and of computing facilities, actual performance and cost. At the end of this chapter we take a glimpse of the extension of the algorithms from two-dimensional imaging to fully three-dimensional volume analysis in the preparation of future medical imaging technologies.

1 INTRODUCTION

1.1. Image reconstruction and medical imaging

Image reconstruction involves a large amount of mathematical methods and numerical implementations in various scientific fields. But it is certainly in medical applications that these procedures are used most intensively. For that reason a lot of advanced research has already been achieved and is still under way for both deeper mathematical insight and for more efficient computation tools.

Nowadays many different medical applications make use of connected mathematical techniques :
- X ray transmission imaging (CT scanners)
- Nuclear medicine using single photons emitting substances or positron emitting radionuclides
- Nuclear magnetic resonance imaging
- Ultrasound tomography

The fundamentals of all reconstruction algorithms are to be found in inversion formulas of the Radon operator. But no single technique could be capable of processing satisfactorily such a wide variety of practical problems; so gradually as the application fields were spreading, the computational aspects and the mathematical developments have rapidly expanded.

This paper reviews some conventional strategies that we might consider as basic approaches. In addition we have included some more sophisticated results as an illustration of new research developments.

1.2. General mathematical frame

The basic formulation of the problem is the following (for simplicity only the 2D case is considered here, see 4.2. for 3D extension).

We want to describe an object by the spatial distribution $f°(x,y)$ of some physical parameter. The domain $|D \subset \mathbb{R}^2$, on which $f°$ is defined as non zero, represents a cross section of the object. For all applications that we are dealing with, $f°$ has a non negative value. $f° : (|D \to \mathbb{R}^+)$.

Using appropriate scaling D may be taken as the unitary disk of $\mathbb{R}^2$ (centre 0 and radius 1).

Any line L in the cross section and intersecting the domain $|D$ can be uniquely determined by giving (Fig. 1) :

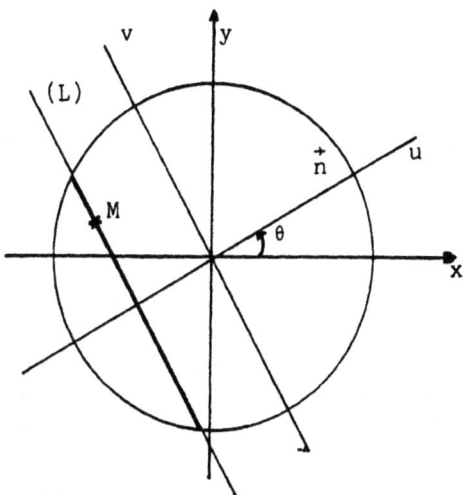

Fig. 1: Parametrization of line integral

$\vec{n}$: a unitary vector of $\mathbb{R}^2$, normal to the orientation of the line ; $\vec{n}$ is associated with an angle :

$$\theta \in [0,\pi]$$

u : $u \in [-1,+1]$ related to the perpendicular distance from the origin

One basic assumption in image reconstruction is that the measurement procedure can give access to the integral value along such a line. This integral is expressed as :

$$p(u,\vec{n}) = \int_L f°(M) dM \qquad (1)$$

where M stands for points belonging to line L.

The explicit formulation in a new coordinate system (u,v) attached to the line L is :

$$p(u,\theta) = \int_{-1}^{+1} f°(u \cos\theta - v \sin\theta, u \sin\theta + v \cos\theta) dv \qquad (2)$$

With fixed θ, $p(u,\theta)$ is referred to as the "parallel-ray projection" of f° at angle θ.

The set of all projections for $\theta \in [0,\pi]$ provides the so-called Radon operator $\mathcal{R}$.

$$\mathcal{R} : f^\circ(\mathbb{D} \to \mathbb{R}^+) \to p = \mathcal{R}f^\circ \quad ([-1,+1] \times [0,\pi] \to \mathbb{R})$$

The inversibility of $\mathcal{R}$ and how it is possible to efficiently compute $\mathcal{R}^{-1}$ are central questions in image reconstruction algorithms.

Formulation of practical problems through the restricted notion of line integral is unrealistic. But it still appears to be a very useful starting point for more sophisticated situations. We now mention a few derivations tractable from basic Radon results:

- Discretness of acquisition through sampling theorems
- Noisy data through optimal filtering results
- Extented integration path
- Non linear context (linearisation by preprocessing)
- Truncated or hollow projections using anlytical extrapolation

However, it is obvious that the analytical approach will exhibit less and less efficiency as the physical context is removed from simple Radon assumptions.

In some cases only the linearity of the relationship between the object and the measure still remains valid without any possible reference on line path. The data collection is then caracterized by a set of weighting functions $\phi_i(x,y)$ and the available set of data is :

$$y_i = \iint_{\mathbb{D}} \phi_i(x,y) \, f^\circ(x,y) \, dxdy \qquad (3)$$

Finding $f^\circ(x,y)$ from a set of such data appears as a pure linear algebra problem very far from Radon transform inversion. Intermediate situations are quite numerous and are thus responsible for a large diversity of algorithms.

1.3. Specificities of data collection

The basic claim needed for mathematical formulation as described by equation (1) is that there is a way to collect data that can be interpreted as linear integration along some well defined domain in the cross section where the imaging device is supposed to work. These domains are preferently rectilinear paths according to the Radon formula, other domains may be accepted in weaker numerical situations. Moreover it is supposed that the geometrical repartition and the total amount of such data is sufficient to insure accurate inversion.

It is therefore convenient to review the data collection systems in medical application in relation to:
- Definition of integration path (collimation effects)
- Linearity of the measure
- Accuracy of the data (statistical perturbations)
- Geometry of the acquisition system

Let us examine two typical examples. X-ray transmission scanners offer the illustration (10), (7) of a system providing a quite good approximation of the Radon assumptions. Strip integrating paths are correctly defined and linear array detectors associated with fan beam geometry give access to an accurately sampled sinogram (typically 10^6 data for one scan). Deviations from linearity due to beam hardening can be corrected. Even when restricting oneself to acceptable doses the number of photons collected is sufficiently important to insure a relative precision of 10^{-3} for each value on a profile. All those reasons explain clearly why algorithms making a direct use of Radon inversion formulas can therefore be successfully implemented.

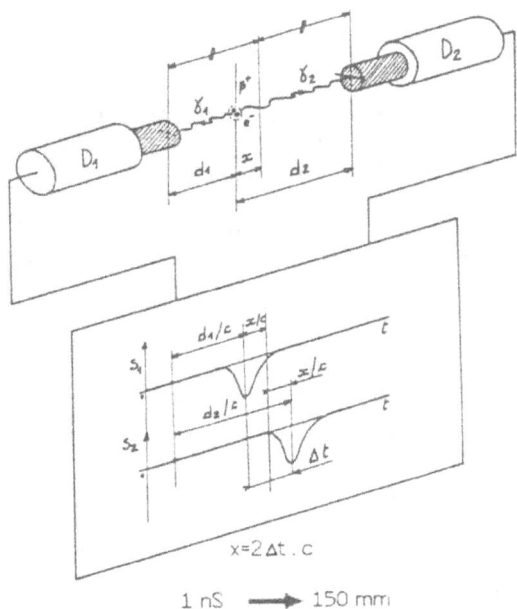

Fig. 2 : Principle of time-of-flight determination in positron tomography

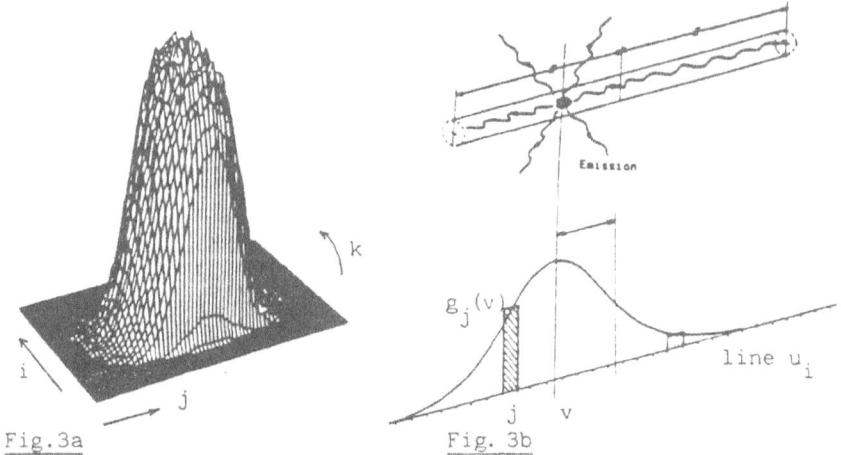

Fig.3a Fig. 3b

Fig.3 : Histoprojection (a) from data histograms (b) in positron emission acquisition with time-of-flight measurement

If we look now at a positron imaging system using time-of-flight information (8), (9) the situation is more complex. The acquisition procedure (Fig. 2) fixes first the direction on which a coincidence has been detected, then associates an estimation of the annihilation position on the line by time-of-flight determination.

The result may be expressed as a collection of counting values that we organize in histo projections (Fig.3a). K = 192 directions covering 360°, J = 64 paths in each direction and I = 64 time-of-flight groupings on each path result in 192 x 64 x 64 observations $y_{k,i,j}$. These data are realisations of Poisson random variables the rate of which is related to the activity f°(x,y) in the object and to the function g(v) describing the error of determination for time-of-flight.

$$y_{k,i,j} = \int g_j(v) \, f_k^o(u_i,v) \, dv \qquad (4)$$

where f_k^o is the expression of f°(x,y) in new coordinates (u,v) related to direction k, $g_j(v)$ is the probability of affectation to the class j of the histogramm of a coincidence appearing at position v on line u_i (Fig. 3b).

As the assumptions are chiefly concerning the statistical properties of the data, it will be important to look for algorithms that fit better into that modeling framework. It has to be noticed that characterisation of the data through (4) is still over simplified for it does not take into account autoabsorption of the emitted photons, geometrical discrepancies in the solid angle within the set of detector pair, calibration, etc...

The survey of all these perturbing features indicate quite well how far we are from the simple line integral model.

1.4. Review of various strategies

There are two main approaches to the problem of image reconstruction.

The first approach is to emphasize analytical developments based on inversion of the Radon integral.

It is thus possible to exhibit many inversion formulas. Next a numerical implementation of the solution is used. This computational step has to take into account the specificities of the problem :

- Sampling of the available data
- Sampling of the reconstructed function
- Statistical properties of noise
- Geometrical description of data collection

All these difficulties induce approximations that are sometimes difficult to quantify.

Commercially available X-ray scanners widely use hardware and software procedures derived from such "transform methods" related to functional analysis, signal theory and digital signal processing techniques.

Some illustrative results concerning these methods are depicted in chapter 2.

An alternative approach is to formulate an a priori discrete version of the problem. A mathematical model relates (most often through a linear operator) the finite set of measured data to another finite set describing the image to be reconstructed. This discrete formulation leads to a system of equations (linear or non linear) to which numerical resolution techniques are applied. In a noisy context the problem has a unique optimum solution highly dependent on the chosen optimization criterion.

The size of the system to be solved is generally very impressive. Either iterative techniques or decomposition in more friendly sub-systems are commonly used for numerical implementation.

This approach is more tightly linked to linear algebra, statistical estimation and optimization theory.

Some illustrative results concerning these methods are depicted in chapter 3.

2 ANALYTICAL APPROACH

2.1. Inversion formula for the Radon transform

The previous discussion about procedures of data collection has shown how idealized the mathematical formulation using the Radon transform is. However it is of great importance to know, through the work of Radon himself (6) that :
$\mathcal{R} : f° \to p = \mathcal{R}f°$ is an invertible operator. Therefore we can expect that if a theoretical solution exists under restricted assumptions there might be some similar ways to approximate a solution in the less restrictive context of practical applications.

The result as established by Radon is :
Any integrable, square, two-dimensional function of compact support is uniquely determined by its Radon transform as defined by equation (2).

Moreover the inversion may be achieved by the following equation :

$$(\mathcal{R}^{-1}p)(x,y) = \frac{1}{2\pi^2} \int_0^\pi \left(\int_{-1}^{+1} \frac{1}{x\cos\theta + y\sin\theta - u} p(u,\theta) du \right) d\theta \quad (5)$$

The integral has to be taken in Cauchy determination.

Direct numerical approximations of integral (5) have been proposed. In the next paragraph we emphasize some fundamental results relating Radon and Fourier transforms from which more convenient algorithms follow in a straightforward way.

2.2. Generalized projection theorems. Back projection operator

Many important and useful mathematical results may be deduced from the following relation :

$$\int_{-1}^{+1} p(u,\theta) g(u) du = \iint_D f(x,y) g(x\cos\theta + y\sin\theta) dx dy \quad (6)$$

This formula is easily proved by substituting p (u,θ) from equation (2) and coming back to the fixed coordinates (x, y). This relation indicates that each dot product in the projection domain has its counterpart as a dot product in the object domain.

Slice projection theorem

The very popular slice-projection theorem is a particular exploitation of (6) with $g(u) = e^{-2\pi i u R}$

This gives us:

$$\int_{-1}^{+1} p(u,\theta) \, e^{-2\pi i u R} \, du = \iint_{\mathbb{D}} f(x,y) \, e^{-2\pi i (x\cos\theta + y\sin\theta)R} \, dxdy \tag{7}$$

We then introduce the useful operator notations:

$$p(u, \theta) \xrightarrow{F_1} F_1(p) = P(R,\theta) \text{ for one dimensional Fourier transform of a projection}$$

$$f(x,y) \xrightarrow{F_2} F_2(f) = F(\mu,\nu) \text{ for two dimensional Fourier transform}$$

$$F(\mu,\nu)(\mathbb{R}^2 \to \mathbb{C}) \xrightarrow{C} C(F) = F(R\cos\theta, R\sin\theta) \quad (\mathbb{R} \times [0,\pi] \to \mathbb{C})$$

for the cartesian to polar coordinate conversion, here applied in the Fourier domain.

Equation (7) is then expressed as :

$$F_1 \circ R = C \circ F_2 \tag{8}$$

This formula gives a straightforward interpretation of the frequency content of the projection in terms of the frequency content of the image.

Back-projection operator

Many inversion formulas make use of the back-projection operator.

$$B : p(\mathbb{R} \times [0,\pi] \to \mathbb{R}) \longrightarrow Bp \quad (\mathbb{R}^2 \to \mathbb{R})$$

Where $Bp(x,y)$ is defined by

$$Bp(x,y) = \int_0^\pi p(x\cos\theta + y\sin\theta, \theta) \, d\theta \tag{9}$$

2.3. Reconstruction by filtered back-projection

This inversion formula is easily deduced by first expressing in polar coordinates the 2.D Fourier relationship between the image f(x,y) and its spectral representation

$$f(x,y) = \int_0^\pi \int_{-\infty}^{+\infty} |R| F(R\cos\theta, R\sin\theta) \cdot e^{2\pi i R(x\cos\theta + y\sin\theta)} \, dR\, d\theta \quad (10)$$

Straightforward use of the slice projection theorem to express C(F) in terms of P(R,θ), followed by definitions of 1-D Fourier transform and the back-projection operator leads to a first inversion expression:

$$\mathcal{R}^{-1} = B \circ F_1^{-1} \circ |R| \circ F_1 \quad (11)$$

This expression is very easy to compute by digital processing and has very useful properties.

F_1 and F_1^{-1} are one-dimensional transformations for which the efficient Fast Fourier Transform (FFT) algorithm is used. The optimal filtering to smooth original data according to signal-to-noise ratio is reduced to one-dimensional problem. The back-projection operation may be restricted to any desired reconstruction domain (zone of interest) and permits geometrical scaling or zooming effects from the same filtered projections.

Moreover it has been demonstrated that an extension of this inversion formula is possible for fan beam geometry (back-projection is in that case a little more complex).(7)

As only one projection is processed at a time it is easy to imagine a pipe-line hardware structure and real time imaging is then conceivable.

2.4. Reconstruction using 2-D Fourier inversion

2.4.1. Estimation in the Fourier domain

The projection-slice theorem suggests a rather direct method for inversion.

From (8) we obtain a precise expression for $\mathcal{R}^{-1}$:

$$\mathcal{R}^{-1} = F_2^{-1} \circ C^{-1} \circ F_1$$

That is :

Step 1 . Take the 1-D Fourier transform of each projection
Step 2 . Change in the Fourier domain the coordinate from polar to cartesian
Step 3 . Take the 2-D inverse Fourier transform

Step 1 and 3 are easily implemented in a numerical way making use of 1-D and 2-D FFT algorithms. But step 2 in spite of an apparent formulation simplicity contains real numerical difficulties. In fact the problem is to construct a good representation on a cartesian grid for $\bar{F_2} f$, being aware of noisy data samples on a polar grid.

A simple way is to compute the cartesian version of $F_2 f$ by local interpolation (nearest neighbor or bilinear interpolation). But important estimation errors may occur chiefly in the high frequency area where the polar sampling is looser and the signal to noise ratio lower. Thus, sophistication of the method is needed to insure as efficient reconstructions as those obtained by filtered back-projection.

2.4.2. Rho-filtered Layergram method

Taking equation (10) and computing the right side double integration without R factor has a two-sided interpretation:

. Taking R away has the effect of producing a filtered version of the image
. Without R factor (10) simply reflects the back-projection operator.

In this way back-projection results in a filtered version of the prior image. A new formula inversion can then be expressed as:

$$R^{-1} = F_2^{-1} \circ C^{-1} \circ |R| \circ C \circ F_2 \circ B \qquad (12)$$

Where F_2 stands for the cartesian version of the Fourier transform and $C^{-1} \circ |R| \circ C$ is the polar expression of the filter with circular symmetry.

Implementation of inversion formulas (12) has two tricky points.

It needs two bi-dimensional Fourier transforms and the computation of the $|R|$ filter in cartesian coordinates requires careful attention.

Moreover the image of Bp (Back-projection of the raw projection data) cannot be restricted to the $|D$ domain so the computation, the smoothing and the first Fourier transform has to be done with at least twice the image size to avoid aliasing effects.

An example of the generalization of that algorithm is given in (8),(9) to reconstruct positron emission images using time-of-flight information. The smoothed "histo-projections" are back-projected, then a bi-dimensional filtering is done using Fourier transform. The filter to be used does of course take into account the spreading value σ in time-of-flight determination. In this case the appropriate filter is:

$$e^{+\pi^2\sigma^2R^2} / I_o(\pi^2\sigma^2R^2)$$

where I_o is the modified Bessel function of the first kind.

3 OPTIMIZATION THEORY AND ITERATIVE TECHNIQUES

3.1. A priori discrete model

We have pointed out previously (paragraph 1.3.) that as soon as linearity is assumed in the measurement procedure a general modelisation for data acquisition may be:

$$y_i = \iint_D \phi_i(x,y) f(x,y) \, dxdy + \epsilon_i \qquad i = 1,\ldots.M \qquad (10)$$

where
- $f(x,y)$ is the function (generally real and positive) to be evaluated on a domain $D \subset \mathbb{R}^2$
- $\phi_i(x,y)$ are known distributions directly related with the measurement procedure (a simple case is to consider $\phi_i(x,y)$ as the indicative function of an integration strip L_i)
- y_i are the M measurements belonging to one acquisition set
- ϵ_i are unknown errors for which statistical properties may be conjectured.

The formulation of the problem is then :
Can we find a "nice" function $f(x,y)$ satisfying the M constraints of equation (10).

"Nice" is a property that is necessary to be precised in order :
- To insure a numerical solution to the system
- To propose a solution with respect to the a priori information on the object $f^o(x,y)$
- To be coherent with the statistical assumptions concerning the physical properties of noise.

Looking for f(x,y) in a numerical way means that we are limiting ourselves to a finite set of parameters describing f(x,y). More formally we look for a discrete decomposition of the form :

$$f(x,y) = \sum_{n=1}^{N} f_n \psi_n(x,y) \qquad n \in 1,2, \quad , N \qquad (11)$$

Some commonly used discrete decompositions are :
a) square pixels
b) polar pixels
c) strip pixels. When using that last sort of decomposition equation (11) determines f(x,y) in terms of back-projections.

Other series expansions are possible for f(x,y) which allow accuracy and a priori properties of the solution to be governed.

Combining equations (10) and (11) leads to the discrete problem :

$$y_i = \sum_{n=1}^{N} (\phi_i, \psi_n) f_n + \epsilon_i$$

We take a matrix notation

y is the M-dimensional data vector
f is the N-dimensional desired picture vector
H is a M x N-elements matrix
e is the M-dimensional vector of statistically known errors

With that notation the system becomes :

$$y = Hf + e \qquad (12)$$

Estimation of f satisfying the constraints of equation (12) for a given data set y is a linear estimation problem for which many approaches exist.

We have to keep in mind that in imaging situations the matrix H contains from 10^4 to 10^5 elements and that it is very sparse. Happily the geometry of acquisition offers rotational invariance that we shall take into account for astute decomposition.

With respect to the pioneer work of Hounsfield we first recall in 3.2. how the first commercial CT scanners dealt with the problem through rather intuitive iterative methods. This approach could be considered now as being completely upset by analytic approaches such as filtered back-projections. But some promising new results in optimization theory (as shown in 3.3 and 3.4.) combined with ever increasing computing power could reverse the actual supremacy of transform methods.

3.2. Principle of iterative techniques

The reconstruction principle used by Hounsfield in the first X-ray CT scanner (10) takes its inspiration from a very intuitive way of solving the system (12) by an iterative procedure: at any step i of the algorithm we predict a set y^i of projections corresponding to the actual estimate of the image f^i at step i by $y^i = Hf^i$.

We examine the infidelity between the data y and the predicted projections y^i by computing for instance the euclidian norm $||y - y^i||$ in R^M. This distance is statistically compared to the assumed accepted error e. The algorithm then stops or proceeds to a next estimate f^{i+1} by back projecting some correcting factor $c^i = g(y^i, y)$. The choice of g specifies the nature of the correction (additive or multiplicative) as well as the amplitude of the corrective contributions, thus :

$$f^{i+1} = f^i + \beta c^i \tag{13}$$

The first step consists in the back projection of the collected data

$f_1 = \beta y$ as $y^0 = y$

Therefore this method may be considered as an iterative approach to carry out the Rho filtering step of the reconstruction algorithm depicted in 2.4.2.

3.3. Non iterative regularized solutions

We have seen in 3.2. that $||Hf - y||^2$ is a measurement of the residual estimation error. The purpose of regularization methods is to realize an agreement between that residual error and a measure of the irregularity of the solution f.

We define the irregularity of f by $||Lf||$ where L is a chosen (N - P) x N matrix and the norm is the usual euclidian norm in R^{N-P}. L is most often a discrete approximation of a derivative operator (gradient or laplacian for instance).

The regularization method produces a set of estimates f_ρ which are the minimizers of :

$$J_\rho (f) = ||Hf - y||^2_M + \rho \, ||Lf||^2_{N-P} \quad \text{with } \rho > 0 \tag{14}$$

This formulation is the so-called Tichonov regularization of the ill-conditioned system Hf = y.

Assuming a weak hypothesis about L, minimization of $J_\rho(f)$ is known (11) (12) to have only one solution f_ρ given by

$$f_\rho = (H^t H + \rho L^t L)^{-1} H^t y \qquad (15)$$

When the applied scheme leading to the numerical image f is suited to the geometrical properties of the collection of data y, one can take advantage of the block-circulant properties of the matrix $H^t H$ to implement efficient computation of (15). See (13) for an illustration of the method applied to positron emission imaging using time-of-flight measurement.

The value of ρ (regularization parameter) is critical to the quality of f_ρ : if ρ is too small the data error induces a solution which is too irregular and if ρ is too large f_ρ is less sensitive to noise but Hf_ρ may be too far from the data.

So the optimum choice for ρ is one of the difficulties of this approach.

Some results reported in (12) give an answer to that problem using generalized cross validation: one omits a single data and studies the validity of the different values of ρ by measuring how the corresponding estimates f_ρ (computed without this data) can predict it. We choose the ρ which gives the best prediction, in the mean, for all possible omissions

The point is that, though theoretically accessible, the solution requires very large computational efforts (much more than computing the solution f_ρ itself by equation (15)).

Fortunately it has recently been shown (14) that the optimum value of ρ could be reached by transforming the expression of the initial problem into an equivalent problem of smaller size. So it is now possible to present algorithms which estimate ρ^* (optimum value of ρ) and compute f_{ρ^*} (the minimizer of J_{ρ^*}) with a cost (number of operations and memory place) nearly identical to the minimum cost of the computation of one estimate for formula (15).

These developments seem to be very promising chiefly when only noisy data are available.

3.4. Maximum likelihood approach

In the applications of emission tomography a basic assumption is the Poisson stochastic model of the counting process. When the counting statistic is low it is no longer possible to use appropriately deterministic models considering noise as an additive perturbation.

It is a distinct advantage of maximum likelihood algorithms (15), (16) to incorporate a proper statistical model. These algorithms estimate iteratively the values of the activity in each pixel from the random vector of experiments by maximization at each step of the likelihood. The model has to be previously described in terms of probability (or something related to the probability that a photon leaving pixel j contributes to the i-th component y_i of the data). The probabilities must be specified in order to take into account physical features such as detector geometry, calibration and attenuation.

The evaluation of the quality of the estimate in terms of likelihood has some nice convergence properties and it allows the inclusion of non-negativity constraints.

4 RECONSTRUCTION METHODS FOR 3-D DISTRIBUTIONS. VOLUDENSITOMETRY

4.1. From 2-D to 3-D imaging

The final purpose of medical imaging is to provide better insight of morphological and physiological properties of human organs ; all these phenomena occur in both time and space so the previous problems are intrinsically 4-dimensional (3 space coordinates and 1 time coordinate).

Dynamic studies are achieved by sequential time sampling of imaging procedures ; but complete 3-D analysis of an organ in medically significant time scales is often incompatible with repeated application of 2-D procedures. So there would be potentially great medical benefits for rapid fully three-dimensional image reconstruction.

Happily the physical phenomena involved in most imaging devices are basically three dimensional ; 2-D data collection is generally the result of geometrical or electronical collimation. For instance cone-beam illumination is the natural use of diverging X-ray sources. Associating such a source with a bi-dimensional detector and selecting proper trajectories provides sufficient conditions for 3-D densitometry.

Gamma emitting radionuclides naturally label an entire volume of interest and, as the photons are emitted on full 4π solid angle, estimation of three dimensional distributions is quite a reasonable goal.

In NMR the great versatility of gradient generation allows an estimation of spin-density integrals to be obtained along any chosen plane. These data are then considered as samples of the 3-D Radon transform of the volumic spin density distribution (17) (18).

So it is an actual trend for all imaging devices to perform computational estimations for the total object (or interesting sub-volumes) and this within a single acquisition reconstruction procedure.

This purpose may only be reached by means of new improvements concerning:
. the technologies of data collection
. the strategies of acquisition modalities including optimization of the trajectories
. the generalisation of reconstruction algorithms
. the techniques for 3-D display

In the next paragraph we present results concerning voludensitometry as an illustration of some new problems occuring in a fully 3-D context.

4.2. Voludensitometry by inversion of estimated 3-D Radon transform

The purpose of voludensitometry is to restitute in one single experiment the absorbance distribution in the whole volume of interest. The acquisition system is composed of an X-ray source providing cone beam illumination and of a bi-dimensional photon detector ; there is a great degree of freedom when defining the trajectories of such an acquisition device in order to insure correct volume reconstruction (19), (20). Once again the Radon transform provides the mathematical frame for that reconstruction.

We suppose that the distribution to be reconstructed $f°(x,y,z)$ is defined on a bounded domain $\mathbb{D}$ (for instance the unit ball of $\mathbb{R}^3$). Each plane P intersecting the domain $\mathbb{D}$ can be parametrized by $\vec{n}$ (a unitary vector of $\mathbb{R}^3$) and u (related to the distance of the plane from the origin). $\vec{n}$ is associated with two angular values $\theta \in [0,\pi]$ and $\phi \in [0,2\pi]$, u is a real value in range $[-1,+1]$.

The 3-D Radon transform $\mathcal{R} : f \rightarrow p = \mathcal{R}f$ is then expressed by

$$p(u,\vec{n}) = p(u,\theta,\phi) = \iint_P f°(M) \, d\vec{M}$$

where $\vec{M}$ stands for the vector of coordinates for points in the plane P.

Just as in the 2-D case some mathematical results exist that provide inversion formulas for the 3-D transform (18).

One very simple formulation is :

$$f(x,y,z) = -\frac{1}{8\pi^2} \int_0^{2\pi} d\phi \int_0^{\pi} P''(u,\theta,\phi) \sin\theta \, d\theta \qquad (16)$$

where $P''(u,\theta,\phi)$ is the second derivative on the variable u. Formula (16) in fact describes a filtered back-projection algorithm. Calculation of the second derivative can be done by a finite impulse response filter; the number of coefficients depends on the noise in the estimation of Radon transform.

The important point concerning X-ray voludensitometry is that a value in the 2-D projection (what we call a radiograph) corresponding to one position of the source, cannot be directly interpreted as a sample value of the 3-D Radon transform. In fact many samples of the 3-D Radon transform may be computed by integration along lines in the 2-D projection.

It has been shown [20] that a good estimate of the Radon transform is possible through numerical approximation of the plane integral using estimated values of the measured lines belonging to the plane.

The different steps of reconstruction can then be summarized as follows:
- Selecting a trajectory amid all admissible trajectories
- Selecting the sampling rate for source positioning on the trajectory
- Selecting the appropriate sampling for evaluation of the Radon transform [21]
- Estimation of the Radon transform from the measured projections
- Computation of the second-derivative on Radon estimates
- Back-projection (using linear interpolation)

5 CONCLUSION

In this article we have proposed a very quick survey of various mathematical aspects of image reconstruction as they are or will soon be widely used in medical imaging systems. Though always referring to a common mathematical formulation a lot of different methods and numerical implementations have arisen, reflecting the particularities of the different measurement procedures and of application fields (X-rays transmission, emission tomography, ultrasound or NMR...).

Although simple and robust algorithms are now at work daily and are commercially available in imaging systems, more and more complex situations are being taken into account, from which difficult new mathematical and computational problems are arising.

So it appears that, in spite of tremendous recent advances, many interesting developments are still to be expected. Moreover image reconstruction from projection appears now to be a motivating research area for image processing, numerical analysis and optimisation theory.

6 ACKNOWLEDGEMENTS

The author is grateful to JL. AMANS, E. CAMPAGNOLO, JJ. CHAILLOUT, D. GIRARD and P. GRANGEAT for stimulating discussions on the subject and for their active research contribution to many aspects of the results presented here.

7 REFERENCES

1. M. Altschuler, Y. Censor, G. Herman...
   Mathematical aspects of image reconstruction from projections. Progress in Pattern Recognition vol. 1 Amsterdam, North Holland 1981
2. Herman GT (ed.) Image reconstruction from projections. Implementation and applications. Topics in applied physics Vol 32. (Springer Verlag, Berlin Germany 1979)
3. Herman GT. Image Reconstruction from projections : The fundamentals of computerized tomography (Academic Press, New York, NY 1980)
4. Herman GT and Natterer F (Ed.) Mathematical aspects of computerized tomography.
   (Springer Verlag, Berlin, Germany (1980))
5. KT. Smith, D.C. Solmon, S.L. Wagner Practical and mathematical aspects of the problem of reconstructing objects from radiography. Bull A.M.S., 83 (1977)
6. Radon J. Uber die Bestimmung von Funktionen durch ihre Integralwerte langs gewisser Mannigfaltigkeiten.
   Berl. Verh. Sachs. Akad. Wiss. Leipzig
   Math - Nature Kl. 69 (1917)
7. Horn B.K.P. Fan beam reconstruction methods
   Proc. IEEE 67 (1979)

8. Ph. Garderet, E. Campagnolo
   Image reconstruction using time-of-flight information in the LETI positron tomography system. Workshop on time-of-flight tomography. IEEE computer society St Louis 1982
9. E. Campagnolo
   Utilisation de la technique de temps de vol pour l'amélioration de l'imagerie en tomographie par positons.
   Thèse de Docteur Ingénieur - Grenoble 1982.
10. GH. Hounsfield. Computerized transverse axial scanning. Br. J. Radio. 46 (1973)
11. G. Wabha Practical approximate solutions to linear operator equations when the data are noisy, SIAM, J. numer. anl. 14 : 651 - 667, 1977
12. M. Stone Cross-validatory choice and assessment of statistical prediction (with discussion), J. Roy. Statist. Soc. Ser. B, 36 : 111 - 147, 1974
13. D. Girard Practical optimal regularisation of large linear system To appear in RAIRO, Anal. Num.
14. D. Girard Les méthodes de régularisation optimale et leurs applications en tomographie : nouveaux algorithmes performants de reconstruction d'images. Thèse Université de Grenoble 1984
15. D. Politte and D. Snyder
    Results of a comparative study of a reconstruction procedure for producing improved estimates of radioactivity distributions in time-of-flight emission tomography.
    IEEE Transactions on Nuclear Science Vol. NS 31 N° 1 (1984)
16. K. Lange and R. Carson
    E.M. Reconstruction algorithms for emission and transmission tomography
    Journal of Computer Assisted Tomography 8(2) April 1984
17. Lauterbur P.C. and Lai C.M.
    Zeugmatography by reconstruction from projections
    IEEE Trans. Nucl. Science NS - 27 (1980)
18. L.A. Shepp Computerized tomography and nuclear magnetic resonance. Journal of Computer Assisted Tomography Vol. 4 N° 1 February 1980
19. Ph. Garderet et P. Grangeat
    Voludensitométrie - Rapports LETI/MCTE/83-106 et 84-016
20. P. Grangeat Methodological study on trajectography GRETSI/CESTA. Premier Colloque Image Biarritz 1984
21. A.K. Louis "Optimal sampling in nuclear magnetic resonance (NMR) tomography". Journal of Computer Assisted Tomography Vol. 6. n° 2 April 1982
22. P. Grangeat. Lecture at the NATO Advanced Study. Institutes Pictorial Information Systems in Medicine. Aug. 27- Sept. 7 1984. Braunlage/Harz, F.R. Germany.
    Voludensitometry : study of the spatial distribution of material density .

Session: Basic Aspects of Medical Imaging

Discussion Summary

As this session was concerned with the basic mathematical problems associated with medical imaging, the discussion was rather limited.

A question asked to Dr. Rescigno was why image processing tended to generate integral equations rather than the differential equations that are often more familiar. Perhaps the most appropriate response is to note that the education of scientists in the area of medical imaging has, in the past, been rather inadequate so that they have had an incomplete mastery of the tools needed for handling many of the problems in this area (for example those required for obtaining numerical solutions to integral equations). Following the paper by Dr. Garderet, the question was raised as to how signal to noise can be optimized from the point of view of selection of an algorithm. Since this is a very general question it was decided that an additional workshop on mathematical techniques in image processing would be held later on in the meeting to allow for more discussion between those participants particularly interested in this issue.

This additional workshop, held two days later, consisted of three presentations: by Aldo Rescigno on "Operational Calculus", by Max Viergever on "Algebraic Reconstruction Techniques (ART) and their Convergence", and by Andrew Todd Pokropek on "Regularized Reconstruction Methods in Tomography". There was considerable interest from the participants of this workshop into the issues of convergence of such algorithms. Additionally there was some extensive discussion as to how such (more sophisticated) algorithms could be implemented, and what computational requirements were needed.

It became evident, during this workshop, that a very considerable armoury of mathematical methods (ranging from ART through Maximum Entropy/Likelihood to Regularized Inverse Methods of parameter estimation) exist without a deep understanding from many of the workers in the field of medical imaging either of the criteria for choosing a given method, or of the details of implementation of such algorithms. As an illustration it was pointed out that many of the implementations of Maximum Likelihood, as presented in current works on this subject, were severely limited by approximations of the stationarity of the point spread function, in order to reduce the size of the matrices involved, and therefore their convergence could not be guaranteed.

It was felt by many of the participants that these mathematical topics could well form the subject of a future NATO conference.

PART II DIGITAL RADIOLOGY: PRINCIPLES, TECHNOLOGY AND CORRELATIVE ASPECTS WITH NUCLEAR MEDICINE

Chairman: Paul H. Heintzen (GFR)

CURRENT STATUS OF DIGITAL RADIOGRAPHY

Robert A. Kruger

Radiology Department, University of Utah Medical Center, U.S.A.

INTRODUCTION

Digital imaging performance is limited primarily by the components constituting the imaging chain and by fundamental physical constraints implicit with x-ray transmission imaging. Undue attention too often is focused on the image processing gymnastics of which a particular system is capable. No amount of image processing, however, could do more to recover information degraded by a faulty or improperly applied imaging component than would improving that component's performance. It is unfortunate that the weakest link in the imaging chain always has the greatest impact on ultimate imaging performance, but if one component is unacceptably poor, then the entire chain will be inferior despite the quality of other components, including the image processor. The greatest improvements in digital imaging performance will be affected either by improvements in the imaging chain or by a fundamentally different imaging approach.

"IDEAL" IMAGING CHAIN

One way to characterize the components of an imaging chain is to compare them to those of a specified ideal system. The ideal system may not be possible except conceptually, but comparison to such an ideal provides a yardstick with which to measure imaging performance. The size of the difference between ideal and actual performance is an estimate of the amount of room for improvement available for each existing component.

The ideal x-ray source would possess three important properties:

1. <u>Arbitrarily high power</u> - The x-ray source should be able to deliver the appropriate number of x-ray photons necessary to image a given amount of tissue: the lower the tissue contrast or the smaller the structure, the greater the x-ray source requirements. It would be desirable to choose an operating procedure based upon the imaging task rather than technical limitations of the source of x-rays.

2. <u>Point source</u> - If all the radiation were created from an infinitesimal "point," the ability to image small structures would not be compromised by the x-ray source. It therefore would be desirable to make the cross-sectional area of the radiation source arbitrarily small.

3. <u>Monochromatic radiation</u> - The ability to produce an x-ray beam consisting of photons having a single energy (monochromatic beam) is desirable. It also would be beneficial to have the ability to "tune" this energy to a particular patient anatomy and imaging procedure. Since imaging performance is x-ray-energy dependent, optimization of image quality is best achieved with x-rays of a single energy.

The properties of the "ideal" detector would include the following:

1. <u>Detection efficiency 100% at source energy</u> - X-ray photons

that strike the detector and are either unabsorbed or utilized inefficiently must be replaced by increasing incident radiation to the patient. It therefore is important that the ideal detector utilize all the x-ray photons produced by the source at some energy (E_s) and which pass through the patient to the detector.

2. *Efficiency 0% at other x-ray energies* - Because of scattering phenomena, x-rays with energy less than E_s emerge from the patient and strike the detector. If the detector were unresponsive to energies other than E_s, scattered x-ray photons would be "invisible" to the detector. Consequently, the deleterious effects of detecting scattered x-rays would be avoided.

3. *Noiseless detection* - The ideal detector would contribute no noise other than that associated with quantum statistics. Detectors that contribute such nonquantum noise sources essentially lower their detection efficiency below 100%.

4. *Unlimited spatial resolution* - This is desirable for exactly the same reasons that a "point" source of radiation is desirable.

5. *Large field of view* - A large field enables all of the relevant anatomy to be seen at once and not in pieces.

6. *Nondistorting* - The detector should provide an accurate measure of anatomic size and shape.

REAL X-RAY SOURCE

The most common type of x-ray source is the rotating anode x-ray tube. While materials have changed and slight modifications have taken place over the years, the basic design has gone unchanged for about half a century. The device is essentially a high-voltage vacuum tube that creates x-rays almost incidentally. Less than 1% of the energy dissipated in such a device produces useful x-rays; most of the rest of the energy results in heat. This heat generation limits tube power.

Besides being capable of delivering only a certain level of x-ray intensity, the contemporary x-ray tube produces x-rays over a broad spectrum of x-ray energies. Not all of these energies are useful for image formation. Some contribute mainly to patient exposure.

In spite of these limitations, an improvement in the x-ray source is not likely to be forthcoming in the foreseeable future. The greatest changes are likely to be in the area of detector technology. For each detector innovation comparison of its characteristics to that of the "ideal" detector listed above will tell us how much progress we are making toward the best we can do.

DATA HANDLING REQUIREMENTS

With what data rates and capacities will our all digital radiography department have to deal in the future if traditional film radiography is to be replaced? The answer, of course, depends on the type of exam being performed. Table I summarizes some educated guesses for a few examination types.

Table I

IMAGE TYPE	IMAGE AREA (mm^2)	RESOLUTION LIMIT (lp/mm)	PIXEL AREA (mm^2)	PIXELS IMAGE	ACQUISITION TIME (sec)	WORD SIZE (bits)	DATA RATE (words/sec)	DATA RATE (bits/sec)	IMAGES PER EXAM	SHORT TERM STORAGE BITS-EXAM
CHEST	1.2×10^5 (30x40cm)	2.5	.04 (.2x.2mm)	3×10^6	1 sec	12	3×10^6	3.6×10^7	2	7.2×10^7
IVA (peripheral)	9×10^4 (30x30cm)	1.5	.09 (.3x.3mm)	1×10^6	.4 sec	10	2.5×10^6	2.5×10^7	60	6×10^8
BIPLANE ARTERIOGRAPHY	9×10^4 (30x30cm)	2.5	.04 (.2x.2mm)	2.25×10^6	.2 sec	8	1.12×10^7	9×10^7	40	3.6×10^9
CINE ANGIOGRAPHY	4×10^4 (20x20cm)	2.5	.04 (.2x.2mm)	1×10^6	$\leq$ .030	8	$\geq 3.3 \times 10^7$	$\geq 2.6 \times 10^8$	10^3	2.6×10^1

A. Chest Radiography

It was assumed that the current chest film size (30 x 40 cm) would constitute the necessary future digital image size. In spite of the high resolution capabilities of film-screen combinations, resolution exceeding 2.5 lp/mm is rarely attained in practical situations. (High contrast resolution phantoms taped to patient chests have verified this finding in our lab.) A pixel dimension of 0.2 mm on a side has a Nyquist resolution limit of 2.5 lp/mm. The image matrix would have dimensions of approximately 1500 x 2000 (3 million pixels). Twelve bit grey scale resolution is assumed, allowing for the increasing dynamic range of such images as scatter rejection techniques and scanning slit (slot) detectors become widespread. Scanning detector arrays promise to reduce imaging time to ~1 second. The data acquisition rate, according to these assumptions, becomes 3.6×10^7 bits/exam.

B. Intravenous Angiography (IVA) - Non-Cardiac

It is assumed that the current film sizes presently used for arteriography (~30 cm x 30 cm) will be necessary for IVA studies in all regions of the body. Lower resolution requirements will be adequate (~1.5 lp/mm) due to the limits imposed by the lower signal to noise ratios achieved compared to selective arteriographic studies. This being the case, each IVA image would be 1000 x 1000 (1 million pixels). Eight to ten bits of grey scale resolution is used currently (10 bits is assumed) and provides adequate results. Imaging rates between one and two per second will be used for a total of perhaps 20 images per projection and an exam may consist of three projections. A data rate of 2.5×10^7 bits per second and a short term storage capacity of 6×10^8 bits/exam will fulfill the future needs of such and IVA study.

C. **Biplane Arteriography**

The requirements for biplane arteriography are increased over IVA studies both because of increased resolution and a doubled rate of x-ray exposures (biplane imaging). Assuming that a piXel size of 0.2 x 0.2 mm is adequate an image matrix of 1500 x 1500 is required. Assuming eight bit grey scale resolution and the generation of 40 images/exam requires a data rate of 9×10^7 bits/sec and a short term storage capacity of 3.6×10^9 bits/exam. An 8 bit grey scale is assumed adequate since intraarterial studies deliver 5-10 times the iodine contrast as intravenous exams.

D. **Cine Angiography**

Heart catheterization procedures will place the severest demands on digital data processing and storage. Even though the image area is the smallest of the four studies considered, both the high imaging rate (> 30 frames/sec) and number of images per exam (>1000) will require data rates of $>2.6 \times 10^8$ bits/sec and short term storage capacity of $>2.6 \times 10^{11}$ bits/exam.

The first question that comes to mind is whether commonly available technology can handle these data rates and storage capacities. Table II lists the properties of several digital processing and storage components which are commercially available at reasonable costs as well as their respective data handling rates and capacities. Comparing Table I with Table II one can answer with an unequivocal "almost". Commonly available technology is very close if one is interested only in short term storage, but not until the much heralded laser disks are available will long term storage needs be met.

Table II. Available Data Rates and Storage Capacities

Component	Rate (words/sec)	(bits/sec)	Capacity (bits)
Analog to Digital Converter (ADC)	3×10^7	2.7×10^8	--
Dedicated Hardwired Processing	2×10^7	3.2×10^8	--
ARRAY Processor	1×10^7	1.6×10^8	
General purpose computer without ARRAY Processor	1×10^6	1.6×10^7	
Winchester Disk	1×10^6	8×10^6	2.4×10^9
Paralleled Disks	1×10^7	8×10^7	2.4×10^9
Digital Tape	1×10^7	1.3×10^8	7×10^{10}

DIGITAL SUBTRACTION ANGIOGRAPHY (DSA)

At present most radiographic studies still rely on film. Digital angiography is an exception. Using DSA a an example we can see the vast number of imaging possibilities that are made possible when radiographic image information is stored in digital form.

The initial motivation for the development of digital subtraction angiography (DSA) was the desire to replace standard intraarterial angiographic procedures with simpler, less invasive (and presumably less dangerous) techniques, specifically intravenous DSA[1-4]. Early clinical success with intravenous DSA[5-11] offered the hope that intravenous DSA would replace intraarterial angiography in the near future. Most of this early DSA work concentrated on the extracranial carotid arteries, aorta, and renal arteries. Today, the technique is being extended to a wider variety of angiographic[12-18] and nonangiographic[19] procedures. In spite of the early success and subsequent proliferation of DSA techniques, however, it is clear that the total replacement of intra-arterial procedures with intravenous DSA is still an unfulfilled promise.

Intravenous DSA as it is implemented today possesses a number of physical and physiological limitations that must be overcome before this promise can be fulfilled. Excessive patient motion artifact, vessel overlap, vessel blurring, or excessive image noise may limit DSA image quality. Perhaps in recognition of these limitations, recent literature indicates an increasing use of intraarterial DSA.[12,20-24] In spite of the fact that it is more invasive than intravenous DSA, it appears that intraarterial DSA offers advantageous reductions in procedure time, contrast material dosage, and patient discomfort compared with film-screen techniques.

A number of investigators are addressing the problems that presently accompany intravenous DSA procedures. Their investigations include the study of DSA-related phenomena such as bolus dynamics[25-28] and alternative DSA image acquisition and processing schemes; temporal integration, recursive filtering, matched filtering, hybrid subtraction, and tomographic DSA. It is the intent of this work to provide an overview of these recent technical developments, describe the differences among them, and point out which problems of DSA each attempts to address and what limitations each of these techniques may have.

CATEGORIZATION OF SUBTRACTION METHODS

As has been pointed out by Mistretta[29], subtraction can be performed with respect to physical variables other than time, such as energy or depth (tomography). A number of recently proposed DSA methods either are new subtraction techniques or are variations on temporal

TABLE III Categorization of Subtraction or Subtraction-Equivalent Techniques Applied to DSA

	Time (t)	Physical Variable Energy (E)	Depth (Z)
First-order subtraction	Conventional DSA Integrated remasking Matched filtering Recursive filtering	Dual-beam energy subtraction (K-edge and non-K-edge)	Tomography
Second-order subtraction	Z Tomographic DSA E Hybrid subtraction t	Three-beam K-edge energy subtraction	

subtraction. A way in which to distinguish the characteristic properties of one technique from another is to note which physical variables (time, energy, or depth) are involved in the subtraction process. Table III categorizes the various subtraction methods that have been studied for DSA applications according to the variable(s) being exploited in the subtraction process.

The first row of the table lists "first-order" techniques. These are methods in which only one physical variable is used in forming the final difference image. The most common form of clinically applied DSA to date is in this row. For noncardiac studies, this technique uses x-ray exposures made once pre second for a total of 15 to 20 exposures spanning the duration of the contrast material bolus arrival and washout. Exposure times are typically in the range of 20 to 200 msec, depending on anatomy. Of the resultant images, two are subtracted from each other to form the final difference image, one taken from among those containing little or no contrast and the second taken at or near peak opacification. Because the two images are acquired at different times, the process is called temporal subtraction. This technique will be designated as "conventional" DSA (CDSA) because it is the temporal subtraction method most commonly used.

Other first-order-subtraction methods also are included in the first row of Table III. Although the processing involved for each method below CDSA (integrated remasking, and matched and recursive filtering) is more sophisticated than that for CDSA, it is still only the physical variable, time, which is being used. Likewise, dual-beam energy subtraction is the first-order difference between two images acquired using two different x-ray spectra, but in a time considered insignificant compared with the phenomenon under study. This particular method still awaits clinical trials.

The lower rows of the table show "second-order" subtraction methods. In these cases the final image is the result of a double subtraction: subtraction first is performed with respect to one physical variable; next, a difference between two of the first-order subtractions is formed to yield the final result. An example is hybrid subtraction, which as described by Brody,[30] is a temporal subtraction of two dual-energy subtraction images, and is listed in the "E" row and "t" column of

Table III. In principle, each physical variable listed (E,Z,t) can be used with itself or either of the other two variables to form a second-order difference image, suggesting six possibilities. Tomographic DSA recently has been studied experimentally, as reported in this issue[31]. Three-beam K-edge energy subtraction has not been used in vivo since the earliest animal studies several years ago[32]. It is possible to go to an even higher order, using three or more variables to form a single difference image.

As detectors become available that meet the resolution requirements listed in Table I, then other areas of radiographic imaging apart from DSA will benefit from digital processing in much the same way that angiography has been enhanced by DSA.

REFERENCES

1. Ovitt TW, Capp MP, Fisher HD, et al. The development of a digital video subtraction system for intravenous angiography. Proc SPIE 1978; 167:61-66.

2. Kruger RA, Mistretta CA, Houk TL, et al. Computerized fluoroscopy in real time for noninvasive visualization of the cardiovascular system. Radiology 1979; 130:49-57.

3. Mistretta CA, Crummy AB, Strother CM. Digital angiography: a perspective. Radiology 1981; 139:273-276.

4. Brenneck R, Brown TK, Bursch J, et al. Computerized video-image processing with application to cardioangiographic roentgen image series. In: Nagel HH, ed. Digital image processing. New York: Springer-Verlag, 1977:244.

5. Strother CA, Sackett JF, Crummy AB, et al. Clinical applications of computerized fluoroscopy: the extracranial carotid arteries. Radiology 1980; 136:781-783.

6. Crummy AB, Strother CM, Sackett JF, et al. Computerized fluoroscopy: digital subtraction for intravenous angiocardiography and arteriography. AJR 1980; 135:1131-1140.

7. Christenson PC, Ovitt TW, Fisher HD, et al. Intravenous angiography using digital video subtraction: intravenous cervicocerebrovascular angiography. AJR 1980; 135:1145-1152.

8. Meaney TF, Weinstein MA, Bounocore E, et al. Digital subtraction angiography of the human cardiovascular system. AJR 1980; 135:1153-1160.

9. Hillman BJ, Ovitt TW, Nudelman S, et al. Digital video subtraction angiography of renal vascular abnormalities. Radiology 1981; 139:277-280.

10. Buonocore E, Meaney TF, Borkowski GP, et al. Digital subtraction angiography of the abdominal aorta and renal arteries: comparison with conventional aortography. Radiology 1981; 139:281-286.

11. Chilcote WA, Modic MT, Pavlicek WA, et al. Digital subtraction angiography of the carotid arteries: a comparative study of 100 patients. Radiology 1981; 139:287-295.

12. Foley WD, Stewart ET, Milbrath JR, San Dretto M, Milde M. Digital subtraction angiography of the portal venous system. AJR 1983; 140:497-499.

13. Pond GD, Osborne RW, Capp MP, et al. Digital subtraction angiography of peripheral vascular bypass procedures. AJR 1982; 138:279-281.

14. Enzmann DR, Brody WR, Riederer SJ, Keyes GS, Collins WF, Pelc NJ. Intracranial intravenous digital subtraction angiography. Neuroradiology 1982; 23:241-251.

15. Wagner ML, Singleton EB, Egan ME. Digital subtraction angiography in children. AJR 1983; 140:127-133.

16. Modic MT, Weinstein MA, Starnes DL, Kinney SE, Duchesneau PM. Intravenous digital subtraction angiography of the intracranial veins and dural sinuses. Radiology 1983; 146:383-389.

17. Buonocore E, Pavlicek W, Modic MT, et al. Anatomic and functional imaging of congenital heart disease with digital subtraction angiography. Radiology 1983; 147:647-654.

18. Ludwig JW, Verhoeven LAJ, Kersbergen JJ, Overtoom TTC. Digital subtraction angiography of the pulmonary arteries for the diagnosis of pulmonary embolism. Radiology 1983; 147:639-645.

19. Brown BM, Enzmann DR, Hopp ML, Castellino RA. Digital subtraction laryngography. Radiology 1983; 147:655-657.

20. Strother CM, Steighorst MF, Turski PA, Sackett JF, Peppler WW. Intraarterial digital subtraction angiography. Proc SPIE 1981; 314:235-238.

21. Crummy AB, Steighorst MF, Turski PA, et al. Digital subtraction angiography: current status and use of intraarterial injection. Radiology 1982; 145:303-307.

22. Miller FJ, Mineau DE, Koehler PR, et al. Clinical intraarterial imaging using recursive digital filtration techniques injecting only small amounts of contrast material or carbon dioxide. Radiology 1983; 148:273-278.

23. Brant-Zawadzki M, Gould R, Norman D, Newton THH, Lane B. Digital subtraction cerebral angiography by intraarterial injection: comparison with conventional angiography. AJNR 1982; 3:593-599.

24. Weinstein MA, et al. Intraarterial digital subtraction angiography. Radiology 1983; 147:717-724.

25. Burbank FH, Brody WR, Hall A, Keyes G. A quantitative in vivo comparison of six contrast agents by digital subtraction angiography. Invest Radiol 1982; 17:610-616.

26. Burbank FH. Determinants of contrast enhancement for intravenous digital subtraction angiography (IV-DSA). Presented at the meeting of the Association of University Radiologists, Mobile, AL, March 22-24, 1983.

27. Mancini GBJ, Ostrander DR, Slutsky RA, Shabetai R, Higgins CB. Intravenous vs. left ventricular injection of ionic contrast material: hemodynamic implications for digital subtraction angiography. AJR 1983; 140:425-430.

28. Modic MT, Weinstein MA, Pavlicek W, et al. Intravenous digital subtraction angiography: peripheral versus central injection of contrast material. Radiology 1983; 147:711-715.

29. Mistretta CA. The use of a general description of the radiological transmission image for categorizing image enhancement procedures. Optical Eng 1974; 13:134-138.

30. Brody WR. Hybrid subtraction for improved arteriography. Radiology 1981; 141:828-831.

31. Kruger RA, Nelson JA, Ghosh-Roy D, Miller FJ, Anderson RE, Liu P-Y. Dynamic tomographic DSA using temporal filtration. Radiology 1983; 147: 863-867.

32. Kruger RA, Mistretta CA, Crummy AB, et al. Digital K-edge subtraction radiography. Radiology 1977; 125:243-245.

CARDIOVASCULAR IMAGING BY ROENTGEN TELEVISION COMPUTER TECHNIQUES

Paul Heintzen

Department of Pediatric Cardiology and Biomedical Engineering
Christian-Albrechts University, Kiel

INTRODUCTION

As a clinical cardiologist I would like to emphasize that the heart is a muscle pump for providing adequate blood flow to the organs and that the understanding of the specific mechanical function of this pump requires knowledge of its dynamic geometry. In particular the SIZE and the SHAPE of the heart chambers and their CHANGES during the cardiac cycle are the immediate, visible expression of the contraction and relaxation of the muscle pump. Dynamic cardiovascular imaging should therefore provide these fundamental geometric aspects of cardiac performance and - if possible - also a measure of the resulting blood flow. At present radiological techniques are still the method of choice for studying the dynamic morphology of the cardiovascular system. Furthermore, radiographic images display the complex information in a way which is optimally adapted to our visual perception.

IMAGE GENERATION

The fundamental process underlying X-Ray image generation is the different absorption of Roentgen rays by material (e.g. bone, tissue, blood, etc...) along the path of radiation (1-7). Although the density differences between the native biological structures of the thorax allow the delineation of the heart and some vessels in plain X-Ray images with a wide and useful clinical application, the essential progress in cardiovascular radiology (which was an indispensable prerequisite for modern cardiovascular surgery) was achieved through the invention of angiocardiography with intravenous or selective contrast material injection into the heart, into the vessels and into the coronary circulation. This conventional angiocardiography or coronary arteriography provides 2-D images of the distribution of X-Ray absorption caused by a 3-D object, specifically marked by a radio-opaque indicator.

The projection of a 3-D object on one 2-D plane has some disadvantages resulting from superimposition. This can, however, be partly compensated for by using biplane or multiplane angiocardiography techniques with angled views for optimizing the projection planes. Furthermore, valuable information from multiple layers are incorporated in one 2-D projection image, since very often structures of interest do not hide or superpose each other. On the other hand, the principal limitations of projection angiocardiography may justify even expensive attempts to achieve a 3-D true spatial and even dynamic spatial reconstruction of the beating heart by radiographic techniques (8). However, these techniques have still to prove of their superiority and clinical relevance.

IMAGING MODALITIES

The 2-D radiation dose distribution behind the object can be transformed into a visible image by various detectors and in the following ways:

1) Images which reproduce the original 2-D radiation dose distribution and thereby reflect the projected cardiovascular anatomical structure;

2) Images which are computed from several exposures of the 3-D object:
   a) taken with different beam directions for tomographic reconstruction of cross sections.
   b) taken at different times for 'functional imaging', thereby reflecting parameters from the cardiovascular system, not represented by any single image.
   c) taken with different radiation exposure (KV, mA, duration, etc...).
   d) the combination of a) and b) or b) and c).

3) Artificial images, obtained by manipulating the original input
   information or combining it with other measures.

IMAGING THE BEATING HEART

Among the detectors which transform the X-Ray radiation into a visible image the invention and continuous improvement of the X-RAY IMAGE INTENSIFIER caused the greatest impact on cardiovascular radiology. It is now the most commonly used instrument for pre-operative cardiovascular investigations. Without considering in details spatial and temporal resolution (optimum between 3 and 4 line pairs/mm) it can be stated that the presently available instruments are of such a high quality that they are almost ideal and superior to any other method with respect to a number of daily required diagnostic decisions to be taken by cardiologists for or against cardiovascular surgery. The main disadvantage from my point of view is the fact that the image at the output screen is not directly available as an electronic signal.

CINE AND VIDEOANGIOCARDIOGRAPHY

Repeated subjective viewing of each angiographic image series is required for the mentioned decision process. Therefore, the dynamic information of the beating heart must be easily reproducible. Roentgen cinematography and videotechniques can meet these requirements.
Although cineangiocardiography has the higher temporal and spatial resolution compared to the conventional video-techniques, one can predict for several reasons that Roentgen television techniques or similar modalities of electronic Roentgen image conversion will replace cinematography more and more within the next decade. One main reason favouring television techniques is the fact that the image information is available as an electronic 'video' signal which facilitates the mixing of biplane information and the combined processing with other physiological reference data (such as ECG, pressure, etc...), as well as the analog to digital signal conversion and consecutive computer processing for QUANTITATIVE PARAMETER EXTRACTION. Although conventional, qualitative angiocardiography is already of indisputable diagnostic value, the extraction of qualitative parameters from angiocardiographic images would give even more insight into the mechanism and

severity of cardiovascular diseases. It is therefore not surprising that the desire for quantitative angiocardiographic image analysis was the strongest stimulus for the development of DIGITAL IMAGING techniques and computer processing independently and even before the advent of computer tomography. What should and can be quantitatively analysed from angiocardiographic image series?
The two main ways for data processing are:
a) the measurement of local DENSITIES and their temporal changes as a special indicator technique;
b) the measurement of single or multiple DIAMETERS, distances or areas, characterizing the dynamic geometry of various cardiovascular structures.

If this is performed by the use of television techniques the procedure is called VIDEODENSITOMETRY or VIDEOMETRY respectively (1, 2, 9-20). It is the purpose of this contribution to describe the principles and essential results of these techniques as well as to outline the path from analog to digital angiocardiographic methods which necessarily led to digital subtraction (DSA) and digital functional angiocardiography (DFA) (Fig. 1).

METHODS

Fundamentals

Quantitative Roentgendensitometric measurements of any kind require the knowledge of the properties of the radiation source, the laws governing the X-Ray absorption by tissue and contrast material and the transfer function of the recording system. With respect to the X-Ray generator, radiation stabilization is imperative and could be achieved by high voltage stabilization via synchronizing the radiation pulses with the cine-and-video chain or by smoothing and controlling the high voltage itself (1).

The application of Lambert-Beer's law to X-Ray attenuation by tissue and contrast material has been tested for continuous and pulsed radiation. With adequate filtering an exponential relationship between the amount of contrast material within the path of radiation and the X-Ray absorption (% transmission) could be established for practically all occurring conditions (4, 7).

Videodensitometry

The most attractive aspects of Roentgendensitometry and in particular of Videodensitometry considered the contrast material as an indicator and applied the principles derived from ordinary dye dilution studies of the circulation, (with some specific adaptations, for example without sampling catheters), to 'radio-opaque' dilution curves. Videosignal processing was initially carried out exclusively by analog means. Later on computerized evaluation of the videodensitometric output signal was the first reason to connect the video-chain to a digital computer (11). The method proved to be useful in a number of applications such as :

1) Determination of circulation times or mean transit times;
2) Determination of cardiac output by applying the STEWART-HAMILTON principle.
3) Determination of ejection or residual fractions from wash-in or wash-out tracings recorded over the central arteries or the ventricles;
4) Determination of endsystolic, enddiastolic or stroke volumes by a double window technique;
5) Qualitative analysis of valvular function;
6) Left to right shunt detection;
7) Flow measurement in different parts of the circulation in absolute and relative terms;
8) The most promising and best establishing clinical application of videodensitometry is its use for QUANTITATION of aortic-, pulmonic- and mitral regurgitation by means of a single or double window, set over the respective heart chambers (19, 20). This procedure was dependent on logarithmic video signal conversion and was facilitated by the use of shaped video sampling windows (1, 21).

The principle of this method is demonstrated in fig. 2 together with its experimental validation. With competent valves, the amount of contrast material injected into the ventricle remains stable during diastole, giving a horizontal plateau in the densogram if the background changes are subtracted. Depending on the degree of regurgitation a diastolic increase of contrast material can be recorded over the ventricle.The increase is proportional to the regurgitant volumes, whereas the systolic loss of contrast material is proportional to the total stroke volume. Densitometric measurements of the regurgitant fraction have been compared to electromagnetic flow measurements and have shown an excellent agreement between both methods in aortic, mitral and pulmonic incompetence (18, 20). This method is routinely applied in our institution for long term follow-up and assessment of the hemodynamic consequences of pulmonic incompetence after surgical correction, in particular in tetralogy of Fallot (22).

Videometry

The second field for useful application of quantitative Roentgen-video-techniques is the automated measurement of distances, diameters or areas. With the progress in electronic technology, it became possible in the late sixties to select from local density differences or gradients of the videoimage the contours of the dye filled cardiovascular structures and to transfer the digitized ventricular border information into a digital computer in real time for further processing. The motivation of a clinical cardiologist for developing these techniques was primarily to facilitate left ventricular volume determination which was too time-consuming by manual procedures and therefore limited to pilot studies. Corresponding biplane diameters of the cardiac silhouettes and an elliptical model with correction factors are used to calculate left or right ventricular volumes. With the appropriate technique and correction procedures even right ventricular volumes can be determined with a degree of accuracy which is not beyond corresponding figures from other physiological methods (15, 23-25). Considering left and right ventricular pump function, it turned out that the right ventricle has a slightly lower normal ejection fraction and ejects its stroke volume from a slightly greater enddiastolic volume level, compared to the left ventricle. The increase in enddiastolic, endsystolic, and stroke volume, normalized for BSA, with increasing age is compensated for by a decreasing heart rate during growth, so that the cardiac index (CI) and in particular the ejection fraction are age-independent 'biological constants', not influenced by the size of the pump (fig. 3). The optimal operating condition of the heart muscle as a whole with normal geometry is reached if about 65% (two-thirds) of the enddiastolic volume is ejected per beat.

CONTRACTION PATTERN ANALYSIS

A two- or pseudo three-dimensional analysis of the overall contraction pattern of both ventricles is possible by a sequential analysis of the ventricular contours and their changes during the cardiac cycle by a semiautomatic analysis of single or biplane angiocardiograms. Irrespective of the detailed geometric fit of any created or assumed 'model' of the real situation, a discrimination between normal and abnormal (pathological) shape changes can be achieved with a comparably small expenditure and extension of the volume programs. The original pseudo three-dimensional model can be sliced into a series of segments, for example, perpendicular to the long axis of the respective ventricle (14). A typical example of an abnormal contracting left ventricle with idiopathic hypertrophic subaortic stenosis, as opposed to the contraction pattern of a failing heart in BLAND GARLAND syndrome, demonstrates the conspicuousness of the contraction disturbances reflected by the geometry and regional contraction velocities shown by this approach (fig. 4).

COMPLETE DIGITAL VIDEO-IMAGE PROCESSING

The above-described techniques for quantitative analysis and data extraction from videoangiocardiography image series, initially carried out only by analog means and not by digital processing of selected image information such as ventricular borders, proved necessary in the procedures for complete digitization of video-image series, as it became technologically feasible (26-29). The rapid progress in semiconductor technology favoured the development of digital video picture memories which allowed real time acquisition of angiocardiographic image series with a spatial resolution of initially 256 x 256 pixels, a grey level resolution of 8 bits and 50 videofields per second (29). In the meantime the spatial, temporal and density resolution could be remarkably increased. The architecture of our system is shown in fig. 5. The interchangeability of the various resolutions and the fields of application is demonstrated in fig. 6. Complete digital image processing procedures allow a maximum flexibility in evaluating a variety of image analysis techniques and the exploration of new biological concepts for circulatory studies. In this context several modes of digital filtering (spatial and temporal), histogram modification image restoration, dynamic - ECG and respiratory gated subtraction and integration techniques as well as on-line subtraction procedures have been worked out in our laboratory since 1975 (15, 26-29, 35-37) and subsequently by other groups (30-34).

CONTRAST ENHANCEMENT IN INTRAVENOUS AND SELECTIVE ANGIOCARDIOGRAPHY

Remarkable contrast enhancement could be achieved not only in non-moving peripheral vessels but also in the central part of the cardiovascular system. The classical example of a left ventricle not visible in the original (best opacified) picture (left) but well-defined after digital background subtraction, image integration and rescaling is given in fig.7. However, satisfactory results from the heart and central vessels require in most cases ECG and respiratory gated sutraction as well as integration techniques (35). We developed programs and functional units which allow selection by cross correlation techniques and subtraction of the optimum background pictures with respect to respiratory background motion (37).

When using these techniques for contrast enhancement, it is possible to obtain adequate opacification of the central cardiovascular structures as well as peripheral vessels even with INTRAVENOUS contrast material injection. Intravenous angiography can also be applied to the peripheral circulation in REAL TIME with or without gating (29). There are many applications for intravenous angio- and cardiography but, as predicted, digital angiocardiography techniques are more and more replacing standard angiocardiography and in particular arteriography. This is possible by performing selective arterial injections and taking advantage of the contrast enhancement by being able to reduce the amount of contrast material to be injected to at least one-third of the dose normally required. Furthermore, important parameters which characterize the pump function of the ventricles - such as ejection fraction (EF) - can be derived from enhanced enddiastolic and endsystolic images alone, so that the X-Ray exposure can be reduced by limiting the ECG gated radiation pulses to the enddiastolic and endsystolic phases of the cardiac cycle. The ejection shell images (fig. 8), obtained with gated or non gated radiation pulses except for ECG gated image selection, also depict some functional aspects of the cardiac motion and contraction (38, 39, 56). If both ventricles and atria are opacified, the enddiastolic - endsystolic subtraction images also allow a better discrimination of the atria from the ventricles, since the increasing and decreasing cavities can be depicted in opposite gray values (e.g. increasing volumes of the atria during ventricular contraction appear brighter compared to the decreasing ventricular cavity from which the ejection shell is dark).

FROM DIGITAL SUBTRACTION TO DIGITAL FUNCTIONAL ANGIOCARDIOGRAPHY

The gain in information by simple or complex subtraction techniques is obtained by using or combining two or more images from an image series, representing the cardiovascular system before or after contrast injection or at various phases of the cardiac cycle (endsystolic/enddiastolic). In any case the resulting images are available as digital electronic signals which can be easily processed with all kinds of programs developed in videometry for a geometric analysis of the cardiovascular system. It could be demonstrated that for left and right ventricular volume determination, calculation or ventricular ejection fractions and contraction pattern analysis, subtraction angiocardiograms offer the same accuracy as conventional angiocardiograms. The method has a high reproducibility, even if the cardiac borders are manually outlined (38-49) (fig. 9). As has been shown by several groups (41, 43, 45) left ventricular function studies before and following physical exercise could be performed with about one-third to one-quarter of the contrast material normally used for each ventriculogram or with the same amount of contrast material used for one conventional levocardiogram to obtain four interventional angiocardiograms. Therefore we conclude that if interventional studies of left ventricular performance are indicated by radiographic techniques, digital subtraction angiocardiography should be applied.

COMPLEX MODES OF FUNCTIONAL IMAGING

If the whole series of videoangiocardiographic images is digitized and stored, any desired combination of pictures can be used to synthesize composite images, whereby the background may be removed and the noise reduced before or simultaneously with the image combination. Useful examples are given elsewhere (50-52, 56). However, the most fascinating aspects of digital angiographic imaging are obtained if the whole series of single or biplane images are considered as a matrix of pixel densograms. This is shown in fig. 10. The digitized data illustrates the simultaneous availability of all pixels wherever or whenever they have been recorded during the angiocardiographic procedure. This allows the nearly unlimited flexibility to select various functional and anatomical aspects from the digitized angiocardiogram or any other time sequence of two-dimensional projection or cross sectional images. The main clinical or physiological problem however, is to elaborate biologically or clinically relevant methods for processing this complex data block. From earlier studies, in particular videodensitometry, several useful principles and methods are known for extracting relevant parameters of the cardiovascular function, such as ejection fraction, regurgitant fraction, cardiac output or arterial blood flow (19, 20). The limitations of this analog technique were mainly due to the small number of measuring windows which have to be set manually. With the whole digitized image series a complete matrix of pixeldensograms is now available. The method for central and regional arterial blood flow measurement; developed in our laboratory (53-56), takes advantage of these experiences and the availability of the whole digitized data block.

BLOOD FLOW DISTRIBUTION MEASUREMENT

The determination of the arterial blood flow is based on the measurement of the progress of the contrast bolus within a branching arterial tree and the videometric or densitometric calculation of the volume of the respective arterial segments. From each pixel densogram - representing the time course of the contrast material passing this image element - several time parameters can be extracted, such as arrival time, time of maximum density, mean circulation time of other values as outlined in figure 11. Experimental studies have shown which time parameters are particularly useful in characterizing the progress of the contrast bolus which in turn is a marker of the blood flow velocity if the geometry of the vessels is taken into consideration. The mean concentration time (fig. 12) and the covariance or cross correlation time are optimally suited for the purpose of time parameter extraction and cardiovascular imaging. The latter is obtained by shifting the sample pixeldensogram with respect to a chosen master-densogram until the max. value of the covariance function is obtained or the cross correlation reaches its highest value. This value can be used as a measure of the similarity between these compared pixeldensograms and the time shift required to obtain this optimum correspondence as the time parameter representing the delay of the sample densogram with respect to the 'reference' or 'master densogram'. If such time parameters for a contrast bolus passing through an arterial level e.g. the thoracic aorta are displayed for each picture element, one obtains a parametric image which is derived from the whole series of original angiocardiographic projection images and thereby represents a new image quality not visible in any single original image. Such PARAMETRIC images may represent functional aspects or any complex geometric measure such as vascular volume. In our method for regional blood flow determination (53) TIME and VOLUME parameters are used. If for example the time of arrival or maximum concentration of the contrast bolus at each pixel is measured and depicted at the respective pixel site as a grey scale level or encoded color, the resulting time parameter images demonstrate the progress of the chosen bolus criterium (Fig. 13). Depending on the velocity of the bolus and the frame rate a TEMPORAL SEGMENTATION can be achieved. It reflects the contrast flow pattern in various ways according to the length of the time segments and the mode of display. The detection and simultaneous two-dimensional display of the flow velocity patterns was not possible previously by any other method. The two-dimensional display of time parameter distribution, however, gives only semiquantitative information about the volume flow or organ perfusion patterns which might however be useful if based on clinical, empirical pattern recognition studies to detect or discriminate normal from abnormal ORGAN PERFUSION. Such studies have been performed to study the kidney, lung and myocardial circulation (18, 29, 56). An example is given in fig. 14.

QUANTITATIVE CENTRAL AND REGIONAL ARTERIAL BLOOD FLOW MEASUREMENT

If the progress of the contrast bolus is quantitated and displayed in the way described above, for example in steps of 20, 40 or 80 milliseconds of the time interval of one cardiac cycle the flow can be calculated if the dimensions of the respective vessels are known. Vessel dimensions can be determined geometrically by videometry calibration or by determining the volume of the individual vessel as obtained by temporal segmentation. The principle applied for vessel volume calculation is taken from indicator dilution techniques well-know in cardiology for many

decades (57) and in an adaptation to Roentgen densitometry
(53-55). With respect to the CONCENTRATION of an indicator, it
is true that the AREA under the time - density curve does not
change along the path of a branching arterial tree. Thus the
passage time increases to the same degree as the concentration is
falling. In Roentgen densitometry the amplitude of the densogram
is not a measure of the concentration but of the MASS, i.e. the
product from concentration and DEPTH and the transradiated
contrast filled space (heart cavity, arterial vessel).
Therefore the complete time-density curves recorded at different
sites of the cardiovascular system cannot have the same area but
differ from each other in a degree which is proportional to the
difference in vessel thickness at the site where the densogram was
obtained. The integration of all areas under pixeldensograms
recorded at a given arterial segment allows the relative or
absolute determination of the volume of this vessel segment. This
concept has been proved experimentally (53-55). By adequate use
of the information of temporal segmentation of the moving contrast
bolus and of volume determination of these vessel segments
relative or following geometric calibration obtained from the
whole matrix of pixeldensograms, absolute flow values can be
determined in central and regional arteries. Together with the
flow pattern analysis these methods open new fields for qualitative and quantitative studies of the cardiovascular system. The
relative blood flow distribution in a branching artery such as the
abdominal aorta or both renal or lower extremity arteries can be
automatically calculated from the volume of the time segments and
the segmentation times. The results can be displayed as percentage
flow by a computer at the corresponding parts of the cardiovascular structure as shown in fig. 15. If this principle is applied
to the central aortic arch as in fig. 15 the segmentation time
should be one or a fraction of the cardiac cycle length. In this
case the pulsatile motion of the cardiovascular structure of the
bolus does not disturb the extraction of anatomically corresponding data for image subtraction and other processing techniques. It
does however reduce the temporal resolution. An example is given
in fig. 16. The first segment represents the spread of the
contrast material during the first heart beat and it is therefore
an indicator of the cardiac output if the volume of the aortic
segment is densitometrically determined as described. In the cases
demonstrated it could be calculated that 14 percent of
the cardiac output goes along a left-right shunt from the central

aorta via a BLOCK TAUSSIG anastomosis into the pulmonary circulation.

References

1. Heintzen PH (ed):
   Roentgen- Cine- and Videodensitometry. Fundamentals and applications for blood flow and heart volume determination.
   Thieme, Stuttgart, 1971

2. Heintzen PH, Bürsch JH (eds):
   Roentgen video techniques for dynamic studies of structure and function of the heart and circulation.
   Thieme, Stuttgart, 1978.

3. Heintzen PH, Bürsch J, Osypka P, Moldenhauer K:
   Röntgenologische Kontrastmitteldichtemessungen zur Untersuchung der Herz- und Kreislauffunktion.
   Elektromed. 12, 82-95 und 145-157, (1967)

4. Heintzen PH, Moldenhauer K:
   The x-ray absorption by contrast material - Theoretical considerations -.
   In: Roentgen-,Cine- and Videodensitometry (PH Heintzen ed.), G.Thieme, Stuttgart 1971, 73-81

5. Heintzen PH, Moldenhauer K:
   X-ray absorption by contrast material using pulsed radiation.
   In: Roentgen-,Cine- and Videodensitometry (Herausgeb. PH Heintzen), G.Thieme, Stuttgart, 85-88, 1971

6. Bürsch JH, Johs R, Heintzen PH:
   Validity of Lambert-Beer´s law in roentgen densitometry of contrast material (Urografin) using continous radiation.
   In: Roentgen-, Cine- and Videodensitometry (PH Heintzen ed.), Thieme, Stuttgart 1971, pp. 81-84

7. Bürsch JH, Johs R, Heintzen PH:
   Untersuchungen zur Gültigkeit des Lambert-Beer´schen Gesetzes bei der röntgenologischen Kontrastmitteldichtemessung.
   Fortschr.Röntgenstr. 112: 259-266, 1970

8. Wood EH:
   New vistas for the study of structural and functional dynamics of the heart, lungs and the circulation by noninvasive numerical tomographic vivisection.
   Circulation 56:506-520, 1977.
9. Wood EH, Sturm RE, Sanders JJ:
   Data processing in cardiovascular physiology with particular reference to roentgen videodensitometry.
   Mayo Clin Proc 39:849-865, 1964.
10. Heintzen PH:
    A simple method for the recording of radiopaque dilution curves during angiocardiography.
    Amer.Heart J., 1965, 69, 720
11. Sturm RE, Wood EH:
    Roentgen image-intensifier, television, recording system for dynamic measurements of roentgen density for circulatory studies.
    In: Roentgen-,Cine- and Videodensitometry (Ed.PH Heintzen) Thieme, Stuttgart, 1971, pp.23-44
12. Heintzen PH, Malerczyk V, Pilarczyk J, Scheel KW:
    On-line processing of the video-image for left ventricular volume determination.
    Comput Biomed Res 4:474-485, 1971
13. Wood EH, Ritman EL, Sturm RE, Johnson S, Spivak P, Gilbert BK, Smith HC:
    The problem of determination of the roentgen density, dimensions, and shape of homogeneous objects from biplane roentgenographic data.
    Proc.San Diego Biomed.Symposium 1972, Vol 11:3-43
14. Heintzen PH, Moldenhauer K, Lange PE:
    Three-dimensional computerized contraction pattern analysis. Description of methodology and its validation.
    Europ J Cardiol 1: 229-239, 1974
15. Heintzen PH, Brennecke R, Bürsch JH, Lange PE, Malerczyk V, Moldenhauer K, Onnasch D:
    Automated video-angiocardiographic image analysis.
    Computer (IEEE) 8 : 55-64, 1975
16. Ritman EL, Sturm RE, Wood EH:
    Biplane roentgen videometric system for dynamic (60/second) studies of the shape and size of circulatory structures, particularly the left ventricle.
    In: Roentgen-,Cine- and Videodensitometry. Edit: Heintzen PH, Georg Thieme Verlag, Stuttgart, 179-211, 1971

17. Heintzen PH:
    Review on the research and some aspects upon modern development of densitometry, particularly roentgen- video- computer techniques.
    Ann Radiol 21: 343-348, 1978
18. Heintzen PH, Brennecke R, Bürsch JH, Hahne HJ, Lange PE, Moldenhauer K, Onnasch D, Radtke W:
    Quantitative analysis of structure and function of the cardiovascular system by roentgen-video-computer techniques.
    Mayo Clin Proc 57: Suppl 78-91, 1982
19. Bürsch JH, Heintzen PH:
    Some principles for circulatory studies using videodensitometry.
    In: Roentgen-Video-Techniques (Ed. PH Heintzen, JH Bürsch) Thieme, Stuttgart 1978, pp. 2-11
20. Bürsch JH, Ostermeyer J, Stelzer E, Heintzen PH:
    Videodensitometric quantification of mitral insufficiency. Concepts and preliminary results.
    In: Roentgen-Video-Techniques (Ed. PH Heintzen, JH Bürsch) Thieme, Stuttgart 1978, pp. 94-100
21. Heintzen PH, Pilarczyk J:
    Videodensitometry with contoured and controlled windows.
    In: Roentgen-,Cine- and Videodensitometry (PH Heintzen ed) Thieme, Stuttgart, 1971, pp.56-61
22. Lange PE, Onnasch DGW, Bernhard A, Heintzen PH:
    The influence of pulmonary insufficiency on right ventricular function.
    Thoracic and Cardiovasc Surg 29/1: 31, 1981
23. Lange PE, Onnasch D, Farr F, Malerczyk V, Heintzen PH:
    Analysis of left and right ventricular size and shape, as determined from human casts. Description of the method and its validation.
    Europ J Cardiol 8: 431-448, 1978
24. Lange PE, Onnasch DGW, Farr F, Heintzen PH:
    Angiocardiographic right ventricular volume determination. Accuracy, as determined from human casts, and clinical application.
    Europ J Cardiol 8:477-501, 1978
25. Lange PE, Onnasch D, Farr F, Heintzen PH:
    Angiocardiographic left ventricular volume determination. Accuracy, as determined from human casts, and clinical application.
    Europ J Cardiol 8: 449-476, 1978

26. Brennecke R, Brown TK, Bürsch JH, Heintzen PH:
    Digital processing of videoangiographic image series using a minicomputer.
    Proc Comp Cardiol, IEEE Computer Society, Long Beach 1976, pp. 255-260
27. Brennecke R, Brown TK, Bürsch JH, Heintzen PH:
    A digital system for roentgen video image processing.
    In: Roentgen-Video-Techniques (Ed. PH Heintzen, JH Bürsch) G.Thieme, Stuttgart 1978, pp. 150-157
28. Brennecke R, Brown TK, Bürsch JH, Heintzen PH:
    Computerized video-image preprocessing with applications to cardio-angiographic roentgen-image series.
    In: Digital Image Processing (Ed. HH Nagel) Springer, Berlin-Heidelberg-New York 1977, pp. 244-262
29. Heintzen PH, Brennecke R (eds):
    Digital imaging in cardiovascular radiology.
    Thieme, Stuttgart, 1983
30. Ovitt TW, Christenson PC, Fisher HD, Frost MM, Nudelman S, Roehrig H, Seeley G:
    Intravenous angiography using digital video subtraction: x-ray imaging system.
    Am J Roentgenol 135:1141-1144, 1980.
31. Ovitt TW, Capp P, Fisher HD, Frost MM, Lebel JL, Nudelman S, Roehrig H:
    The development of a digital video subtraction system for intravenous angiography.
    Proc SPIE 167:61-65,1978
32. Mistretta CA, Crummy AB, Strother CM, Sackett JF (eds):
    Digital subtraction arteriography: An application of computerized fluoroscopy.
    Year Book Medical Publ., Chicago, 1982.
33. Höhne KH:
    Digital image processing in medicine.
    Lecture Notes in Medical Informatics Vol.15, Springer, Berlin Heidelberg New York, 1981.
34. Nudelman S, Capp MP, Fisher HD, Frost MM, Roehrig H:
    Photoelectronic imaging for diagnostic radiology and the digital computer.
    Proc SPIE 164:138-146, 1978

35. Brennecke R, Hahne JH, Moldenhauer K, Bürsch JH, Heintzen PH:
    Improved digital real-time processing and storage techniques with applications to intravenous contrast angiography.
    Proc Comp Cardiol, IEEE Computer Society, Long Beach 1978, pp. 191-194
36. Brennecke R, Hahne HJ, Moldenhauer K, Bürsch JH, Heintzen PH:
    A special purpose processor for digital angiocardiography. Design and applications.
    Proc Comp Cardiol, IEEE Computer Society, Long Beach 1979, pp. 343-346
37. Brennecke R, Hahne HJ, Bürsch JH, Heintzen PH:
    Optimization of generalized subtraction operations for digital fluorography.
    In: Digital imaging in cardiovascular radiology (PH Heintzen, R Brennecke eds), Thieme, Stuttgart, 1983, pp.67-80
38. Mancicni GBJ, Higgins CB, Norris SL, Slutsky RA:
    Cardiac imaging with digital subtraction angiography.
    Cardiovasc Intervent Radiol 6:252-262, 1983
39. Engels PHC, Ludwig JW:
    Digital subtraction arteriography of the left ventricle using time interval difference mode.
    In: Digital Subtraction Arteriography (Ed.: Mistretta CA, Crummy AB, Strother CM, Sackett JF), Year Book Med Publ, Chicago, 1982, pp.123-124.
40. Tobis J, Nacioglu O, Johnston W, Seibert A, Iseri LT, Roeck W, Elkayam U, Henry WL:
    Left ventricular imaging with digital subtraction angiography using intravenous contrast injection and fluoroscopic exposure levels.
    Am Heart J 104:20-27, 1982
41. Tobis JM, Nalcioglu O, Henry WL:
    Cardiovascular applications of digital subtraction angiography.
    Mod Concepts of Cardiovasc Disease 53:31-36, 1984
42. Heintzen PH, Bürsch JH, Hahne HJ, Brennecke R, Budach W, Lange PE:
    Assessment of cardiovascular function by digital angiocardiography.
    JACC 5 Suppl 1:150-157, 1985
43. Spiller P, Jehle J, Lauber A, Pölitz B, Schmiel FK:
    Digital subtraction Angiocardiography: A semiinvasive method to study left ventricular regional and global function.
    In: Ventricular Wall Motion (U.Sigwart, P.H.Heintzen, eds), Thieme, stuttgart, 1984, pp.34-39

44. Norris SL, Slutsky RA, Mancini GBJ, Ashburn WL, Gregoratos G, Peterson KL, Higgens CB, Einsidler E, Dillon W:
Comparison of digital intravenous ventriculography with direct left ventriculography for quantitation of left ventricular volumes and ejection fractions.
Am J Cardiol 51: 1399-1403, 1983

45. Nichols AB, Martin EC, Fles TP, Stugensky KM, Balancio LA, Casarella WJ, Weiss MB:
Validation of the angiographic accuracy of digital left ventriculography.
Am J Cardiol 51:224-230, 1983

46. Engels PHC, Ludwig JW, Bruschke AVG, Plokker HW:
Cardiac digital video substraction angiography emphasizing left ventriculography.
In: Digital Imaging in Cardiovascular Radiology (P.H.Heintzen, R.Brennecke, eds), Thieme, Stuttgart, 1983, pp.192-204

47. Engels HC, Ludwig W, Verhoeven AJ:
Left ventricle evaluation by digital video subtraction angiocardiography
Diagn Radiol 144:471-474, 1982

48. Sasayama S, Nonogi H, Kawai C, Fujita M, Eiho S, Kuwahara M:
Automated method for left ventricular volume measurement by cineventriculography with minimal doses of contrast medium.
Am J Cardiol 48:746-753, 1981

49. Higgins CB, Norris SL, Gerber KH, Slutsky RA, Ashburn WL, Baily N:
Quantitation of left ventricular dimensions and function by digital video subtraction angiography.
Radiology 144:461-469, 1982

50. Bogren HG, Bürsch JH, Brennecke R, Heintzen PH:
Choice of projection in intravenous digital angiocardiography.
In: Digital imaging in cardiovascular radiology (PH Heintzen, R Brennecke eds), Thieme, Stuttgart, 1983, pp.212-215

51. Bogren HG, Bürsch JH, Brennecke R, Heintzen PH:
Intravenous angiography using digital image processing. 1.Experience with axial projections in normal pigs.
Invest Radiol 17:216-223, 1982

52. Bogren HG, Bürsch JH, Brennecke R, Heintzen PH:
Intravenous angiography using digital image processing. II.Detection of left-to-right shunts in an animal model.
Invest Radiol 18:11-17, 1983

53. Bürsch JH, Hahne HJ, Brennecke R, Grönemeyer D, Heintzen PH:
    Assessment of arterial blood flow measurements by digital angiography.
    Radiology, 14: 39-47, 1981
54. Bürsch JH, Hahne HJ, Brennecke R, Eicker C, Heintzen PH:
    Arterial blood flow analysis by digital angiography.
    In: Digital imaging in cardiovascular radiology (PH Heintzen, R Brennecke eds), Thieme, Stuttgart, 1983, pp.115-123
55. Bürsch JH:
    Use of digitized functional angiography to evaluate arterial blood flow.
    Cardiovasc Intervent Radiol 6: 303-310, 1983.
56. Heintzen PH:
    Digital Angiokardiography.
    In: Cardiac imaging and image processing (Collins SM, Skorton DJ, eds.), in press
57. Bloomfield DA:
    Dye curves.
    University Park Press, Baltimore 1974
58. Lange PE, Ewert B, Budach W, Onnasch DGW, Radtke W, Heitzen PH:
    Right and Left Ventricular Digital Subtraction Angiocardiography Global and Regional Accuracy.
    In Premier Colloque Image: Traitement,Synthese, Technologie et Applications (Eds: Feldmann M and Gillet JP) Cesta, Paris, 791-796,984

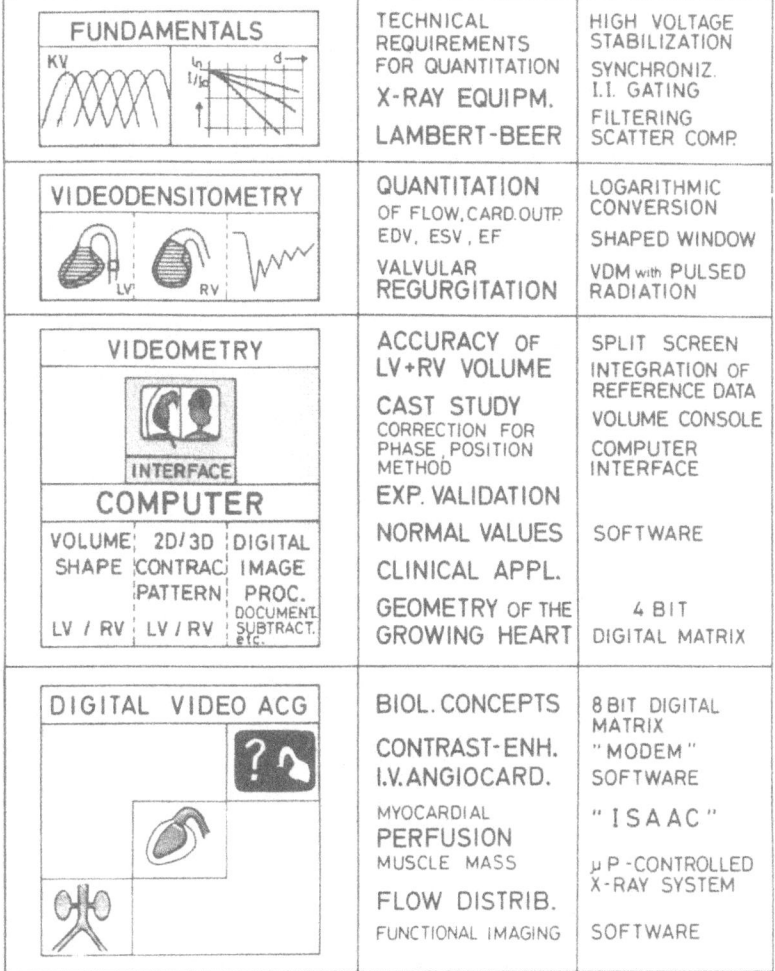

Fig. 1
Survey on the evolution of digital angiocardiography from videodensitometry and videometry after having worked out the fundamentals for using the X-Ray equipment as a measuring tool. Middle column: experimental and clinical concepts and goals. Right column: bioengineering efforts and development to meet the targets.

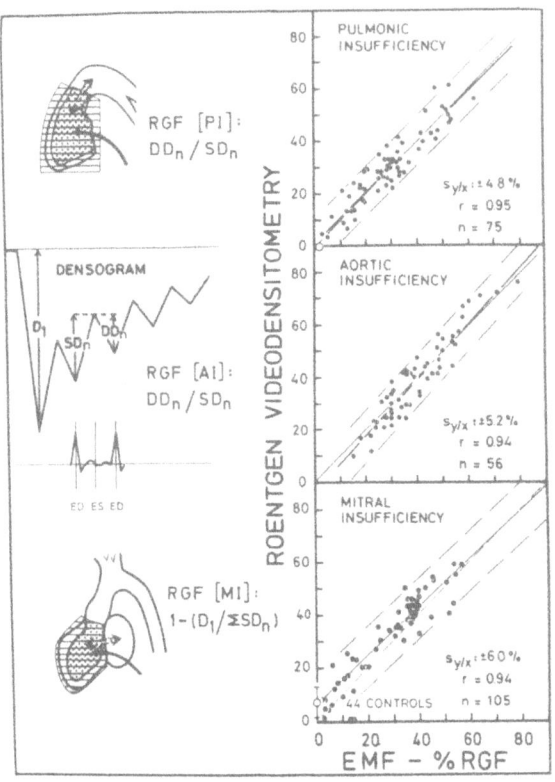

Fig.2
Principle for videodensitometric determination of the regurgitant fraction in pulmonic, aortic and mitral insufficiency (left) and results of the experimental validation of the methods. D_1 = maximum deflection of the densitogram; SD_n = systolic change of the densitometric signal; DD_n = diastolic change of the densitometric signal; ED = enddiastole; ES = endsystole. RGF = regurgitant fraction; EMF = electromagnetic flowmeter.

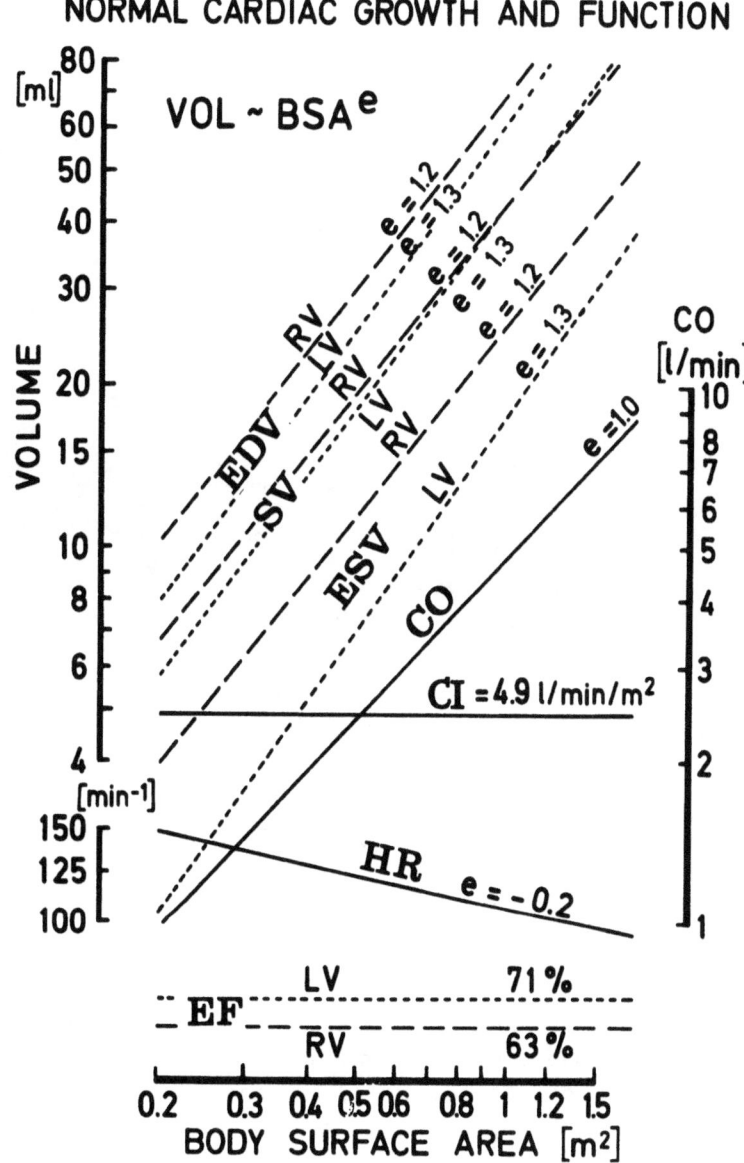

Fig. 3
Normal left (LV) and right (RV) ventricular enddiastolic (EDV) and endsystolic (ESV) volumes and derived parameters during the period of growth plotted on a double logarithmic scale. Volumes increase as a power function with a mean exponent (e) of 1,2 in relation to body surface area (BSA). As a result of the decreasing heart rate (HR) with growth, cardiac output (CO) increases in proportion to BSA. Ejection fraction (EF) and cardiac index (CI) are independent of BSA. SV = stroke volume.

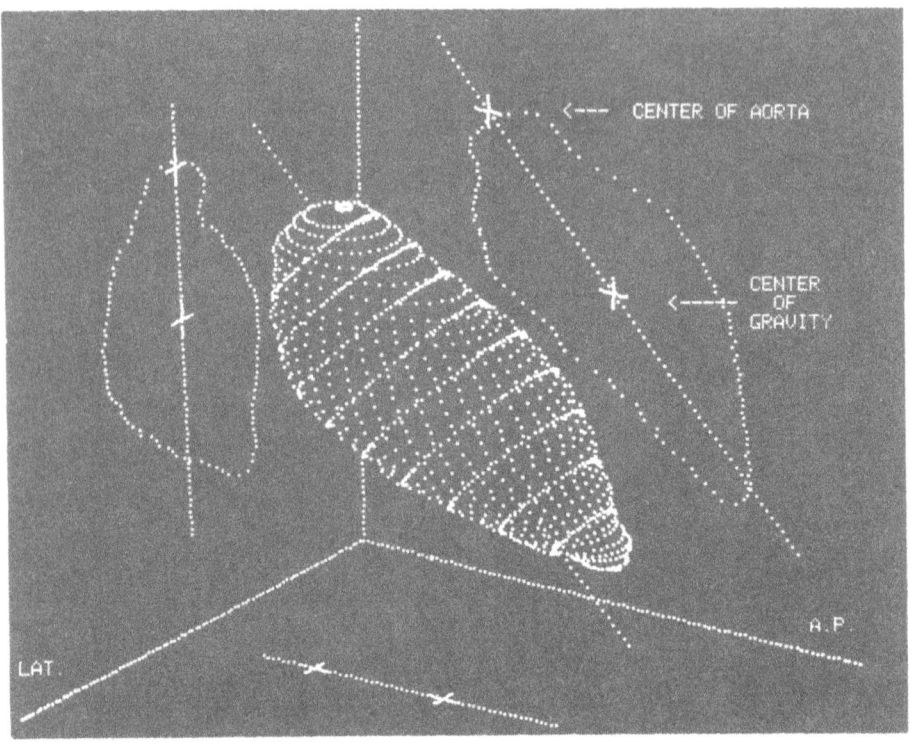

Fig.4a
Three-dimensional model of the left ventricle derived from biplane projection ventriculograms, assuming elliptical cross sections. The long axis can be calculated by connecting the center of the aortic valve with the center of gravity or with the manually-defined apex.

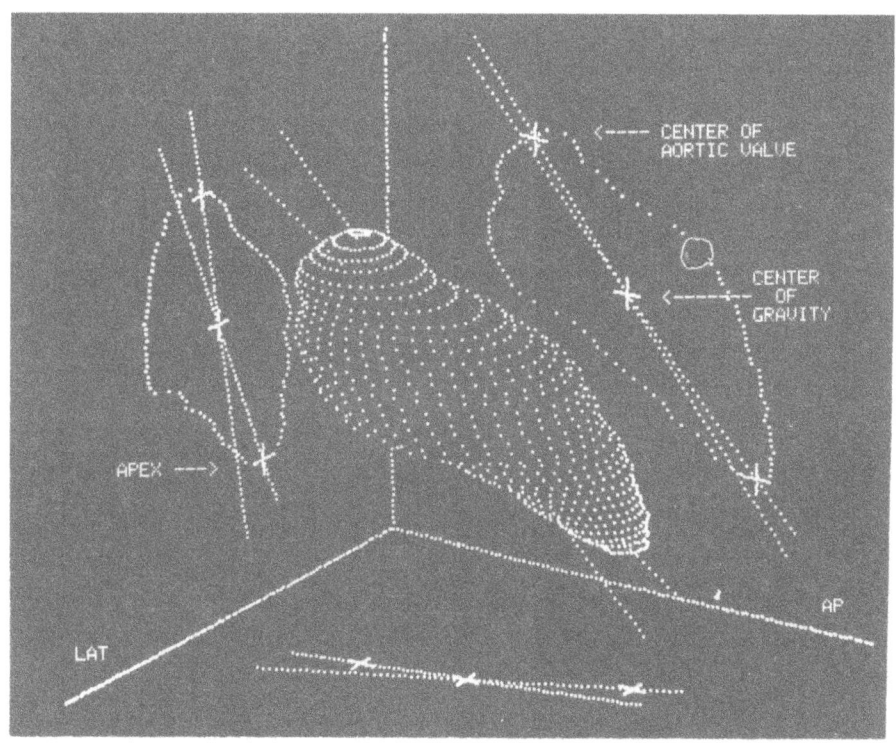

Fig. 4b
The computer-generated 3-D model can be cut into any desired number of cross sections perpendicular to the defined long axis. The circumference of these (in our case nine) cross sections can be followed during contraction. Their changes in circumference length or velocities (see fig. 4c e 4d) can be measured and displayed in various modes.

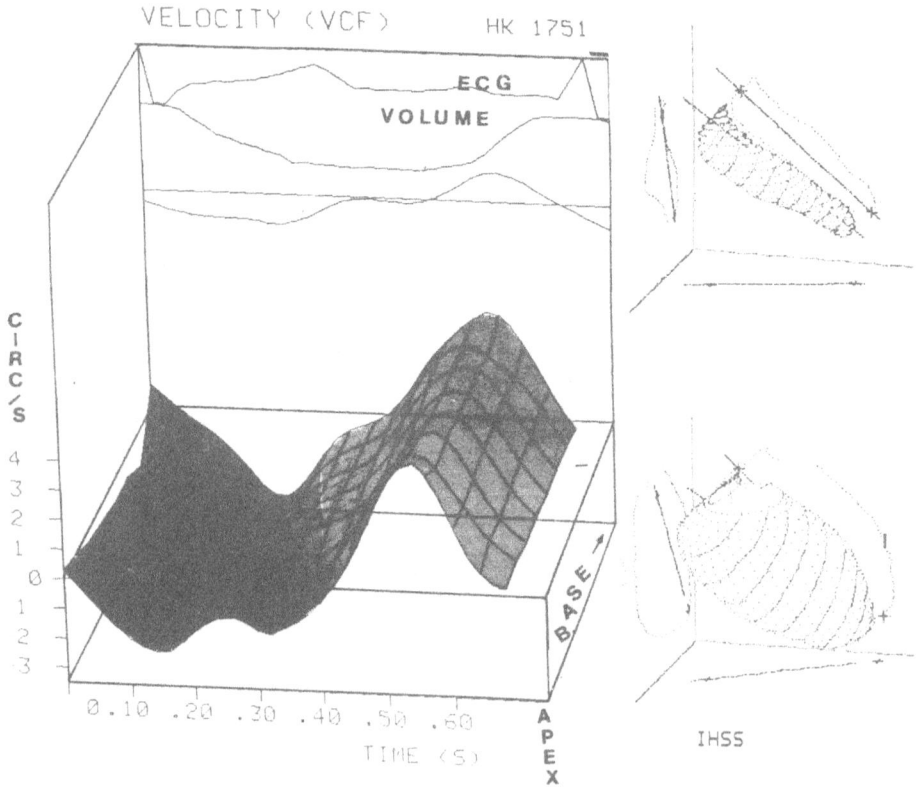

Fig. 4c
Three-dimensional display of the changing contraction velocities of nine cross sections (according to figures 4a e 4b) during cardiac cycle in a case of idiopathic hypertrophic cardiomyopathy.

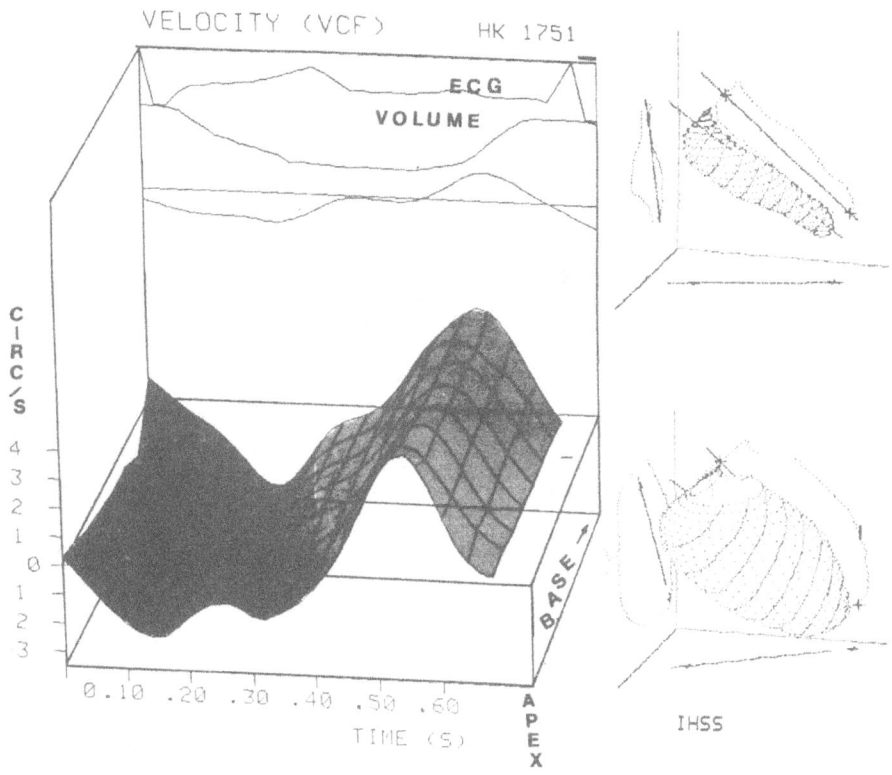

Fig. 4d
Three-dimensional display of the changing contraction velocities of nine cross sections during cardiac cycle of a child affected by Bland-White-Garland syndrome. The display shows a homogeneous reduction of circumference fiber shortening velocities compared to the increased short axis contraction velocity shown in fig. 4c.

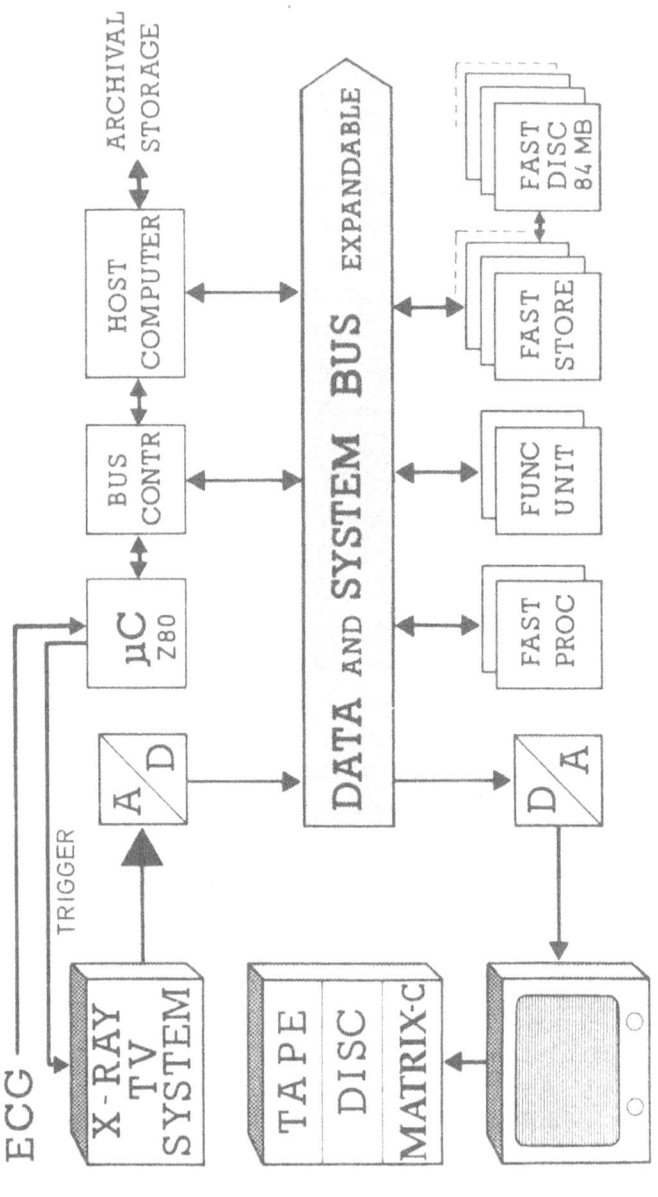

Fig. 5
Architecture of a fast and flexible bus: Image Sequence Acquisition Analysis oriented Computer (ISAAC) for real time digital processing of angiocardiograms and various options for post processing (29, 36).

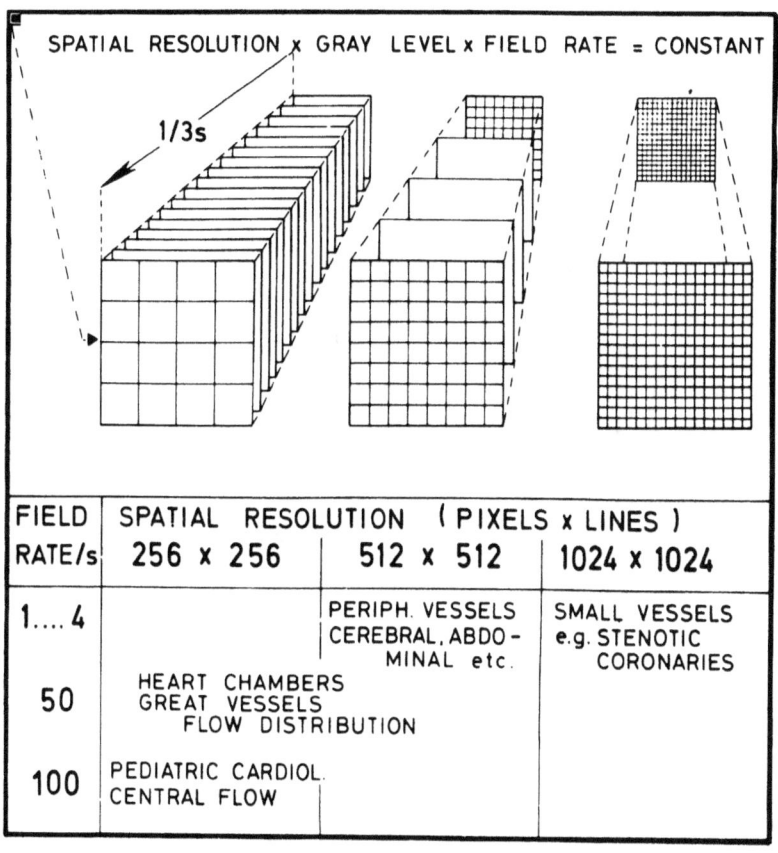

Fig. 6
Schematic representation of the relation among spatial, temporal and density resolution for a given maximal data rate. The three boxes correspond to the small pixel in the upper left corner of the frame of the picture. Possible indications for the chosen matrix size and frame rate are given in the lower part of the figure.

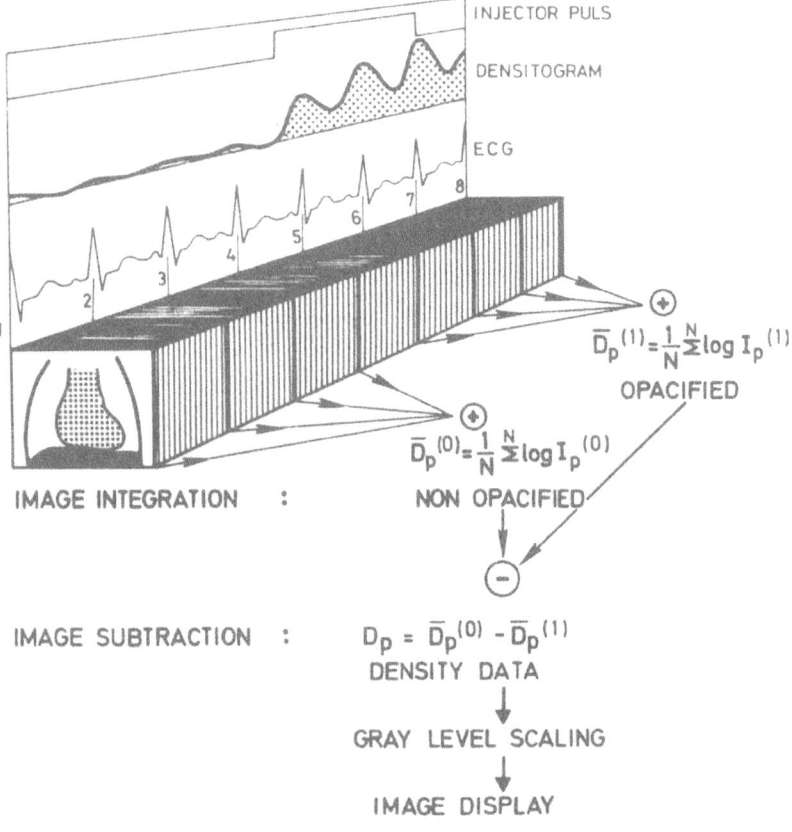

Fig. 7a
First example of the effect of digital subtraction angiocardiography on contrast enhancement. Left: best opacified levocardiogram with low dose contrast injection into the left ventricle. Right: result from digital image processing techniques according to fig. 7b.

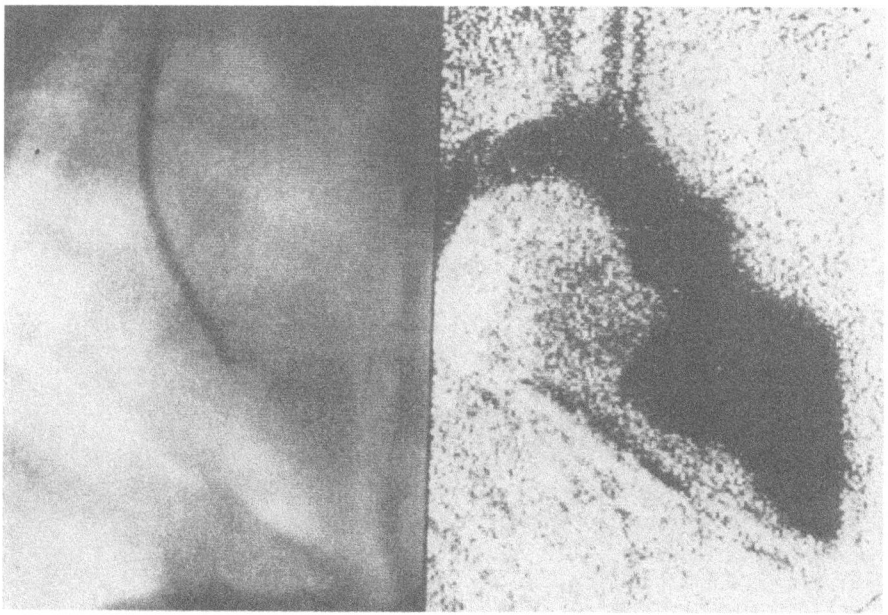

Fig. 7b
ECG gated enddiastolic images from angiocardiographic series are selected and summed up (integrated) before contrast injection providing the averaged background image. After logarithmic signal conversion, this background image is subtracted from a number of enddiastolic images, similarly obtained, following contrast injection.
The subtraction image can be amplified and optimally scaled for display (From Brennecke et al. 26).

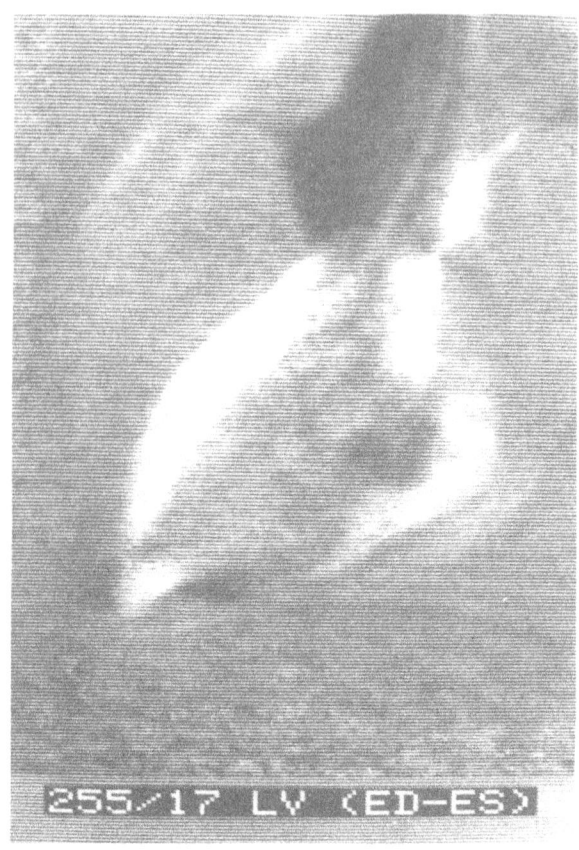

Fig. 8
Ejection shell image of the left ventricle following the creation of an experimental infarction of the circumflex coronary artery of a pig. Subtraction of systolic pictures from diastolic ones shows the internal motion of the left ventricular endocardial wall as a bright shell. Whereas in the infarcted region there is no motion (gray) or an inverse outward motion (dark area) close to the diaphragm.

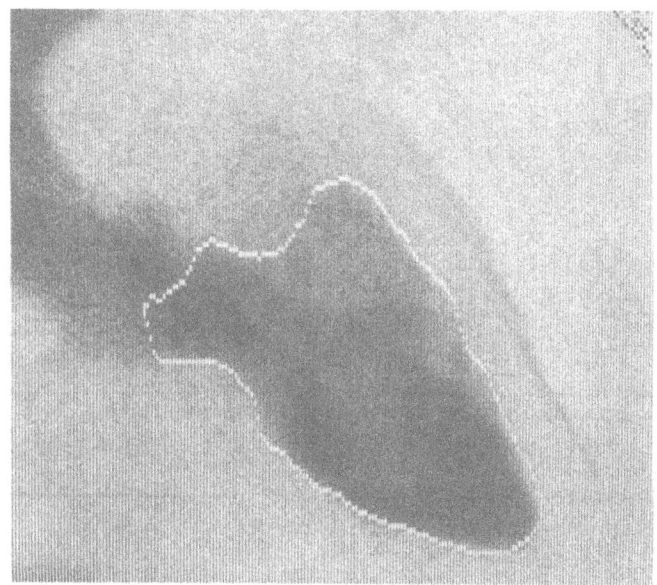

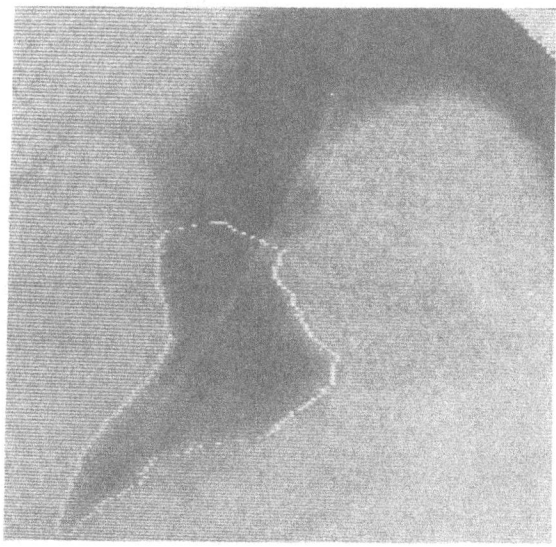

Fig.9a
Digital subtraction angiocardiograms from the left ventricle in enddiastole and endsystole with the endcardial borders traced manually.

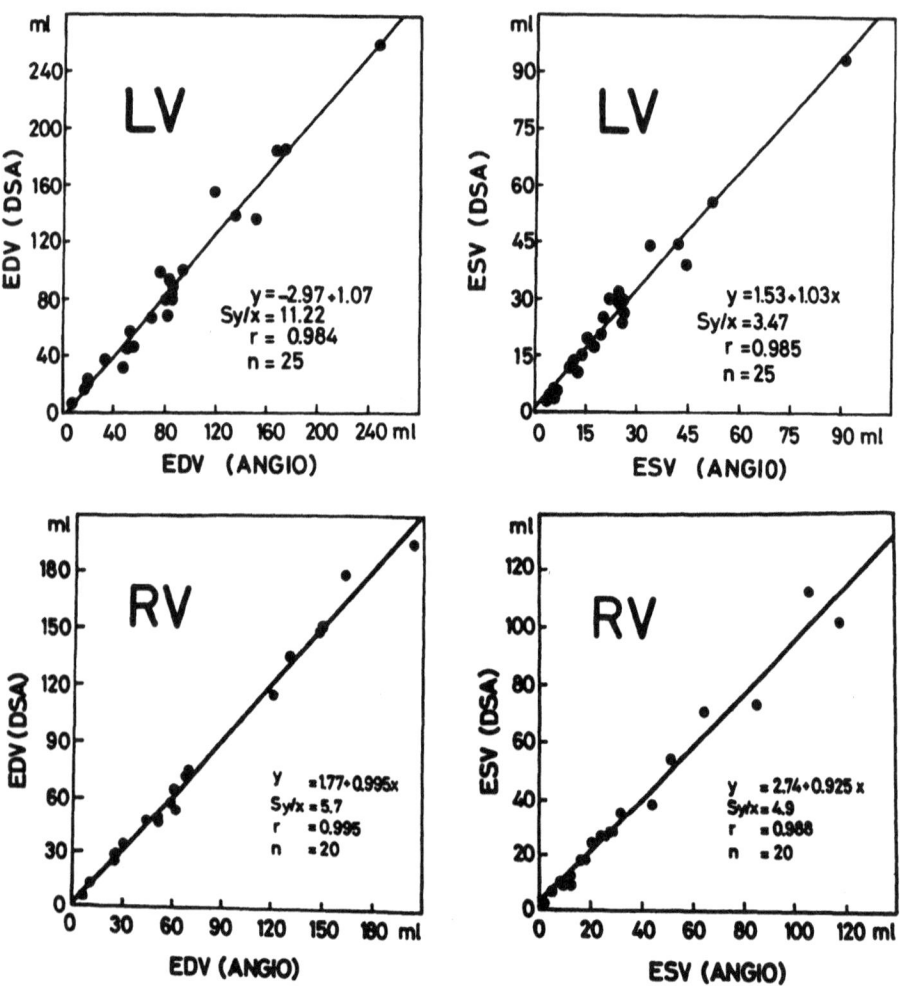

Fig.9b
From ventriculograms of the left and right ventricle, volume determination has been carried out, as in conventional videometry and compared to volume values, obtained from the same patients by standard left ventriculography as the best available reference. The statistical parameters for the left and right ventricles, obtained from these studies are given respectively in the upper and lower rows (58).

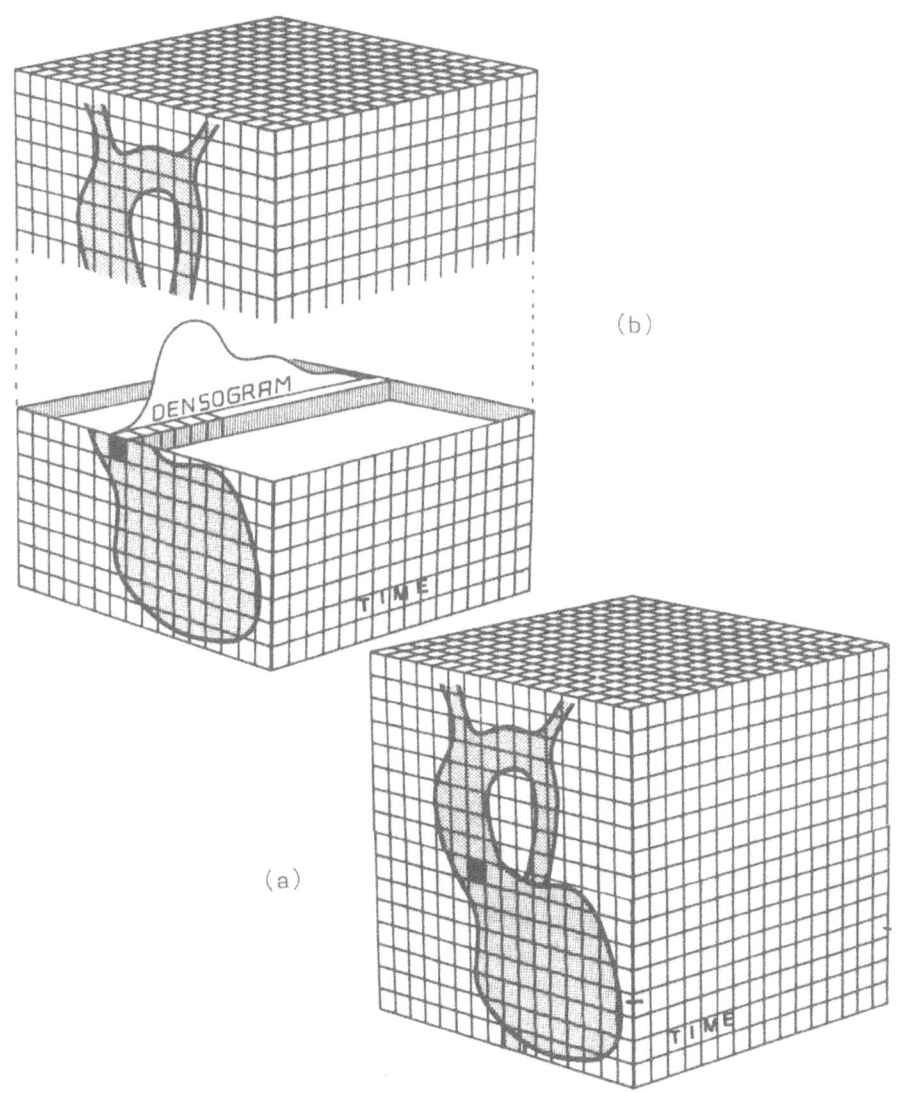

Fig.10
Schematic demonstration that in a digitized image series each picture element (pixel) can be considered as a densitometric window (a) so that the density changes at each pixel with time constitute a matrix of 'pixeldensograms' (b).

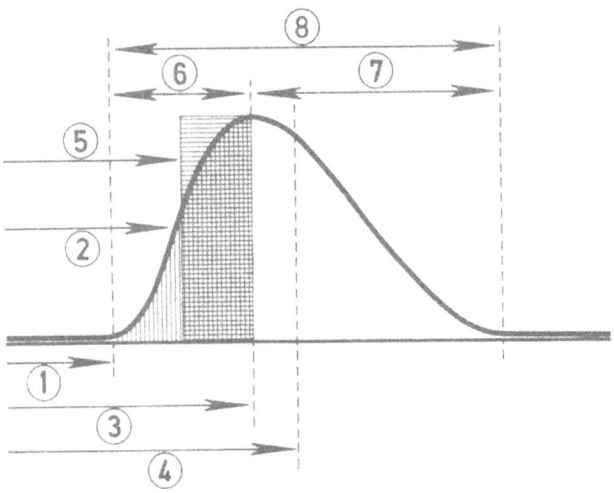

TIME PARAMETER

Fig.11
Schematic diagram of the time parameters which can be extracted from an ideal pixel-densogram. (1) Appearance time, (2) 'half max' time, (3) time of maximum, (4) mean circulation time, (5) mean concentration time, (6) wash-in time, (7) wash-out time, (8) total passage time.

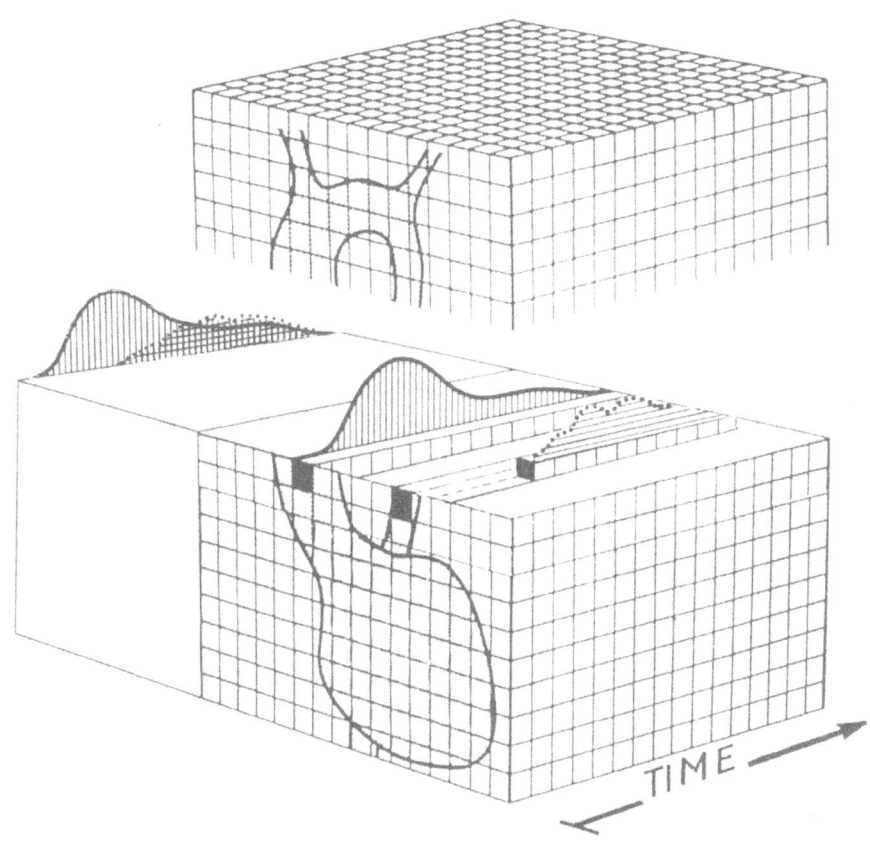

Fig. 12a
Demonstration of the principle according to which parameter images can be obtained. The densogram recorded at the descending aorta has a different shape and amplitude. It is delayed with respect to the 'reference-densogram' recorded over the ascending aorta. All digitized densograms can be shifted in the time axis until the optimum correspondence between both densograms is obtained by applying cross correlation techniques or determining the maximum covariance.

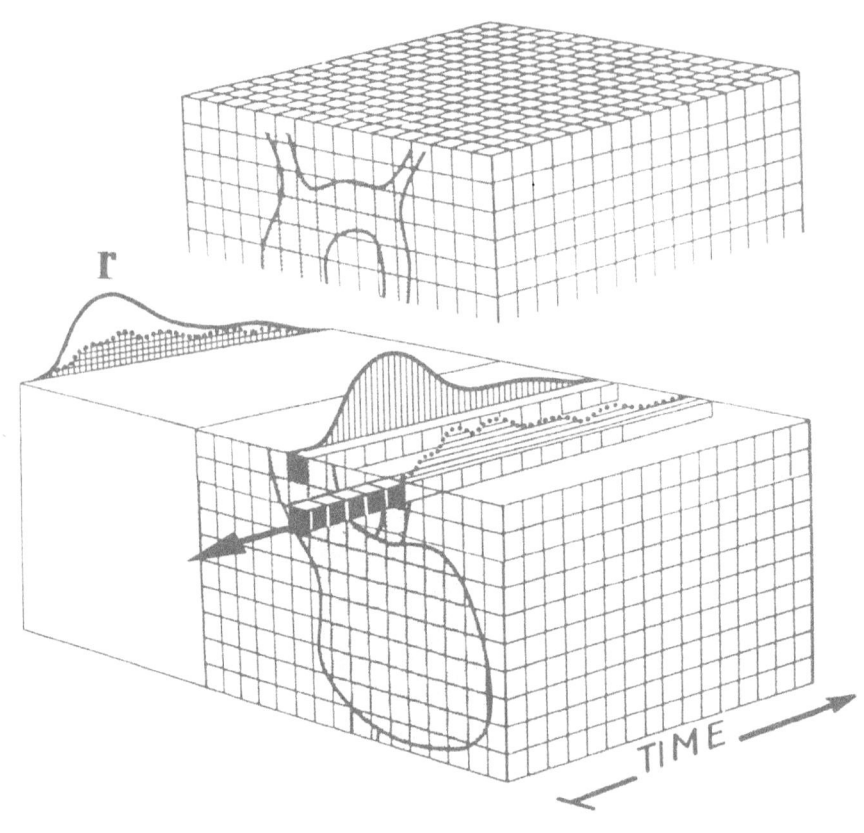

Fig.12b
The time shift required to reach the highest degree of similarity between both densograms (expressed by the cross correlation coefficient. r) is a measure of the bolus temporal delay compared to the reference-densogram. This time value can be displayed as grey or colour value at each given pixel. In this way the time parameter image is obtained. If the r values are displayed at each pixel site, the image obtained is an expression of the similarity between the various densograms with respect to the shape and amplitude. It allows discrimination between typical and artificial bolus wave forms or any other density change with time.

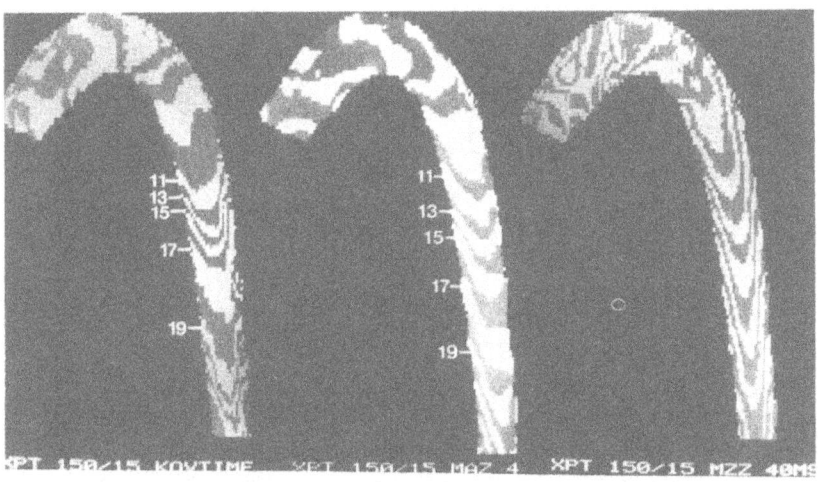

Fig. 13
Three examples for the temporal segmentation and analysis of a thoracic aortogram. Time segments of 40 milliseconds are alternately displayed in dark and light. Various time parameters have been chosen for the analysis. Left: covariance time. Middle: mean concentration time (MAZ) and mean circulation time (MZZ) in the right example. Note the different sensitivity of the methods for the detection of pulsatile flow (From Buersch et al (58) with permission).

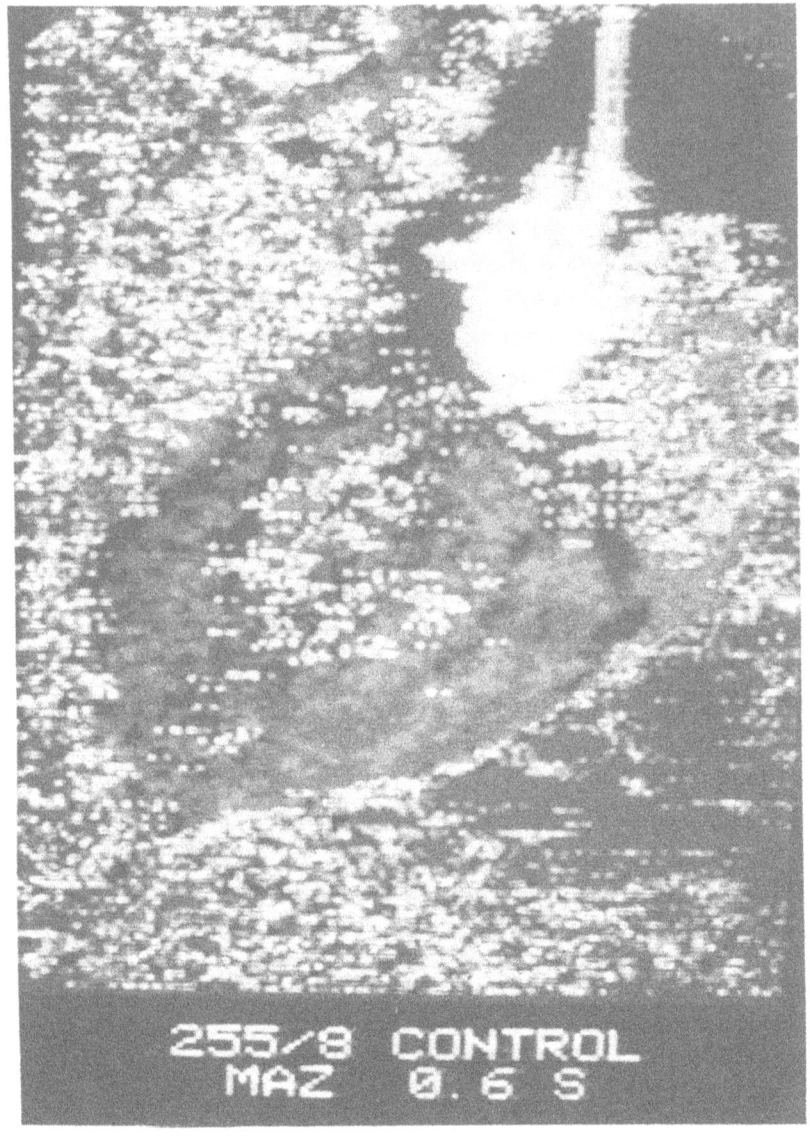

Fig. 14a
Segmented time parameter image of the coronary arteries and circulation in an animal study following contrast injection into the ascending aorta. Each of the differently coloured segments from red to orange, yellow, green and blue indicate flow propagation within 0,6 seconds, corresponding to one cardiac cycle length. ECG gated image acquisition is required in such studies. The figure shows the control image with rapid opacification of the coronary arteries and myocardium.

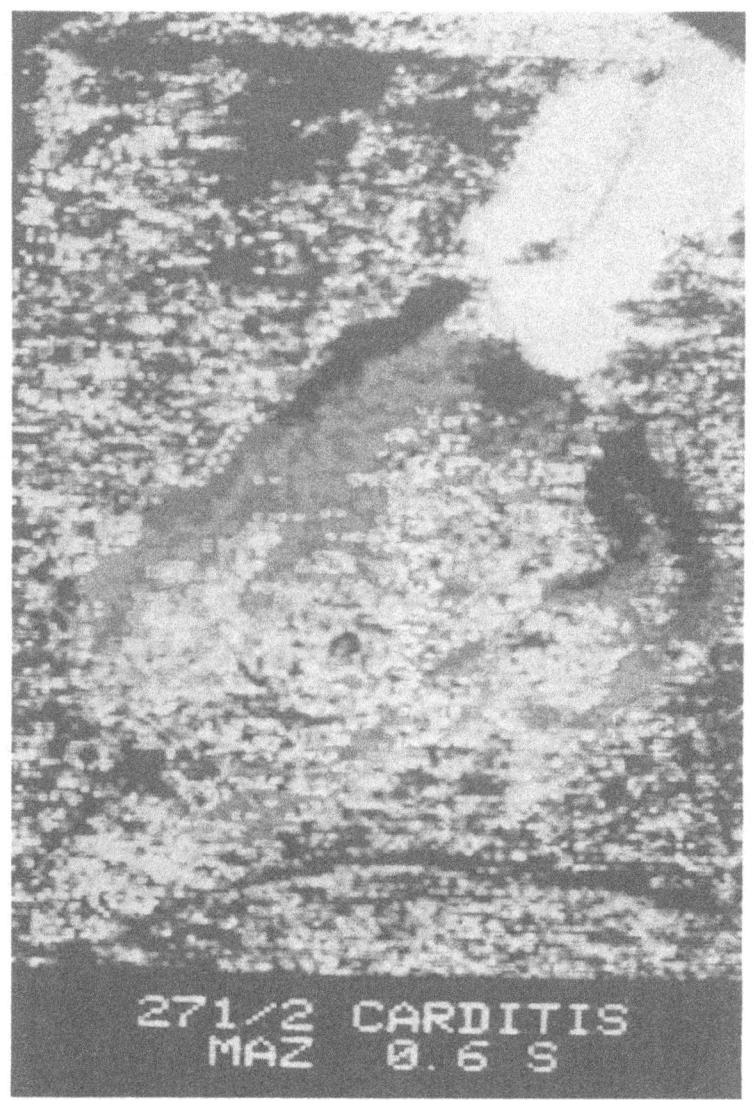

Fig.14b
Global delay in contrast propagation in the coronary arteries as well as into the myocardium so that three-colour segments can be distinguished in the coronary arteries.

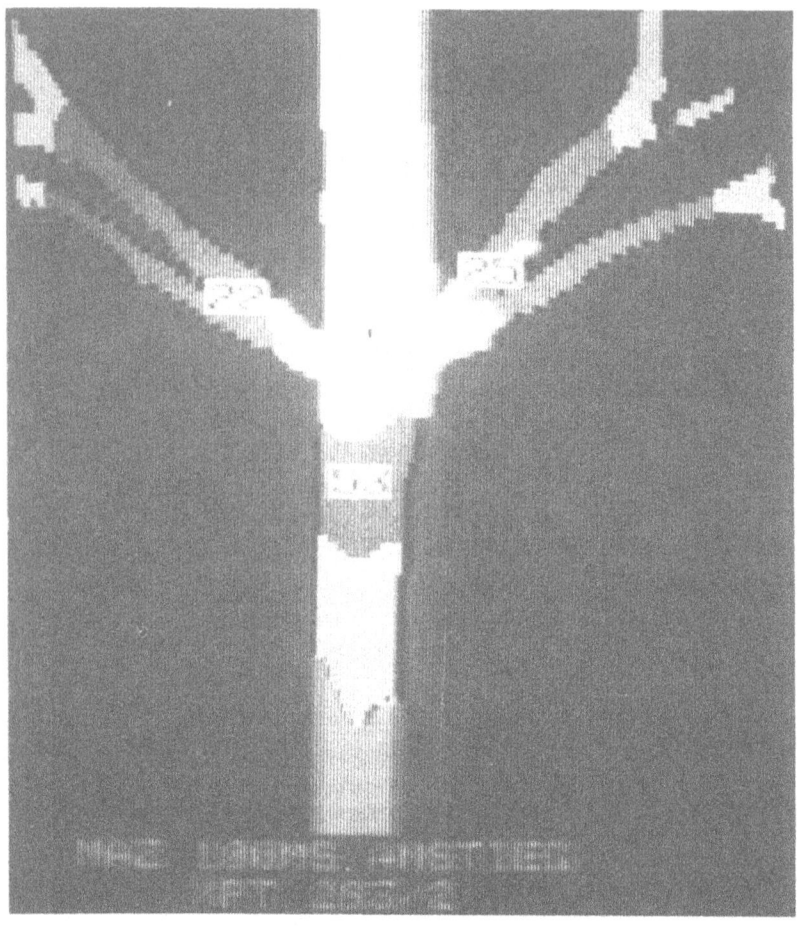

Fig. 15
Flow distribution image showing volume flow data (percent of the sum of the three vessels). The flow distribution can be calculated from the coloured time-segments depicting the progress of the bolus within 100 milliseconds and from the integrated volume of these segments. The flow distribution can be calculated and converted into the absolute flow value if a dimensional calibration is performed.

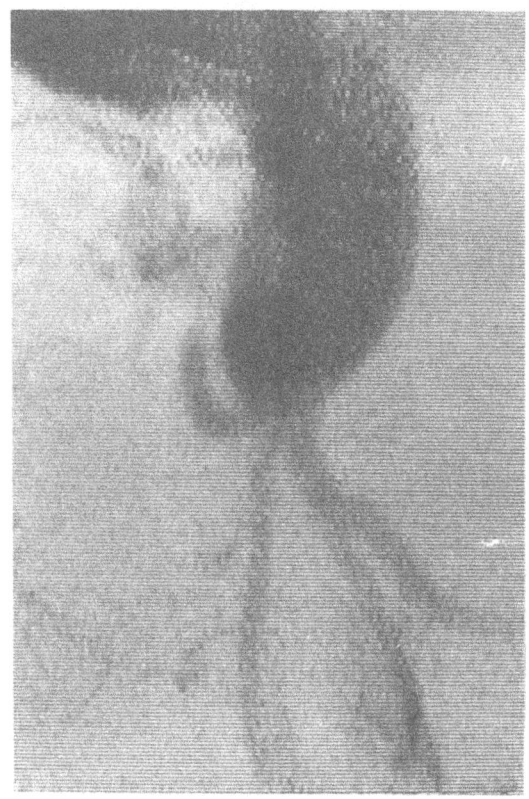

Fig.16a
Result of flow parameter calculation in the AP view from a patient with a Blalock-Taussig anastomosis. Original low contrast angiocardiogram.

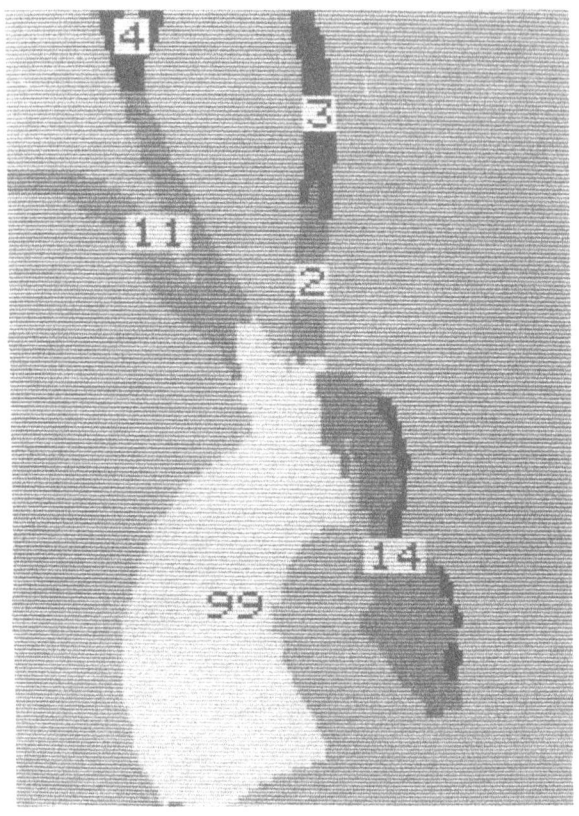

Fig. 16b
Digitally processed image with temporal segmentation visualized by various gray levels. Length of time segment: one cardiac cycle. Numbers refer to the relative volume flow. As can be seen, 99% (100%), that is the stroke volume, is distributed to the central arteries in such a way that 14% of the stroke volume enters the pulmonary circulation via the Blalock-Taussig anastomosis. Other parts of the circulatory system are removed by a mask. (From Buersch et al (54) with permission.)

ADVANCED TECHNIQUES FOR DIGITAL ANGIOGRAPHY OF THE HEART

K.H. Höhne, U. Obermöller, M. Riemer, G. Witte

University Hospital Eppendorf
Institute for Mathematics and Computer Science in Medicine
and Department of Radiology
Martinistr. 52
D-2000 Hamburg
F.R.G

ABSTRACT

Digital angiography is widely considered as being simply a method in which images taken at different times are subtracted from each other. This paper presents some techniques which are performed in the frequency domain after the application of the Fourier Transform. Nonselective bypass angiograms and intravenous ventriculograms are taken as examples to show that simple procedures utilizing these techniques exhibit the advantages of improved signal to noise ratio in the subtraction images, reduction of motion artefacts, easy application of phase-synchronous subtraction, integration and quantitative visualization of blood propagation. Furthermore it is shown that the storage of the angiographic image sequence as Fourier-coefficients leads to data compression and convenient data access in an image database.

1 INTRODUCTION

Digital Angiography is an imaging modality which is increasingly being applied in clinical work because it allows less invasive procedures than conventional techniques. Its principle is simple: instead of imaging the original organ, only intensity changes with time or with radiation energy are visualized. The result is an enhancement of interesting structures. The most trivial method of visualizing changes is simple image subtraction. Subtraction, however, is only a special case of a larger class of temporal filter operations resulting in parametric images or enhanced image sequences as shown in earlier publications [1-6]. Fig. 1 shows as an example of a time of arrival image of the lungs of a child [7]. It is now well known from signal processing theory, that the design and investigation of temporal filters is very suitably done in the frequency domain. The aim of this paper, which is an updated version of an earlier publication [8], is to show that also in the case of digital intravenous angiography the processing and storage in the Fourier domain exhibits advantages for the extraction of morphological and functional information as well as for data compression and the convenient storage of data. This will be demonstrated with the examples of nonselective bypass angiograms and intravenous ventriculograms.

2 MATERIAL

2.1 Ventriculograms

After central venous injection of 25 ml of 76 % contrast medium (CM), a fluoroscopic sequence was taken at $10 \mu R$ per video frame using a Siemens high resolution image intensifier video unit. The image sequence was stored on video tape. Subsequently a quarter of the full screen, containing the left ventricle, was digitized with a gray scale resolution of 256 and a spatial resolution of 128 x 128 pixels at a rate of 50 images/s. Up to 10 heart cycles (about 500 images) were taken without synchronisation with the cardiac cycle.

2.2 Nonselective bypass angiograms

Continuous mode fluoroscopy was performed here at 10 µR/frame after arterial injection of 30 ml of 76 % contrast medium into the aortic root. The image sequence was stored on video tape. A region of interest was digitized as described above. Images were taken without synchronization with the cardiac cycle.

Digitization was performed in real time with the CA-1 (Computer-Angiography One) system [3,8], which incorporates an 8 Mbyte random access image sequence storage. The subsequent computations have also been done both with this system, and with our VAX 11/780 image processing computer which is linked to the CA-1 System in the Department of Radiology.

3 METHOD

Fig. 2 shows one frame of a low contrast angiographic sequence produced as described in paragraph 2 showing three coronary bypasses. By looking through the whole image sequence in the time direction at the depicted regions of interest we obtain typical intensity-time curves (ITC) as show in fig. 3. In the case shown six heart cycles are observed. Their structure is produced both by the motion of the contrast medium (slowly varying component) and the periodic movement of the heart (cyclic component). The extraction or enhancement of such characteristic patterns will probably lead to images or image sequences in a semiquantitative, more compact or at least in an enhanced form.

It is now very well known from signal processing that curves with such sinusoidal patterns are analyzed best in the frequency domain after application of the Fourier transform. With the discrete Fourier transform the original curve F(t) is approximated as a sum of sine and cosine functions with frequencies $i\omega$ and corresponding coefficients a_i and b_i, where $\omega = 2\pi/T$, T is the basic period length (in units of images) and i is the harmonic number.

$$F(t) \approx F_R(t) = \frac{a_0}{2} + \sum_{i=1}^{n} a_i \cos i\omega t + \sum_{i=1}^{n} b_i \sin i\omega t$$

where t is the discrete time $t_1 \ldots t_N$.

This equation may also be written in terms of an amplitude A_i and a phase φ_i for the ith frequency:

$$F(t) = \frac{a_0}{2} + \sum_{i=1}^{n} A_i \sin(i\omega t + \varphi_i)$$

where

$$A_i = \sqrt{a_i^2 + b_i^2}, \quad \tan \varphi_i = \frac{a_i}{b_i}$$

Since the A_i and φ_i are better suited for interpretation than a_i and b_i, they are used throughout the following discussion. The idea of filtering the angiographic sequences in the time domain has already been used by the authors for data compression and for the enhancement of morphology in angiographic image sequences. The aim of this paper is to show that nearly all procedures of digital subtraction, functional imaging and data compression can be performed most conveniently through simple manipulations of the coefficients A_i and φ_i.

4 RESULTS

When the ITCs are subjected to the Fourier transform, spectra of the amplitudes A_i are obtained as shown in fig. 4. Spectrum 1 is derived from a pixel on a bypass, whereas spectrum 2 is in a region through which a ring belonging to an artificial valve moved. In both cases a high amplitude at frequency zero, representing the static component, is observed. In the case of the bypass high amplitudes are also observed in the adjacent low frequency bins. These are due to the CM-motion. They are absent in the case of the moving ring. In both regions maxima at the heart frequency and its multiples are observed. These are due to motion. Structure is typically no longer observable beyond four to five multiples of the heart frequency (A_{24}, A_{30} in the shown case). We now proceed to discuss these manipulations in detail.

4.1 Noise suppression

The most simple procedure is to omit the high frequencies and to retransform the image sequence into the time domain. In the retransformed sequence noise is suppressed without blurring of spatial detail. In an earlier publication [10] we have shown for intravenous ventriculograms that including four multiples of the heart frequency leads to less noisy images without loss of diagnostic information. This application alone, of course, would not justify the transformation into the Fourier domain, since filters with similar properties can be implemented very easily in the time domain.

4.2 Data compression

However, if only the amplitudes A_i and phases φ_i of the contributing frequencies are stored an appreciable compression of the data is also achieved. A sequence of 6 heart cycles taken at 50 images/sec may have 300 images. If the reconstruction from all frequencies up to the 4th multiple of the heart frequency is performed, the value of n in formula (1) is 4*6 = 24. We therefore need only 49 coefficients, which results in a compression factor of 6 [10].

4.3 Phase synchronous integration

If the motion of the CM is not of interest, a further compression is possible by just neglecting the frequencies between the heart frequency and its multiples. The result is a phase synchronous integration, which can be applied e.g. for noise reduction in wall motion studies. A necessary condition, of course, for the success of this method is that the heart frequency must be stable during the observation period.

4.4 Blurred mask subtraction

It is known that the amplitude A_0 is the mean intensity over the observation time. Presented in image form it is nothing else but a "blurred mask". Omission of A_0 and retransformation therefore automatically leads to a blurred mask subtraction image sequence.

4.5 Phase synchronous subtraction

Exact subtraction of angiographic image sequences of the heart can only be obtained by phase synchronous subtraction of sequences taken before and after the application of the contrast medium. In the time domain this works only if the heart rate is the same in both sequences. This is not necessary if the subtraction is done in the frequency domain. Here only the number of cycles has to be equal. Although this method is quite elegant, the practical experience gained so far indicates that the blurred mask subtracted sequences of the A_1 image are better diagnostically. This is obviously due to the inherent irreproducibility of the heart motion between two consecutive cycles. Another source of error is that the individual motion characteristics do not all scale identically with a varying heart rate.

4.6 Selection of CM-motion

If we look at the A_1 image, we see that it is a very good approximation of a subtraction image (fig. 5). This is due to the fact that A_1 represents the slowly varying part of the bolus curve as shown in fig. 3. But there are at least two advantages compared to simple subtraction: since A_1 is the result of a fitting of the whole ITC, its signal to noise ratio is better than that from simple subtraction. The ripple due to the heart motion is also filtered out, which suppresses motion artefacts to a certain extent. For example the ring of the artificial mitral valve which is visible in the original image disappears in the A_1-image. The A_1-image is closely related to the images gained by matched filtering [11] or cross correlation techniques [6]. The φ_1-image is nothing else but a CM-arrival time image [1-4].

4.7 Selection of heart motion

If we are interested only in wall motion, we can select the amplitude and the phase of the heart frequency. This method has already been applied in nuclear medicine [12]. Due to its superior spatial and temporal resolution digital angiography seems to be a much more valuable technique. Fig. 6 shows as an example the amplitude image of the heart frequency of a patient after pacing and after the application of nitroglycerine. In the first case a severe amplitude drop near the apex can be recognized, in the latter case a minor drop of amplitude near the anterior wall is visible. They are scarcely detectable from the native intravenous sequence.

The phase of the heart frequency is shown in fig. 7. A phase jump is visible at the apex of the paced heart, indicating a paradoxical motion. In the absence of pacing a slight non-synchronization at the apex and the anterior wall can be seen,

4.8 Combined presentation of amplitudes and phases

An even more compact pictorial description of the image sequence is obtained when amplitude and phase are represented in a single image, as shown in fig. 8. Here the amplitude A_1 is coded as intensity and the phase φ_1 is coded in color. Besides enhancing morphological structures, simultaneous visualization of the propagation times through color reflects the different functions of the bypasses. Fig. 9 shows the same type of image derived from a selective arteriogram. The perfusion of the myocardium can be visualized. Since the subjective impression of intensity and color are not independent of each other such images present certain problems in their interpretation.

Nevertheless this method shows a superior temporal differentiation as compared to methods where the arrival time is only measured at a fixed heart phase [13].

4.9 Special properties concerning application in an image database

The storage of the image sequences as the coefficients of a set of basic functions not only leads to a high data reduction, but also implies some interesting data-technical properties for the access of medical image databases, which may become increasingly relevant [14,15,16]. One such property is that different views of the data as described above, can be obtained simply by retrieving a portion of the coefficients or through simple manipulations.

Another aspect concerns the limited transmission speed of conventional data links. Let us assume that we have a hardware system which performs the additions and refers to look-up tables necessary to reconstruct the sequence from the Fourier coefficients in real time. An image sequence with blurred image quality can be displayed as soon as the first three coefficient matrices (A_0, A_1, φ_1) have been transmitted from the database. As the endless film loop proceeds and more coefficients become available, the quality improves. The radiologist thus first has an overview of the organ and can then concentrate on special regions of interest, which become sharper in the course of time. Even with modest transmission speeds the radiologist is not forced to wait.

CONCLUSIONS

We have shown that the Fourier-transformation of the intensity-time curves of digital angiograms of the heart leads to some striking advantages over conventional techniques of digital angiography. Fig. 10 summarizes the results. We obtain subtraction images with an improved signal to noise ratio and reduced motion artefacts. Functional images of the blood propagation in bypasses and coronary arteries are produced, which, to a large extent, exclude artefacts due to heart motion. Phase synchronous subtraction and integration can be performed in a simpler way than in the time domain. Finally storage and retrieval of different "views" of the image sequences is greatly facilitated. Special hardware is, of course, required to implement the algorithms for routine utilization. The expenses, however, will drop, as special processors capable of performing the Fourier-transform become standard devices for signal and image processors.

ACKNOWLEDGEMENTS

The authors wish to express their gratitude to Prof.Dr. Rödiger (Department of Cardiovascular Surgery) and F. Böcker (Institute for Mathematics and Computer Science in Medicine) for valuable hints and to Dr. R. Kellogg (University of Maryland) for his help in preparing the manuscript.

REFERENCES

1. K.H. Höhne, M. Böhm, W. Erbe, G.C. Nicolae, G. Pfeiffer, B. Sonne: ˜Computer Angiography - A New Tool for X-Ray Functional Diagnostics.˜ Med. Progr. Technol. vol.6, pp.23-28, 1978.

2. K.H. Höhne, M. Böhm, W. Erbe, G.C. Nicolae, G. Pfeiffer, B. Sonne, E. Bücheler: ˜Die Messung und differenzierte bildliche Darstellung der Nierendurchblutung mit der Computer-Angiographie˜ Fortschr.Röntgenstr. vol.129, pp.667-672, 1978.

3. K.H. Höhne, M. Böhm, G.C. Nicolae: ˜The Processing of X-Ray Image Sequences˜ in P. Stucki (ed.): ˜Advances in Digital Image Processing˜, Plenum Press, 1979, pp.147-163.

4. K.H. Höhne, U. Obermöller, M. Böhm:˜X-Ray Functional Imaging - Evaluation of the Properties of Different Parameters˜. Proc. Conf. on Digital Radiography, Stanford, Proc. SPIE 314, 1981, pp.224-228.

5. R.A. Kruger, J. Nelson: ˜A Method for Time Domain Filtering Using Computerized Fluoroscopy˜, Med. Phys. vol.8, pp.466-470, 1981.

6. R. Brennecke, H.J. Hahne, J.H. Bürsch, P.H. Heinzen: ˜Optimization of Generalized Subtraction Operations˜ in P.H. Heintzen, R. Brennecke (eds.): ˜Digital Imaging in Cardiovascular Radiology˜, Georg Thieme Verlag, pp.80-88, 1983.

7. G. Riediger, G. Grävinghoff, K.H. Höhne, E.W. Keck: Bestimmung der Lungenankunftszeiten von Kontrastmittel bei Ventrikelseptumdefekten mit Hilfe der Computerangiographie", Zeitschr. für Kardiologie, in press.

8. K.H. Höhne, U. Obermöller, M. Riemer, G. Witte: "Fourier Domain Techniques for Digital Angiography of the Heart", IEEE Trans. on Med. Imag., Vol. MI-3, pp.62-67, 1984.

9. M. Böhm, G.C. Nicolae, K.H. Höhne: "PROFI.11: A Simple Dialog Language for the Processing of Image Sequences". Proc. 1st Int. Symp. on Medical Imaging and Image Interpretation, Berlin, IEEE Publ., pp.386-391, 1982.

10. K.H. Höhne, U. Obermöller, M. Riemer, G. Witte, M. Böhm: "Data Compression in Digital Angiography using the Fourier Transform", Med. Phys, vol.10, pp.899-905, 1983.

11. R.A. Kruger, P. Liu: "Digital Angiography using a Matched Filter", IEEE Trans. on Med. Imag., Vol. MI-1, Nr.1, 1982.

12. W.E. Adam, A. Tarkowska, F. Bitter, M. Strauch, H. Geffers: "Equilibrium (Gated) Radionuclide Ventriculography", Cardiovasc. Radiol. vol.2, pp.161-173, 1979.

13. M.T. LeFree, R.A.Vogel: "Digital Goes to the Heart", Diagnostic Imaging vol.5, pp.62-66, 1983.

14. K. Aßmann, K.H. Höhne: "Investigation of Structures and Operations for Medical Image Databases" Proc. 2nd Conf. on Picture Archiving and Communication Systems (PACS II), Proc. SPIE 418, pp.282-286, 1983.

15. K. Aßmann, R. Venema, M. Riemer, K.H. Höhne: "The ISQL Language - a Uniform Tool for Managing Images and non-Image Data in an Image Database System." Proc. Internat. Symposium on Medical Images and Icons, Arlington 1984, IEEE Publ. pp.42-45.

16. K.H. Höhne (ed.): "Pictorial Information Systems in Medicine", NATO-ASI-Series, Springer, Berlin, to be published 1985.

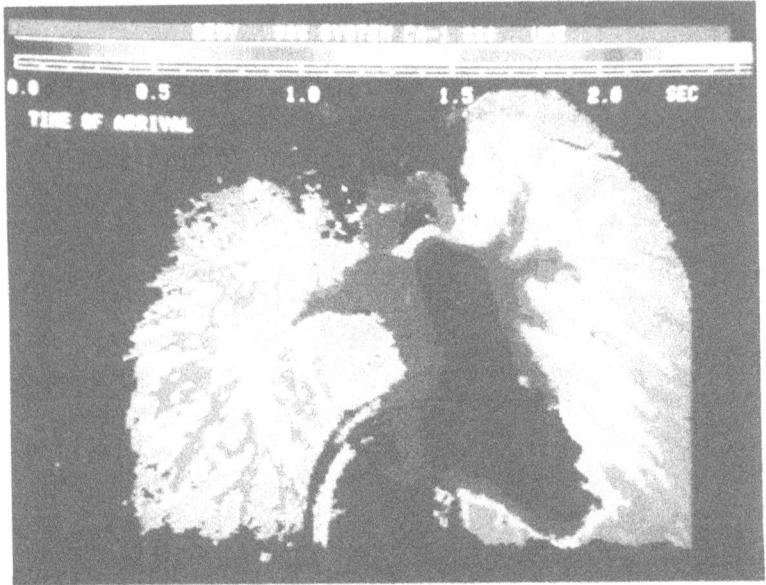

Fig. 1. Time of Arrival image of the lungs of a child

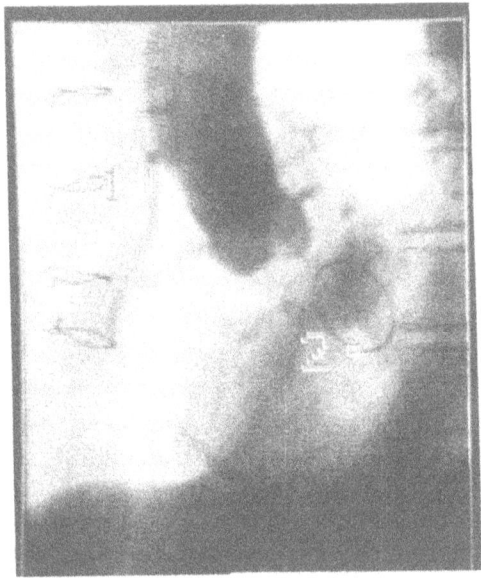

Fig. 2. Frame of a nonselective arteriogram of a heart with two regions of interest: a bypass (1) and an artificial valve (2)

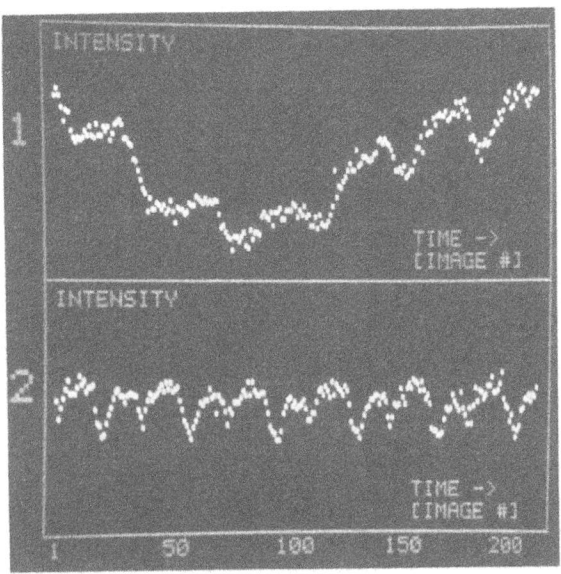

Fig. 3. Intensity-time curves (ITC) at the regions of interest of fig. 1.

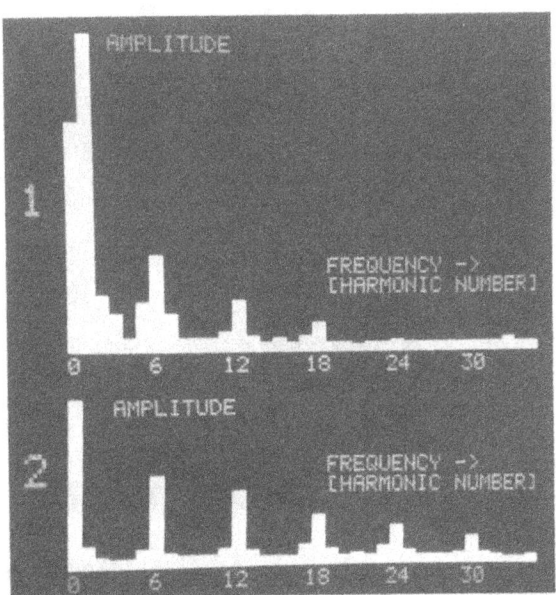

Fig. 4. Frequency spectra of the sample ITCs at the regions of interest in fig. 1.

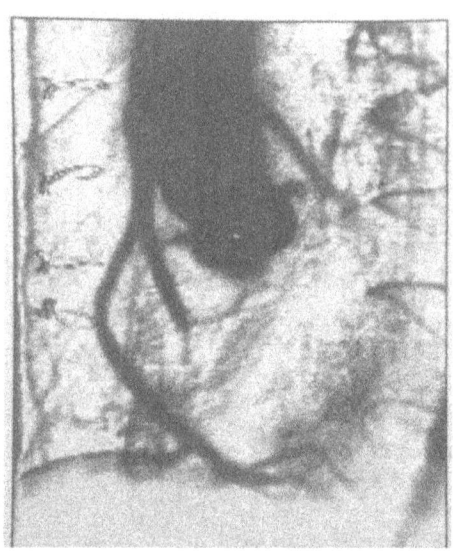

Fig. 5. A_1-image of the image sequence of fig. 1.

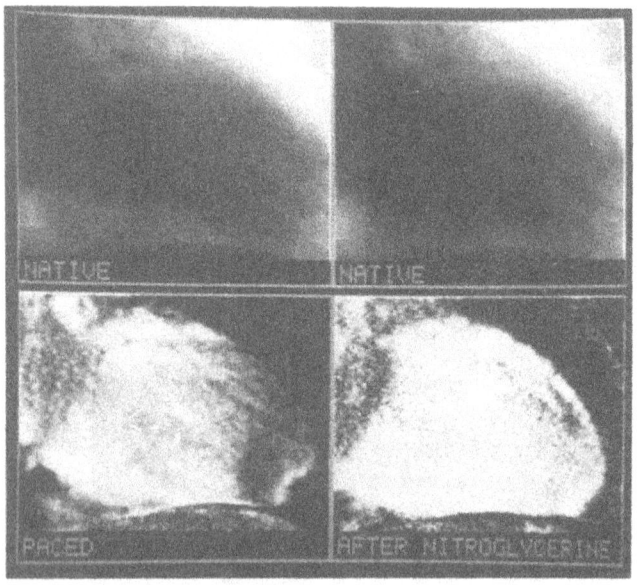

Fig. 6. Native images (top) and A_H (=amplitude of heart frequency)-image of two intravenous ventriculograms of the same heart taken after pacing (left) and after nitroglycerine (right).

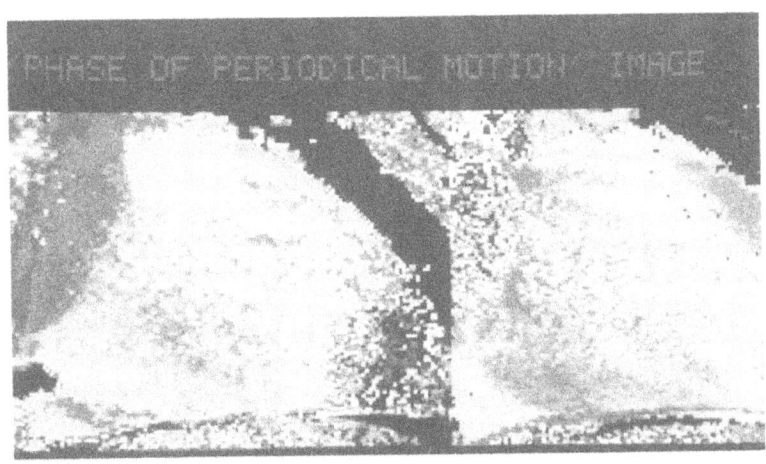

Fig. 7. φ_H (=phase of heart frequency)-image of an intravenous ventriculogram as in fig. 7.

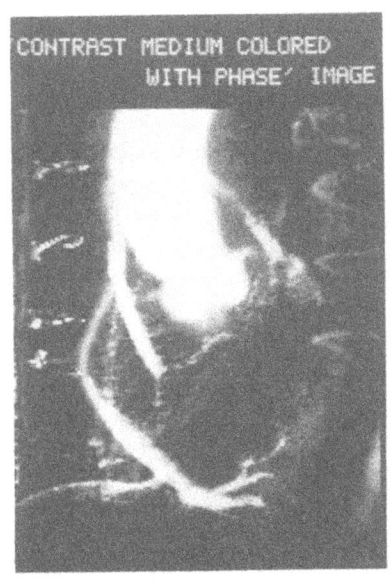 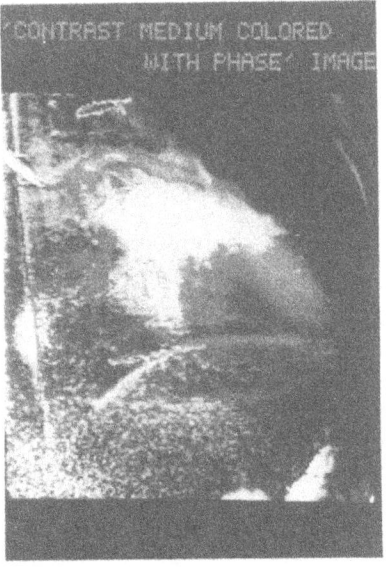

Fig. 8.
Fig. 9. Combined image of A_1 and φ_1 of the image sequence of fig. 1. A_1 is coded as intensity, φ_1 is coded as color.

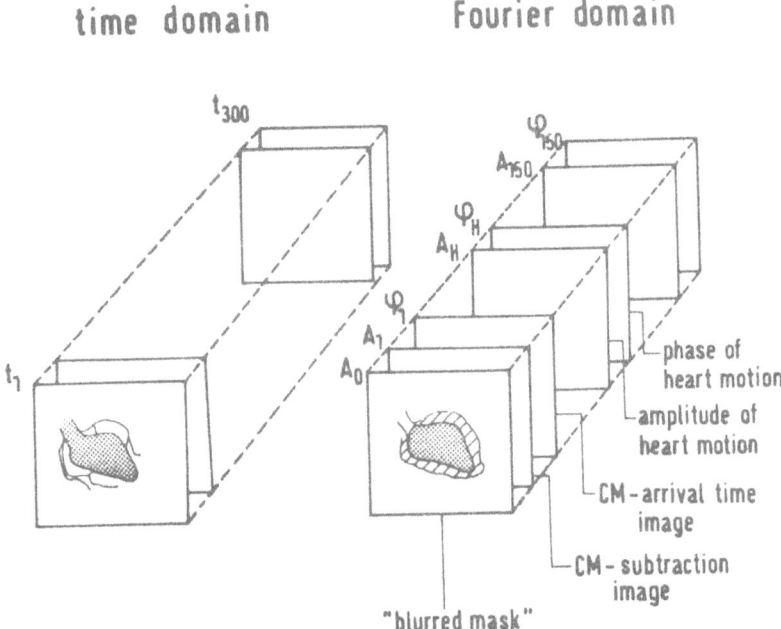

Fig. 10. Demonstration of the different meaning of Fourier images as compared to the original image sequence.

CARDIOVASCULAR NUCLEAR MEDICINE AND FUNCTIONAL IMAGING

Paolo Marzullo, Oberdan Parodi, Calogero R. Bellina, Claudio Marcassa, Danilo Neglia, Antonio Benassi, Alessandro Riva, Antonio L'Abbate
CNR Institute of Clinical Physiology and Istituto di Patologia Medica, University of Pisa, Italy

INTRODUCTION

In the last few years it has been clearly demonstrated that the evolution and prognosis of cardiac disorders are strictly correlated with residual ventricular function (1,2).

The need for early detection of myocardial segments "at risk", as revealed by provocative tests, and prevention of irreversible injury through medical or surgical treatments has stimulated the development of new non-invasive procedures. Among them, cardiovascular nuclear medicine provides qualitative and quantitative information on regional and global ventricular function which can be monitored and/or followed-up because of their good reproducibility and high diagnostic accuracy.

Radionuclide Angiography (RNA)

RNA is a well established non-invasive technique able to provide vast information on ventricular function (3). RNA allows global, regional and systo-diastolic evaluation of ventricular function in coronary artery disease (Tab. 1). The technique is safe, non-invasive and highly reproducible; it provides useful clinical information on the clinical course of different cardiac disorders by short and long-term monitoring of ventricular function.

Qualitative analysis. Cine-mode display of RNA implies the same diagnostic basis of conventional contrast ventriculography. More than one projection is always acquired and evaluated; this approach allows the study of all myocardial segments as well as of the right ventricle (Fig. 1). Like many qualitative techniques, well experienced observers are required.

All other qualitative data derived from RNA are characterized as "functional".

A functional image is a single, color coded, static image, derived from dynamic series, providing information on sequence and/or entity of regional wall motion.

Stroke image is the easier way to produce a functional imaging; the image itself is generated by substracting the end-systolic frame from the end-diastolic one. Akinetic regions, that means regions without systo-diastolic excursion, will generate a "hole" in the stroke image as compared to normokinetic areas (Fig. 2).

Although frequently generated for conventional qualitative analysis, the most widely used computer algorithm to generate functional imaging is phase analysis.

What is meant by phase analysis? The computer algorithm used is a Fourier fit of the time/activity curve in each pixel and calculation and color-coding of phase and amplitude values from the fitted curve.

The derived images, called "phase" and "amplitude" images, strictly related to onset and progression of mechanical systole and to stroke volume respectively, are used for evaluation of wall motion abnormalities in cardiac disorders (4,5) (Fig. 2) or in ventricular conduction abnormalities (6,7).

Why phase analysis? Phase analysis uses the information from the whole cardiac cycle and consequently represents the actual systolic and diastolic events. It is a pixel-by-pixel analysis, which means that phase analysis may be considered more regional than other types of computer analysis.

It does not require background subtraction and contributes to enhanced precision in delineating atrioventricular borders. It allows, through its color coding, the clear delineation of areas of various degrees of abnormality also demonstrating, if present, abnormalities of electrical activation. It is not influenced by adjacent structures and contributes to the quality control of RNA

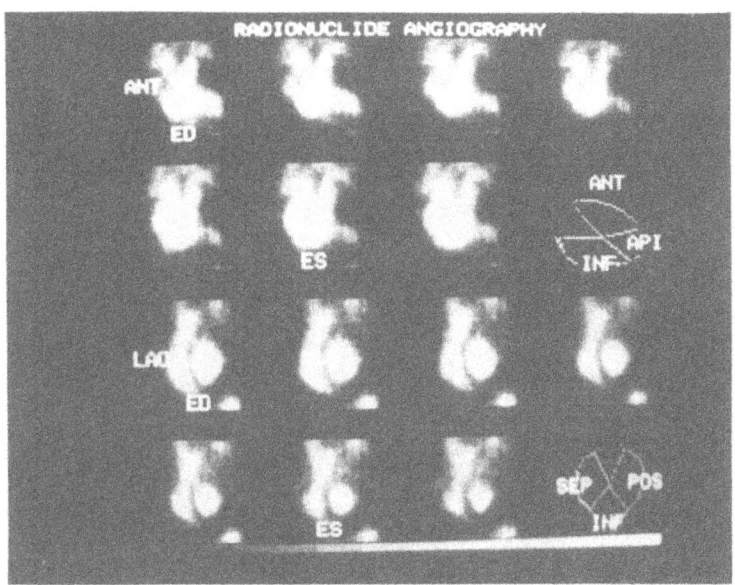

Fig. 1: Radionuclide angiography obtained in anterior (ANT) and left anterior oblique (LAO) projections following in vivo red blood cell labeling with 99m Tc. Cardiac function is represented in different phases of cardiac cycle, e.g. end-diastolic and end-systolic (ED, ES). Radionuclide angiography, utilizing different views, allows the study of all myocardial segments.
The three main coronary territories are always visualized: anterior (ANT), septal (SEP), inferior (INF), apical (API) and postero-lateral (POS).
This approach allows the identification of regional wall motion abnormalities in patients with coronary artery disease.

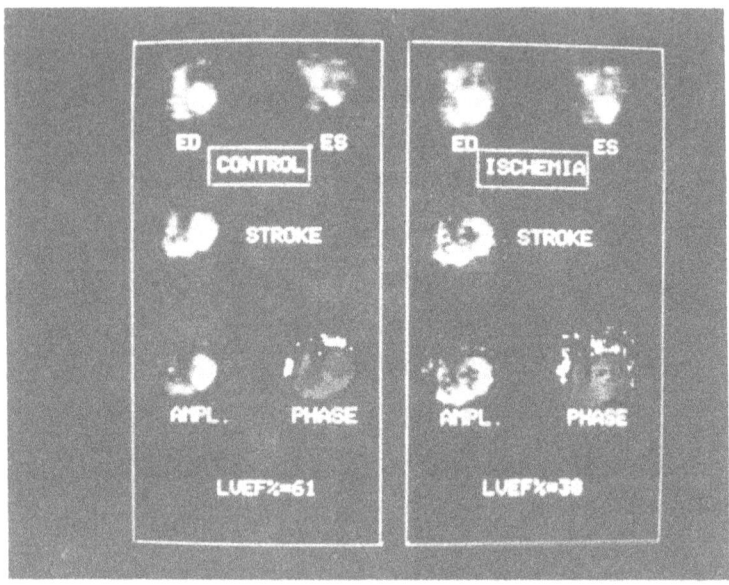

Fig. 2: Conventional radionuclide angiography obtained in left anterior oblique projection in the same patient during ischemia (ischemia, right panel) and in control conditions (control, left panel). Stroke (STROKE), amplitude (AMPL.) and phase (PHASE) images are shown as an example of functional imaging.
The basal state is characterized by normal systo-diastolic excursion, uniform stroke and amplitude images and homogeneous phase image. During ischemia, systo-diastolic excursion decreases in the septal region, ventricular volume increases, stroke and amplitude images reveal a "hole" in the septal region and phase image shows asynchronous wall motion in the same area.
As reference, the evident decrease in global left ventricular ejection fraction (38%) is also represented.
Functional imaging provides a "first impression" information to be subsequently validated by quantitative analysis.

studies.

Furthermore, all qualitative analysis of RNA must be considered as biventricular, which is very useful in various types of cardiovascular disease.

Quantitative evaluation. Global ejection fraction represents a well established and a helpful clinical non-invasive quantification of left and right ventricular function. Since the ejection fraction is a global index of ventricular function, (Tab. 1), a regional impairment in coronary artery disease may be masked and its effect offset by a compensatory hypermotility of normal segments. Increased motility of control segments has been demonstrated to be a compensatory mechanism during ischemia in both animal (8) and human (9) studies.

Despite these limits, global ejection fraction still represents the most widely used quantitative index of left and right ventricular function.

Determinations of regional ejection fractions may overcome limitations of global measurements. Yet, as previously demonstrated (10), long acquisition times are needed to obtain statistically adequate counts, a requirement difficult to meet during transient ischemia.

Quantitative phase analysis (Tab. 1), obtained by quantifying the phase distribution histogram (Fig. 3) of the number of pixels with each phase value, has been demonstrated to be a more sensitive index than global ejection fraction in detecting transient ischemia in man (Fig. 4) (4,11). Furthermore, quantitation of biventricular phase images allows an easy comparison with previous studies or with different populations of patients with cardiovascular disorders.

Diastolic indices. Asynchronous wall motion during ischemia or after myocardial infarction is frequently related to delays in the onset of regional diastolic relaxation or slower relaxation rates as observed in animal experiments (12) and in patients during episodes of angina (13). To overcome the limits of ejection fraction as a systolic index of ventricular function, diastolic indices such as time and peak filling rate may be complementarily used in the assessment of diastolic function. Furthermore, it is important to remember that phase analysis, relating to both systolic and diastolic events, may detect isolated diastolic abnormalities.

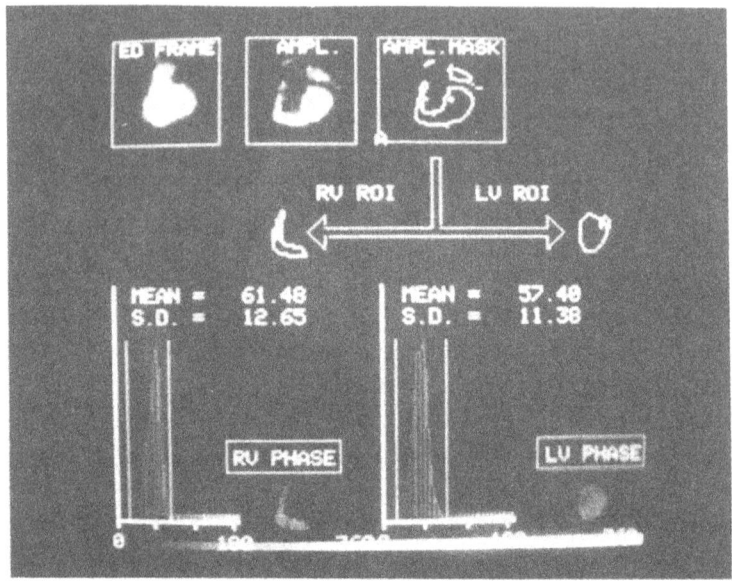

Fig. 3.: Computer algorithm used to provide quantitative information from qualitative amplitude/phase analysis.
From radionuclide angiography amplitude image is generated via a Fourier fit of the time-activity curve in each pixel. Using an amplitude mask right and left ventricular regions of interest are generated (RV ROI, LV ROI).
Subsequently, the number of pixels with each phase value is represented as a histogram; the histogram is quantified by the value of its standard deviation (S.D.) from the mean of the peak.
S.D. is then used as an index of regional wall motion.

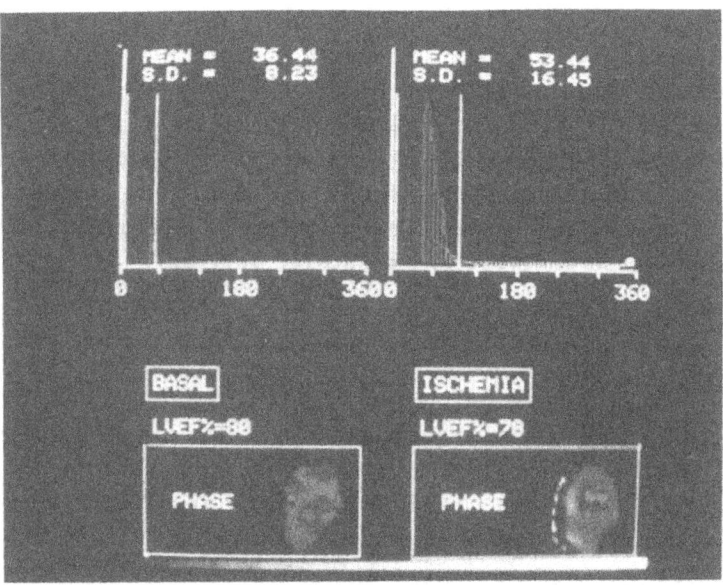

Fig. 4: Left ventricular phase histograms and phase images derived from radionuclide angiography performed in the basal condition (BASAL) and during transient ischemia (ISCHEMIA).
Although the left ventricular ejection fraction remained virtually unchanged, the phase images reveal regions of delayed phase corresponding to the infero-apical and septal walls (dotted line in the phase image).
In addition, the left ventricular histogram considerably widens during ischemia.
Despite limitations of the Fourier fit of the time/activity curve, the method nevertheless is highly accurate in detecting transient wall motion abnormalities.

What are the limitations of phase analysis? The limits of phase analysis are mainly those which affect RNA, that means spatial and temporal resolution.

Although the fit of the time/activity curve using the first Fourier harmonic may be considered as approximative, multiharmonic techniques are growing (14).

In conclusion, when considering qualitative and quantitative information derived from RNA, we can say that functional imaging could provide a "first impression" image to be subsequently refined by cine-mode display, calculation of ejection fraction, quantitative phase analysis and diastolic indices.

Correlative Aspects of Cardiovascular Nuclear Medicine and Digital Angiography

Digital subtraction angiography (DA) is a technique which utilizes a high-speed digital computer to enhance conventional radiographic images (15), resulting in high resolution images of the left ventricle and allowing visualization of wall motion abnormalities at rest (16) or following exercise (17). Moreover, DA has been completely validated in the assessment of ventricular volumes and ejection fractions, the results of which were virtually indistinguishable from those obtained with standard left ventricular contrast angiography (18). When comparing DA and RNA, several technical and clinical considerations must be examined (Tab. 2).

DA is primarily characterized by a high temporal and spatial resolution; its main limits are represented by the low possibility to obtain multiple views and by possible contrast reactions and inhomogeneities of contrast material. Dynamic studies, such as the effort test, are not feasible as a step-by-step study and pharmacological interventions (e.g. dypiridamole and ergonovine) are limited to two or three acquisitions. In addition, functional imaging in DA is still limited to a few computer algorithms. In this field, the theoretical basis of the pixel-by-pixel analysis is based on the analysis of the time attenuation (time/intensity) (19) curve as compared to the time/activity curve of RNA.

Other approaches have been used; the endocardial edge displacement and the average amplitude of excursion (20) have provided excellent functional images which well correlate to clinical data.

TABLE 1 · INDICES OF VENTRICULAR FUNCTION PROVIDED BY RADIONUCLIDE ANGIOGRAPHY.

QUALITATIVE	QUANTITATIVE
CINE-MODE (2V)	EJECTION FRACTION (GLOBAL, 2V)
STROKE IMAGE (2V)	EJECTION FRACTION (REGIONAL, LV)
PHASE/AMPLITUDE (2V)	PHASE (REGIONAL, 2V)
EJECTION FRACTION (2V)	DIASTOLIC INDICES (GLOBAL, LV)

(FUNCT connecting qualitative items)

2V=EVALUATION OF LEFT AND RIGHT VENTRICLE, LV=EVALUATION OF LEFT VENTRICLE, GLOBAL=INDEX OF GLOBAL VENTRICULAR FUNCTION, REGIONAL=INDEX OF REGIONAL VENTRICULAR FUNCTION, FUNCT=FUNCTIONAL IMAGING.

TABLE 2 · HOW TO COMPARE DIGITAL ANGIOGRAPHY AND RADIONUCLIDE ANGIOGRAPHY

	DA	RNA
SPATIAL RESOLUTION	+++	+
TEMPORAL RESOLUTION	++++	+
DEGREE OF INVASIVENESS	++	-
RADIATION DOSE	+++	++
MULTIPLE VIEWS	LIMITED	+++
CONTRAST REACTIONS	POSSIBLE	-
INHOMOGENEITY OF CONTRAST MATERIAL	POSSIBLE	-
FUNCTIONAL IMAGING	LIMITED	++++
SOURCE OF ERROR	HIGHER	LOWER
DYNAMIC STUDIES	LIMITED	++++

DA=DIGITAL ANGIOGRAPHY, RNA=RADIONUCLIDE ANGIOGRAPHY

Conclusions

Although both DA and RNA are still affected by technical and clinical limitations they offer to the cardiologist a good diagnostic tool for a non-invasive functional study of the ventricular performance.

In recent years cardiology has become more and more dynamic, which means that cardiologists want to know how and to what extent ventricular function changes during acute myocardial infarction, during episodes of effort or resting angina or following drugs administration.

Studies performed in control conditions are nowadays considered insufficient; for this reason, when compared to DA, cardiovascular nuclear medicine and its functional imaging still offer the only capability of short and long term monitoring of ventricular function in different clinical conditions. A technological and clinical cross-fertilization of these two techniques is still in course.

Acknowledgments

The Authors are very grateful to Mrs. Daniela Banti for her secretarial assistance in preparing this paper.

REFERENCES

1) Schulze, R.A., Pitt S., Griffith L.S., Ducci H.H., Achuff S.C., Baird M.G., O'Neal Humphries J. Coronary angiography and left ventriculography in survivors of transmural and non transmural myocardial infarction. American Journal of Medicine 64 (1978) 108-113.
2) Borer, J., Rosing D., Miller R., Stark R., Kent K., Bacharach S., Green M., Lake C., Cohen H., Holmes D., Donohue D., Baker W., Epstein S. Natural history of left ventricular function during 1 years after acute myocardial infarction. Comparison with clinical, electrocardiographic and biochemical determinations. American Journal of Cardiology 46 (1980) 1-12.

3) Adam, W.E., Torkowska A., Bitter F., Strauch M., Geffers N. Equilibrium (gated) radionuclide ventriculography. Cardiovascular Radiology 2 (1979) 161-173.
4) Marzullo, P., Parodi O., Schelbert H.R., L'Abbate A.: Regional myocardial dysfunction in patients with angina at rest and response to isosorbide dinitrate assessed by phase analysis by radionuclide ventriculograms. Journal of the American College of Cardiology 3 (1984) 1357-1366.
5) Ratib, O., Henze E., Schon H., Schelbert H.R. Phase analysis of radionuclide ventriculograms for the detection of coronary artery disease. American Heart Journal 104 (1982) 1-12.
6) Botvinick, E., Dunn R., Frais M., O'Connell W., Shosa D., Herfkens R., Scheinman M. The phase image: its relationship to patterns of contraction and conduction. Circulation 65 (1982) 551-560.
7) Swiryn, S., Pavel D., Byrom E., Bavernfeind R., Strasberg B., Palileo E., Lam M., Wyndham C., Rosen K. Sequential regional phase mapping of radionuclide gated biventriculograms in patients with sustained ventricular tachicardia: close correlation with electrophysiologic characteristic. American Heart Journal 103 (1982) 319-332.
8) Savage, R.M., Guth B., White F.C., Hagan A.D., Bloor C.M. Correlation of regional myocardial blood flow and function with myocardial infarct size during acute myocardial ischemia in the conscious pig. Circulation 64 (1981) 699-707.
9) Distante, A., Rovai D., Picano E., Moscarelli E., Palombo C., Morales M.A., Michelassi C., L'Abbate A. Transient changes in left ventricular mechanics during attacks of Prinzmetal angina: an M-mode echocardiographic study. American Heart Journal 107 (1984) 465-474.
10) Maddox, D.E., Holman G.L., Wynne J., Uren R., Parker J., Idoine J., Siegel L., Neill J., Cohn P., Holman L. Regional ejection fraction: a quantitative radionuclide index of regional left ventricular performance. Circulation 59 (1979) 1001-1029.
11) Parodi, O., Marzullo P., Neglia D., Galli M., Distante A., Rovai D., L'Abbate A. Transient predominant right ventricular ischemia caused by coronary vasospasm. Circulation 70 (1984) 170-177.
12) Théroux, P., Ross J., Franklin D., Kemper W.S., Sasayama S. Regional myocardial function in the conscious dog during acute coronary occlusion and responses to morphine, pro-

pranolol, nitroglycerin and lidocaine. Circulation 53 (1976) 302-314.
13) Mancini, J., Slutsky R., Norris S.L., Bhargava V., Ashburn W.L., Higgins C.B. Radionuclide analysis of peak filling rate, filling fraction and time to peak filling rate. American Journal of Cardiology 51 (1983) 43-51.
14) Goris, M., Briandet P., Kriss J. Decomposition of the information content of first harmonic phase images, vol. 1 (Proceedings of the 3rd World Congress of Nuclear Medicine and Biology, Paris, Raynaud C. Editor, 1982) 46-49.
15) Baily, N. Video techniques for x-ray imaging and date extraction from roentgenographic and fluoroscopic presentations. Medical Physic 7 (1980) 472-478.
16) Higgins, C., Norris S., Gerber K., Slutsky R., Ashburn W., Baily N. Quantitation of left ventricular dimensions and function by digital intravenous ventriculography. Radiology 44 (1982) 461-469.
17) Goldberg, H., Moses J., Borer J., Fisher J., Tamari I., Skelly N, Cohen B. Exercise left ventriculography utilizing intravenous digital angiography. Journal of the American College of Cardiology 2 (1983) 1092-1098.
18) Goldberg, H.L., Borer J.S., Moses W.L., Fisher J., Cohn B., Skelly N.T. Digital subtraction intravenous left ventricular angiography: comparison with conventional intravascular angiography. Journal of the American College of Cardiology 1 (1983) 858-862.
19) Widmann, T.F., Ashburn W.L., Higgins C.B., Peterson K.L. Assessment of left ventricular wall motion by regional phase analysis of digital intravenous contrast fluoroangiography. Computers in Cardiology, (IEEE Computers Society, 1982) 105-108.
20) Ratib, O., Righetti A. Multiharmonic fourier analysis of ventricular wall motion for the detection of regional alterations in contraction and relaxation. Computers in Cardiology, (IEEE Computers Society, 1983) 423-426.

DIGITAL RADIOGRAPHY AND NUCLEAR MEDICINE: CORRELATIVE ASPECTS AND TECHNOLOGICAL CROSS-FERTILIZATION

C.L. Partain, M.D.,Ph.D, M.V. Kulkarni, M.D., R.R. Price, Ph.D, M.P. Sandler, M.D., J.A. Patton, Ph.D, D.R. Pickens, Ph.D, J.J. Erickson, Ph.D, A.E. James, Jr, J.D., M.D.

Department of Radiology & Radiological Sciences, Vanderbilt University Medical Center, Nashville, Tn, U.S.A.

INTRODUCTION

The term "digital radiography," for practical purposes recently has adopted several meanings. These include intravenous contrast angiography, scanned projection radiography (CT based radiography), dynamic computed tomography, multi-regional digital radiographic flow studies, and digitized ultrasound and radionuclide images.

In addition, the newer modalities involve digital image processing and display, nuclear magnetic resonance imaging, positron and single photon emission tomography, scatter radiography, micro-wave and infra-red imaging, and x-ray fluorescence tomography. All of these modalities represent the general term "digital radiography" (1-10).

The term, however, usually refers to peripheral intravenous angiography. This technique is relatively non-invasive and may be used to assess most of the vessels studied conventionally by catheterization methods. The technique utilizes real time digital processing of x-ray transmission data from a standard image intensifier, one component of a video fluoroscopy system. A block diagram of the Vanderbilt Digital Radiography System is shown in Figure 1 (3).

CHARACTERISTICS OF DIGITAL RADIOGRAPHY

There are a number of advantages and potential patient benefits of digital radiography. The method has essentially the same mild risk as intravenous renography and, thus, it permits evaluation of high risk and asymptomatic patients. Other advantages include a reduction in number of catheterizations; cost reduction by allowing angiography on an outpatient basis; an increase in effectiveness of conventional angiography; allowance of processed temporal subtraction in real-time; and provision for hard copy of subtracted images using a multiformat camera. In addition, digital radiography is a straightforward procedure requiring minimal computer or basic science expertise for technical performance or maintenance. Operational benefits also include energy subtraction; low contrast detectability; flexible display for rapid, accurate and interactive processing of detected information; digital control; digital storage/retrieval; high speed; and procedure flexibility.

Digital radiography is not an ideal modality. Its limitations include patient motion artifacts, sensitivity to registration errors, decreased anatomical resolution, and decreased vascular selectivity.

CORRELATIVE ASPECTS WITH NUCLEAR MEDICINE

Many digital radiographic (DR) studies are complementary to nuclear medicine. These include dynamic brain scanning and carotid DR, as well as dynamic liver-spleen scanning and aortic DR. Other studies are likely to be directly competitive, and future efficacy and cost benefit evaluation will determine which procedure, or combination of procedures, will be performed in various diagnostic situations.

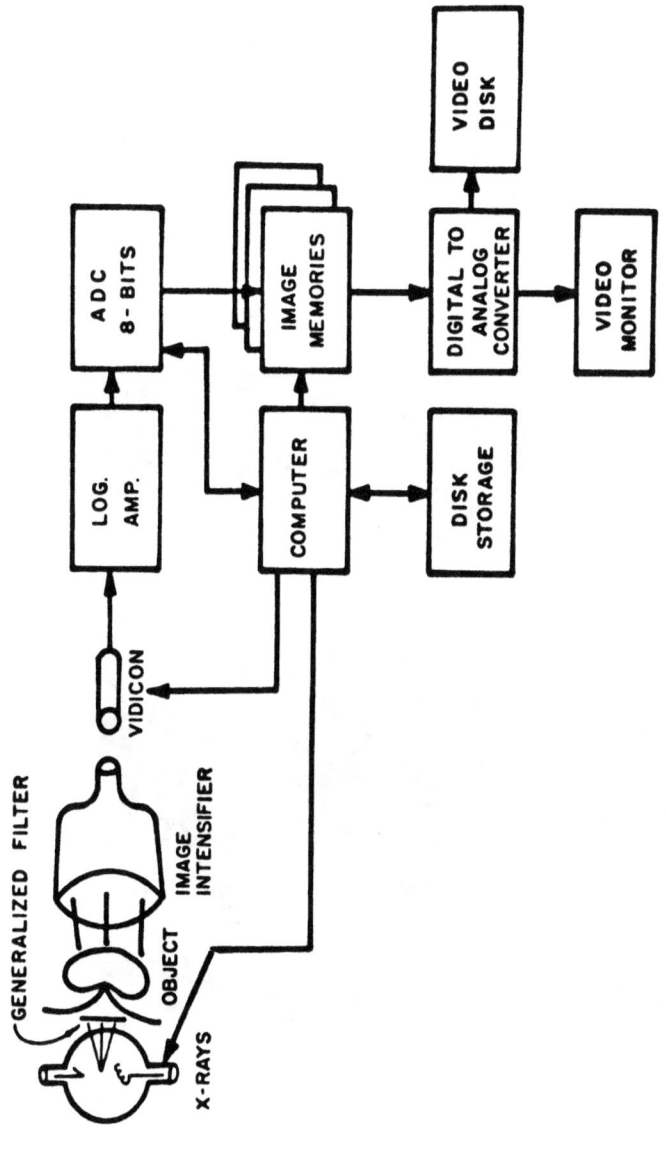

Fig. 1. Schematic diagram of the Vanderbilt University Digital Radiography System. (Reproduced by permission of Grune & Stratton, ref. 11, and Raven Press, ref. 12.)

TECHNICAL CROSS-FERTILIZATION

Vascular Studies

Figure 2 demonstrates the excellent visualization of the abdominal aorta, renal arteries and kidneys from a normal patient using the intravenous digital angiography technique. Notice that significantly improved anatomic resolution is available compared to conventional radionuclide flow studies and may be the study of choice when anatomical detail is needed unless the patient is allergic to contrast material.

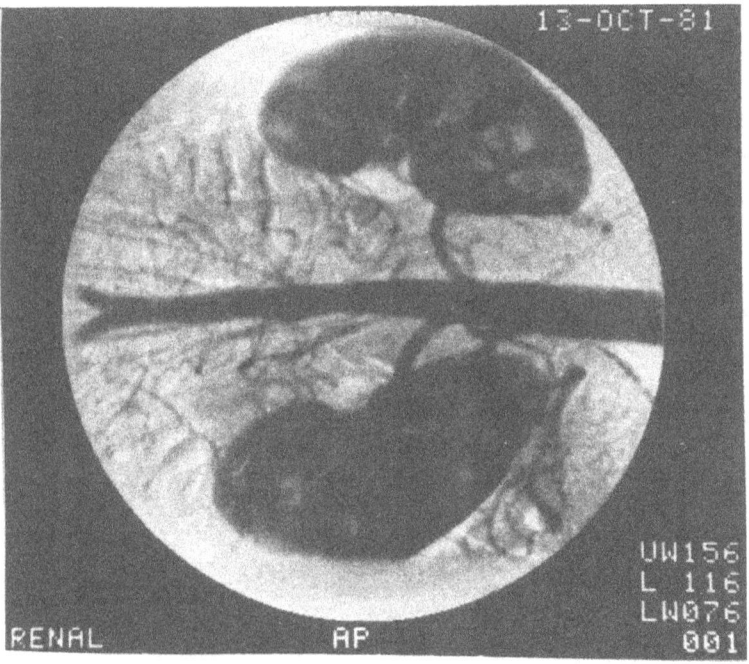

Fig. 2. Digital radiography following intravenous contrast injection demonstrating patient aorta, renal arteries, and kidneys, where a mask image was subtracted from the contrast radiography image and serial contrast-enhanced images were added.

Figure 3 correlates a radionuclide lung scan in a dog before and after embolization, with a contrast digital radiographic study in the arterial and parenchymal phases. In our series of ten dogs, we were able to diagnose pulmonary emboli accurately due to the combination of vessel occlusion, intraluminal clot, and parenchymal perfusion defect.

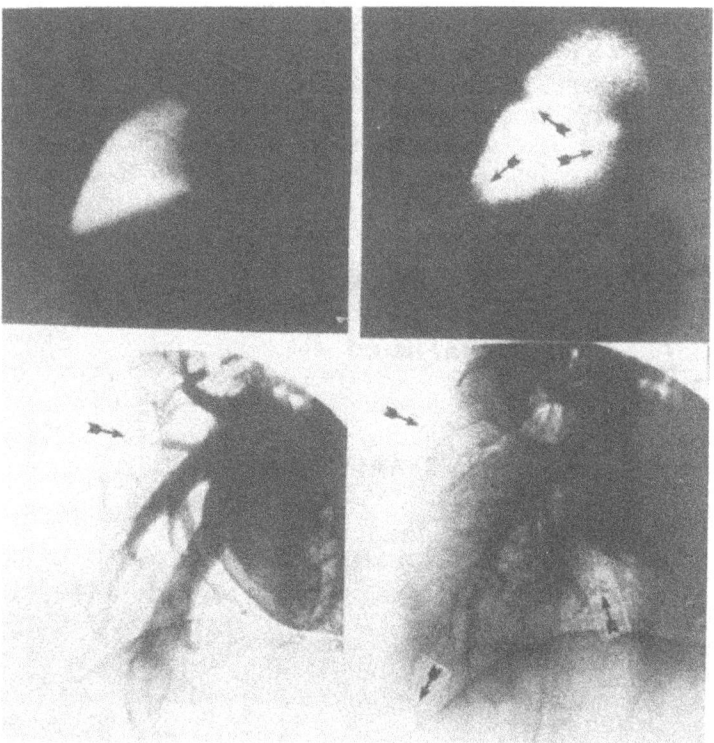

Fig. 3. Comparison of radionuclide lung scan and digital radiography in pulmonary emboli in a dog. UPPER LEFT. Lung scan, right lung, normal, before embolization. UPPER RIGHT. Lung scan, after embolization, multiple peripheral defects indicated by arrows. LOWER LEFT. Arterial phase DR study, occluded vessel at arrow. LOWER RIGHT. Parenchymal phase DR study, peripheral perfusion defects noted at arrows. (Reproduced by permission of Raven Press, ref. 12.)

Funtional Renal Imaging

This study may be performed by both DR and nuclear medicine. Note the regional organ perfusion time-density curves in Figures 4 and 5. Figure 4 represents a digital radiographic renogram in a monkey using Renograffin-60 and stable (cold) ortho-iodinated-hippuran, and the curves are seen to resemble very closely comparable Tc-99m DTPA and I-131-OIH curves in a normally functioning kidney. The Tc-99m DTPA and Renograffin 60 dynamic curves are measures of glomerular filtration. The hippuran curve is a measure of tubular secretion. In Figure 5, Conray-400, an agent which is handled by the kidney by glomerular filtration, is utilized to demonstrate the ability of DR to evaluate differential renal function time-density curves in multiple regions.

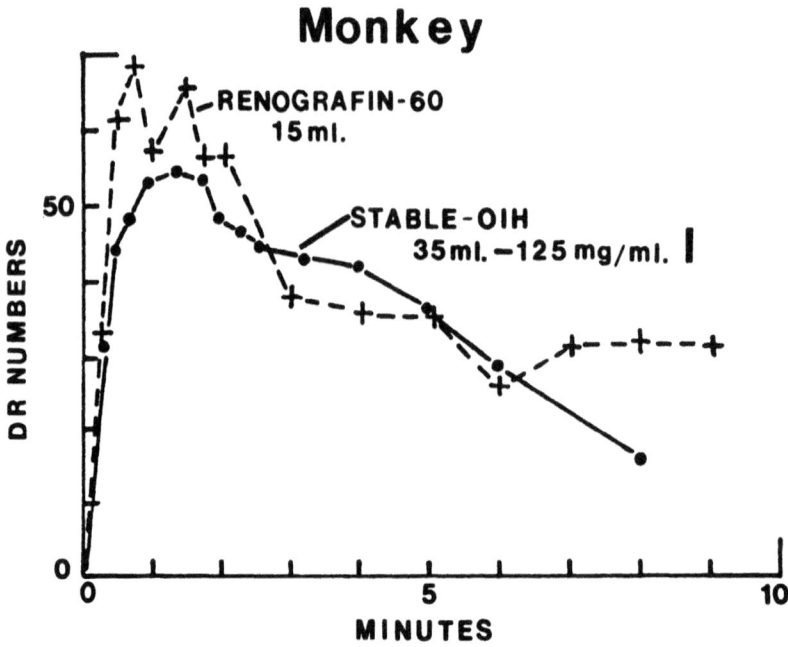

Fig. 4. Time-density curves from DR study in monkey comparing Renograffin-60 and stable OIH clearance. (Reproduced by permission of Raven Press, ref. 12.)

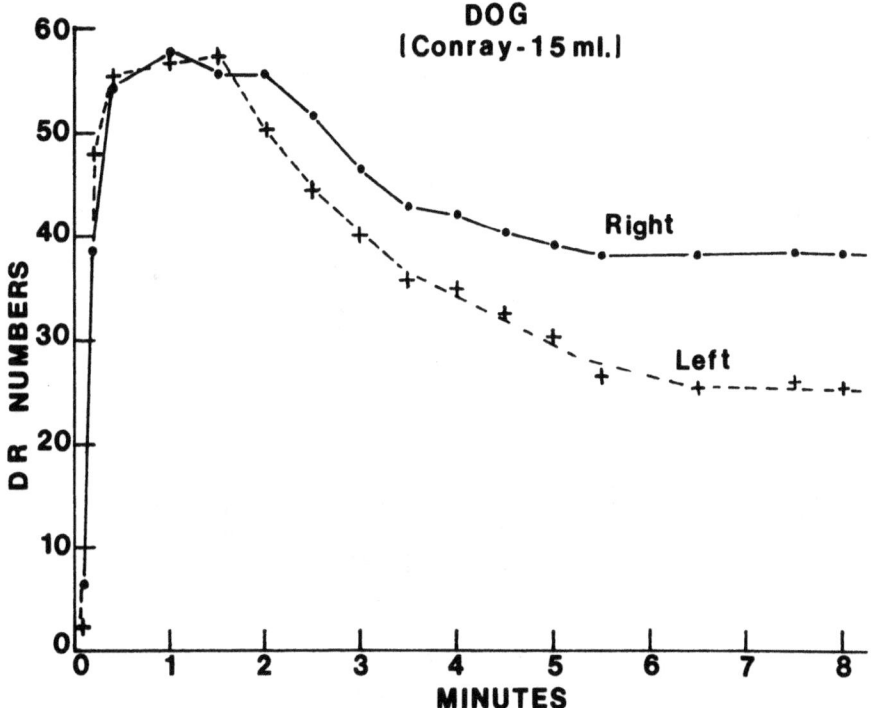

Fig. 5. DR time-density curves in a dog with region-of-interest analysis from each renal cortex. Notice that the right kidney demonstrates decreased renal clearance. (Reproduced by permission of Raven Press, ref. 12.)

Human DR renal kinetics studies with Conray-400 are shown in Figures 6 and 7. The prompt blood flow is demonstrated in Figure 6 for the first 25 seconds after injection. In Figure 7, the time-density renogram is shown for the first 10 minutes after injection. This is very comparable data to renal nuclear medicine studies using Tc-99m DTPA and Tc-99m glucoheptonate.

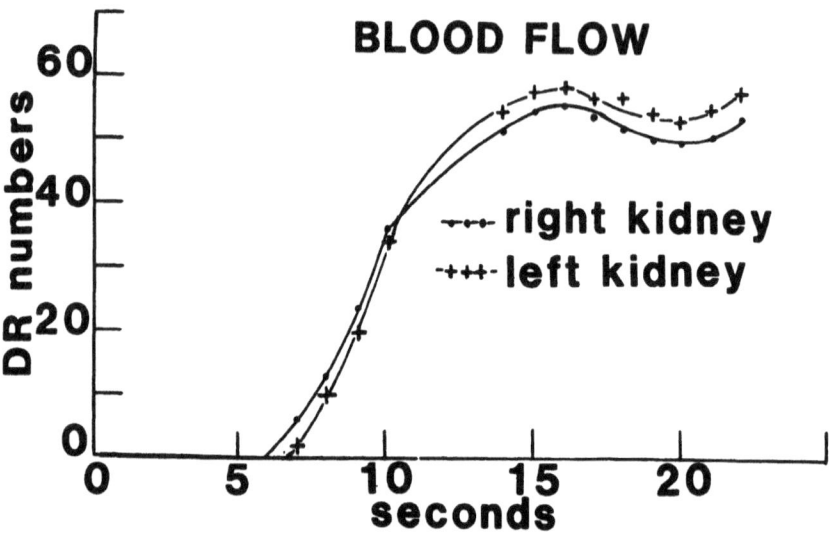

Fig. 6. Prompt renal DR in normal patient showing symmetrical blood flow to each kidney.

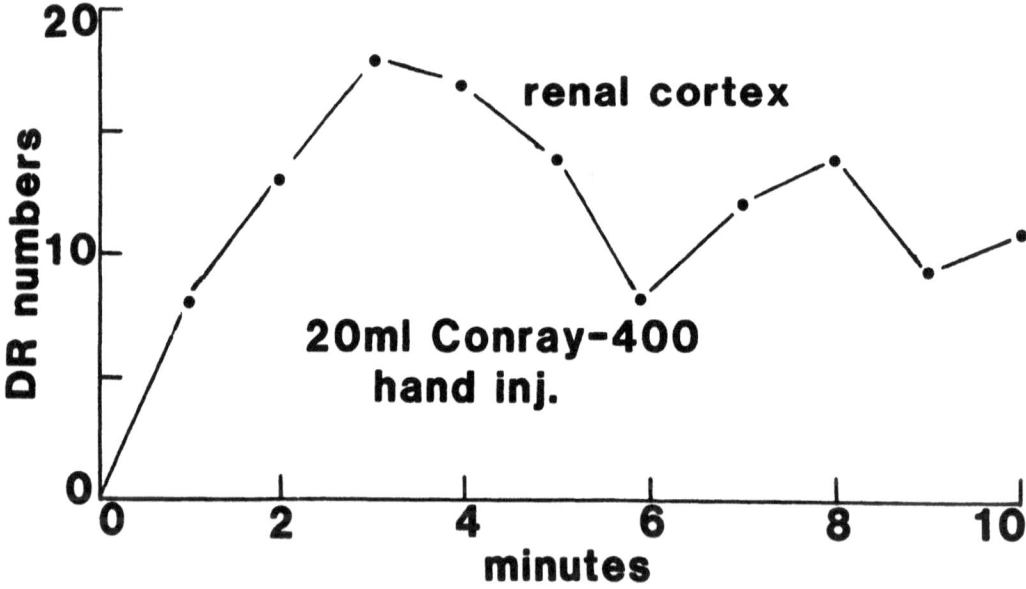

Fig. 7. DR renogram in same patient as in Fig. 6 demonstrating the kinetics of Conray-400 for 10 minutes after injection.

CONCLUSION

Digital radiography is a reasonably economical system that helps diagnostic imaging physicians to develop increasingly less-invasive procedures, obtain maximal information at a given dose and increase the flexibility and convenience involved with diagnostic workups.

The range of applications of DR has not been fully established at this time. Comparison of its properties with those of conventional nuclear medicine may suggest areas of potential application. Compared to nuclear medicine techniques, DR in general provides improved anatomical resolution, improved contrast resolution, sometimes equivalent functional information, and decreased imaging time. On the other hand, some functional nuclear medicine studies provide information not available by DR; these include the gallium scan, bone scan, hepatic-biliary scan, and lung scan.

Therefore, nuclear medicine procedures will be complementary in some instances to digital radiography procedures and competitive in others. The proper roles of each modality in various clinical settings await future detailed and comprehensive efficacy studies.

Acknowledgments

The editorial and photographic assistance of Margaret Moore and John Bobbitt respectively are gratefully acknowledged.

REFERENCES

1. Price RR, Rollo FD, Monahan WG, James AE: Digital Radiography: A Focus on Clinical Utility. New York, Grune & Stratton, 1982.

2. Erickson JJ, Rollo FD: Digital Nuclear Medicine. Philadelphia, J. B. Lippincott, 1983.

3. Erickson JJ, Price RR, Rollo FD, Pendergrass HP, Gerlock AJ, James AE and Partain CL: A digital radiographic analysis system. RadioGraphics 1(2):49-60, 1981.

4. Partain CL, Price RR, Patton JA, Erickson JJ, Pickens DR and James AE: The potential impact of digital radiography on the specialty of nuclear medicine. Clinical Nuclear Medicine Supplement, Vol. 6, 105, P2-P4, 1981.

5. Crummy AB, Strother CM, Sackett JF, et al: Computerized fluoroscopy: digital subtraction for intravenous angiocardiography and arteriography. AJR 135:1131, 1980.

6. Ovitt TW, Christenson PC, Fisher III HD, et al: Intravenous angiography using video subtraction: x-ray imaging system. AJR 135:1141, 1980.

7. Christenson PC, Ovitt TW, Fisher III HD, et al: Intravenous cervicocerebrovascular angiography. AJR 135:1145, 1980.

8. Meany TF, Weinstein MA, Buonocore E, et al: Digital subtraction angiography of the human cardiovascular system. AJR 135:1153, 1980.

9. Mistretta CA, Crummy AB. Computerized fluoroscopy. In Coulam CM, Erickson JJ, Rollo FD, et al (eds): Physical Basis for Medical Imaging. New York, Appleton-Century-Crofts, 1981.

10. Mistretta CA, Hillman J, Buonocore E, et al: Digital subtraction radiography. Radiology 139:273, 1981.

11. Price RR, Rollo FD, Monahan GW, James AE: Digital Radiography: A Focus on Clinical Utility. New York, Grune & Stratton, 1982.

12. Price RR, Partain CL, Kulkarni MV, Patton JA, Pickens DR, Waddill WB, Jolles H, Diggs J, Reilly R, Winfield AC, James AE: Digital radiography and its potential impact on radionuclide imaging. In Freeman LM and Weissmann HS (eds): Nuclear Medicin Annual 1984, New York, Raven Press, 1984.

DISCUSSION SUMMARY

PANEL ON:
DIGITAL RADIOLOGY: PRINCIPLES, TECHNOLOGY AND CORRELATIVE ASPECTS
WITH NUCLEAR MEDICINE

A. Todd Pokropek:

There has been much discussion about 'the numbers game'. What are the spatial and temporal requirements in Digital Radiology? Given the present poor 'press' given to DR (DSA in particular) is this primarily a result of technological problems, or a result of the misuse of the technique by clinicians?

P. Heintzen:

I do not think that Digital Radiology DR in general has a 'poor press'. Furthermore, the 'press' - at least a certain press - is no valid indicator of the usefulness or significance of a new method. With respect to your question, one has to consider that DR is still a rapidly evolving field. Under such circumstances, it happens that overestimation of the benefits, uncritical use and, on the other hand, overlooking of the specific potential of such a new method often occurs. Furthermore, radiology is such a broad field with a very wide spectrum of problems - the solution of which requires various spatial, temporal and density resolutions as well as image generation and processing techniques - so that Digital Radiology has many faces. Digital subtraction angiography is only a small field. However - besides tomographic reconstruction - the desire for contrast enhancement and quantitative data extraction from angiocardiographic image series very much stimulated electronic and digital imaging techniques. The equipment developed to achieve these goals was and still is not perfect or of comparable quality. Most commercially available instruments allow at present only a simple digital subtraction angiography. They do not provide the specific potential of processing angiographic image series, that gives access to various aspects of cardiovascular anatomy and function. There are certainly specific benefits of 'simple DSA', if the indications are made critically. However, at least in the initial optimistic phase, some gain in contrast resolution had been obtained by more contrast material injected intravenously and a reduced spatial resolution. This might be responsible for the poor 'press'. In the meantime it became clear that the appropriate use of contrast enhancement with selective injections is becoming the broader invasive field of DSA and functional imaging offers the real advantages in DR.

D.P. Boyd:

What is the conceptual basis for processing of digital-subtraction-angiographic pictures with Fourier analysis variations since the X, Y and Z spatial coordinates are also varying with time in cardiac images?

P. Heintzen:

The contrast bolus in conventional angiocardiography is a 'first pass' phenomenon, not a periodic function. However, depending on the site of contrast injection and densitometric recording there are heart-rate related waveforms superposing the basically monophasic waveform, which depends mainly on the injection mode (duration, amount, site of contrast injection) and pathophysiology of the cardiovascular system. It is obviuosly one goal to separate these various waveforms by Fourier analysis, to characterize the shape of the bolus and to come to a physiologically meaningful interpretation of the frequency components. One can also deduce from the phase shift of the fundamental frequency the time delay of the bolus at various places of the circulatory system. We found this approach not very useful in most cases and had the impression that Fourier analysis was mainly applied, because the programs were at hand and successfully applied in nuclear medicine (where, however, the conditions were quite different in gated blood pool studies). But also in these applications the interpretation appears, to me, questionable in many instances since - as you mentioned - the X, Y and Z coordinates are varying with time, therefore not allowing particularly when applied to the heart and cardiac borders, discrimination between thickness changes or lateral motion of the cardiovascular structure.

Y.Z. Ider:

Excluding coronary diagnosis, can radionuclide imaging do everything that is possible with Digital Subtraction Angiography? (Ejection Fraction, etc...)

P.Heintzen:

It is generally accepted, that nuclear medicine can provide ejection fractions with a degree of accuracy which is adequate to the clinical requirements. However, most of the limitations in this respect compared to angiocardiography (analog or digital) are due to the lower spatial and temporal resolution. With respect to 'subtraction' of the 'background' there is no way to do this similar to digital subtraction angiocardiography since the radiation source is at the same time the indicator and inside the circulatory system; the background cannot be measured independently (without indicator) and non invasively. It might however be of minor importance.

Y.Z. Ider:

Do Fourier methods offer any advantages for detecting cardiac walls and therefore for automatic determination of cardiac volume? To your knowledge, has this possibility been tested?

P. Heintzen:
We do not believe that Fourier analysis is a useful method for ventricular border definition from angiocardiograms. As already pointed out by D.P. Boyd, the density changes around the ventricular borders can be due to thickness changes or lateral movements of the ventricles alone or a combination of both.

R. Kruger:

Is cardiac study complete for the imaging of coronary vessels?

P. Heintzen:

Depending on the various types of cardiovascular anomalies, different angiocardiographic and or coronarographic approaches are indicated. A very large group of (mainly adult) patients needs a coronary angiography and left ventriculography. In most of the congenital and valvular heart diseases a coronarography or even an angiocardiography is not needed.

M. Waller:

Could you please explain more fully how dual energy subtraction is used to remove motion artifacts.

P. Heintzen:

In dual energy subtraction, slow changing background structures (soft tissue, bone, etc...) are eliminated since in short time intervals (20 - 40 milliseconds) 2 exposures with different KV's are taken for which the absorbtion differences caused by these moving tissues are small . Therefore they cancel out. If the two energies are, however, just below and above the so called K-edge of the contrast material, even in small time intervals the contrast material does not cancel out. A combination of dual energy subtraction and temporal subtraction - so called hybrid subtraction digital angiocardiography - is also described. (References: Guthaner, Brody et al. Cardiovasc. Intervent. Radiol. 1983, 6: 290-294. Mistretta et al.: Digital subtraction arteriography: 1982 Year Book Medical Publ., Chicago/London).

P. Marzullo:

In our Institute we spent some years in the study and quantification of myocardial blood flow using Xenon gases or microspheres in man. The experimental basis of this technique is surely well known. Have you any experimental model comparing microsphere distribution and Digital Radiology perfusion images?

P. Heintzen:

We have not used microspheres, nor have we tried to quantify myocardial blood flow. We have however compared perfusion defects in animal experiments with the postmortem determined infarct size.

POSTER SESSION

DIGITAL RADIOGRAPHY USING THE INDIVIDUAL PHOTON COUNTING TECHNIQUE

R. Bellazzini, A. Brez, A. Del Guerra,
M.M. Massai and M.R. Torquati
Dipartimento di Fisica dell'Università di Pisa
and INFN - Sezione di Pisa

1   INTRODUCTION

In the last ten years the field of medical imaging has been revolutionized by the introduction of new methodologies (CAT, Digital Radiography, NMR, etc...) combined with powerful digital techniques. On the other hand, the field of medical radiation detectors has remained more steady. Almost all of the existing devices are still of the integrating type, which are often hampered by linearity, noise or dynamic range problems. In this respect, a detection system counting individual photons should have several advantages: i) low noise, given by definition by the photon statistics; ii) high linearity and dynamic range limited only by dead-time losses (which can be accounted for). A MultiWire Proportional Chamber (MWPC) is a poissonian, electronic, area detector and for this reason since its introduction it has received great attention for its possible application in the biomedical field. However, to be suitable for medical imaging a MWPC should satisfy the following stringent requirements: 1) good detection efficiency; 2) good spatial resolution; 3) high-rate capability. To satisfy the first requirement one has to use a gas with a high atomic number (Xenon), possibly at high pressure. For the second requirement, the use of a monochromatic X-ray source with energy just above the K-edge of Xenon (=34.6 KeV) can greatly help to achieve a submillimeter spatial resolution. Until a few years ago, the speed of the electronic data acquisition system was the most severe bottleneck for the solution of the third problem. The recent introduction of very fast TDC's and of Histogramming Memories has greatly simplified the problem, allowing a data capability of more than 1 MHz to be reached in a straightforward way. The modern generation of MWPCs seems to be competitive with the existing imaging devices, especially when quantitative studies on stationary objects must be performed (i.e. bone or lung densitometry).

2 THE MONOCHROMATIC X-RAY SOURCE

A quantitative study of radiation transmission through matter requires the use of a monochromatic source. Important parameters like attenuation coefficient, thickness, or mass can be measured only by using a source with a well defined energy. We have developed a monochromatic, fluorescent, X-ray source by using a conventional tube with targets and filters of various elements. The advantages of this solution are: i) it is inexpensive because an x-ray generator is available in every diagnostic center; ii) the energy of the source can be selected by simply modifying the target-filter combination; iii) patient and operator exposure is limited to the examination time. A scheme of the fluorescent X-ray source is shown in fig. 1 . The detector is exposed to the fluorescent X-rays which pass first through a filter and then through the exit aperture. The filter material, with a K absorption edge between the K_α and K_β lines of the target, removes most of the K_β as well as scattered radiation.

Consequently, nearly monoenergetic K_α X-rays are obtained. The whole system was carefully alligned with a laser beam. For the selection of three different X-ray energies (40, 42, and 45 KeV), we have used three combinations of four elements (Samarium, Neodymium, Dysprosium, and Gadolinium) for the target and filter (see Table 1). The target was a foil 25 mm x 25 mm with a thickness of 700 μm.

The spectra generated from a Samarium target with and without the Neodymium filter are shown in fig. 2a and in fig. 2b , respectively. The use of the Neodymium filter reduces the number of the K_β X-rays from the Samarium target and improves the purity of the beam. The spectrum shown contains 96% K_α X-rays; it is, therefore, highly monoenergetic. The flux incident on the whole chamber placed at a distance of 70 cm from the target was $\simeq 2 \times 10^6$ photons/second. The X-ray tube used for these measurements was a very simple, portable, instrument with half-wave rectification and a current limit of 5 mA at the maximum accelerating voltage of 80 KV. A flux greater by at least one order of magnitude can be obtained by using a modern three-phase X-ray generator with full wave rectification, 110-120 KVp and a current output of 10 mA. If we assume a 10% detection efficiency and, for example, a 20% X-ray transmission through an arm we can estimate a data rate of $\simeq 10^6$ counts/second that corresponds well to the speed of the electronic data acquisition system (see sec. 4). It should be noted that an equivalent data rate could be obtained with a ^{153}Gd source of, at least, 1 Ci strength.

3 THE MWPC

The chamber we built is a thin chamber (6.4 mm total active thickness). To counteract the decrease of efficiency we built a chamber that could be operated at pressures of up to four atmospheres. Increasing the pressure gives the further advantage of reducing the range of the photo - and Auger - electrons thus improving the spatial resolution and allowing for the use of sources with higher energies (up to ~ 70 KeV). The main geometrical parameters of the MWPC are listed in Table II. The area of the chamber (128 mm x 128 mm) was selected to fit the present size of the CAMAC memory (128x256 pixels). The spatial sampling is therefore 0.5 mm in the direction parallel to the anode wires and 1 mm in the orthogonal direction. Since Xenon is a very expensive gas, the MWPC must be sealed or flushed at a very low rate (< 0.3 bubble/second). The MWPC has been operated for six months with the same gas filling without any significant modification of the working conditions.

4 THE READ-OUT ELECTRONICS

A short examination period is imperative in order to avoid loss of resolution due to patient movements.

Therefore, a primary goal of the read-out system design was to reach a rate capability of a few hundreds kilohertz.

The position read-out system that we adopted is based on cathode-coupled delay-lines (50 ns/cm specific delay), and very fast Time to Digital Converters (LeCroy 4202, ~ 500 ns typical conversion time). The signals at each end of the delay-lines are preamplified with "electronic cooling" of the noise temperature, amplified, and discriminated with a Constant Fraction Technique (CFD ORTEC 583). A very attractive feature of the 4202 TDC is the possibility of measuring positive (the start before the stop) as well as negative (the stop before the start) times. The total delay of the delay-lines is thus reduced by one-half. A pile-up inspector aborts the acquisition of any event which is followed by a second event within a time window of 1 μs. A gateable, presettable timer and counter measure the system dead-time. The anode signal is used only as a gate for the TDCs. A Single Channel Analyzer permits a pulse-height analysis of the anode signal to select the energy window of interest. To by-pass the slow CAMAC cycle and to efficiently store the great amount of data collected in a short time, the most significant seven bits of the first TDC and the most significant eight bits of the second TDC are hardwired on the same output bus to form a 15 bit data word containing the x,y coordinates of an accepted event. The output bus addresses a Fast CAMAC Histogramming memory (Le Croy 3588). This module acts, in this case, as a two-dimensional Multichannel Analyzer. The read-increment by one-write cycle of the memory takes only 1.2 μs allowing a data rate of up to 800 KHz. When the acquisition is started, it proceeds independently, so that the computer (Digital LSI 11-02) can be used to read-out the CAMAC memory and to display the data.

A gray or color real-time image of the x-ray transmission pattern through the object is displayed by means of an image processing system consisting of a matrix of 256x256 pixels, each 10 bits deep. A detailed description of the MWPC performance is reported elsewhere (1).

5   THE IMAGING CAPABILITY OF THE SYSTEM

To study the imaging capabilities of the system we have imaged several objects with high and low contrast. Figure 3 shows the reconstructed image of two steel nuts of 1 cm outer diameter, separated by 700 μm. Figure 4 shows an example of the possibilities offered by the digital nature of the reconstructed images. In this case, the wrench image was pixelwise divided with a normalization exposure obtained immediately after the first one with the wrench removed and the results logarithmically scaled down. In this way the original image was corrected for inhomogeneities of the system response function and, more significantly, was transformed into an image with a different information content (i.e. the two-dimensional distribution of the wrench thickness). A more difficult problem is to image an object with a very low contrast. Figure 5 shows an image of a shell that was interposed between the source and the detector. All the significant morphological structures are well resolved.

6 APPLICATION OF THE MWPC TO BONE DENSITOMETRY STUDIES

A natural application of this system is in the field of quantitative studies of stationary objects (i.e. body extremities). In this case the measurement can take several seconds without too much discomfort for the patient. At a rate of 100 KHz, 5-10 seconds are more than sufficient to collect statistically significant data, thus minimizing the problem of patient movements.

An interesting application is the direct measurement of bone mass as already introduced by Horsman et al. (2). In short, the technique is as follows: take a transmission image of a human wrist surrounded by a water bolus; then take a second image of the same water bolus with the sample object removed; divide the two images and take the logarithm of the result. The bone mineral content M is proportional to the sum of the contents of each pixel of the resulting image. The advantages of this technique relative to a scanning arrangement are: i) it is faster; ii) the repositioning accuracy is higher. Figure 6 shows an image of the bone mass distribution of the wrist of a human skeleton.

7 CONCLUSIONS

The described system has shown interesting promise for medical imaging applications. It has a submillimiter spatial resolution and a rate capability that can reach the 1 MHz level with faster delay- lines. The digital nature of the resulting images allows extraction of quantitative information from the data and the capability of reaching a much higher sensitivity than conventional X-ray film.

References

1) R.Bellazzini et al., Nucl.Instr.Method (1984, in press.)
2) A.Horsman et al.,Phys.Med.Biol. 22,1059 (1977)

TABLE I - X-ray Energy selection.

Target	Samarium	Gadolinium	Dysprosium
Filter	Neodynium	Samarium	Gadolinium
Energy	40 keV	42 keV	45 keV

Active area	128x128 mm^2	Gas filling	Xe-CO_2
Anode-cathode gap	3.2 mm	Window thickness	0.18 g/cm^2
Anode wire spacing	2 mm	Detection efficiency	10%
Anode wire diameter	20 μm	Spatial resolution	500 μm
Cathode strips width	2.7 mm	Energy resolution	30%

TABLE II - The MWPC parameters.

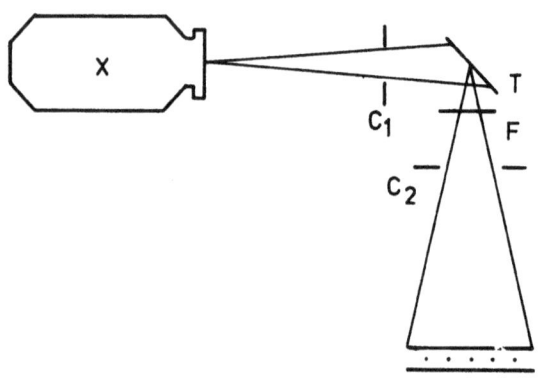

FIG.1 - A scheme of the fluorescent X-ray source.

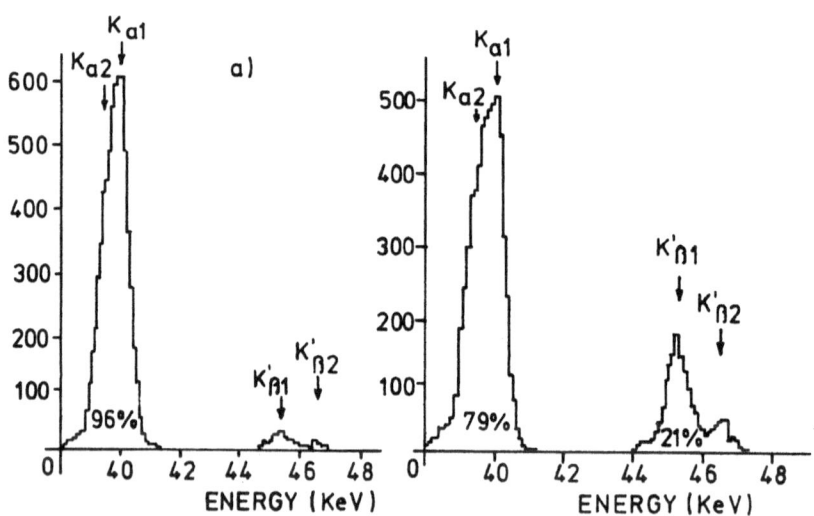

FIG.2 - a) Spectrum generated by a Samarium target with the Neodymium filter; b) The same of a), without the Neodymium filter.

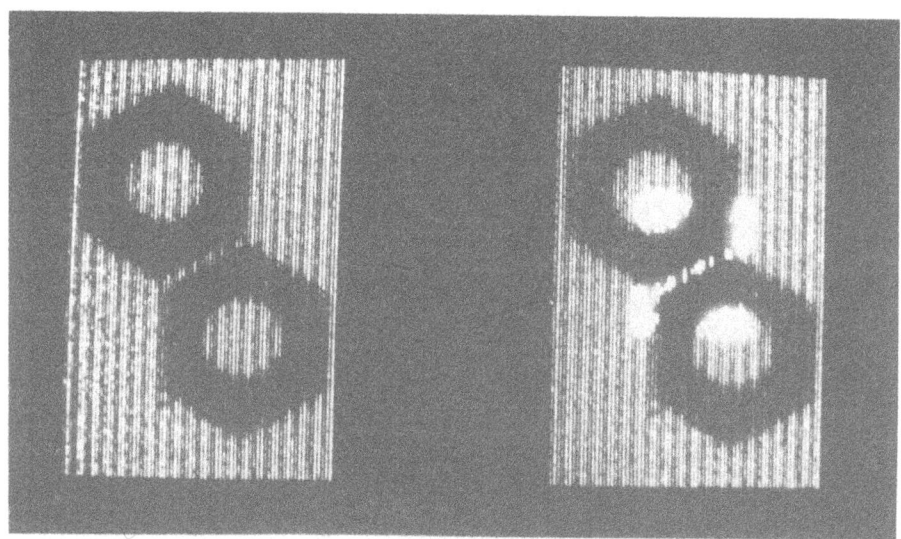

FIG.3 - The reconstructed image of two steel nuts separated by 700 μm obtained at 45 keV energy.

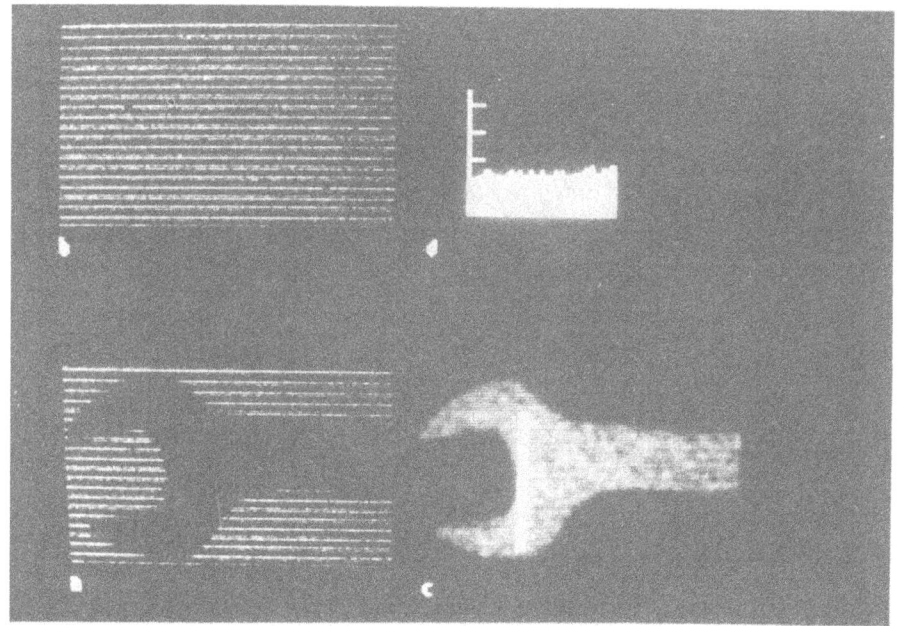

FIG.4 - An example of digital image processing.

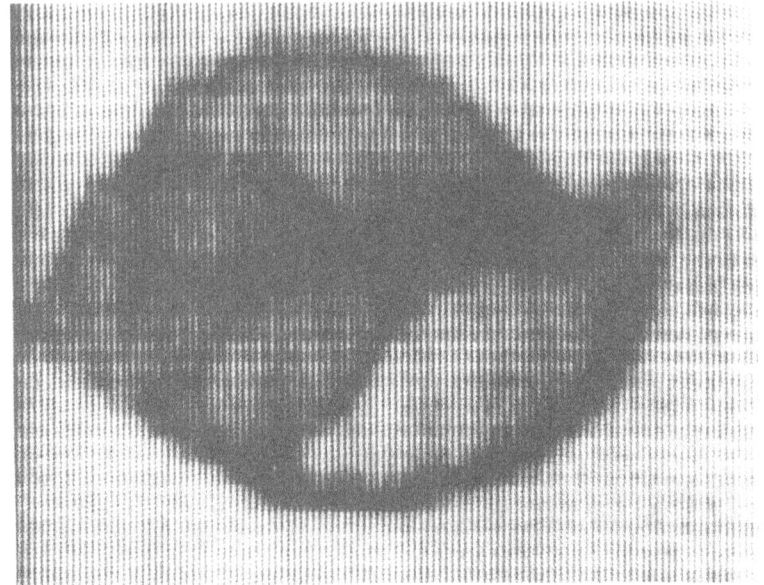

FIG.5 - A MWPC shell radiography.

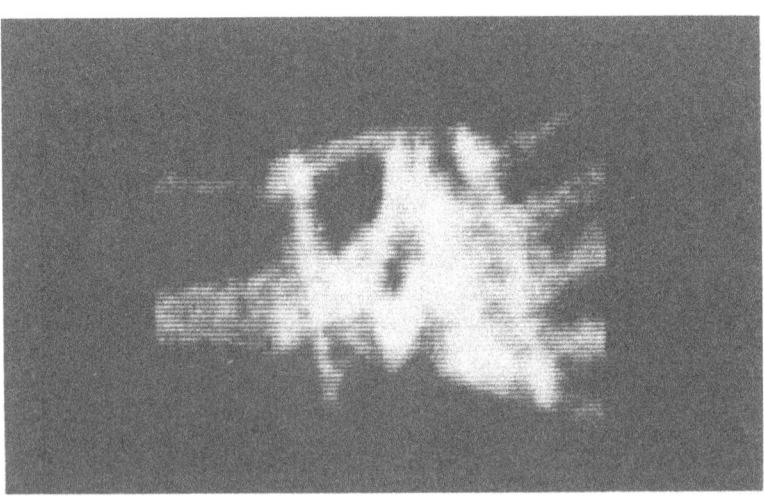

FIG.6 - The two-dimensional bone mass distribution of a wrist of a human skeleton.

PART III X-RAY COMPUTED TOMOGRAPHY

Chairman: Douglas P. Boyd (U.S.A.)

BASIC TECHNOLOGICAL ASPECTS AND OPTIMIZATION PROBLEMS IN X-RAY COMPUTED TOMOGRAPHY (C.T.)

R. ALLEMAND

CEA - CENG LETI/MCTE - 85 X 38041 GRENOBLE CEDEX FRANCE

1 INTRODUCTION

The principles of Computed Tomography (C.T.) have been widely reviewed in published works, no parts of which are reproduced in this paper.

Very important efforts have been made in this field over the last decade, so that several generations of C.T. machines have been successively proposed to the radiologist community.

The main sources of image artefacts have been investigated, and now, it can be assumed that most of the machines are capable of producing good image quality in routine clinical examinations. However, this does not mean that new technical advances could not take place in the near future. Physical limitations have not yet been reached for several characteristics and new improvements can be expected in different fields: more powerful X-ray tubes, new types of high resolution mono and multi-slice detectors, integrated technology for high density data acquisition systems, fast reconstruction processing systems, etc... Nevertheless, competition will take place in the near future between C.T. imaging and N.M.R. imaging and it is clear that new efforts in C.T. technology will be accepted by the manufacturers, provided that X-ray C.T. continues to play its significant role.

The current status and future prospects of physical performance are analysed here and the optimization problems are approached.

2. C.T. ARCHITECTURE EVOLUTION

The original system for the brain, developed by Hounsfield (1973), employs a translate-rotate movement in which the X-ray tube and a single detector scan the patient along a large number of sets of parallel rays. Very good image quality is obtainable with this basic method as long as the object to be imaged is stationary. The scattered radiation rejection rate is excellent, the source-detector combination can be moved in small steps involving a very good linear sampling, and the level of artefacts is lower than with one-motion machines.

The second scanning mode has been introduced to speed up the data collection process without losing the advantages of the first one. It uses an array of detectors and a translate-rotate motion for the source-detector system. For each linear scan, data is collected for many sets of parallel rays (typically 20 to 60). Such scanners have been built with a typical exposure time of several tens of seconds. The image quality is excellent and that type of C.T. remains of great interest for brain imaging. The "fan beam" method involves only one motion and it represents a widespread solution (third generation machines). The array of detectors is large enough to enclose the whole reconstruction area and the X-ray source multidetector combination rotates around the object. For each slice, the data collection process can be achieved in a few seconds. That type of C.T. is well suited for whole-body imaging since organ motion artefacts are considerably reduced. This arrangement requires a very high stability for the detector and data acquisition electronics. Each detector cell images a circular path around the center of rotation and a very small difference in response between adjacent cells can generate circular artefacts. Great efforts have been made by most manufacturers and that difficulty is now overcome. This architecture is the most widespread one because it can now be used for brain as well as for whole body imaging, and it represents a trade off between the performance and the technological complexity.

An alternative solution consists in employing a stationary circular array of detectors and a rotating X-ray source. This is a good approach for reducing motion artefacts. An exposure time of one second can be reached, but this scanning mode requires a larger number of detectors than the fan beam method and it needs very thin detectors since each cell has to detect on a large range of angular directions. Also, the scattered radiation contribution is higher than for the previous method.(1)

One second exposure time is approximately an upper limit for C.T. with mechanical motion. C.T. imaging for fast moving organs, such as the heart, requires new technological and data collection solutions. Several approaches have been investigated, but it is not the purpose of this paper to describe this topic.

3 MAIN CHARACTERISTICS OF C.T. MACHINES

3.1. Physical Characteristics

The density resolution and the spatial resolution are the two major physical characteristics.

3.1.1. The density resolution. The basic limitation to the density accuracy is due to the statistical nature of X-ray photons. Therefore, a comparison between two machines has to be made with the same radiation dose. The physical limitation is reached when all the incident photons, emerging from the object, are detected and when the scattered radiation rejection by the detector is total. Therefore the density resolution test is an indirect measurement of the detection efficiency (including collimation, edge effects,...) and of the capability of the detector to reject the scattered radiation from the object and from the detector itself. With normal testing conditions, the density resolution is currently 0.2 - 0.3 % for a modern C.T. machine.

3.1.2. The spatial resolution. The spatial response is typically of 12 to 15 pairs of lines per centimeter (pl/cm) for high performance machines and 7 to 8 pl/cm for conventional machines. This value does not represent a physical limit. It is a trade-off between technological, electronic and data processing complexity.
The slice thickness is currently of 8 to 10 mm, in order to image a complex organ with a reasonable number of slices. Each voxel is, therefore, a long parallelepiped and that shape generates image artefacts, as it will be discussed later. Furthermore, the detector technology becomes more difficult when the number of cells increases. Also, data collection and data processing requires faster electronics.

3.2. Operating Characteristics

Exposure time per slice represents a major characteristic in minimizing the image artefacts, due to the organ motion.

The data collection does not exceed a few seconds in most machines.

Furthermore, it is essential to be able to collect 10 to 20 successive slices, in order to image an entire organ. This means that the image reconstruction time must be reduced to a few seconds and that the heat load of the X-ray tube must be large enough to accept such a cadence. X-ray tubes with large rotating anodes using the thermal properties of the bulk material have been specially designed for C.T.

3.3. Radiation Dose Utilization

It is essential to minimize the dose to the patient for a given quality of image. This means that the number of incident photons which do not participate in the data collection must be as low as possible.

The X-ray beam has to be carefully filtered to minimize the low energy photon contribution from the X-ray spectrum. These photons increase the patient's dose but they do not yield a useful signal because they are absorbed inside the patient.

The shape and the size of the focal spot of the X-ray tube are also very important factors. A large focal spot is required to maximize the radiation output, but the radiation dose utilization coefficient is reduced because of the fan beam collimation. This effect is particularly important for thin slice imaging, and also because the spatial resolution in the transverse plane decreases.

The stopping power of the multidetector is of course an essential factor for radiation dose utilization. Each cell of the detector has to be collimated in order to minimize the scattered radiation contribution from the organ. So the number of useful photons is reduced by this collimator, and the overall efficiency, which is the product of the quantum efficiency and the geometric photon efficiency, does not exceed 60 % in practice.

The radiation dose is maximum at the level of the skin. It is currently of 2-3 Rads for a conventional machine.

Many possible improvements in X-ray C.T. are restricted by the radiation dose. For instance, to decrease the pixel width (spatial resolution) by a factor of 2 with the same signal to noise ratio (in terms of statistical noise), the dose has to be increased by a factor of 8. Also, to improve the density resolution by a factor of 2, the dose has to be increased by a factor of 4.(2)

3.4. Parameters to Be Considered for C.T. Imaging

Besides the above-mentioned physical and operating characteristics, different parameters have to be taken into account in evaluating C.T. image quality. (3)

3.4.1. "Beam hardening" effects. Because the photon attenuation is lower when the energy is increasing, the energy distribution spectrum of the X-ray beam changes as it passes through the object. It is the phenomenon of "beam hardening". A calibration procedure, using several attenuation phantoms, is necessary in order to determine the detector response to a polychromatic X-ray beam for different attenuation thicknesses.

3.4.2. Scattered radiation contribution. For large objects (40 cm), the scattered radiation contribution can reach the same order of magnitude as the useful signal itself. It is a low spatial frequency spurious signal, which degrades the signal to noise ratio and the image contrast. In order to reject it, it is essential to put a fan beam collimator just in front of the multi-detector. Its geometrical accuracy, its positioning and its stability in rotating motion require very stringent demands. To illustrate this statement, it is useful to recall that each measurement has to be made with an accuracy, of 2-3% in the whole dynamic range, which can reach about 500 for large objects. Therefore, a very small geometrical distortion can generate strong circular artefacts since each cell images a circular path around the centre of rotation.

3.4.3. "Partial volume" effects. 10 mm thick slices are currently used to scan a complete organ which requires 10 to 20 successive slices. These values correspond with a reasonable exposure time for the patient (problems of motion artefacts) and they are compatible with the heat load of the present X-ray tubes. The size of each voxel is about 1 x 1 x 10 mm . As the anatomical structures present complicated shapes with strong gradients (bones and soft tissue), it means that the measured attenuation is not the true one. This phenomenon is called " partial volume " effect; it can be emphasized by the focal spot size of the X-ray tube. One way of reducing this effect is to choose smaller slice thicknesses, currently employed to image complex structures with strong attenuation gradients, particularly in brain imaging.

3.4.4. Technological parameters. Mechanical stability is of major importance. C.T. imaging requires very accurate measurements ($\sim$ 2-3 %) on a large dynamic range ($\sim$ 500). This data has to be collected from a heavy X-ray source-detector combination rotating around the patient, assuming that certain, very difficult problems have first been overcome.

X-ray tube: the thermal performance requires a large rotating anode with a heavy bulk material and the measurement accuracy needs a very stable focal spot. These two conditions are very difficult to obtain and special tubes for C.T. have been designed. Rotating anode wobble and filament vibrations, in particular, generate severe artefacts on the reconstructed image. The HV supply must also be very stable ($\sim 10^{-4}$).

Detector: the detector is the main factor of C.T. design and performance. It operates in current mode because the photon flux is too high to work with pulse methods. (The direct flux is about 10^{10} events/cell). Its design must take into account several major factors:
- high stopping power
- good linearity on a large dynamic range ($\sim$ 500)
- good packing fraction
- negligible cross-talk between adjacent cells.
- high stability of response

Two types of detectors have been designed for C.T.. (1)

Linear array of solid state detectors: each cell is made up of a scintillator, optically coupled to a low leakage current photodiode, working in photovoltaic mode. This arrangement shows a good packing fraction and a high stopping power. It is essential to choose a scintillator, which does not yield a long period light emission component, in order to avoid pile-up effects between successive measurements. Bismuth-Germanate (BGO) and Caesium-Iodide (CsI) have been employed but now Cadmium Tungstate ($CdWO^4$) is preferred because it combines three major advantages: the light emission is well suited to the photodiode sensitivity, it is not hygroscopic and it has no long period light component. This solution is well adapted to the fourth generation machines (a complete ring of stationary detectors) because thin and efficient detectors can detect on a large range of angular directions. Is has also been employed for the third generation machines (fan beam method).

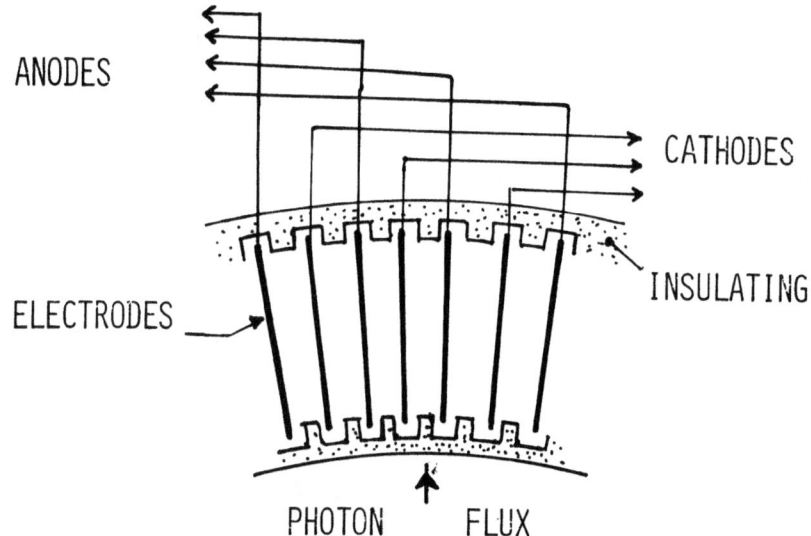

Figure 1 : Principle of an ionization multidetector

- Ionization multichamber : the figure 1 shows a typical arrangement of such a detector. The electrodes are focused on the X-ray focal spot and they have a triple function :
  . collimation for the scattered radiation from the object
  . collimation for the scattered radiation and fluorescent X-rays produced inside the detector itself
  . collection of the charges created by ionization in the gas

Xenon is the best choice for this application because of its high stopping power. No purification system is required since the chamber operates in ion collection mode. The time response is compatible with the time sequence of the data. For instance, for a 1 mm interelectrodes space, a 30 atmospheres pressure and a 1 KV HV supply, the collection time is about 1,5 ms.

This solution exhibits major physical advantages :
- a good linearity of response on a large dynamic range
- a very good stability
- no pile-up effects
- a good quantum efficiency

Nevertheless, extreme mechanical and electrical care is required for the insulating, the positioning and the mechanical holding of the electrodes. Small deviations from the ideal mechanical and electrical conditions generate severe artefacts.

Now, most of these technological difficulties have been overcome, and this solution has been chosen for a large number of fan beam machines.

Whatever the detector may be, the usual value is about 0.5 mm aperture, and a one thousand cell linear array has currently been manufactured.

3.4.5. Other parameters

Several other parameters have to be considered for a C.T. design such as :

- The measurements calibration method
- The X-ray beam monitoring
- The linear and rotating sampling problems
- The X-ray energy optimization as a function of the organ to be imaged

Their discussion is beyond the scope of this paper.

4 CURRENT STATUS AND FUTURE PROSPECTIVES OF C.T. PHYSICAL PERFORMANCE

The current physical and operating characteristics of the commercially available high level C.T. are :

- spatial resolution : 12 to 15 pairs of lines per centimeter
- minimum exposure time : 1 to 2 seconds
- slice thickness : adjusting from 1 to 10 mm
- number of sequential slices : 15 to 30

4.1. Density Resolution

The density resolution is difficult to characterize since it depends on many factors : the radiation dose, the X-ray energy, the slice thickness, ... A typical value of 2 to 3 $^o/_{oo}$ is currently obtained on brain imaging.

This characteristic exhibits a physical limit which is given by the number of photons needed to obtain a given density resolution due to the statistical nature of X-ray photons. The present performance is close to this physical limit. For the photons emerging from the object, the overall detection efficiency presently reaches 60 %. For the incident photons entering the object, some advances can be expected in using smaller focal spot tubes, but that approach is very difficult to obtain because of the anode heat-load limitations.

An alternative solution for improving the density resolution consists in using contrast material and this method is widely employed in clinical routine.

Another promising approach to reaching the absolute density measurement has been investigated by different groups, using a dual energy X-ray beam. For soft tissue, the C.T. number is proportional to electron density since compton interactions represent a very large amount of the total interactions. Due to photoelectric interactions, it is not the case for bone material. A dual energy data collection allows these two contributions to be separated and the absolute density measurement can be reached both for soft tissue and for bone materials.

4.2. Spatial Resolution

The spatial resolution in the transverse plane is presently limited by technological problems, but there is no fundamental reason which prevents future improvements.(4)

The expected advantages of a better spatial resolution are very important :
- An improvement for small size and high contrast structure imaging (internal ear structures for instance)
- A reduction of spark artefacts close to the high gradient structures, and consequently a better density resolution in these regions
- A lower expansion of the quantum noise due to the reconstruction process

The ideal detector should be in the millimeter range, typically 0.3 to 0.4 mm cell width, and the dead space should not exceed 20% of the useful area. Such a detector would require new techniques for high density data collection to be simultaneously developed in order to reduce the complexity and the cost.

A first step can be expected with the conventional technologies to achieving 20 pairs of lines per centimeter.

The spatial resolution along the longitudinal axis also needs to be improved. Major advances can be expected:

- A better image quality for small structures with a high contrast
- A more accurate density resolution by reducing the partial volume effect
- A better image contrast for organ edge regions

Beam thickness of 1 to 1.5 mm can be used with the present machine but the useful photon fraction is then significantly reduced, and consequently, the exposure time increases in the same proportion with the drawbacks already mentioned.

The development of multi-line detectors will be a major advance in C.T. (4). So several slices (approximately 10) will be stored simultaneously with the same exposure time as for a present large thickness slice, and this method will provide a much better photon flux utilization. It is a very promising way of reaching a true three-dimensional imaging.

This three-dimensional approach assumes that efforts can be made in several fields:
- More powerful X-ray tubes since photon statistics will be the physical limitation of the image quality for each slice
- The development of multilinear array detectors providing a good packing fraction (in order to minimize the dose to the patient) and a good rejection of scattered radiation. A stack of 10 to 12 linear arrays of one thousand cells each with 0.4 to 0.5 mm aperture seems to be a good trade-off between the performances and the cost and complexity.
- The development of high density, fast and low cost data collection electronics. Integrated technology seems to be a very promising way
- The development of fast digital process systems in order to reduce the reconstruction time since the image matrix size and the number of slices will be larger.

5 CONCLUSION

A competition is arising between C.T. and NMR in the field of medical diagnostic imaging, and it is clear that the interest of the medical community is presently focused on NMR imaging.

Nevertheless, it appears reasonable to assume that the clinical interest of C.T. for different pathologies will continue. As long as this statement is confirmed, new technical advances can be expected in the near future in order to improve the main characteristics which are : the density resolution, the spatial resolution and the X-ray exposure time.

Since this paper only concerns the technological aspects, the major advances can be expected in the field of photon flux production and detection.

C.T. requires very stringent demands on X-ray tubes. Special tubes have already been developed for that application but further improvements are needed for high spatial resolution multislice machines.

Multi-linear array detectors seem to be the major technological advance to be accomplished in the near future in order to significantly improve the image quality and to reach true three-dimensional imaging.

REFERENCES

(1) R. Allemand : Les méthodes de détection en tomographie par rayons X. p. 72-96; colloque sur les techniques tomographiques par rayons X et par émetteurs gamma et positons. Grenoble - Juin 1978
(2) B.M. Moores, R.P. Parker, B.R. Pullan. Physical aspects of medical imaging 1981. John Wiley-Sons Lt.
(3) G.T. Herman. Image reconstruction from projections. p. 40-54. 1980 - Academic Press
(4) E. Tournier, R. Allemand. Perspectives de l'imagerie par scanner X.
5e Congrès Européen de Radiologie - Bordeaux Septembre 83.

CLINICAL APPLICATION OF X-RAY CT: RESULTS, LIMITATIONS AND FUTURE
NEEDS

L. Di Guglielmo, A. Villa, L. Biazzi

Institute of Radiology, University of Pavia, Pavia, Italy

   Computer tomography (CT) has produced such enormous progress in the clinical field that its realization has been compared to X-ray discovery. It is impossible to summarize here all the clinical applications of CT. But we can state, from a very schematic viewpoint, that up to now the clinical evolution of CT has followed three main, different ways: Morphology, Densitometry, Dynamics.

1. Morphology. This is the field in which the most important realizations have been reached. A wide variety of structures and organs have been examined, even those which are very small and difficult to investigate. Some examples: the pancreas has always raised the greatest difficulties to traditional roentgenologic investigations, and in the majority of cases only indirect information could be obtained. CT, however provides a direct, simple and complete visualization of the pancreas in all its sections (fig. 1), and when dilated, even the pancreatic duct can be visible. A correct evaluation of the suprarenal glands has always been very difficult to obtain by means of the traditional X-ray investigations and invasive and complex techniques such as retropneumoperitoneum or superselective angiography had therefore to be employed. CT now clearly shows shape, size and volume of both suprarenal glands. Further patent examples of organs or regions previously difficult or impossible to investigate

and now easily demonstrated by means of CT are: the spinal canal and its content, the orbit (fig. 2), the intervertebral disk (fig. 3) the pericardium, the soft tissues of the limbs and so on. Such an accurate morphological study has made possible the definition of a normal CT anatomy. As a consequence, the knowledge of normal patterns has made it possible to point out pathological findings and thus to build up a true pathological CT semeiotics (fig. 4).

2. **Densitometry.** In this field progress has not been proportional to that of morphology. However densitometric evaluation acquires a decisive value in a great number of situations. A typical example is that of paracardiac opacities, the nature of which cannot be defined by traditional X-ray methods. However, CT densitometry provides a correct differentiation of fluid collections (cysts or pericardial diverticula) from paracardiac fatty collections (lipomas) or from solid masses such as pericardial or lung tumors. In the same way densitometry is of basic importance in differential diagnosis of pericardiac effusion (fig. 5) and fibrous adhesions (fig. 6). The pericardiac fluid itself may exibit different values, thus rendering possible the differentiation of exudative effusion from hemopericardium and kilopericardium. Furthermore, densitometric evaluation of pericardiac fluid may be the only way to detect solid formations that would otherwise go unrecognized such as primary or metastatic pericardiac tumors (fig. 7). Another example of the great capacity of densitometry is provided by the different findings of hyperdensity in liver cirrhosis and very low density in liver steatosis. The use of iodinated contrast media produces changes in densitometric values and this can be decisive for diagnosis. Sometimes, even severe pathological conditions may exhibit the same density as the surrounding tissues. After contrast medium injection, since vascularization is different, there is also a different enhancement, and thus a different densitometric coefficient that allows the lesion to be detected. Moreover the enhancement modalities can be different in various pathological conditions. A typical example is the peripheral enhancement of abscesses.

3. **Dynamics.** In dynamics, CT implies the use of iodinated contrast media and the fast recording of tomograms. Many interesting investigations have been carried out concerning the enhancement-

curves of various organs, both in normal and pathological conditions. A good example of the clinical application of these investigations is the demonstration and evaluation of hepatic metastases. In fact metastases enhancement is quite variable. This variability is obviously related to vascularization and we know from angiography that the degree of vascularization of liver metastases is quite variable. This accounts for such CT behaviour. There are some cases where the metastases, very poorly or not at all visible under basal conditions, become more and more evident after rapid contrast injection: these are non vascularized metastases. In other patients metastases become even more dense than the liver: these are hypervascularized metastases. Finally, in poorly vascularized metastases the enhancement of the liver and of the metastases is not simultaneous: in the early phases the liver becomes more dense and the metastases are better visible; subsequently the metastases also become opaque and isodense with the liver and therefore they can no longer be seen. But the most important applications of dynamic CT concern the study of the heart and vessels.

CT without contrast medium clearly demonstrates the cardiac shape, the calcifications (valvular, coronaric, myocardial, thrombotic, pericardial) and the pericardium. The pericardium is always clearly visible because of the presence of epicardial fat inside and pericardiac fat outside. However the visualization of the cardiac cavities requires the administration of contrast medium (100-200 ml) and two essential techniques are availble: a) Angio-CT or "sequential dynamic CT" (fig. 8): the fast administration of the contrast bolus and rapid sequence scanning.

Seven tomograms can be made in 1 minute; the information of each tomogram can be split into 3 consecutive images and 21 images can therefore be obtained in 1 minute. This technique provides a good demonstration of the progression of contrast medium through the heart and great vessels and of the morphology of single cavities and vessels (fig. 9). Moreover, rapid displacements of the bed allow a complete examination of the heart at different levels. b) Cardio-CT or ECG gated CT (fig.10). The scan information is synchronized with the ECG. The interval between two R-waves is conventionally divided into 100 points. It is possible in this way to obtain information concerning single points corresponding to various stages of the cardiac cycle. In our routine, we usually take into consideration four stages: diastole, end-diastole, systole and end-systole. Images are sharp and well defined. Myocardial wall, septa, single heart cavities and their changes from diastole to systole are clearly visible. Moreover, this technique provides the possibility of measuring the changes in thickness of the ventricular wall and the septum from diastole to systole (fig. 11), and evaluating diameters, areas (fig. 12) and volumes of the ventricles. A pre-shaped software programme allows various hemodynamic parameters such as the ejection fraction and the segmentary ventricular dynamics to be obtained.

Finally, it is possible to evaluate the rotation of the heart on its longitudinal axis: in normal conditions the septum forms an angle of about 40° with the median sagittal line. Right ventricular hypertrophy produces a left-rotation of the heart with widening of the angle. Left ventricular hypertrophy produces, to the contrary, a right rotation and reduction of the angle. The clinical indications of cardiac CT are very numerous and in our experience they prove to be more and more important. We are only able to recall a few examples here. In acquired valvular diseases CT is the best technique for the demonstration and evaluation of intra-atrial thrombi, especially if localized in the auricular appendage. Moreover CT allows a good demonstration of pressure or ventricular volume overloading. In primitive cardiomyopathies it is possible to differentiate the various types: dilatative (fig. 13), restrictive, hypertrophic obstructive and non obstructive (fig. 14). CT can be decisive in the differential diagnoses of other secondary cardiomyopathies (ischemic heart diseases) and of constrictive pericarditis. In ischemic heart diseases a good demonstration is obtained of: diffuse or regional changes of ventricular and septal dynamics, myocardial thinning and calcification, aneurysms, even the smallest ones and those localized on the inferior ventricular aspect, intracavitary thrombi, pseudo-aneurysms.

Cardiac tumors are precisely demonstrated with a good evaluation of their size, localization and extension. Both primitive and metastatic lesions can be described, as well as benign and malignant types. CT is essential in differential diagnosis of pericardiac and mediastinal tumors.

Hydatic cysts are well diagnosed and their intramyocardial, intracavitary, pericardial localizations are found. All pericardial diseases are potentially indications for CT investigation: congenital anomalies, such as pericardial absence, effusions, fibrous adhesions, traumatic lesions with pericardial rupture and pneumopericardium, primitive and metastatic tumors.

Post-operative controls, essentially concerning: a) aorto-coronary by-pass; although results are inferior to those of traditional selective angiography, CT is considered the best non-invasive method now available in evaluating the by-pass patency; b) aneurismectomy and septal reconstruction; c) complications, such as aortic dissection, localized pericardial effusion, abscesses, fistulas.

The limits of the CT method are quite few and consist essentially of the use of X-rays and iodinated contrast media. On the other hand, the potential evolution of CT may still lead to important developments and these will not so much concern morphology but rather densitometry and dynamics. Investigations are already in progress on a <u>more precise definition of tissues</u>. Physical techniques have been developed with the aim of evaluating atomic number and electron density of tissues by means of a double energy method (1,2) or by means of a simple energy method, provided that the chemical composition of the structure is approximately known. In the field of dymanics the aim is to obtain real-time images of moving organs and thus their cinematography registration. This goal has also been partially obtained already. A cine-CT scanner system has been realized (3) in which a focused electron beam and a stationary detection array are employed. The extremely short scan time (33 msec) allows blood flow and wall motion study. In addition, to image the heart in motion, a three-dimensional high speed scanner was constructed (4). Multiple contiguous simultaneous transverse sections are obtained by means of multiple X-ray sources. Although three-dimensional studies still have an investigational research role, they demonstrate significant promise for practical clinical application.

In the future, efforts to improve CT technology will have to take into account the important new advent of magnetic resonance. Nevertheless our opinion is that, although magnetic resonance will certainly improve our knowledge and increase our ability to investigate the human body, the basic morphological semeiotics, both in normal and pathological conditions, will remain, as we have described, by means of CT.

REFERENCES

1. Brooks R.A. A quantitative theory of the Hounsfield unit and its application to dual energy scanning. J. Comput. Ass.Tomogr. 4, 1977, 487-493.
2. Brooks R.A., Mitchell L.G. and Di Chiro G. On the relationship between computed tomography numbers and specific gravity. Phys.Med.Biol., 26, 1981, 141-147.
3. Boyd D. Computerized transmission tomography of the heart using scanning electron beams. CT of the heart and the great vessels. Futura Publ. Comp. New York, 1983, 45-55
4. Sinak L.J. and Ritman E.L. Dynamic spatial reconstructor. CT of the heart and the great vessels. Futura Publ.Comp. New York, 1983, 61-73 .

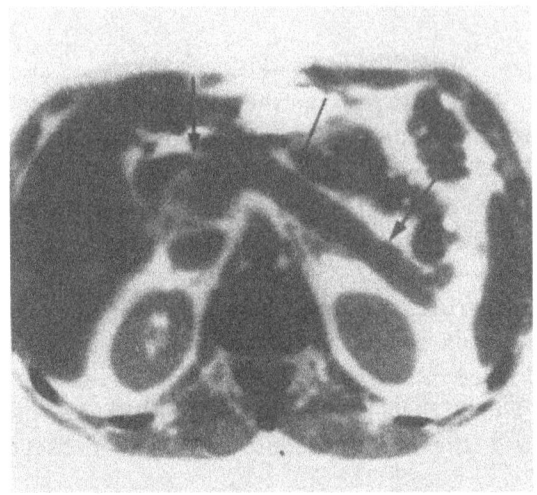

Fig. 1 Complete visibility of the pancreas (arrows)

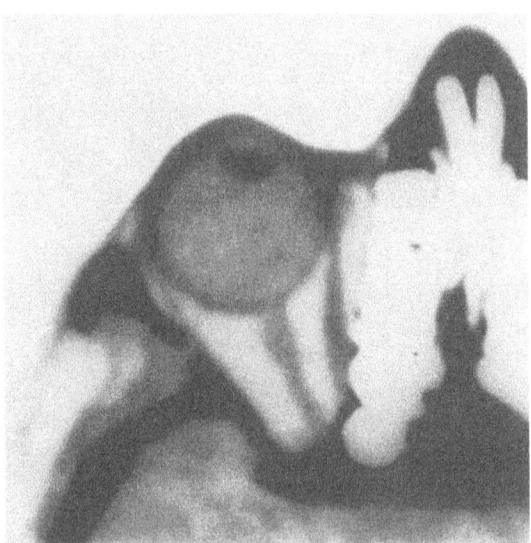

Fig. 2 The orbit under normal conditions. The ocular bulb with its crystalline lens, the optic nerve and muscles are visible.

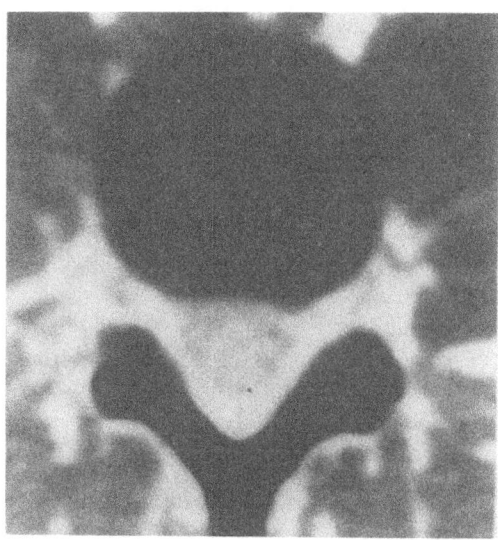

Fig. 3 Tomogram of the vertebral spine at the level of the intravertebral disk.

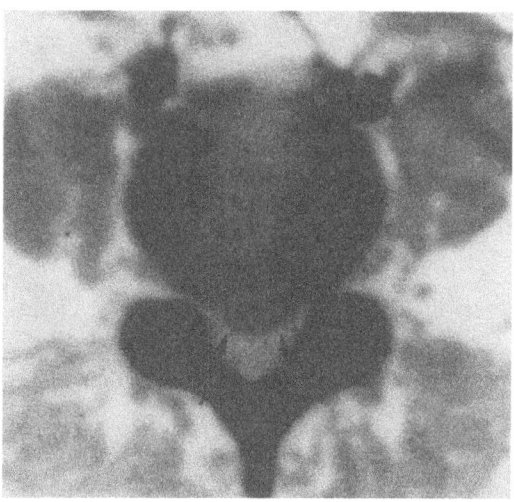

Fig. 4 Herniated intravertebral disk (arrows)

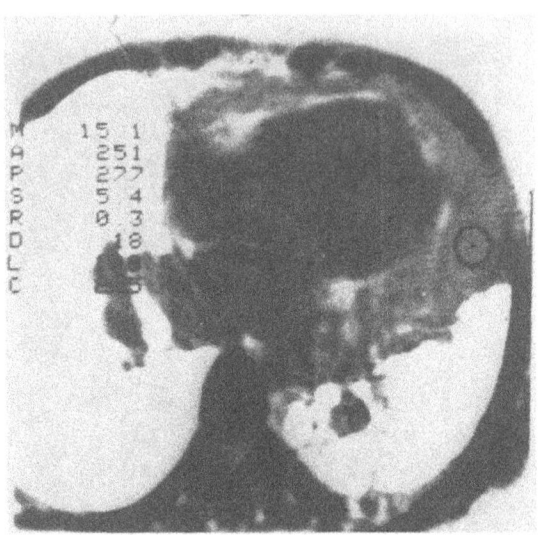

Fig. 5 Severe pericardial effusion. Densitometric value (O) of liquid.

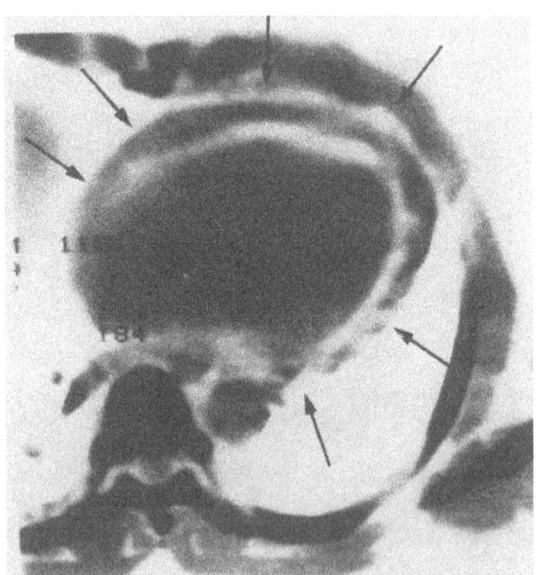

Fig. 6 Diffuse pericardial thickening (arrows) as a pericarditis sequela. Densitometric value of fibrous tissue.

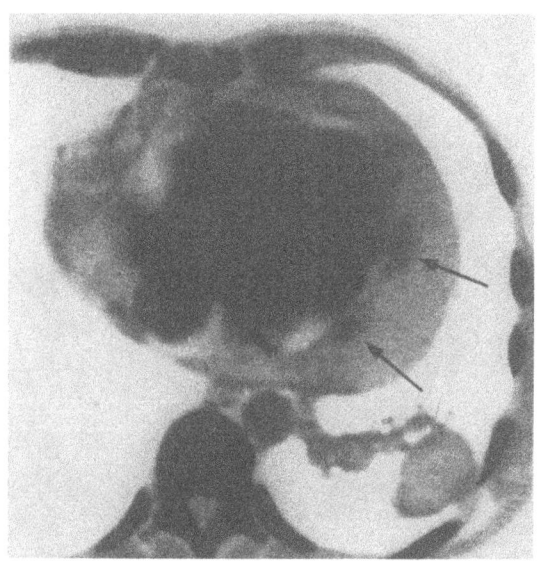

Fig. 7 Pericardial effusion in a patient with bronchial carcinoma. Multiple nodular metastases (arrows) are directly visible on the visceral pericardium.

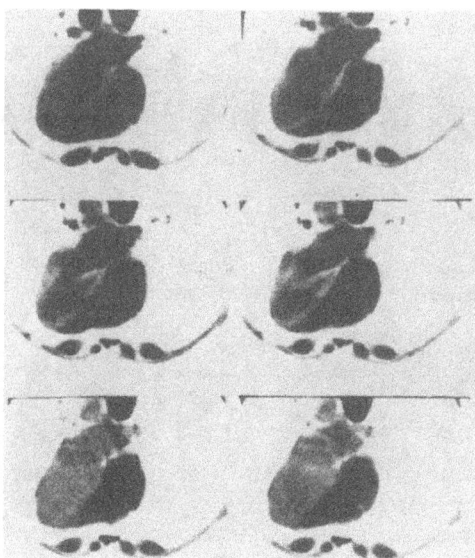

Fig. 8 Angio-CT of the heart. Sequential progression of the contrast bolus through the heart cavities.

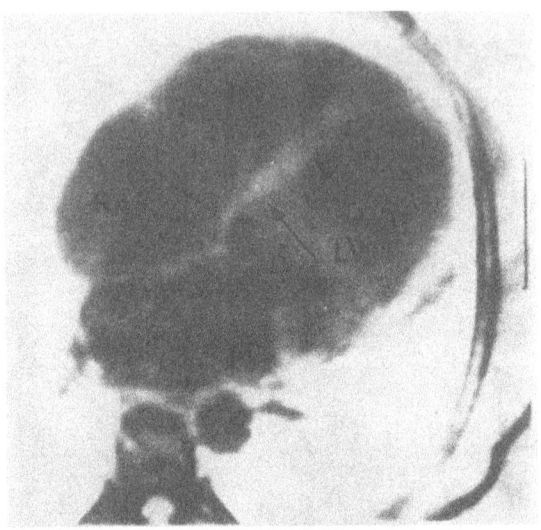

Fig. 9 Normal morphology of the heart cavities. RA = right atrium, RV = right ventricle; LA = left atrium; LV = left ventricle. Good visibility of intraventricular (arrows) and interarterial (arrow heads) septa.

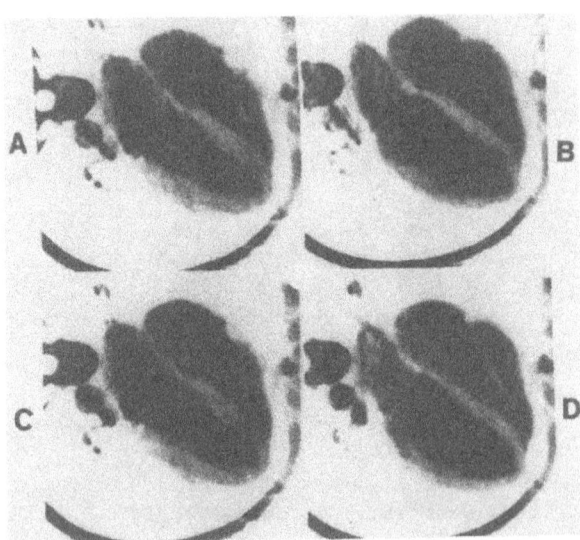

Fig. 10 Cardio-CT. A, B = diastole, end-diastole; C, D = systole end-systole.

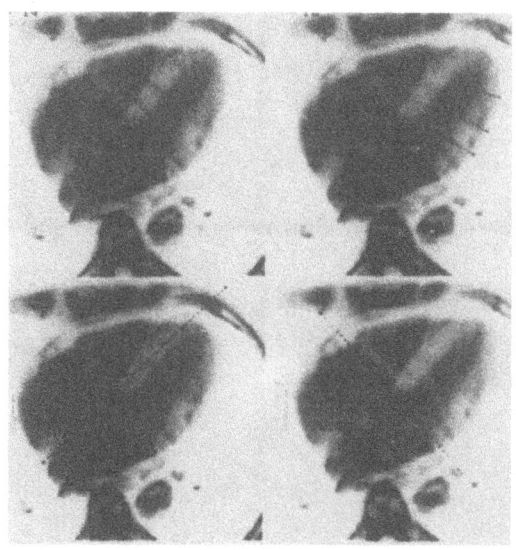

Fig. 11 Evaluation of septal and myocardial wall thickness and of short and long left ventricular axes.

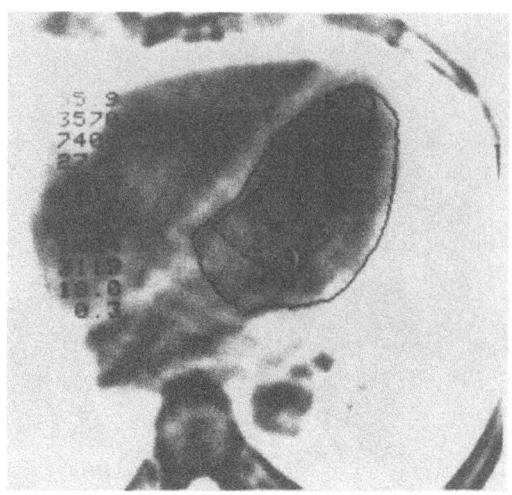

Fig. 12 Evaluation of left ventricular areas in diastole and systole.

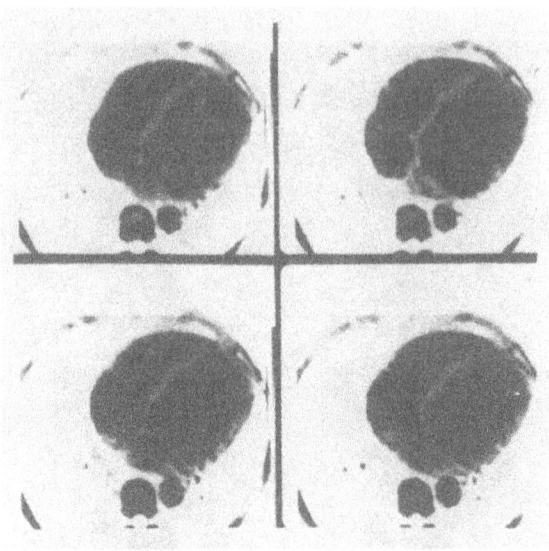

Fig. 13 Primitive dilatative cardiomyopathy. Changes of wall thickness and of ventricular volumes from diastole to systole are insignificant.

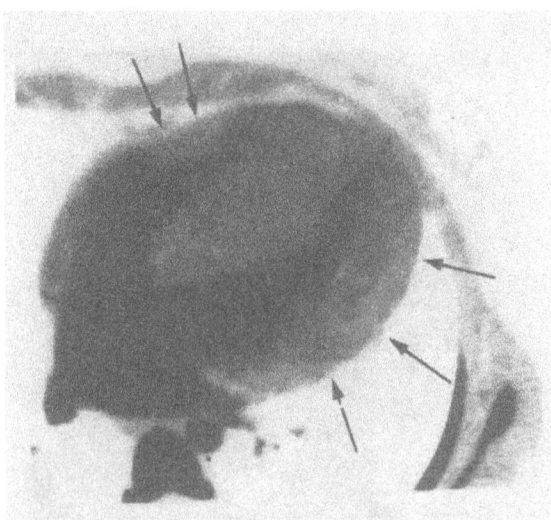

Fig. 14 Primitive hypertrophic non-obstructive cardiomyopathy.- The myocardial wall of both ventricles (arrows) and the intraventricular septum (arrow heads) are enormously enlarged.

CINE CT: A NEW TECHNOLOGY FOR CARDIAC COMPUTED TOMOGRAPHY

D.P. Boyd[1,2], K.R. Peschmann[1,2], R.E. Rand[1,2], J.L. Couch[2],
S.A. Napel[1,2], R. Gould[1], D.W. Farmer[1], M.J. Lipton[1], and
C.B. Higgins[1]
Department of Radiology, University of California, San Francisco[1]
and Imatron Inc, South San Francisco, CA[2]

Introduction

Despite its major impact on diagnosis in other organ systems [1,2], CT has yet to play a distinct diagnostic role in the clinical evaluation of the heart due to the rapid cardiac motion which degrades image resolution. Despite limitations, however, conventional whole-body CT scanners have a number of useful cardiac applications [3-10]. ECG-gated reconstructions on whole-body scanners have increased the temporal resolution of such systems, but they are still limited by their single slice configuration which does not permit an integrated picture of the heart during the same phases of the cardiac cycle [11-14]. Nonetheless, feasibility studies in cardiac patients using modified conventional body scanners showed considerable promise and prompted research into the development of a dedicated cardiac device.

The technical requirements for adequate evaluation of cardiac anatomy and physiology, namely scan speeds in the 33-100 msec range, simultaneous multi-slice capability, 15-20 multi-level scans/second and a repeat multi-slice study at one per second, have been realized with the inception of the Cine-CT scanner (C-100 Imatron Inc.). This scanner acquires scan data in 50 milliseconds by eliminating moving parts and using a scanning electron beam to produce a high speed x-ray source. [15] In this device the x-ray source consists of a single bend scanning electron beam that is magnetically focused and deflected onto a semi-circular tungsten target ring, (figs 1,2). X-rays are detected in a stationary double array of 864 scintillation-photodiode crystals. The detectors are arranged in two side-by-side rings enabling dual-slice scans simultaneously. Using successive scans on four tungsten target rings up to eight slices can be scanned in a little over 200 milliseconds. Using a single target ring cine scanning at speeds of up to 17 dual-slice scans per second are available.

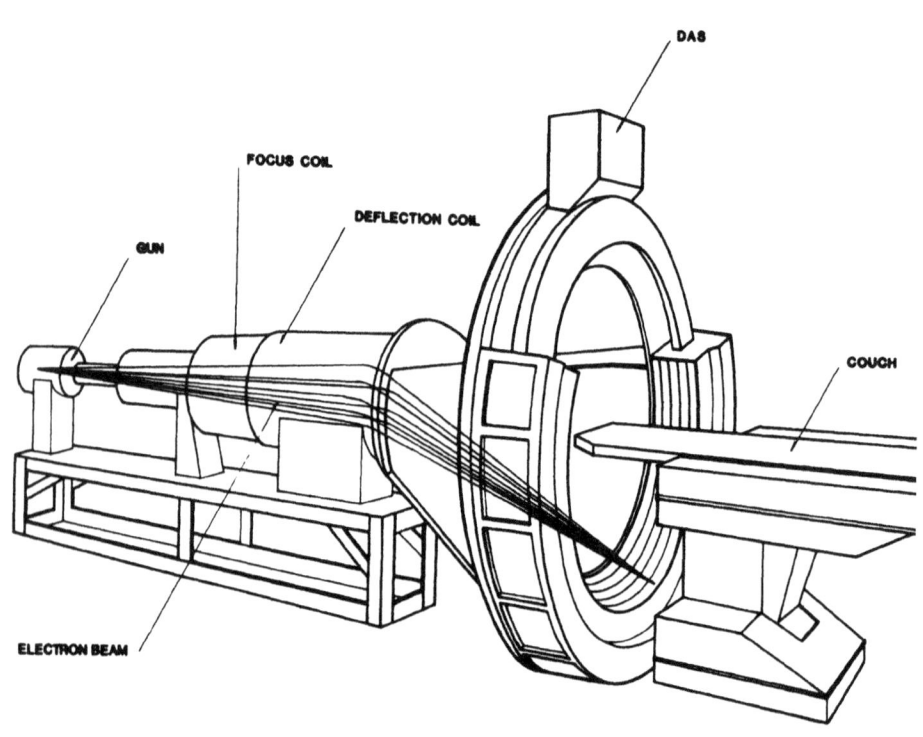

Figure 1: Schematic illustration of Imatron C-100 scanner. The 800 mA electron beam, accelerated at 130 kV, is focused and deflected at an angle of 33-37°, then swept 210° along one of the four fixed tungsten target rings, as pictured. The fan beam of radiation produced then passes through the patient, impinging on the two rows of stationary detectors above the patient. Detector output is then accumulated in the DAS (data acquisition system).

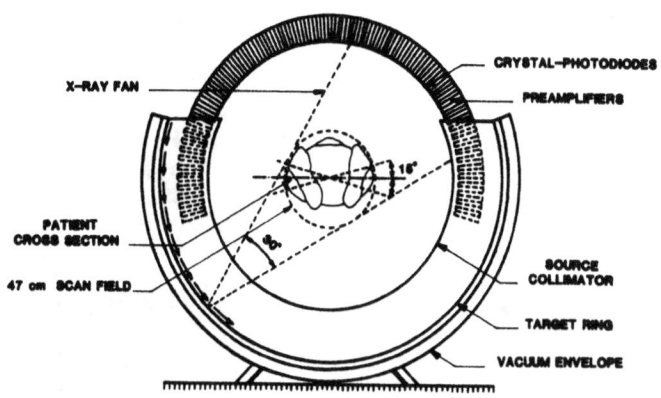

Figure 2: End-view of the cine scanner illustrating the moving x-ray fans and stationary detector array. Approximately 15% of overscan data is obtained in a full 210° scan.

The research that led to the development of Cine-CT began in 1976 at UCSF as a University-based project to study the feasibility of achieving fast scanning speeds for cardiovascular applications. After evaluating several alternative approaches to ultra-fast CT, the scanning electron beam approach was selected as offering the most promise. At that time, high-power electron beams operating in the space-charge-limited region were not well understood and a great deal of development both theoretical and practical was needed. By 1981, the first prototype electron beam was produced in a test bed device. In 1982, the Cardiovascular CT (CVCT) scanner prototype was demonstrated. The commercial version now referred to as Cine-CT, was completed by Imatron in 1984 and is now installed in four research hospitals for clinical evaluation, (fig 3).

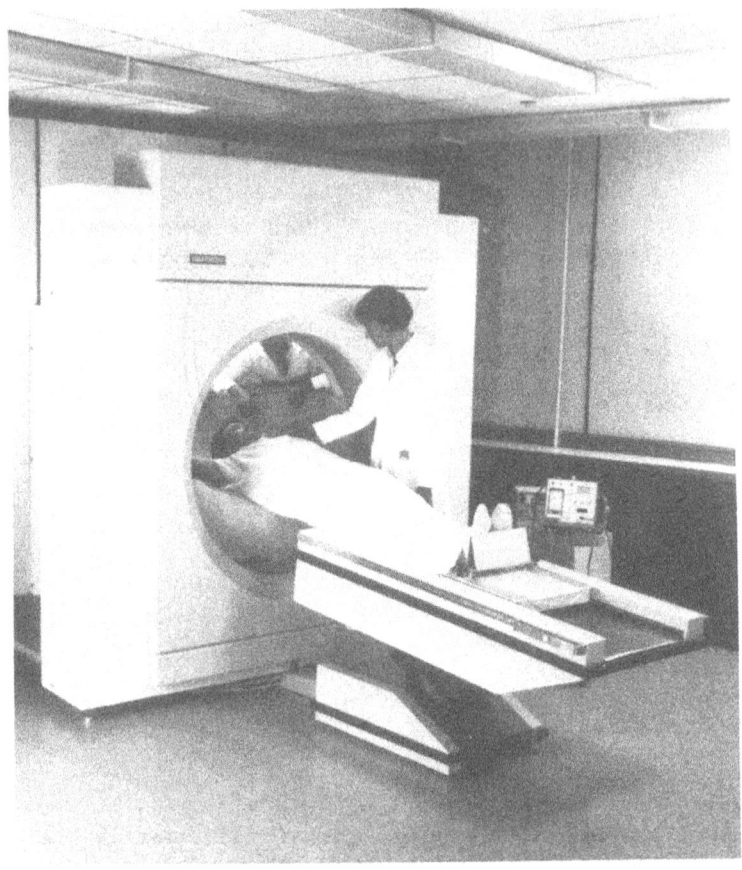

Figure 3: C-100 Cine-CT scanner installation at UCSF. Overall system dimensions are comparable to conventional CT scanners. The couch can be tilted vertically and slewed in the horizontal plane for scanning oblique slices. This capability is facilitated by the large gantry aperture.

Three scanning modes are possible with the Cine-CT system. In the continuous or cine mode, the scanning sequence can be performed without interruption for one or more heartbeats in order to image the heart and evaluate cardiac motion. The flow or triggered mode repeats the millisecond exposures at a slower rate, with the interscan delay determined by the patient's electrocardiogram. A full resolution mode provides an enhanced look at cardiac anatomy and extends the utility of the scanner in more traditional CT applications.

Continuous or Cine Mode

Following a peripheral venous injection of a high iodine concentration contrast media, two contiguous 8 mm slices are obtained simultaneously with each 50 msec exposure, at the rate of 17 exposures per second. The acquired images demonstrate various phases of systole and diastole during the same heart cycle (fig 7). Segmental wall motion and cavity dynamics can be assessed from the cinematic display of individual scans on the video monitor. When compared with cineangiographically demonstrated wall motion abnormalities, the cine tomographic method of analysis had an accuracy of 87% in 20 patients with previous myocardial infarctions [17].

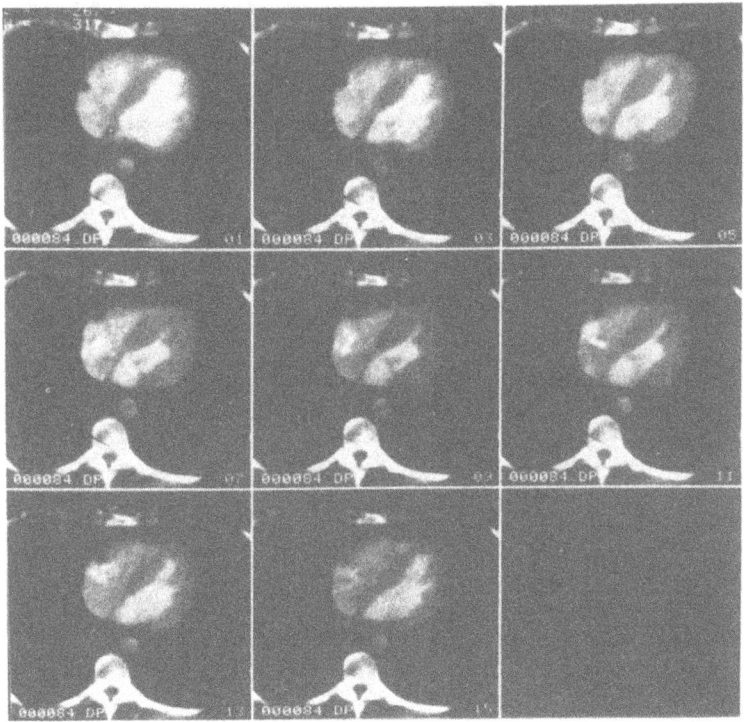

Figure 4: Eight sequential images from a cine-mode study in a patient with hypertrophic cardiomyopathy. The upper left image represents end-diastole with the sequence progressing through systole and back to diastole of the next heart beat.

Due to the Cine-CT system's hundred-fold increase in temporal resolution compared to third or fourth generation whole-body scanners, and spatial resolution of 1.5 mm, the endocardial and epicardial walls are well demarcated, permitting an accurate measurement of myocardial wall thickening during systole. Furthermore, boundary detection can be enhanced with the aid of the half contour edge analysis method described recently [18]. Briefly, half contour CT numbers are derived between the myocardium and chamber and the myocardium and the lung. The computer identifies these numbers and defines the endocardial and epicardial boundaries.

By comparing the change between end-diastolic and end-systolic stress at the levels examined, a fractional ejection fraction can be calculated. Utilizing a brisk peripheral intravenous infusion combined with cine acquisition at all eight levels (all four target rings scanned sequentially), it is possible to accurately calculate the ventricular ejection fraction. At the current scanning speed of 50 msec., it is possible to scan the entire left ventricular volume at a rate of 4.5 eight-slice volume images per second.

The ability to accurately quantify dynamic myocardial thickness is of paramount importance, as the correlation between wall-thickening abnormalities and myocardial ischemia is well documented, and has been further demonstrated with animal work utilizing the Cine CT system [18,19]. Figure 5 illustrates a typical myocardial wall thickening analysis.

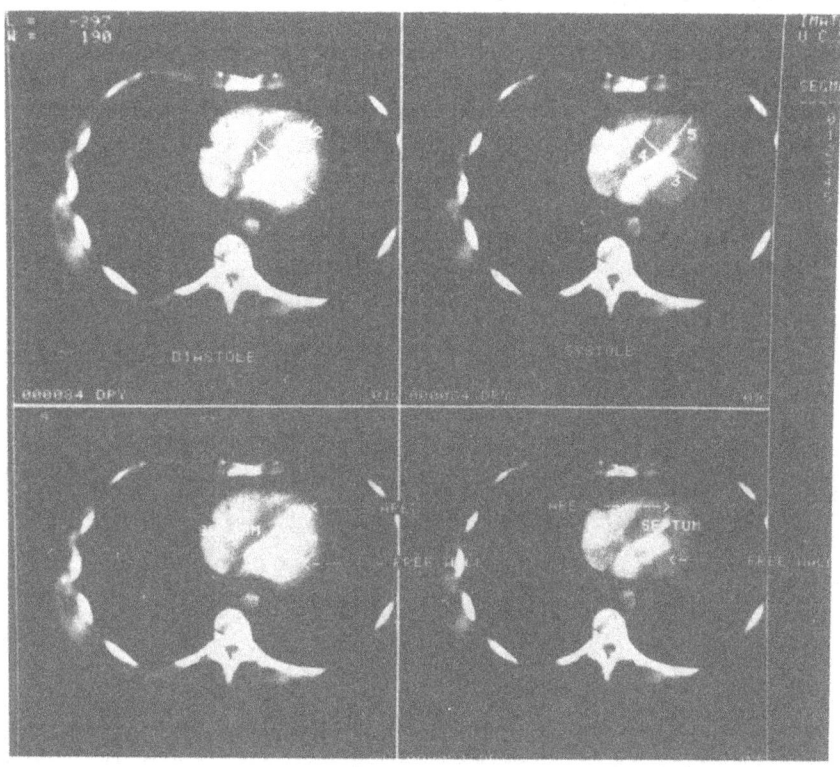

Figure 5: Wall thickness has been measured for the diastolic and systolic cardiac phases. Regions, the intraventricular (1,4), left ventricular apex (2,5), and lateral free wall (0,3), have been selected for analyses.

Flow (Triggered) Mode

In this mode of operation, two contiguous 8 mm slices are again obtained simultaneously for each 50 msec exposure, but each exposure is triggered by the patient's ECG so as to occur at a specific phase of 20-40 sequential cardiac cycles. This mode provides the transit time of the contrast agent through the vascular structures in the tissue planes scanned and samples each cardiac cycle at a particular phase, usually end-diastole. Using multiple target rings, it is also possible to image the ventricular volume with the passage of a single contrast bolus.

By utilizing time vs. density (CT number) analysis, parameters such as cardiac output and coronary artery bypass graft patency can be determined (fig 6). Conventional whole-body units showed considerable promise in these areas [3,21], but with the increased sampling rate of the cine system there are considerably more data points available and curve fitting is thus potentially more accurate.

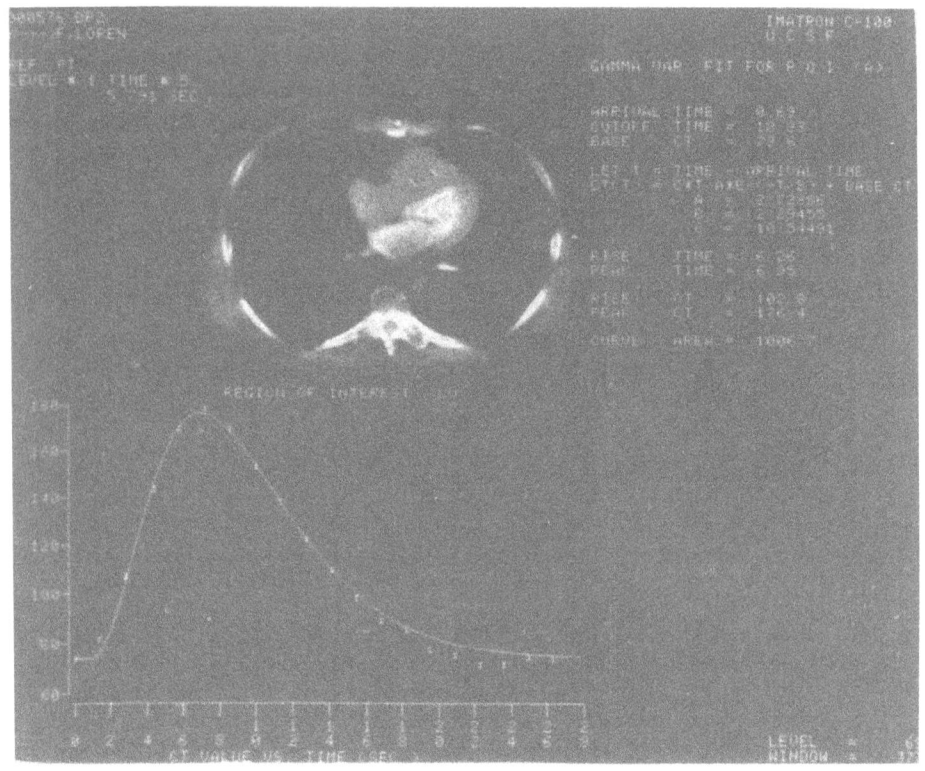

Figure 6A: Single axial 50 msec image from a triggered or flow sequence when the contrast bolus is present in the left ventricle. Following the placement of a region of interest over the left ventricular cavity, the computer plots a time vs. mean CT number (density) curve. These points are then fit to a standard theoretical curve (gamma variate), which corrects for a secondary recirculation peak if present. This curve has the general form $ate^{-bt} + C$, where a,b, and c are parameters determined by the least squares fit and t is time in seconds. After performing the fit, the computer calculates various bolus parameters, including the rise time, peak time, and area under the curve. The dashed lines indicated an ischemic region in the septum.

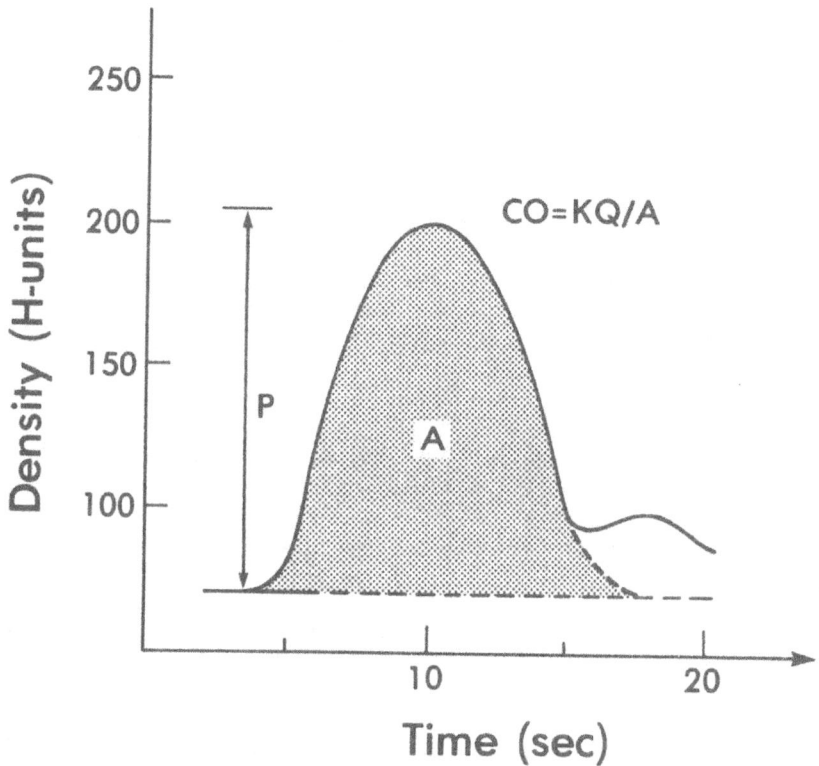

Figure 6B: Cardiac output (CO) can be determined from the area under the left ventricular curve (A) as in figure 5A, if the quantity of iodinated contrast medium injected (Q) is known, according to the equation CO = KQ/A. K is a factor representing the density valve of the injected contrast medium.

During contrast enhanced conventional CT, regions of myocardial ischemia present as perfusion defects, suggesting that delineation of infarcted and at risk areas of myocardium following coronary artery occlusion might be possible [4,5,7]. Furthermore, if blood flow measurements could be obtained in conjunction with exercise, coronary artery reserve as well as collateral flow could be assessed.

Utilizing the flow mode of image acquisition, such measurements of relative myocardial perfusion have been possible (fig 7). Because the images are triggered at end-diastole of each cardiac cycle, the effect of cardiac motion on these measurements is minimized. Absolute myocardial blood flow can be derived by interpreting the relative myocardial time/density curve in concert with the cardiac output, both of which are determined by indicator dilution. For any given contrast injection, measurement of the area under the time/density curves of the aorta and left ventricle is constant and representative of cardiac output [21]. Absolute flow can then be calculated for any myocardial region as the ratio of peak enhancement of the time/density curve in that region to the area under the aortic or ventricular time/density curves.

$$F/V = P/A$$

F/V = blood flow per unit volume of tissue (ml/min/ml)

P = peak of the tissue flow curve (H)

A = the area under the aorta or left ventricular time/density curve (H.min)

This formula assumes that the myocardial contrast washout time is longer than the width of the aortic or ventricular time/density curve. This is true in the myocardium, because transit time through the capillary bed is longer than the duration of the systemic venous contrast bolus injection. Figure 7 demonstrates a lack of flow in an infarcted region of myocardium (A points). Current animal studies are being conducted in order to corroborate this method.

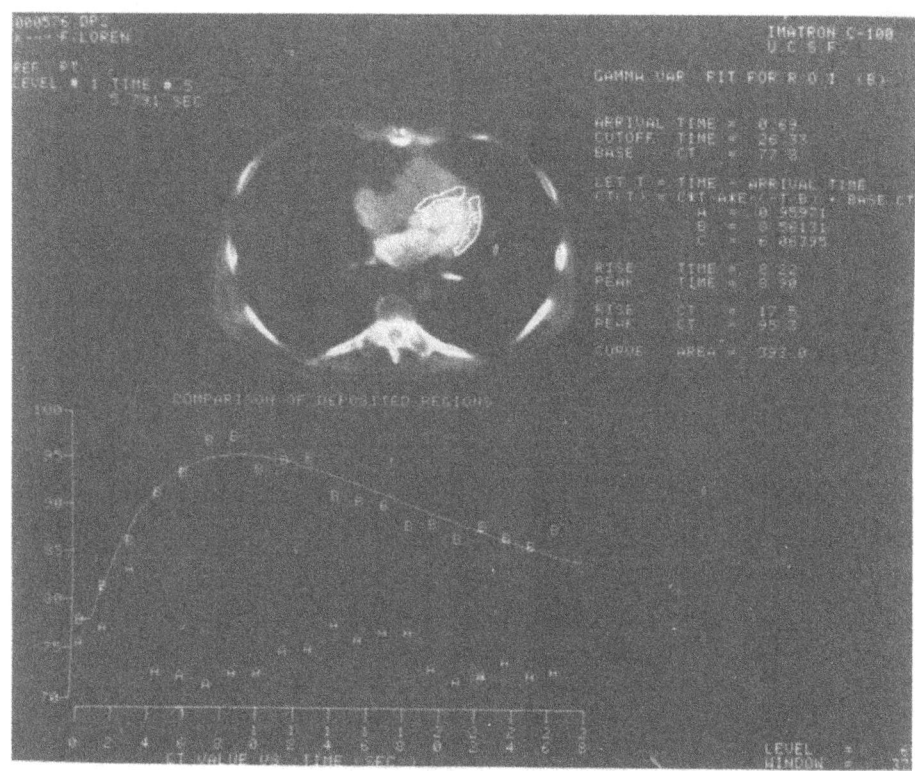

Figure 7A: Myocardial perfusion curve generated over the lateral wall (B) and septum (A) from the patient of (fig 6) with a previous myocardial infarction. Curve analysis provides the peak height which can be used to calculate myocardial flow in the lateral wall. Flow is absent in the infarcted septal region.

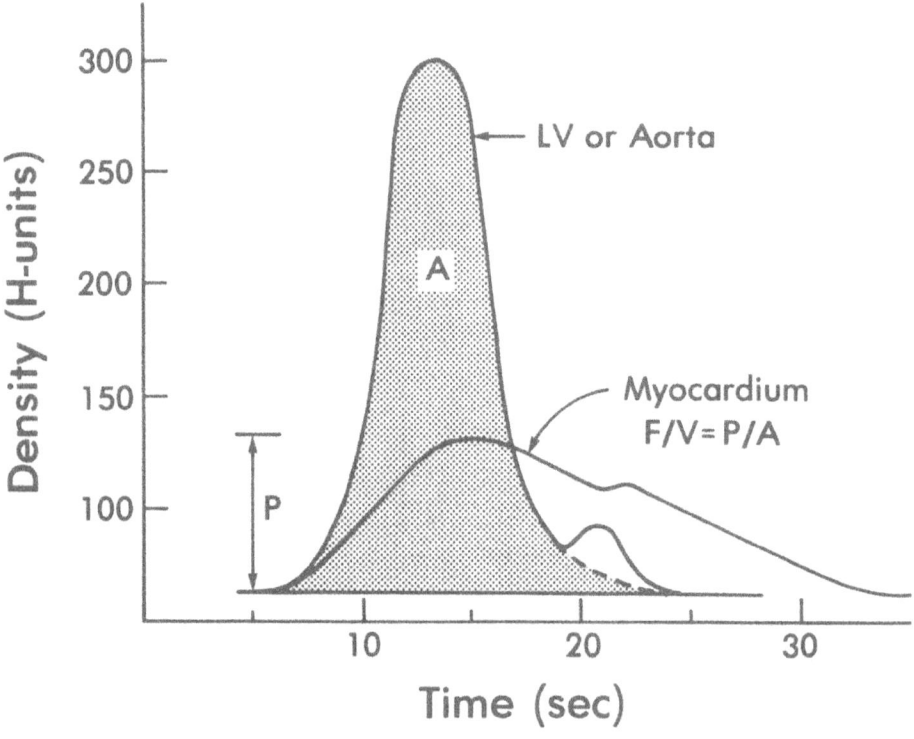

Figure 7B: Blood flow (F/V) in any myocardial region can be calculated as the ratio of the peak of the time density curve in that area (P) to the area under the aorta or left ventricle time-density curve (A), which is representative of cardiac output.

Using the flow acquisition mode and time/density analysis, our clinical experience has indicated that it may be possible to quantify relative valvular insufficiency over time. The potential to assess shunt fractions in various intracardiac shunts has been indicated by recent animal experience. [22]

Full Resolution Mode

This acquisition mode employs an averaging technique coupled with a limited cine acquisition. Four to eight 50 msec exposures at the same level are averaged together providing a relative exposure time of 232-464 msec (fig 8). With the slightly longer exposure time, the contrast resolution of anatomic structures is enhanced, providing more detail in situations where increased temporal resolution is less critical. By scanning all four target rings, producing an eight slice volume sequence, eight centimeters of the thorax can be scanned in just under three-quarters of a second, virtually eliminating the problem of slice registration due to the patient's inability to suspend respiration for the scanning interval. Anatomic surveys of the thorax to evaluate aortic abnormalities of pericardial disease can be easily conducted in under 10 seconds, while quantitation of left and right ventricular mass can be performed in a fraction of the time required by conventional CT scanners. [23]

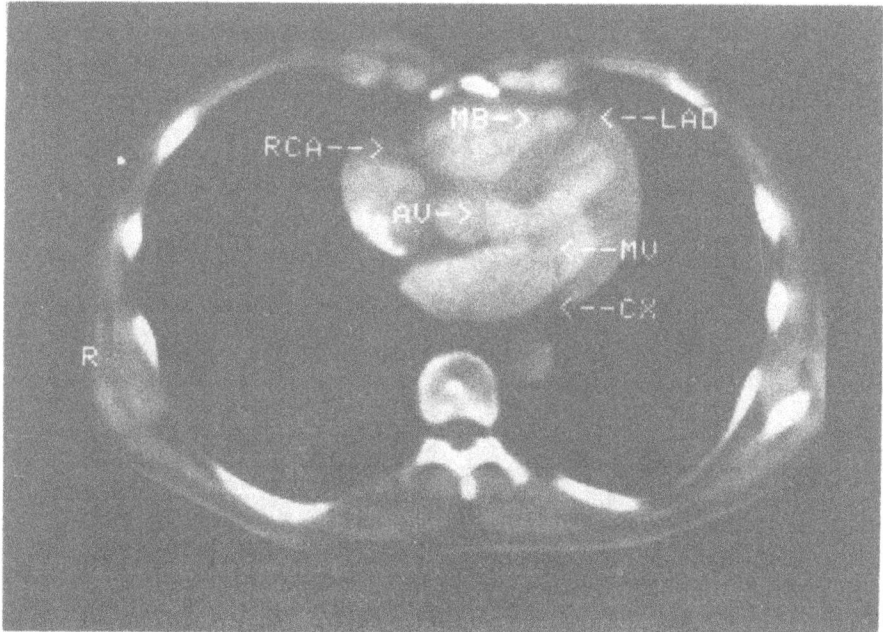

Figure 8: A four frame average from a cine study of a patient with hypertrophy and myocardial infarction. The increased resolution offered by the mode reveals small anatomical features not normally seen in CT. This slice is at the level of the four cardiac chambers with the left ventricular outflow tract at the center. All three major coronary arteries (RCA, LAD, CX) are well seen in cross section. The leaflets of the mitral valve (MV) and aortic valve (AV) are resolved. The moderator band in the right ventricle (MB) is seen.

Using the full resolution mode, the utility of the scanner has also been extended into more traditional whole-body CT applications. Although the Cine-CT system is not yet optimized for scanning in these areas, there is considerable enthusiasm regarding the clinical experience with scanning of the abdomen (fig 9). Head scanning offers even further challenges which have recently been undertaken.

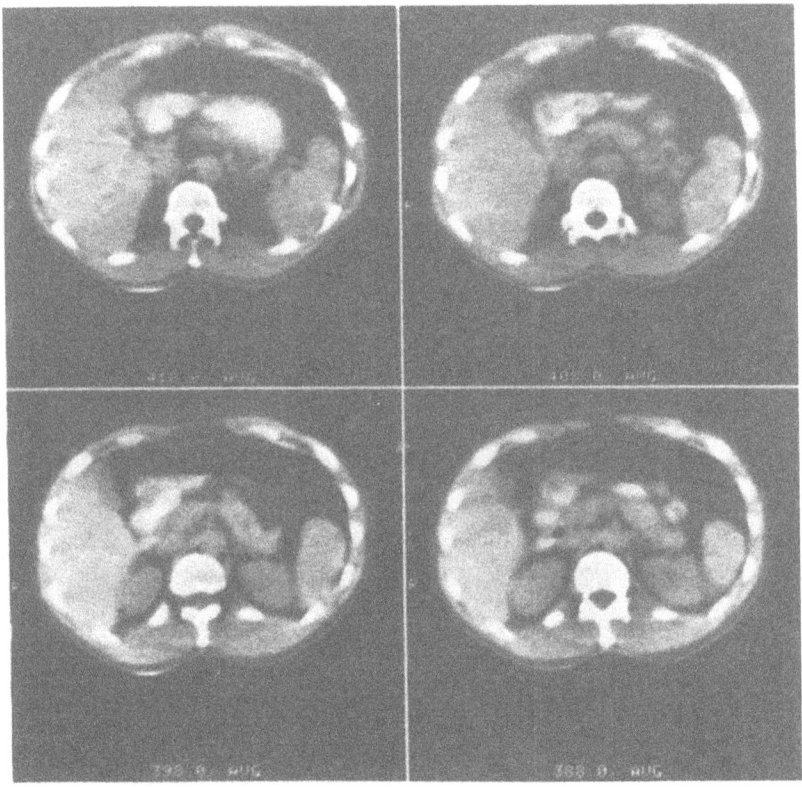

Figure 9: Four contiguous, 8 mm, full resolution images in an abdominal sequence. The image on the upper left is most cephalad and the lower right most caudad. These images were obtained in 0.8 sec of imaging time yet provide excellent visualization of the abdominal viscera.

A Look to the Future

The potential impact of the C-100 Cine-CT system on conventional diagnostic x-ray imaging is being explored as the initial production units are installed at various locations across the United States: University of California, San Francisco; Deborah Heart and Lung Institute, Browns Mills, New Jersey; University of Illinois, Chicago, IL; University of Iowa, Iowa City, Iowa; Health Care Affiliates, Inc., Laguna Hills, CA.

As the spatial resolution of the C-100 system increases, not only will Cine-CT display improved capability in imaging the heart, but better visualization of all regions of the body may be possible. Pediatric applications of CT will also be widened by added scanning flexibility and millisecond scan speed. Body surveys conducted in the emergency setting following trauma could be performed in moments relatively unaffected by patient movement, and yield a valuable adjunct to patient triage.

Another soon to be exploited capability of Cine-CT is the development of volume images. Rapid scanning combined with high-speed table motion can permit acquisition of 80 successive levels in a few seconds. Three dimensional display software and hardware could be used to view the resulting volume image. the Mayo Clinic's DSR group has previously demonstrated the power of tissue dissolution and reprojection methods. [24] Surface display algorithms are another possibility. The excellent slice registration inherent in a short scanning interval are key to this exciting future capability of Cine-CT.

Clinical evaluation of the C-100 Cine-CT system will continue in the near future with additional controlled studies comparing the CT findings with established angiographic, echocardiographic, and nuclear medicine techniques. These studies will help further determine the sensitivity and specificity of Cine-CT for cardiac diagnosis. If the promising clinical experience thus far continues, the Cine-CT system should reach its anticipated potential. Cine-CT may replace current third- or fourth-generation CT scanners for general diagnostic purposes and become the primary cardiac imaging technique of the future.

REFERENCES

1. Hounsfield GN: Computerized Transverse Axial Scanning (tomography): Part I. Description of system. Br J Radiol 46: 1016, 1973.

2. Hounsfield GN: Nobel prize acceptance speech. Med Phys 7: 283, 1981.

3. Brundage BH, Lipton MJ, Herfkens RJ, et al: Detection of Patient Coronary Bypass Grafts by Computed Tomography: A preliminary report. Circulation 61: 826, 1980.

4. Higgins CB, Carlson E. Lipton MJ (Eds): CT of the Heart and the Great Vessels: Experimental evaluation and clinical application. Mount Kisko, New York: Futura, 1983.

5. Lipton MJ, Higgins CB: Evaluation of Ischemic Heart Disease by Computerized Transmission Tomography. Radiol Clin North Am 18: 557, 1980.

6. Moncada, R, Baker M, Salinas M, et al: Diagnostic Role of Computed Tomography in Pericardial Heart Disease: Congenital Defect, Thickening, Neoplasms and Effusions. Am Heart J 103: 203, 1982

7. Lipton MJ, Brundage BH, Doherty PW, et al: Contrast Medium Enhanced Computed Tomography for Evaluating Ischemic Heart Disease. Cardiovasc Med 4: 1219, 1979.

8. Masuda Y, Yoshida H, Morooks N, et al: ECG-Synchronized Computed Tomography in Clinical Evaluation of Total and Regional Cardiac Motion: Comparison of postmyocardial infarction to normal hearts by rapid sequence imaging. Am Heart J 103: 230, 1982.

9. Berninger WH, Redington BW, Doherty P, et al: Gated Cardiac Scanning in normal and Experimentally infarcted Canines. J Comput Assist Tomogr 32: 155, 1979.

10. Farmer DW, Lipton MJ, Webb WR, et al: Computed Tomography of Congenital Heart Disease. J Comput Assist Tomog (in press).

11. Ringerty HG, Skioidebrand CG, Refsum H, et al: A comparison Between the Information in LCG Gated and Nongated Cardiac CT Images. J Comput Assist Tomogr 8: 933, 1982.

12. Mattrey RF, Higgins CB: Detection of Regional Myocardial Dysfunction During Ischemia with Computerized Tomography: Documentation and Physiologic Basis. Invest Radiol 17: 329, 1982.

13. Lipton MJ, Napel S, Brundage BH, et al: Electrocardiographic Gated CT for Regional Myocardial Motion Analysis. Circulation 64: 220, 1981.

14. Lacknu K, Thurn P: Computed Tomography of the Heart: ECG-Gated and Continuous Scans. Radiology 140: 413, 1981.

15. Boyd DP: CTT of the Heart Using Scanning Electron Beams in CTT of the Heart: Experimental Evaluation and Clinical Application. C. Higgins (Ed), Mt. Kisco N.Y., Futura Publishing Co., 1983.

16. Boyd DP, Lipton MJ: Cardiac Computed Tomography. Proc IEEE 71 (3): 298, 1983.

17. Lipton MJ, Farmer DW, Killebrew E, et al: Evaluation of Regional Myocardial Function with Cine-CT in Patients with Prior Myocardial Infarction. To be presented at the Radiological Society of North America, Scientific Assembly and Annual Meeting. Nov. 1984.

18. Farmer, DW, Lipton MJ, Ringerty RG et al: In Vivo Assessment of Left Ventricular Wall and Chamber Dynamics During Transient Myocardial Ischemia Using Cine Computed Tomography. Am J Cardiol (in press).

19. Mattrey RF, Slutsky RA, Long SA, et al: In Vivo Assessment of Left Ventricular Wall and Chamber Dynamics During Transient Myocardial Ischemia Using Prospectively ECG-Gated Computerized Transmission Tomography. Circulation 67: 1245, 1983.

20. Thompson HH, Starmer CF, Whalen RE, et al: Indicator Transit Time Considreed as a Gamma Variate. Circ Res 14: 502, 1984.

21. Axel L, Herfkens RJ, Lipton MJ: Cardiac Output Determination by Dynamic Computerized Tomography. Invest Radiol 14: 389, 1979.

22. Ringertz HG, Lipton MJ, Breznock EM, et al: Cine CT Scanning in Congenital Heart Disease, presented at the Association of University Radiologists' 32nd Annual Meeting, May 1984.

23. Reiring AJ, Rumberger JA, Higgins CB, Lipton MJ, Skorton DJ, Collins SM, Ell SR, Marcus MD: Determination of Left Ventricular Mass by Rapid Acquisition Computed Tomography. Clin Res, 1984 (in press) (Abstract).

24. Ritman EL, Kinsey MJ, Robb, RA et al: 3-Dimensional Imaging of Heart, Lungs, and Circulation. Science 210: 2/3, 1980.

DISCUSSION SUMMARY

SESSION ON X-RAY COMPUTED TOMOGRAPHY

This session consisted of a thorough review of the technical progress in CT (Allemand), the success of CT in clinical radiology (Di Guglielmo) and an example of a recently introduced high-speed, multi-slice CT scanner (Boyd). During the discussion, several technical questions were raised by the participants in order to clarify various points.

The subject of dual-energy CT was raised as a method of characterizing the electron density and atomic number of tissues. Commercial dual-energy CT scanners using correct preprocessing methods have been introduced by two companies. Calibration difficulties and insufficient computer power limit the Cine-CT scanners' capability in this direction. This area has been discussed in the proceedings of the International Workshop on Bone and Soft Tissue Densitometry, published every 18 months in the Journal of Computer-Assisted-Tomography.

Several questions regarding the specifications and current performance of Cine-CT (C-100) scanner were raised, including spatial resolution (Masotti), radiation dose (Allemand), cost and throughput (Kettschau) and focal spot size (Allemand). The current spatial resolution is 1.75 mm resolving power and 2.8 mm FWHM. The radiation dose is 0.25 Rads per 50 millisecond scan; this gives 5-10 Rads for a typical patient study. The Cine-scanner is quoted at $ 1.6 M and will cost $ 400-500 per patient study. Patient throughput, as high as 6 patients/hour may be possible for conventional studies. The electron beam focal spot size is 3 mm FWHM and relatively independent of beam energy. The current resolution is 1.5-2 less than that achieved by state-of-the-art fourth generation conventional CT systems but is expected to improve in the near future.

The future of cone beam systems (Todd Pokropek) and scanning beam methods in radiography (Guzzardi) was discussed. Fully 3-dimensional cone beam CT systems will await the development of a cost-effective 2-dimensional detector array and data acquisition systems. Such systems are prohibitive in cost today. Scanning electron beam methods will not be generally used in X-ray imaging, since such tubes have a moving X-ray source and are therefore limited to tomographic applications.

Finally, participants pointed out that other dynamic imaging methods, such as echo-planar NMR (Guilfoyle) and digital radiography (Heintzen) are currently undergoing rapid development and may become competitive with Cine-CT in cardiac imaging.

THE ACCURATE 3-D RECONSTRUCTION OF THE GEOMETRIC CONFIGURATION OF VASCULAR TREES FROM X-RAY RECORDINGS

D.J. Hawkes[1]   A.C.F. Colchester[2]   C.R. Mol[3]

1 Department of Medical Physics, St. George's Hospital, Tooting, London, SW17, UK.

2 Department of Neurology, Atkinson Morley's Hospital, Wimbledon, London, SW20 UK.

3 IBM Scientific Centre, St. Clement Street, Winchester, UK.

1 INTRODUCTION

We describe here our method for the accurate reconstruction and display of the three dimensional (3-D) configuration of a vascular tree from two X-ray views. In order to achieve this, the precise location and orientation of the X-ray equipment must be known for both views. Each vessel segment of the vascular tree is identified and located in each view and the calibre of each vessel segment is calculated and, from the resulting 3-D data set, a 2-D image of the vascular tree, from any chosen viewpoint is reconstructed. The blood vessels are represented by cylinders joined by spheres and shaded to give the impression of depth, the third dimension.

2 METHOD

We have adapted the method of MacKay et al (1) for the geometric calibration of the X-ray systems. An 8cm perspex cube was constructed. This cube contained 14 steel balls, 1.5mm diameter, accurately positioned at the apices and at the centre of each face. The cube must be imaged with the X-ray system in the same position as that used for the images of the patient. In simultaneous biplane angiography, first the patient and then the cube are imaged without moving the X-ray equipment. When only one X-ray set is available, the patient is imaged from one view and the position of the X-ray equipment is noted. Without moving the patient the X-ray equipment is moved to the second position and an image is recorded. The patient is then removed, the cube positioned in the field of view and images are recorded for both positions of the X-ray system. The identification and location of six or more markers in each view permits the derivation of the transformation matrices between the 3-D object space and the X-ray images.

For the images of vascular trees which are presented here, simultaneous biplane angiography was performed on a CGR Angiomax biplane X-ray system. The same exposure factors and volumes of contrast material were used as for conventional cine angiography. Cine frames were viewed with a Plumbicon camera and the video signal digitised to yield an image of 1024 x 1024 pixels at 8 bits/pixel. The images were transmitted to an IBM 4341 computer. Background subtraction was performed using a 'mask' image obtained from a film taken before the arrival of contrast material in the region of interest. Pincushion distortion in the image intensifier was removed by applying a correction derived from an image of a 2cm grid.

The reconstruction technique relied on the unambiguous identification of each segment of the vascular tree in each view. The computer provided assistance in the identification of key features, or landmarks, in each view, as follows: When the user had identified a landmark in one view the computer superimposed the locus of the projection of that landmark, the 'auxiliary line', on the other view. This considerably simplified the task of identification.

We have extended this principle in the following way. If a vessel was located in each view the operator traced each projection of the vessel. Starting from the first point on one projection, the intersection of the auxiliary line of this point and the projection of the vessel in the other view, the image co-ordinates of the point in the second view, were derived by the computer. Hence the 3-D location of the point can be found. This process was continued for each point on the projection of the vessel. Where ambiguity arises the lines were assumed to be drawn in the same direction, e.g. in the direction of flow, in each view. Certain ambiguities were still theoretically possible but in the vascular structures studied so far we have been able to identify all vessels with a diameter greater than 1.5mm.

The diameter of each vessel was determined from one of the X-ray views by an adaption of the method of Kooijman et al (2). The profile of the film density was plotted perpendicular to the direction of the vessel centreline. A background value for every point along the profile was estimated by linear interpolation between the background values well outside the vessel. After background subtraction the profile was differentiated twice. The vessel edges were defined as the points, on each side of the centreline, were the sums of the moduli of the first and second derivatives reached a maximum. The vessel width was the distance between these points in the 3-D object space. The operator was then given the choice of accepting or rejecting this value and inserting an estimated value.

The reconstruction of the vascular system was displayed as a 2-D image giving the visual impression of three dimensions. Each straight element of a vessel was represented by a cylinder with a diameter proportional to the vessel width. The cylinders were joine by spheres with a diameter equal to that of the larger cylinder and shaded to give the impression of solidity and depth (3). A curved vessel was represented by a series of short cylinders joined by spheres.

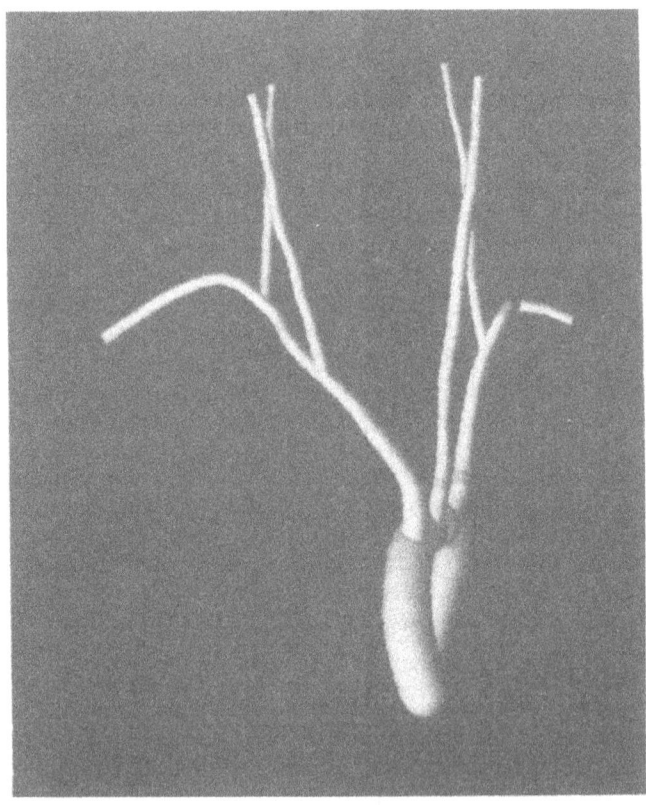

Figure 1: Anterior view of the major vessels branching from the arch of the aorta.

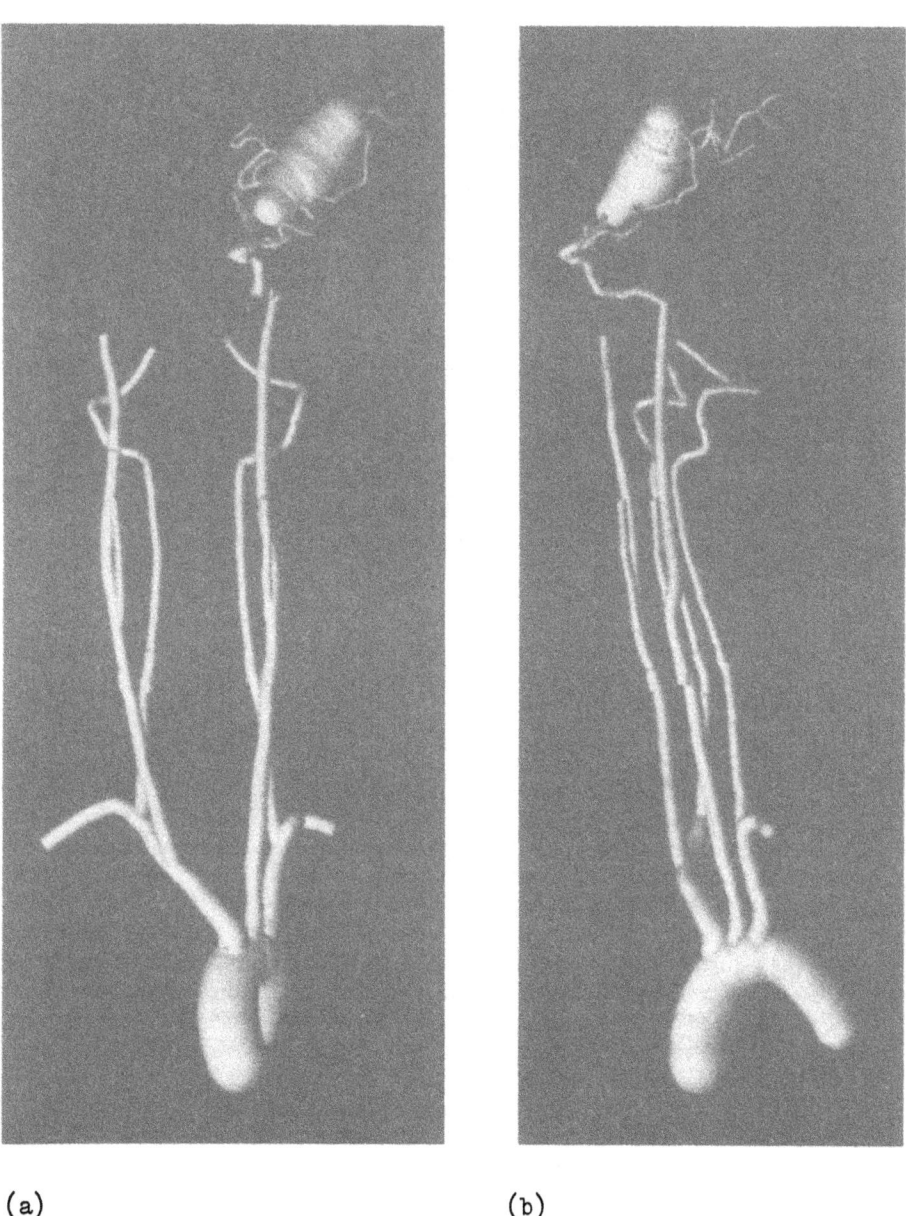

(a) (b)

Figure 2: (a) Anterior and (b) left lateral view of the major vessels of the head and neck of a patient with an AVM

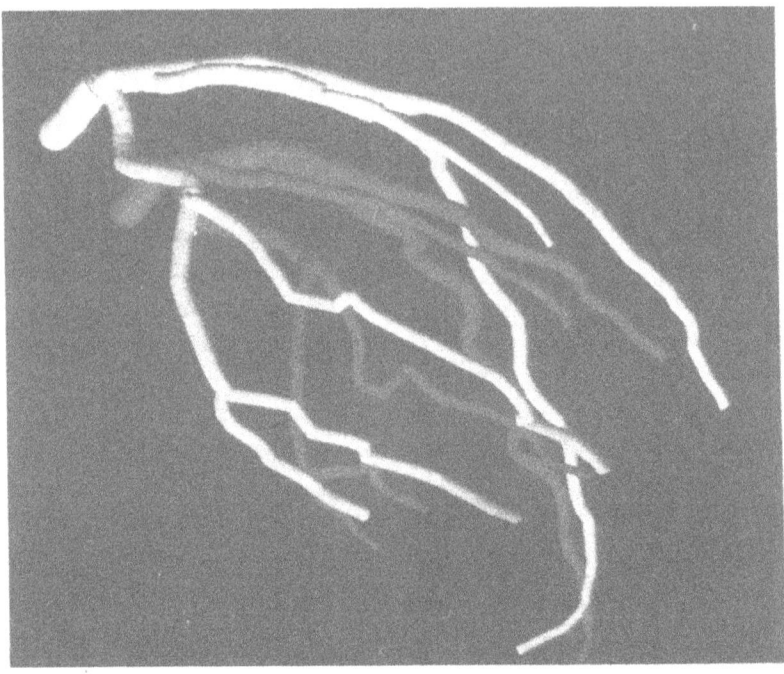

Figure 3: Superimposition of the coronary arteries at systole (yellow) and diastole (white).

3 RESULTS

Figures 1, 2 and 3 show examples of images obtained from the 3-D reconstruction technique using simultaneous biplane angiography. Figure 1 shows a view of the major vessels branching from the arch of the aorta. Figure 2 shows the major vessels leading from the arch of the aorta to the neck and head of the same patient who had a large cerebral arterio-venous malformation (AVM). Three different sets of angiograms were used in this reconstruction: one biplane pair from the aortic region, one pair from the neck region and one pair from the head. The composite 3-D image was obtained by interactively rotating and translating each 3-D image on the computer display. Individual tiny vessels constituting the AVM could not be resolved and this region was represented by a single solid cylindrical structure. However, the major feeding vessels to the AVM are clearly seen.

Figure 3 shows a superimposition of the coronary arteries at systole and diastole from a left mainstem injection. Tracing the 3-D position of coronary artery landmarks provides an accurate method of measuring true epicardial wall motion (1).

The accuracy of the reconstruction technique has been assessed by imaging the cube in the same position as for the calibration and reconstructing the positions of the markers. For simultaneous biplane angiography the standard deviation of the error in the reconstructed positions of the markers was $\pm$ 0.7mm. There was an angle of 90° between the two X-ray axes. For reconstructions from a single X-ray system the standard deviation of the error in reconstruction was 1.05mm, 0.96mm, 1.56mm and 1.70mm for angles between the two positions of the X-ray axes of 90°, 40°, 20° and 10°.

4 DISCUSSION

We have developed a technique for generating 3-D images of vascular systems from X-ray recordings in two planes. Our method combines accurate geometric calibration of the X-ray system with a high quality 3-D graphics display system. This technique is accurate both for simultaneously acquired views using a biplane X-ray system and for sequential views in two planes using a single X-ray system. The error tends to increase as the angle between the two views decreases. However, even at 10° the technique is adequate for our applications and at small angles the task of vessel identification is considerably simplified and automatic techniques become feasible.

These images will be useful as a diagnostic aid; as an aid to the planning of surgery; for the selection of the optimal radiographic views for visualising a particular vessel segment; as a teaching aid; and for combination with data from other 3-D imaging techniques such as X-ray CT, ultrasound, MRI, PET and ECAT.

Having accurately determined the 3-D structure, we may determine the magnification and orientation of vessel segments for absolute calibre and length measurements; convert contrast bolus transport time to velocity and volume blood flow; measure path lengths between features such as stenoses and bifurcations, which is important when identifying lesions in serial quantitative studies or when combining data from two views; and tracing the movement of blood vessels in the analysis of cardiac ventricular wall motion.

Further work is required to automate the analysis of the images of the cube, improve vessel centreline location and develop methods for the automatic identification of vessel segments in each view.

REFERENCES

1. MacKay, S.A., Potel, M.J. and Rubin, J.M. Graphics Methods for Tracking Three-Dimensional Heart Wall Motion. Computers and Biomedical Research 15 (1982) 455-473

2. Kooijman, C.J., Reiber, J.H.C., Gerbrands, J.J., Schurrbiers, J.C.H., Slager, C.J., den Boer, A. and Serruys, P.W. Computer-Aided Quantitation of the Severity of Coronary Obstructions from Single View Cineangiograms. Proc ISMII '82 (1982) 56-64

3. Burridge, J. submitted for publication.

POSTER SESSION

APPLICATION OF COMPUTER-TOMOGRAPHY IN INDUSTRIAL PROBLEMS

A. Kettschau, J. Goebbels

Federal Institute for Materials Testing, Berlin, Germany

INTRODUCTION

After the fast development of X-ray-computer-tomography in medicine a wide range of applications of CT in industry is expected, as was the case with conventional X-ray techniques.

In particular, the fact that practically no dose limitations exist and in most cases much more measuring time is available, seemed to make CT in materials testing much easier than in medicine. Additionally, the regular and well-known shapes of most objects are considered to be an essential advantage.

On the other hand, industrial problems are demanding in some aspects high improvements to a CT-scanner, in order to obtain valuable information from a CT-picture.

These problems are:

- high absorption coefficients for some materials and large diameter objects resulting in absorption factors of up to five or six orders of magnitude;
- the combination of different materials with high contrast cause artefacts in many cases;
- the large variety of objects, object sizes (from 10 mm to several meters), and the high variety of structures to be detected (e.g. cracks, voids with size down to 0.1 mm, inhomogeneous material) resulting in difficulties in optimizing system lay-out

and minimizing measuring time.

CT-SCANNER DESCRIPTION

At the Federal Institute for Materials Testing a CT-scanner is under development, which shall fit a wide range of possible applications.

The radiation sources are a 400 Ci Co-60 nuclide and X-ray sources up to 420 KV at 10 mA. The use of a linear accelerator (at 3 MeV) for thick walled components has been planned. The detector system consists of 31 photomultipliers with plastic scintillators with an angular difference of 1 degree mounted to a lead collimator. The collimator channels have a length of 210 mm, the width is 1 mm, the height ranges from 8 to 1 mm. The size of the scintillators is 190 x 8 x 12 mm. The maximum object circle is 1 m, the distance between source and collimators is 1400 mm. The scanning motion is performed at the object. The object table is capable of vertical and horizontal motion and full-circle rotation. Its maximum load is 1000 Kg, the mechanical accuracy is better than 0.1 mm.

Compared to medical CT-systems the following details may be outlined:

- due to the high radiation energies needed (1 MeV), thick-walled collimators must be used;
- because of the low numbers of detectors, a translation-rotation movement is still necessary;
- spatial resolution given by collimators and source size fixed to 1 mm, variable thickness of investigated layer from 1 to 8 mm.

Due to the fixed geometric parameters and the wide range of possible applications, the tomograph cannot be optimized in measuring time and costs. However a set of different programs for image reconstruction and image processing can be tested. Experiments with this CT scanner can give the information necessary for constructing tomographs suited to special problems.

SELECTED EXAMPLES

The following pictures are tomograms of two objects investigated with a CT-scanner: 1) a container for radioactive waste containing a glass matrix and 2) a plastic insulator.

Defects of the waste container are cracks (increasing the effective surface), voids, inhomogeneous material, insufficient mixing of the components, segregation of components.

Primary defects of the high voltage insulator are inhomogeneities in the material, due to the insufficient mixing of the components in the production process. Secondary defects are the cracks and a discharge channel from top to bottom due to electric failure.

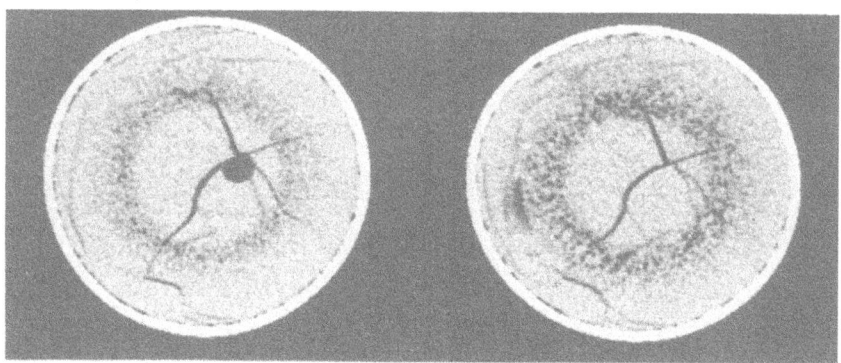

Fig. 1 Tomograms of a radioactive waste container.

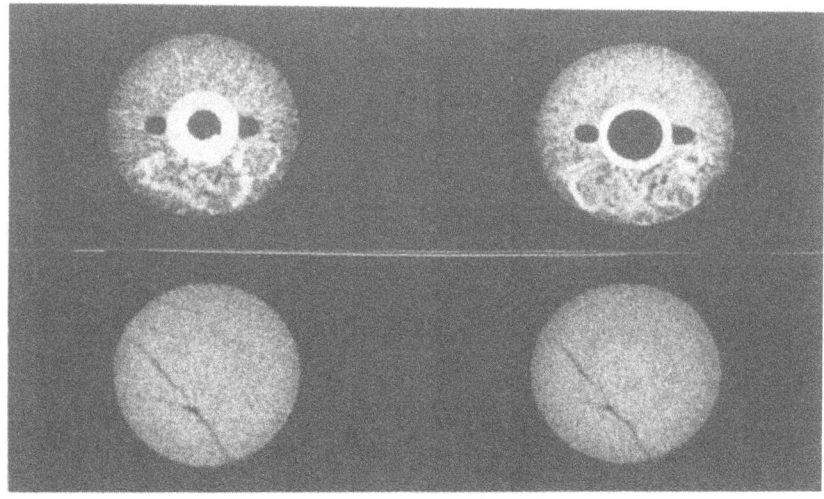

Fig. 2 Tomograms of a high voltage insulator.

PART IV ULTRASOUND IMAGING: CURRENT TRENDS AND CLINICAL APPLICATIONS

Chairman: Peter N.T. Wells (U.K.)

BASIC PRINCIPLES AND ADVANCED TECHNOLOGICAL ASPECTS OF ULTRASOUND IMAGING

Leonardo Masotti

Dipartimento di Ingegneria Elettronica, University of Florence, Florence, Italy

Introduction

In modern medicine there is an ever increasing tendency to make use of images for diagnostic purposes. In a general sense these images constitute concise illustrations of the information supplied by an energy source which is either generated by the object under examination or made available by a suitable source.

For the human body, images can be formed of organs or their activity using the natural energy emitted by the body itself: electrical signals (electrocardiographic and electroencephalographic maps and tracings), magnetic signals (magnetocardiograms), infrared rays (thermographs), sound signals (phonograms) or by using injected energy (scintigraphy). Other systems such as endoscopy, radiography, echography and nuclear magnetic resonance examinations require the intervention of external sources of energy.

In examinations using external energy sources such as X-rays, ultrasound and injected radioactive substances, the information contained in the images is produced by the interaction between the energy and the organ under examination. This interaction can be visualized in two different ways: an image may be formed by the energy which manages to pass through the organ or its parts, or the energy reflected or scattered from portions of the structure under examination may be transferred into images. The two techniques are respectively termed visualization by transmission and visualization by reflection.

In the visualization by transmission technique, the energy is propagated through the object, i.e. the biological tissues: the energy which is not absorbed, scattered or reflected by the tissues is visualized. Traditional radiology makes use of this technique.

The visualization by reflection method uses the energy which has been scattered back from or reflected by the tissues. In most cases, diagnostic ultrasound currently uses the technique of formation of images by reflection.

1. The properties and nature of ultrasound tomographic images

The ultrasonic energy required to form an image must be supplied from an external source which can be continuous or impulsive. The formation of images by reflection makes use of impulsive ultrasound energy.

Ultrasound diagnosis, which has developed over the last thirty years, is in routine use in obstetrics and gynaecology, ophthalmolog internal medicine, cardiology and neurology.

The special characteristics of ultrasound include visualization of the interfaces between soft tissues without contrast medium; a no invasive and atraumatic examination for the patient: depth and strat graphic measurements of organs; creation of images of organs in motion, and information on blood flow.

The term ultrasound describes the general form of mechanical ene gy emitted by the mouth during speech, but at a frequency above the limit of human audibility. The maximum frequency audible to man is 16,000 cycles per second, called Hertz (Hz), whereas clinical echography now uses frequencies from 1 to 15 million Hz (MHz).

One of the characteristics of ultrasound is that of propagating through soft biological tissues at a sufficiently low speed, around 1500 metres per second and very close to that of water propagation (Table 2.1.1.). In this way, electronic systems can be used to follo the progress of the echo signals in time and supply an image which represents the morphology of what the ultrasound is revealing within the human body.

Ultrasound waves, at energy levels which are harmless to both patient and operator, are transmitted into the human body by means of a piezoelectric transducer, also called a probe, i.e. an element which, after the application of an electrical signal, vibrates and transmits these vibrations (Fig. 1.1.) into the object in contact with it, and reciprocally after the application of vibrations reflec ed or scattered by the tissues, supplies to the electronic receiver an electric signal.

In most echographic applications, ultrasound is emitted in the form of pulses, i.e. mechanical vibrations of short duration (Fig. 1.2.). When the mechanical vibration encounters an obstacle (the interfaces between one tissue and another, discontinuity in the biological tissue, cavities full of fluid, calcification, air bubbles or foreign bodies) as the wave front advances part of the energy is reflected and the rest continues. The same transducer used to emit the ultrasonic pulse responds to mechanical vibrations by generating a corresponding electric signal.

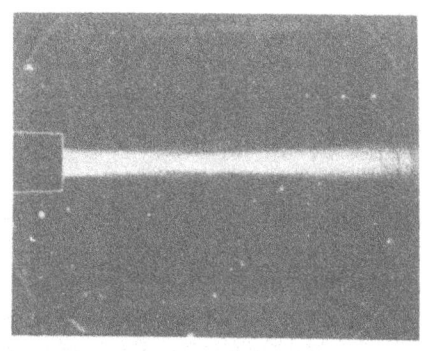

Fig. 1.1 - Ultrasound beam emitted by a focused probe operating at 3.5 MHz, displayed according to the Schlieren method, as used at the non-Destructive Testing Laboratories of the CCR at Ispra (Italy).

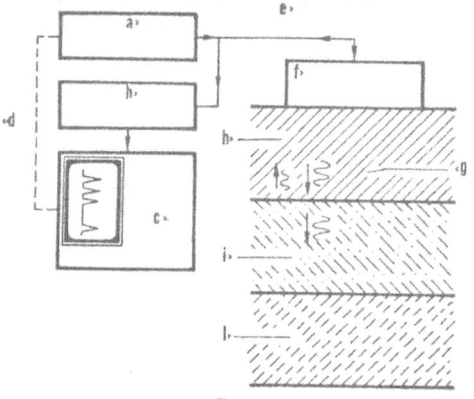

Fig. 1.2 - Simplified diagram of echographic equipment with A-mode display. a) transmitter; b) receiver; c) oscilloscope; d) trigger signal; e) pulse electrical signal; f) piezoelectric transducer; g) pulse mechanical signals; h) medium 1; i) medium 2; l) medium 3; m) medium 4.

The electric signal is transmitted to a series of electronic circuits and frequently presented as a luminous signal on the screen of an oscilloscope. By making a correlation between the luminous point on the screen and the distance travelled by the ultrasonic waves advancing within the tissues, an image is formed of the organization of the layers encountered by the ultrasound beam in the direction in which the transducer is pointing.

A similar principle, i.e. displaying the echo signals to form images of the region explored by the probe, is adopted by sonar equipment which uses the same type of mechanical waves as clinical echography. On the other hand, radar equipment which is also an echographic system, is based on the use of electromagnetic waves.

The images used in clinical echography, as seen in detail in § 5.1, may be of the tomographic type (B-mode), or appear in the form of descriptive tracings of the movement of organs or their parts in relation to time (TM-mode) along a single interrogating position of the probe. Other tracings provide images of the amplitude of the echo signals in relation to the distance from the probe along a single observation direction (A-mode). Finally, tracings or images may be displayed showing the amplitude of Doppler signals or the variation of their relative frequency spectrum in relation to time (§ 5.2).

2. Characteristics of ultrasound waves

Elastic waves at ultrasonic frequency are generated by a perturbation which causes the particles* of a given medium to vibrate. The vibration of the particles of the medium is a basic characteristic of the propagation of elastic waves. It is therefore impossible for such waves to advance in a vacuum.

Different modes of propagation are possible and in diagnostic applications longitudinal waves are used. In this type of waves the par ticles which make up the propagation medium vibrate forwards and back wards around their intermediate position, so that the energy is trans mitted through the medium as a perturbation without transfer of matte and the vibrations of the particles are in the direction of propagation of the wave.

This is the origin of the term "longitudinal". When the direction of movement of the particles is perpendicular to the direction of propagation of the wave the terms "transverse" or "shear" are applied

Longitudinal waves can pass through all kinds of media, whilst transverse waves can only advance in solids. This is due to the fact that fluid and gaseous media cannot withstand shear stress under normal conditions.

The presence of an acoustic perturbation in an elastic medium is characterized by the change of a certain number of physical variables which describe the state of the system or medium. Examples of these variables include pressure, temperature and density.

For a sinusoidal plane wave propagating along the direction x (when there is no attenuation of the wave, due to absorption of energy by the medium, or to other mechanisms which will be examined further on), the changes of physical variables can be expressed in the form (2.1), in cases in which linear response of the medium to stress occurs,

* By particles we mean an elementary volume sufficiently small for the variable amounts within the medium (e.g. pressure) to be constant.

$$q = Q \cos\omega(t - \frac{x}{v}) \qquad (2.1)$$

In this equation, q stands for one of the variables which undergo sinusoidal variations due to the presence of a perturbation in the medium. Q indicates the amplitude of the cyclical changes of such variable; t and x are time and the spatial coordinate, ω is the "angular frequency" (linked to the frequency f by the relation $\omega = 2\pi f$) and v is the velocity of wave propagation.

The wavelength λ* and the frequency f are linked to the velocity of propagation v by the well-known equation:

$$v = f \cdot \lambda \qquad (2.2)$$

The velocity at which the energy is transmitted through the medium, which coincides with the velocity of propagation v, depends on the elastic properties of the medium, i.e. on how the force is linked to displacement of the medium, and on the average value, ρ_o, of the density, which links the force to acceleration of the medium.

The velocity of ultrasound waves in soft tissues, as mentioned above, is that of longitudinal waves, as only this type of wave can propagate, and is calculated by the expression valid for fluids:

$$v = \sqrt{\frac{k}{\rho_o}}$$

where v is the velocity of propagation, k is the coefficient of elasticity which links local pressure to the relative variation in size of the elementary small volume due to dilatation or elastic compression.

As the modulus of elasticity and the density for a given material vary with temperature, the speed of sound also varies with temperature, usually increasing with a rise in temperature to a maximum, and then decreasing.

The velocity of propagation can be roughly considered constant in the frequency interval used in diagnostic applications.

Other important characteristics of ultrasonic waves include acoustic pressure p, speed of particles u, intensity I and displacement of particles y.

Acoustic pressure is the variation of pressure with respect to resting conditions at a given point of the medium at a given moment,

---

* Length λ is the distance in the medium between the two consecutive particles which assume the same displacement value at the same time: the period T is the time necessary for the wave to advance by a distance λ in the medium (Fig. 2.1).

which gives rise to a compression (or expansion when negative) as the result of an acoustic perturbation. Speed u is the speed of a vibrating particle in a given point of the medium at a given time; this should not be confused with the velocity of wave propagation v. Both p and u vary according to a law of the type represented by the equation (2.1).

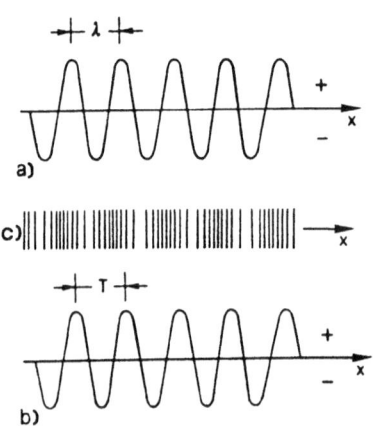

Fig. 2.1 - Amplitude of particle displacement with respect to the point of equilibrium for longitudinal waves. a) Pattern space at a certain time; at a subsequent time the figure would be transferred towards the direction x, being moved at the velocity of propagation; b) Pattern in time of particle displacement at a certain point in space; c) Density of particles as a function of the propagation distance at a certain time.

Characteristic impedance of the medium. The ratio p/u is termed specific acoustic impedance and for plane waves it is numerically equal to the product $\rho_0 \cdot v$, and better known as the characteristic impedance of the medium. For other configurations of the acoustic field including the case of stationary plane waves, specific acoustic impedance differs numerically from $\rho_0 \cdot v$.

Intensity. The intensity at each point of a wave is defined as the energy flow per unit of time through the unit area perpendicular to the direction of propagation at the point considered. It is linked to the peak value of acoustic pressure, p_p, the peak value of the displacement of the particle y_p, the peak value of the speed of the particle u_p, and to the characteristic impedance $\rho_0 \cdot v$, by the following relation:

$$I = \frac{1}{2} p_p u_p = \frac{1}{2} p_p^2 / \rho_0 \cdot v = \frac{1}{2} u_p^2 \rho_0 v = \frac{1}{2} \omega^2 y_p^2 \rho_0 v \qquad (2.3)$$

with $u_p = 2\pi f y_p = \omega y_p$.

The intensity can be expressed in Watts per cm². The maximum value of ultrasonic intensity is important in relation to possible biological effects and the minimum value in relation to the capacity of an echographic system to reveal the presence of the smallest forms of discontinuity in the tissues examined. It is often advantageous to measure the ratio between pairs of values of intensity, especially if the level of one is taken as a point of reference.

Decibel. In practice it is convenient to use the decibel scale defined as follows:

$$\text{number of decibels (dB)} = 10 \log (I/I_o) \qquad (2.4)$$

where I_o is taken as the reference point of intensity.

The logarithm is the number representing the index which is given to 10 to obtain the given ratio.

The dB or decibel is derived from the combination of *Bel* (from the surname of the researcher Bell) defined as the logarithm of root 10 of a relation and *deci*, i.e. a tenth. The number n which expresses attenuation or amplification values in decibels is therefore 10 times greater than that expressing attenuation or amplification values in Bel.

It should be kept in mind that:

$$\log \frac{I}{I_o} = - \log \frac{I_o}{I}$$

When a comparison is made between the amplitude of two echo signals, this can still be expressed in dB, but as intensity is proportional to the square of the amplitude, as described by formula (2.3), the ratio of amplitudes in dB is obtained from:

$$\text{number of decibels (dB)} = 10 \log \frac{A_2^2}{A_1^2} = 20 \log \frac{A_2}{A_1}$$

where A_2 is proportional to the amplitude of the second echo signal and A_1 is proportional to the amplitude of the first signal.

The value of amplitude A with respect to a reference amplitude A_o is given in dB from $20 \log A/A_o$.

It should be noted that an attenuation of 20 dB therefore means a reduction in intensity of 100 to 1 and a reduction in amplitude of 10 to 1.

2.1 Absorption and attenuation

In biological tissues the intensity I, at a given frequency, decreases with distance x along the propagation direction of ultrasound, according to the ratio:

$$I = I_o \exp[-2\mu \cdot x] = I_o e^{-2\mu \cdot x} \qquad (2.1.1)$$

e being the number of Neper, base of natural Neperian logarithms, I_o the intensity at x = 0, and 2μ the coefficient of intensity absorption. The corresponding expression for the amplitude is thus:

$$A = A_o \exp[-\mu \cdot x] = A_o e^{-\mu x} \qquad (2.1.2)$$

where A_o is the amplitude at x = 0 and μ is the coefficient of amplitude absorption. Hence from (2.1.2)

$$\mu = -\frac{1}{x} \ln(A_o/A) = \frac{1}{x} \ln(A/A_o) \qquad (2.1.3)$$

As ln is the symbol for the natural logarithm of root e, in this way μ is expressed in nepers per centimetre (Np/cm). Absorption is usually expressed also in terms of a coefficient of absorption α expressed in decibels per centimetre (dB/cm) so that:

$$\alpha = 20 \log \frac{A}{A_o} = 20 \log \frac{A_o e^{-\mu \cdot 1}}{A_o} = 20 \log_{10}(e^{-\mu \cdot 1}) \qquad (2.1.4)$$

the logarithm of root 10 being written in the more explicit form $\log_{10}$ rather than log,

$$|\alpha| = 20(\log_{10} e)\mu = 8.686\mu \qquad (2.1.5)$$

similarly:

$$|\alpha| = 10 \log \frac{I_o}{I} = 10(\log_{10} e)2\mu = 4.343 \cdot 2\mu = 8.686\mu \qquad (2.1.6)$$

With this definition of absorption coefficient it follows that if the medium introduces an attenuation of 40 dB, between two points, this means that the intensity is reduced from 10000 to 1 and the amplitude from 100 to 1. In fact, it should be kept in mind that the intensity is proportional to the square of the amplitude (§ 2 Decibel).

For an echo signal reflected by a discontinuity occurring at a di tance of L = 10 cm from the probe, with a homogeneous tissue interpos for which the absorption coefficient is 1 dB/cm MHz, the attenuation to absorption alone, is given by:

$$(\alpha \cdot f_o \cdot L \cdot 2) dB$$

where the factor 2 takes into account the course of transmission (probe-discontinuity) and return (discontinuity-probe) of the ultrasonic wave. Assuming that the probe is operating at $f_o = 2$ MHz, and substituting the values we have:

(1 . 2 . 10 . 2) = 40 dB

i.e. the amplitude of the signal is reduced by a factor of 100 due to this cause alone.

Acoustic absorption is strong in all biological tissues and is mainly due to the transformation of ultrasonic energy into thermal energy.

Attenuation of ultrasonic intensity of the ultrasound beam is not only due to absorption, but also to divergence of the beam, scattering and reflection by small discontinuities and mode conversion (whereby the energy is divided into vibrations in several different directions, each having a different velocity of propagation).

In soft tissues, absorption is roughly proportional to the frequency according to the law: $\alpha(f) = \alpha \cdot f$; the attenuation due to absorption, for the outward course alone, is usually between 1 and 2 dB/cm MHz (i.e. between 1 and 2 dB per centimetre per MegaHertz). Absorption in biological tissues is mainly linked to the protein content, although a component of absorption does depend on other factors [6],[7].

The values of the absorption coefficient α for various media, are listed in Table 2.1.1.

Absorption is very low in fluid media, intermediate in soft tissue and very high in bone and gas at the frequencies used in diagnostics.

The absorption trend in relation to the frequency could be one of the elements for classification of tissues [30] at least "in vitro". Numerous research studies in this field are currently underway in different laboratories all over the world (§ 2.2.4.1).

It should also be kept in mind that when structures fall in the far field of a transducer the acoustic intensity decreases as the inverse of the square of the distance. This attenuation is known as attenuation due to divergence of the beam, or "diffraction loss".

2.1.2 Choice of frequency

Information on the absorption of different tissues and the depth of the organ to be studied allows a choice of probes for various applications. The highest frequencies give better resolution, i.e. better display of detail, but unfortunately cannot be used unless, for a given power emission by the probe, a sufficient intensity reaches the organ to be examined. The following frequencies are currently in use: 1.5; 2.25; 3.5 MHz for the abdomen; 5; 7; 10 MHz for the breast, thyroid and other superficial organs; 2.25; 3.5 MHz for the heart; 5; 7 MHz for newborns; 1; 2.25 MHz for the brain and 10 MHz and over for the eye.

2.2 Propagation across interfaces

When an ultrasonic wave, propagating in an acoustically uniform medium, reaches an interface with a medium of differing characterisstic mechanical impedance, reflection and refraction of the wave occur.

2.2.1 Normal incidence

For incidence of a wave over a theoretically plane surface, along the direction of the perpendicular to the surface, i.e. normal incidence, the fraction of incident energy reflected is obtained from the equation:

$$R = \frac{(z_2 - z_1)^2}{(z_2 - z_1)^2} \qquad (2.2.1.1)$$

in which z_2 and z_1 are the characteristic impedances of the two media (§ 2 and Fig. 2.2.1.1). The fraction of incident energy transmitted in medium 2 is equal to $1 - R$.

The characteristic impedance values of different media are reported in Table 2.1.1.

If we take the case of passage through soft biological tissue for which it is assumed: $z_1 = 1.5 \times 10^5$ g/cm² x s, and air for which: $z_1 = 0.0004 \times 10^5$ g/cm² x s, from (2.2.1.1) we obtain $R \simeq 1$ i.e. $1 - R \simeq 0$, i.e. there is no transmission of ultrasonic energy in medium 2, i.e. air. This explains why gas spaces (e.g. lung, gut) along the path of the ultrasonic wave may prevent visualization behind them, unless they are comparable in size to or smaller than the wavelength at the frequency used. In the latter case the ultrasonic wave passes beyond the obstacle due to diffraction.

Similarly, if we consider propagation from a fluid medium 1 (e.g bile, urine) with $z_1 = 1.5 \times 10^5$ g/cm² x s, to a medium 2 made up of a lithic formation with $z_2 \simeq 10 \times 10^5$ g/cm² x s, we obtain $R \simeq 0.5$ and $1 - R \simeq 0.5$, so that the ultrasonic energy which penetrates the calculus is a low fraction of that being incident. There is also an absorption of the energy transmitted which propagates in the calculus and finally a low fraction of the energy which reaches the other interface, i.e. the exit, between the calculus and the underlying medium, can propagate into the underlying tissue. The part of this energy reflected by possible discontinuities encountered by the ultrasound beam below the calculus meets this obstacle again on its return to the transducer.

As a whole, the above description accounts for the typical acoustic shadows present behind the calculi, due to the lack of signals reflected by possible structures below the calculi.

2.2.2 Refraction

For oblique incidence (Fig. 2.2.2.1) the wave is deflected if the velocity v_1 in medium 1 is different from velocity v_2 in medium 2. The ratio between the angle of incidence and that of refraction is governed by Snell's law:

$$\frac{\sin \theta_i}{\sin \theta_t} = \frac{v_1}{v_2} \qquad (2.2.2.1)$$

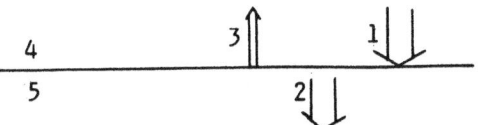

Fig. 2.2.1.1 – Reflection by normal incidence of the ultrasound wave over the surface of separation between two different media 4 and 5: part of the incident energy (1) is transmitted (2), whilst the rest is reflected (3).

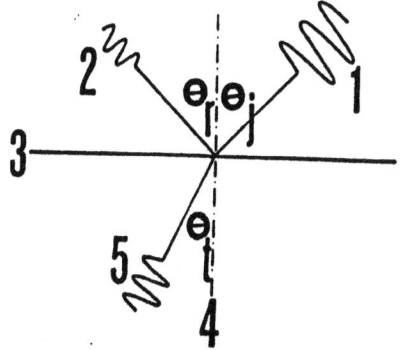

Fig. 2.2.2.1 – Refraction of the ultrasound wave along the pathway with oblique incidence between two media with different propagation velocities: 1) Incident wave, 2) Reflected wave, 3) Discontinuities between the two media, 4) Normal line at the margin, 5) Refracted or transmitted wave.

Table 2.1.1 Data on several inert materials and biological tissues. For water, aluminium, mercury and perspex the data refer to a frequency of 1 MHz.

MATERIAL	T(°C) (temperature)	z (g/cm^2·s·10^5) (characteristic impedance)	v (m/s) (velocity of sound)	α (dB/cm) (absorption coefficient)	F (MHz) (frequency)
Steel	20	47.6	5810		
Water	20	1.48	1430	0.0022	
Aluminium		18.0	6400	0.018	
Araldite		3.0		6.0	
Air	37	0.0004	331	12.0	
Bakelite		3.63	2590		
Iron		40.7	5850		
Mercury		19.7	1450	0.0004	
Castor-oil		1.43	1500	0.37	
Brass		38.0	4490		
Perspex		3.20	2680	2.0	
Lead		27.3	2130		
Polystyrene		2.90	2670	0.35	
PVC		3.30	2400		
Copper		41.1	4600		
Tin		19.9	3320		
Glass		13.6	5420		

BIOLOGICAL TISSUE

					F (MHz) (frequency)
Fat	24	1.38	1476	0.6	1.8
Blood	22	1.67	1570	0.3	2
Liver	24	1.64	1585	0.8	1.8
Kidney	24	1.62	1560	1.3	1.8
Brain	24		1560		1.8
Breast	in vivo		1450-1570	0.5-1.1	1.76
Skull	in vivo	≃ 4.0	3370	2.7	0.1
Skeletal muscle (parallel to fibres)	26	≃ 1.6	1592	2.5	1
Skeletal muscle (perpendicular to fibres)	26	≃ 1.6	1610	1.1	1
Spleen	18	1.63	1578	0.3	1

The difference in velocity between various soft tissues is relatively small, as seen in Table 2.1.1. When bone is present along the ultrasound path, marked refraction occurs.

This is the reason why ultrasound tomographic images of the human body, using transmitted energy and reconstruction techniques similar to those of CAT scan and X-rays, are being developed for the breast and not for other organs which include bone along the ultrasound path.

In fact, refraction due to the presence of bone prevents correlation between the degree of absorption in the transmitter-receiver direction with that of the intervening tissues which is possible with X-rays. On the other hand, as already mentioned, ultrasound tomographic images can be formed directly as in echography, thanks to the low propagation speed of ultrasound which allows direct use of the energy reflected. The usefulness of computed tomography with ultrasound, when theoretically possible, as in the breast, lies in the prospect of reconstructing maps of absorption and velocity of propagation of the organ in the plane of exploration. In this way further information could be added to that on the morphology and distributed reflectivity contained in the echographic image.

2.2.3 Reflection by oblique surfaces

When the incidence is not normal, the amplitude of the echo signal picked up by the transducer is very much dependent on the difference in angle, with respect to normal incidence. For an angle of incidence of a few degrees, the amplitude decreases below the value of a tenth of that obtained for normal incidence (angle 0°); this occurs at both short and long distances from the transducer. The qualitative explanation for this observation is fairly simple: close to the transducer the portion of the receiving surface that collects the reflected beam decreases with an increase of the angle of incidence. For disstances in which the beam is formed the transducer is illuminated almost evenly by the reflected beam, but the sensitivity of the transducer is reduced on deviation from the axial direction in accordance with the directivity function of the transducer (§ 4).

2.2.4 Scattering

In cases of interfaces which are large with respect to the wavelength, reflection is specular, as seen in paragraphs 2.2.2 and 2.2.3, and is accompanied by a shadow effect over the structures lying below, dependent in size on the state and nature of the tissue. When the obstacle is much smaller than the wavelength the radiation is scattered uniformly in all directions and the incident wave envelops the obstacle by diffraction with limited disturbance.

To ultrasound, the parenchyma of biological tissues behaves as a matrix of scattering centres, some larger than others and spaced according to the state and nature of the tissue.

Scattering within biological tissues reduces the propagating energy so that it contributes to attenuation together with reflection, refraction, divergence of the beam and absorption due to transformation of acoustic energy into thermal energy.

Scattering by the internal structures of soft tissues is particularly important in the differentiation of the tissues displayed in the tomographic image. In fact, the internal structure of soft tissue is inhomogeneous both in organization and type of cells so that the amplitude, shape and spatial distribution of the internal echo signals are dependent on the nature and state of the tissue examined. It has been reported that scattered energy is dependent on the orientation of the transducer with respect to the tissue [29],[52].

2.2.4.1 Interaction between ultrasound and biological tissue

According to many authors, and as pointed out in our discussion of the physical characteristics of ultrasound, it is already possible to establish a rough identification of tissue characteristics, listed schematically in the following Table.

Table 2.2.4.1

Tissue	Internal echoes	Attenuation	Characteristics
Calcification	Strong	Very high	Opaque for underlying structures.
Fibrous	Large	High	Reduced penetration.
Soft	Medium	Medium	-
Fat	Low	Low	Some intensification of posterior echoes.
Fluids	None	Negligible	Intensification of posterior echoes and acoustic shadow due to refraction at margins.

3. Transducers

3.1 Construction

The basic transducer which transmits and receives the ultrasonic pulses is made up of a piezoelectric disk, usually from 1 to 2 cm in diameter, or of rectangular or annular elements in the case of arrays, which will be dealt with further on. These elements are electrically stimulated by means of two electrodes in the form of two parallel metallized faces (Fig. 3.1.1). By applying a voltage variation (a short pulse for pulsed equipment or a continuous wave for some Doppler devices) between the electrodes, the inverse piezoelectric effect causes a synchronous variation in the thickness of the transducer. Reciprocally, a mechanical disturbance (an ultrasonic pulse) applied to the transducer and making its thickness change, generates a difference in potential (an electrical signal) between the electrodes due to the direct piezoelectric effect. The thickness of the piezoelectric disk is made equal to half a wavelength in the ceramic device, at the central frequency at which the transducer is intended to operate. This condition is called 'resonance' so that under these conditions variations in thickness of the disk are at maximum. Similarly, the transducer presents maximum sensitivity as a receiver when it interacts with acoustic energy at its own frequency of resonance. The piezoelectric element is connected from behind to an acoustically absorbent material designed to absorb the wave which is emitted from its back face. This posterior structure helps to muffle the resonant element so that it can operate on a wider frequency band (bands at 3 dB up to 40% of the central frequency are typical) and so that damped oscillation, i.e. short pulses, can be emitted to obtain good axial resolving power (§ 4.1) in pulsed echographic systems.

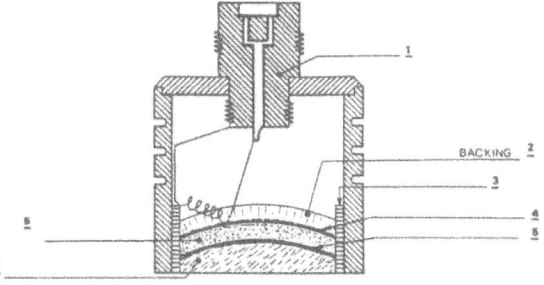

Fig. 3.1.1 - Schematic section of a focussed transducer for echotomography.
1) connector; 2) backing material; 3) acoustical insulator ring; 4) posterior electrode; 5) anterior electrode; 6) curved piezoelectric ceramic; 7) anterior matching material.

Between the piezoelectric element and the anterior surface of the transmitter an impedance matching layer is formed. In its simplest form, the layer has a thickness of λ/4, or its uneven multiple, at the central frequency of resonance of the piezoelectric element and depending on the speed of longitudinal waves in the medium of which this layer is composed. This material is obtained by loading epoxy resin with tungsten powder to approximate the value of characteristic impedance of about 6.7×10^5 g/cm^2 x s which represents the theoretical value of geometric mean impedance between that of the ceramic surface and that of water or soft biological tissues. This allows maximum transfer of energy between the two media. In more recent transducers several superimposed layers are used each with λ/4 with closer differences in impedance value to pass from the ceramic impedance value ($\simeq 30 \times 10^5$ g/cm^2 x s) to that of water or biological tissues ($\simeq 1.5 \times 10^5$ g/cm^2 x s).

This transducer, also called a probe, is connected to the patient's skin by means of a watery or oily gel to guarantee mechanical continuity without an air gap which would lead to reflections of energy returning towards the transducer and thus prevent the formation of images or tracings. The whole system is fitted with a casing which acts as an electric screen as well as a container.

Fig. 3.1.1 shows a transducer for manual scanning equipment. The disk appears concave with the concavity towards the part to be placed in contact with the patient or liquid in the case of probes with a connecting tank. This curvature of the surfaces is due to the need to focus the ultrasound beam to improve lateral resolution (§ 3.2.1).

In other devices, the piezoelectric element has flat surfaces and a converging lens is attached to the transmitter face of the transducer. Other models use mirror focussing, or multiple elements controlled by delay lines which can be programmed electronically to provide electronic focussing (§ 3.2.1.2).

3.2 Ultrasonic field

If acoustic intensity is plotted along the axis of the flat disk transducer without a lens the dependence illustrated in Fig. 3.2.1 is obtained. The upper part of the figure shows a diagram of the plots of acoustic intensity in planes perpendicular to the axis of the transducer at various distances from the transmitter surface.

On the axis the intensity increases, on approaching the transducer, reaching a maximum at a distance x', called characteristic distance, from the source, given by:

$$x' = \frac{a^2}{\lambda} \qquad (3.2.1)$$

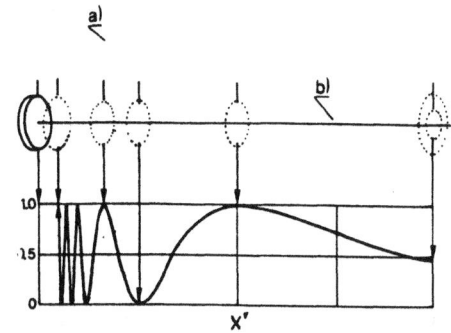

Fig. 3.2.1 - Variation of acoustic intensity in relation to distance from the transducer. a) Acoustic intensity on the emitting face of the transducer; b) Central axis of the acoustic beam. The upper part shows a diagram of the variation of acoustic intensity on planes perpendicular to the transducer axis. Below: the variation of intensity along the axis.

In (3.2.1) a is the radius of the piezoelectric disk and λ is the wavelength in the medium in which the ultrasound propagates.

From this point, continuing towards the source, the axial maxima and minima follow each other at short distances; the intensity in planes perpendicular to the acoustic axis also undergoes considerable variations over short distances.

Two regions in the beam can be distinguished, that between the source and the last axial maximum in x' is called the near zone (or Fresnel zone); the region from distance x' from the source theoretically up to infinity is called the far zone (or Fraunhofer zone). In the near zone the beam is approximately cylindrical; in the far zone it is conical and diverges by an angle $\pm\theta$ with respect to the central axis, obtained from:

$$\sin\theta = 0.61\lambda/a \qquad (3.2.2)$$

where a and λ have the meaning specified in (3.2.1).

In the near zone the considerable variations due to slight movements are caused by the interference of waves transmitted by various points of the source (flat disk) which escape, due to differences along the path equal to uneven multiples of half wavelength, creating points in which the intensity has minimum values, whilst path differences equal to a wavelength or its whole multiples interfere constructively giving maximum intensity values.

In the far zone, path differences due to waves transmitted by various points from the source are small, especially around the acoustic axis, so that acoustic intensity has a much more regular behavior and decreases as the inverse square of distance (§ 2.1) (conical shape which the beam assumes while it diverges).

As can be seen in (3.2.1) the shape of the beam mainly depends on the diameter of the transducer and the wavelength in the tissues in which the ultrasound propagates. For a transducer with a disk 20 mm in diameter, working at a frequency of 1.5 MHz, the beam formed in water can be considered cylindrical up to a distance of 10 cm from the piezoelectric crystal surface (near zone); beyond this distance the beam is conical with an overall aperture of about 7 degrees.

The length of the near field increases with the increase in diameter of the transducer and the ultrasound frequency. On the other hand, in the far zone, the divergence decreases with the increase in diameter and frequency.

3.2.1 Focussing

As stated above, in the near zone the beam has an irregular profile and is thus unreliable for reproduction of the structures examined with echography. As previously mentioned, it is possible to focus the ultrasonic beam so that the beam is formed at a slightly shorter distance from the transmitter face, compared with a non-focussed beam and with less divergence within a certain range of distances. The width of such a beam will then however increase with respect to the non-focussed beam, but at greater distances which are no longer useful for echographic examination.

3.2.1.1 Lens focussing

As previously mentioned, the ultrasonic beam can be focussed by placing acoustic lenses in front of the piezoelectric crystal (Fig. 3.2.1.1.1.). The target is "in focus" in the zone where the waves emitted by the various parts of the transducer arrive at the same time, i.e. in phase and thus interfering in a constructive fashion. Conversely, the echo signals from the focussed target reach each poin of the transducer at the same time, and hence in phase.

The lens material is usually absorbent and the increase in thickness towards the edges also has the effect of reducing the amplitude of the wave emitted from near edge points. This leads to alterations of the ultrasonic field, with a decrease in the focussing power of the system but with a useful reduction of the lateral lobes.

Fig. 3.2.1.1.1 - Transducer focussed using a superimposed acoustic lens (1) over the emitting face of the piezo-electric ceramic (2) surface.

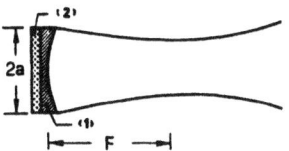

Lateral lobes. The lateral lobes of the ultrasonic beam are undesirable because, in the region of the useful central beam, they correspond to false directions, more or less differing from those of the main axis, in which the transducer emits and receives, though with less sensitivity.

Highly reflecting objects present in these spurious directions give reception signals which are added to those of objects present along the beam axis, i.e. along the sensing direction of the transducer, and hence along the line of sight displayed in the visualization screen. Confusing images can therefore be produced, as a result of this type of artifact.

3.2.1.2 Electronic focussing

In ultrasound diagnostics the target is a continuous object and optimal resolution requires focussing, i.e. good lateral resolution (§ 4.2) over the whole field of vision.

This can be achieved with a system which allows a focal distance varying continuously, or by small steps, as occurs in practice because the focal zone of the beam is of a certain finite extent (§ 3.2.1.3). In reception it is necessary to make sure that the focus is formed at gradually greater distances at a rate corresponding to the arrival of the signal returning from interfaces further and further away. The shift of focus towards greater distances, cyclically repeated at each excitation of the transducer, must take place at half the velocity of the returning ultrasonic signals in biological tissues. This is only possible using a system in which the focus is varied by an electronic control. As focussing of the emitted beam can only be fixed at the time of excitation of transducer, for transmission a focal distance is pre-arranged cyclically for each excitation. The whole distance to be explored is divided into a finite number of focal zones and a different zone is covered by each pulse emitted. In some equipment only one focussing is made in transmission for each line of sight.

Dynamic programmed focussing is obtained electronically using transducers made up of an array of several concentric rings (Fig.

3.2.1.2.1) or by an array of radiating linear elements and programmed delay lines operating in transmission and reception in a fashion similar to electronic sector scanning of the ultrasound beam (§ 6.2.2.1). By intuition the formation of a focussed beam can be imagined as being obtained from the convergence of rays emerging perpendicularly from a concave surface. Assuming we create a transmitting surface which is not continuous, but made up of discrete elements (Fig. 3.2.1.2.2a), the focal distance could be changed by altering the curvature of the surface on which the transmitting elements are placed.

It is possible to create electronically the delays corresponding to the physical distances to be travelled by the ultrasonic waves emitted by the individual elements when placed on a flat surface. If, as shown schematically in Fig. 3.2.1.2.2b, a linear array of elements is available, the difference in the path of the various waves for constructive interference to distance F, can be created electronically by delaying even further the excitation pulses which feed the transducers closest to the centre, as outlined in Fig. 3.2.1.2.2b, with a symmetrical law of delay with respect to the central element. In reception the signals received by the individual elements will be delayed by the same law and then summed up.

However, even in the case of the lens in Fig. 3.2.1.1.1. for fixe focus, the focussing mechanism can be intuitively understood bearing in mind that the lens material is characterized by a higher velocity of ultrasound propagation than that of the medium in which focussing is obtained, i.e. water or biological tissues. Hence the components of the wave front emitted at the same time from the various points of the flat ceramic surface reach an ideal flat surface parallel to the disk emitting face, with different delays (less for those nearer the margins as they have crossed a greater thickness of material at high speed) and they tend to arrive simultaneously on the axis at distance F as if they had been emitted from a curved surface such as that in Fig. 3.2.1.2.2a.

Fig. 3.2.1.2.1 - Annular ceramic array realized by laser cutting a piezoelectric ceramic disk (L. Masotti).

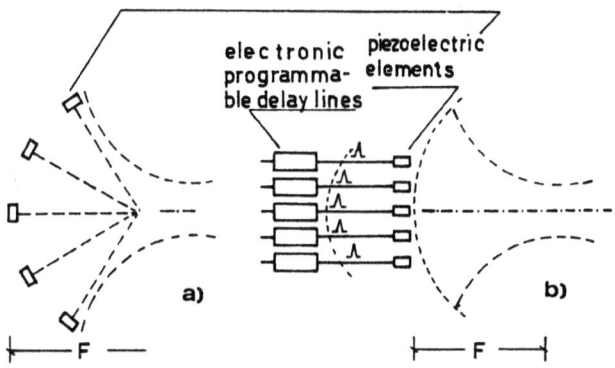

Fig. 3.2.1.2.2 - Multielement probe with focussed ultrasonic beam.
a) Curved surface array; b) Flat array with delay adjustment between signals of various elements.

The change in focal distance, which requires a change in the curvature of the surface of the components of Fig. 3.2.1.2.2a, is thus obtained by varying the law of delays in transmission and reception. In practice, different laws are used in transmission and reception. More specifically, a limited number of poorly defined and hence more extended focuses are used in transmission. The corresponding portion of the line of sight is formed for each corresponding element of the image by dynamic focussing made up of denser more pronounced focal segments in the zone of interest, using the law of delays in reception (Fig. 3.2.1.2.3).

In Fig. 3.2.1.2.1 a probe is shown for electronic focussing by an array of annular elements. The differences between the two systems mainly lie in the shape of the beam. For annular arrays the focussed beam has the same shape in all planes passing through the axis of the beam (this depends on the rotation symmetry of the structure). For linear arrays, the beam is focussed dynamically only in the plane containing the beam axis and perpendicular to the narrow side of the emitting elements. The beam is thus dynamically focussed only in the scanning plane for linear arrays with lateral linear scans.

Similarly, for electronic sector scan arrays (§ 6.2.2.1) we shall see that electronic focussing is only possible in the scanning plane. In the plane perpendicular to that, only a fixed focus using a lens can be achieved at the present time.

Fig. 3.2.1.2.3 - Linear array probe with electronic dynamic focussing. A) Qualitative pattern of signal delay; B) Qualitative pattern of focussed beam shape. a) Focussing zones; b) transmission beam shape; c) reception beam shape.

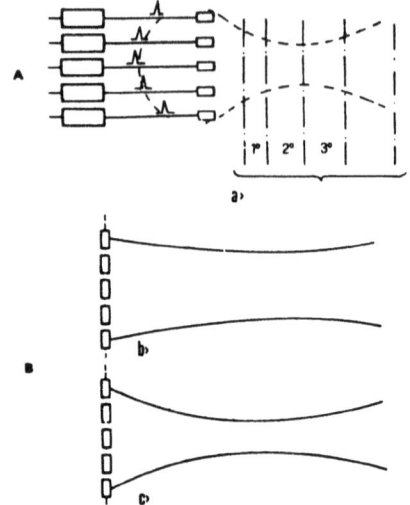

3.2.1.3 Characteristics of the focussed beam

There are three different types of focussing for fixed focus transducers: long, medium and short.

The first produces a narrow beam over a useful, rather wide range and, together with the medium type, is widely used in diagnostics. The size and shape of the focal region depend on the wavelength in the medium, the diameter of the transducer and the focal distance F from the lens; the greater the diameter of the transducer, the more defined the focus.

For a circular transducer the focal volume is an ellipsoid with a dimension D_y, according to Fry and Dunn*, in a perpendicular direction to the acoustic axis, between the points where the intensity is reduced by 3 dB with respect to the maximum:

$$D_y \simeq k_y \, F/2a \qquad (3.2.3)$$

with k_y roughly equal to 1 as long as ψ is less than 50 degrees (Fig. 3.2.1.3.1).

The length of the focal volume along the direction of the acoustic axis is obtained from:

---

* Fry W.J. and F. Dunn. Ultrasound: analysis and experimental methods in biological research. Physical Techniques in Biological (ed. W.L. Nastuk), vol. IV, 261-394, Academic Press N.Y. 1962.

$$D_x \simeq K \cdot D_y \tag{3.2.4}$$

if ψ is less than 50 degrees, K is given by 15 (1-0.01ψ) with ψ expressed in degrees.

It should be noted in (3.2.3) that the greater the diameter 2a of the piezoelectric disk, other conditions being equal, the smaller the D_y, i.e. the focal spot. Furthermore, from (3.2.4) it emerges that the smaller the focal spot, the smaller the depth of focus. These concepts are summarized in Fig. 3.2.1.3.2.

Finally it should be emphasized that the stronger the focussing, the higher the energy density in the focal zone and the echo signals reflected by objects in this zone are therefore more intense.

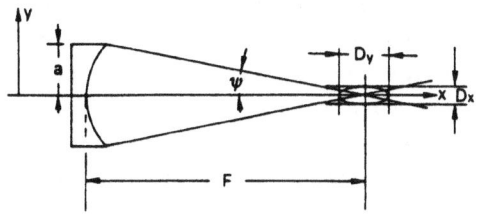

Fig. 3.2.1.3.1 - Diagram of the focal zone of a focussed transducer.

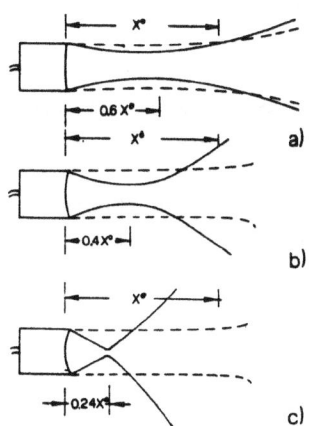

Fig. 3.2.1.3.2 - Diagram of the ultrasonic beam for long (a), medium (b) and short focussing (c). The continuous line represents the focussed beam profile, the dashed lines show that of the non-focussed beam.

4. Resolution

There are two types of resolution: *axial or range resolution* and *angular or lateral resolution*.

As is seen further on, it should be kept in mind that the resolutions obtainable by a system are highly dependent on the position of the controls of the equipment and on the display system. Therefore the following definitions are provided for potential resolutions and the causes of deviation from those obtainable in practice. It should also be pointed out that good resolution for the purpose of displaying images gives an improvement in terms of revealing details in the structures examined and clarity of contours.

4.1 Axial resolution

Axial resolution is the capacity to resolve two point reflectors in the direction of the axis of the ultrasound beam. In current systems axial resolution is better than the lateral resolution obtain able in practice.

Axial resolution depends on the duration of the ultrasonic pulse. In fact, the shorter the pulse, the shorter the distance between two adjacents objects which produce two echo signals which are only partially superimposed. Fig. 4.1.1 demonstrates that for a given pulse direction the signals of two objects (in this case, wires) tend to become superimposed and hence indistinguishable (i.e. not resolvable) as the wires move closer together.

If we assume (according to a broadly accepted standard) that for the distance x_2 the two signals are at the limits of distinguishibili ty, we can link axial resolution to the duration τ, measured between the two points on opposite sides of the peak, at which the amplitude is decreased by 6 dB (i.e. half value) compared with the maximum value. Generally the corresponding temporal distance between the peaks will also be τ and this distance can be calculated as the difference between wire 1 and wire 2 in the round-trip travel time of the ultrasound pulses.

The link between the two measurements: x_2, taken as the axial resolution, and τ, the duration of the pulse, is given by:

$$2x_2 = v \cdot \tau \qquad (4.1.1)$$

from which:

$$x_2 = \frac{v \cdot \tau}{2} \qquad (4.1.2)$$

where v is the ultrasound propagation velocity in the medium. From (4.1.2) it can be deduced that, for a given v, the better the axial resolution, i.e. shorter x_2, the shorter the duration of the pulse; this duration depends on how much the transducer is damped (§ 3.1), i.e. the number of vibrations emitted by the transducer when it is excited during transmission.

At a given central operating frequency, axial resolution improves when the transducer is more damped (Fig. 4.1.2).

Fig. 4.1.1 - Diagram of A-mode display of an echographic signal in three different situations for wires parallel to each other and perpendicular to the beam axis, struck by ultrasound in the direction of their alignment. The echographic signals are more or less distinguishable depending on the reciprocal distance of the wires.

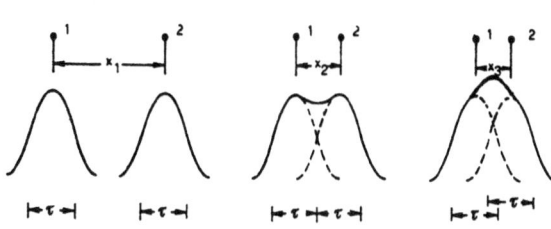

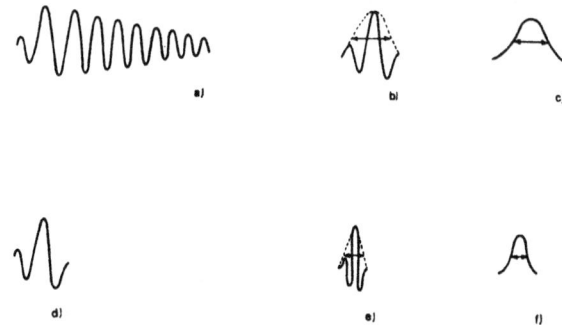

Fig. 4.1.2 - At the same frequency a non highly damped transducer: d) emits and receives shorter pulses and hence allows better axial resolution than a low damped transducer a). At the same dampening, i.e. number of oscillations in the pulse b), c), a higher frequency transducer, e), allows shorter impulses and hence better axial resolution c), f).

Axial resolution also depends on the frequency, improving with an increase in frequency. This dependence on frequency follows from the fact that for transducers with the same damping (resonance coefficient Q) the number of significant oscillations contained in the pulse is practically the same for different frequencies. As the frequency increases, there is a decrease in the duration, i.e. the period of time of the single oscillation, and hence the duration of the pulse.

4.2 Lateral resolution

Lateral resolution signifies the capacity for resolving two point reflectors at an equal distance from the transducer but situated in two different directions from it.

This resolution *depends on the width of the ultrasonic beam at the distance under consideration, i.e. on the point at which the objects to be resolved are situated*. In practice how can you tell whether lateral resolution is more or less good? We imagine moving an ultrasonic beam as in Fig. 4.2.1, by moving the transducer either manually or mechanically, depending on automatic scanning, or by making an electronic commutation of the active elements of an array, or finally by operating an electronic scan (§ 6.2.2.1).

In this way we can explore the objects situated along the various lines of sight and observe the result presented on the screen. Ideally, only the objects present along a single orientation of the ultrasound beam should appear in the image on the corresponding line of sight displayed on the screen. In practice, since the ultrasonic beam is wider than the width corresponding to a single line of vision, the objects are displayed in a distorted fashion, i.e. a sort of lengthening of the objects in a transverse direction, perpendicualr to the orientation of the ultrasonic beam. In this way, objects which are in fact separate may appear attached in the image (cf. Fig. 4.2.1).

The maximum lateral resolution of a focussed transducer occurs in the focal region of the ultrasonic beam. The narrower the focal spot, the shorter the transverse distance between two point reflectors at which they can still be distinguished in the image. Lateral resolution can be evaluated by knowing the acoustic pressure profile of the ultrasonic beam impinging on an object. Taking a small sphere as the object, Fig. 4.2.2 illustrates the profiles of acoustic intensity at a generic distance from the transducer.

At various distances from the transducer a width y_0 at -3 dB, or at -6 dB with respect to the maximum, can be defined in the profile of acoustic pressure and linked to lateral resolution. If we assume that the display system, possibly using suitable chromatic codes, allows adjacent levels with small differences to be distinguished, in a situation such as that illustrated in Fig. 4.2.2, we can attribute to the transducer (simple or array) a resolution equal to the width of the beam y_0 at -6 dB at the distance considered from the transducer. For a different distance, the profile of acoustic pressure changes and hence the value y_0 (Fig. 4.2.2).

Fig. 4.2.1 - Diagram of data loss in the echographic image due to poor lateral resolution. In fact wires 1 and 2 struck perpendicularly to their axis by the ultrasonic beam cannot be distinguished in the echographic image.

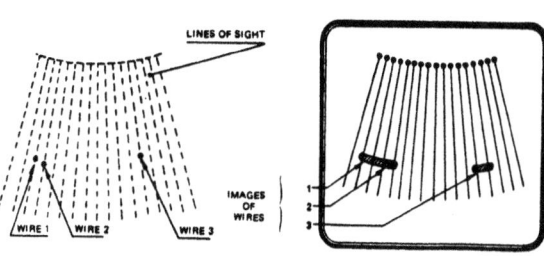

Fig. 4.2.2 - Relative pattern of acoustic pressure in a direction perpendicular to the axis of the ultrasonic beam which strikes the two wires 1 and 2 at the reciprocal distance y_o, moving the transducer parallel to itself. At different distances from the transducer different values of the distance between the points are obtained at which acoustic pressure has been reduced by -6 dB with respect to maximum.

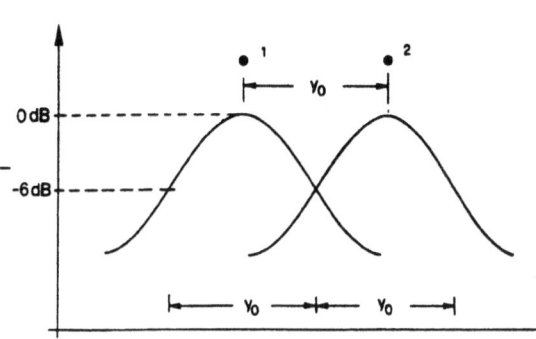

It should be kept in mind that other values can be given for lateral resolution, defining it as the width of the beam measured at -20 dB or at -40 dB with respect to the maximum rather than referring to -6 dB as above.

It should also be emphasized that if the profile of acoustic pressure impinging on the single wire during the movement of the transducer is that shown in Fig. 4.2.2, the amplitude of the signal received for objects along the directions at a distance of $y_o/2$ with respect to the maximum direction, is not at -6 dB but at -12 dB compared with that received from objects along the maximum direction, i.e. acoustic axis. This occurs because the transducer emits an amplitude 6 dB lower in directions at $y_o/2$ and in reception it is also 6 dB less sensitive along these directions with respect to the maximum direction, so that the total amplitude received is 12 dB lower. This makes the possibility of distinguishing point targets more convincing, having defined the lateral resolution as corresponding to the width of the beam at 6 dB. Further on, we shall see that lateral resolution is degraded by the effect of compression on signals, performed in order to enable adequate screen display (Fig. 5.3.1.2).

4.3 Influence of amplification on resolution in B-mode display

Accurate adjustment of amplification is important for both axial and lateral resolution. A threshold exists in all B-mode display systems above which the signal is displayed.

As seen in Fig. 4.3.1, different images are obtained by varying the amplification control of the ultrasonic device. Different images are obtained for the same objects, at the same distance, with the sam transducer and hence with the same potential lateral resolution, measured as width of the signal at -6 dB from the maximum. An increase in amplification leads to a greater width of displayed signal. The B-mode display shown in Fig. 4.3.1 is of the bistable type, with grey scale this effect is less pronounced but still important due to the compression of the signals and non-linear response of the display system.

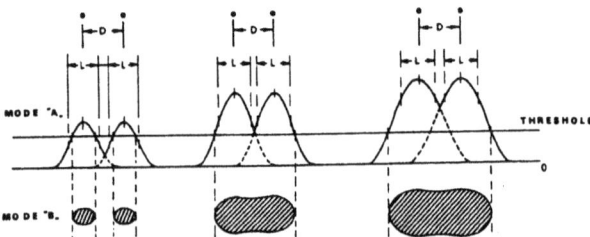

Fig. 4.3.1 - Diagram of the influence of gain adjustment of echographic equipment on the resolution obtained in B-mode display. As the gain increases (right-hand figure) the rendering of details in the images deteriorates.

5. Equipment

Mention was made in section 1 of the principle of displaying echo signals so as to create images corresponding to the region explored by the sensor. Let us briefly go over the concepts in order to illustrate several characteristics of the equipment.

Fig. 5.1 shows a diagram of a piece of manual scanning echotomographic equipment. The probe is made up of a single transducing element which is made to be replaceable in order to provide a choice of the most suitable size, frequency and focal distance for the examination required. The probe is moved manually across the skin surface of the patient in the section plane to be examined.

In automatic scanning, single element probes may be arranged to undergo rapid mechanical vibration, or rotation for sectorial exploration. Alternatively, there are probes made up of several transducing elements (in technical terms the group of elements is referred to as an "array") placed one next to the other and electronically activated in a suitable sequence. This subject will be further explored in the following paragraphs.

Fig. 5.1 shows the trigger-pulse generator which simultaneously synchronizes the transmitter, the sweep generator and the time-gain compensation amplifier (which compensates for the increase in attenuation with range). The probe contains a piezoelectric material, usually constructed using piezoelectric ceramic of lead zirconate titanate or lead metaniobate.

As stated earlier, the laws governing the reflection of ultrasound are similar to those of optics, so that the echo signals from interfaces more or less perpendicular to the axis of the ultrasonic beam return to the transducer which converts them into electrical signals. The arrival time of these signals depends on the distance from the interfaces and the speed of ultrasound.

In soft human tissue the speed can be taken as approximately 1500 m/s so that a thickness of one centimetre travelled by ultrasound on a return journey corresponds to a delay of about 13.3 μs (microseconds) for all soft tissue. If the transmission is repeated with the transducer pointing in the same direction at a sufficiently high repetition rate (with a frequency over 50 Hz) the image of the single line of sight, obtained by sending the received signals to a cathode-ray tube, is persistent.

Most equipment used for pulse ultrasound diagnosis has a repetition frequency between 300 and 3000 Hz with an ultrasonic pulse duration of a few microseconds. As stated earlier, the carrier-frequency of the pulse varies between 1 and 15 MHz depending on what the equipment is used for. On the one hand, the highest frequencies allow better resolution of the details of the internal organs of the human body, on the other there is less penetration as they involve greater absorption of ultrasound by living tissue (around 2 dB per MHz per cm of tissue thickness crossed on a return journey).

Time depth compensation (TDC) or time gain compensation (TGC).
In order to improve interpretation of the signals displayed on the cathode-ray tube, they are received by an amplifier whose magnification increases in time starting from the moment of synchronism of the driver rate, i.e. from the moment of transmission. Ideally this should make sure that the echo signals from deeper structures, hence more attenuated, are more amplified and thus give similar images for similar structures, independent of their depth.

Fig. 5.1 - Block diagram of a static scanner. 1) Rate driver or generator of the pulse repetition rate; 2) Transmitter; 3) Controller of gain compensation as a function of depth; 4) Sweep generator; 5) Receiver; 6) Cathode-ray tube; 7) Generator of position data of the ultrasonic beam.

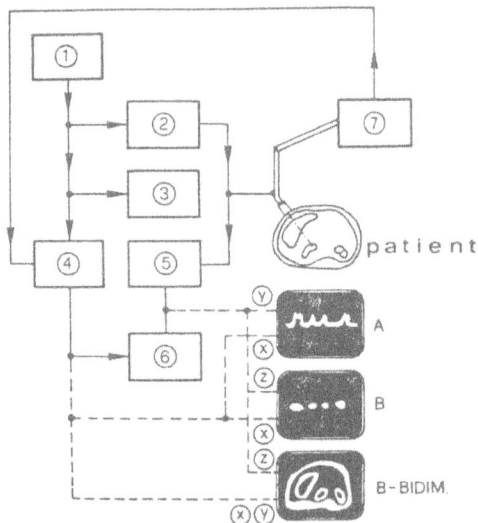

The display of echo signals on the cathode-ray tube varies according to the diagnostic use of the equipment.

In ultrasound echographic equipment various adjustments are possible such as variations in the amplitude of the ultrasonic pulse transmitted, adjustment of the law of gain variation in time, variations in a circuit threshold to eliminate lower signals and possible pre- and post-processing controls as well as several ordinary controls of an oscilloscope.

5.1.1 A-mode display

By transmitting the echo signals to vertical deflection plates of the oscilloscope and the sweep generator output to horizontal deflection plates a type A display is obtained (from the word amplitude (Fig. 5.1.4.1).

This display mode is used when diagnostic information can be obtained by studying the amplitude of the echo signals. This type of display is limited by the fact that it supplies time-amplitude information in the direction of a single ultrasonic line of sight and is therefore highly dependent on the angle and position of the probe, but nevertheless it provides useful information for tissue typing studies.

5.1.2 B-mode display

By causing the echo signals to modulate the brightness of the cathode-ray tube and connecting the sweep generator output to deflection plates a type B display is obtained (from the word brightness) (Fig. 5.1.4.1). In this way each echo signal is displayed at an appropriate point along an otherwise invisible time base.

The image is formed on the screen by the display of luminous dots corresponding to ultrasonic echoes. The brightness of the point increases with the amplitude of the echo signal according to a law which is not necessarily linear. Type B display is mainly limited by the low dynamic range provided by the brightness modulation of the cathode-ray tube. However, this system is the basis of two-dimensional type B imaging and TM display systems (time-motion).

5.1.3 Two-dimensional B-mode display

B-mode systems, in which echo signals are displayed as illuminated dots, allow the screen to display several lines of sight at the same time, i.e. a number of sensing directions of the manual or automatic scanning probe. In this way the examination can be carried out with a hand-held or mechanical scanning probe.

The illuminated dots are displayed on the screen in the same sequence of time and geometry according to which the ultrasonic signal encounters a differing acoustic impedance along its path, whilst the ultrasonic beam moves in the scanning plane.

A mechanical arm can be fitted to the probe of a manual scanning device which permits movements within one plane and electronically transmits to the display system the required information about the position and orientation of the probe. In automatic scanning the reference points of the ultrasonic beam are electronically formed in succession.

By transmitting the echo signals to the brightness modulation of the cathode-ray, and the position data together with the time base signals to the deflection system, a two-dimensional B-mode display is obtained. The data on the position of the probe and the direction of the ultrasonic beam in the patient's body are used to determine on the screen the location and direction of the time base, modulated in brightness. This system permits two-dimensional imaging of a section (tomography) in the scanning plane with continuous recording of echo signals as the probe is moved around the patient by hand or as the ultrasonic beam is moved automatically.

Fig. 5.1.4.1 - A-mode display, B-mode display and diagram of TM tracing.

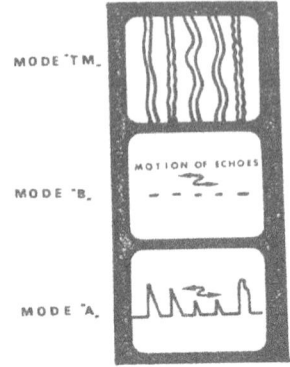

In order for the eye to see the whole image as the ultrasonic beam is moved during scanning, the brightness at individual points has to persist sufficiently to accomodate manual or slow automatic scanning. In other words, the echo signals successively received fro the interfaces encountered by the ultrasonic signal from different orientations of the probe are stored in a memory. In early types of equipment this image storage was obtained with storage tubes and, later, electronic scan converters were used to form the image.
More recently, digital storage systems have been introduced, based on principles similar to those used in computers (§ 5.3). In automat ic scanning systems with a high number of images per second, the images from all lines of sight in a predetermined sequence are formed in rapid succession so that the eye of the observer can follow its development directly on the screen of the cathode-ray tube without a scan converter system. However, in the latest equipment it is possible to "freeze" an image of particular interest using digital stor age devices. Automatic systems with high line density, and thus having a low image frame rate, also require scan converters by which to display the image.

5.1.4 Time motion

This is a fairly special type of screening mode widely used in echocardiography but which is also arousing interest in obstetrics for the monitoring of fetal movements and cardiac pulsations.
The probe is kept fixed along a chosen line of sight and the ech signals are displayed on the screen as illuminated dots along a vert cal (or horizontal) line which runs slowly (several centimetres a se ond) in a horizontal (or vertical) direction, remaining parallel to itself. The echo signals, from moving anatomical structures such as

valves and cardiac walls, correspond to illuminated dots which move nearer or further away with respect to the illuminated dot corresponding to the transmitter face of the probe. The dimension of the display line parallel to itself allows the display of the progress in *time* of this motion depending on the scaling factor due to the running speed of the illuminated tracing (Fig. 5.1.4.1).

In this way a tracing is formed which marks the course in time of the various positions assumed by the reflecting surfaces or scattering tissue discontinuities encountered by the ultrasonic signal on its course. Apart from the screen of a cathode-ray tube, the tracing can also be recorded on light-sensitive paper with a fiberoptic recorder, or photographed as a "frozen" image on the screen using digitized scan converters.

5.2.1 Doppler technique

If an ultrasonic wave travels between two transducers along a path of varying length in time, the frequency at the receiver differs from that at the transmitter (Doppler effect) by an amount $f_D = 2v_r(\cos\gamma) f/v$, f being the frequency transmitted, v_r the velocity of the reflector, v the velocity of ultrasound propagation in the medium considered and γ the angle between the direction of the ultrasonic beam and the direction of the reflector's movement.

In many applications use is made of frequency shift of a continuous wave ultrasonic beam reflected by a moving structure, to collect information on its velocity. The objects of this study are the movements of red corpuscles of blood vessels and the displacement of valve flaps of the fetal heart. In the latter applications the measurement obtained is the frequency of the fetal heart beat.

The frequencies used in obstetrics and gynaecology are 2 - 5 MHz, whilst frequencies up to 10 MHz are adopted in the study of superficial vessel blood flow.

5.2.2 Continuous wave Doppler systems

The transmitter emits continuous vibrations; the probe contains a receiving and a transmitting transducer. The signals at different frequencies at the mixer output (obtained from the beat of signals from moving structures with signals from fixed structures or from the reference signal emitted) are filtered, amplified and transmitted to a loudspeaker or headphones in order to aid interpretation through the ear of the operator, and to a recording and processing device, the latest models of which also supply spectral analysis.

5.2.3 Direction sensitive Doppler systems

Data on the direction of movement of the structure under examination are supplied by the sign of f_D; by more complex processing, based on multiple frequency conversions, it is also possible to extract information on the sign of f_D and separately to display the spectrum of frequency shift corresponding to positive and negative flow velocities.

5.2.4 Pulsed Doppler systems

Continuous wave Doppler systems do not supply information on the distance of the different reflectors from the probe, whereas pulsed transmission systems do provide such data.

Doppler signals can be separated by means of the "distance gate" technique in which the frequencies of isolated echo signals at an interval of distance are compared with those of a pulse modulated continuous wave oscillator which supplies a constant transmitted frequency. Some types of equipment display tracings of the progress in time of the speed of small blood volumes revealed in dynamic sonographic images of both the heart and body sections, including the vessels. Recently, maps of blood movements across the heart valves have been obtained.

5.3 Grey scale tomographic images

For images displayed as representations of echo amplitude, i.e. B-mode, use of a storage tube does not provide good data on the different amplitudes of echo signals, due to the very limited range of the brightness obtainable. The conventional storage tube permits imaging of organ contours but does not include information on the amplitude of echo signals, due to the very low dynamic range of the signals displayed. Variations in the amplitude of echo signals due t the weak reflection of the internal structure of tissues, typical of their internal architecture, contain information on the type and sta of tissues. In order to better exploit the information on the interaction between ultrasonic energy and tissues, imaging has been force to display signals formed both by the energy reflected and that scat tered by microstructures.

The use of non-linear amplification results in a change in the ratio between the amplitude of echo signals so that within the dynamic range of grey scale, or chromatic shading of the screen it is possible to display the effects of both reflected energy and much weaker diffuse energy. In particular, most of the dynamics of grey or chromatic scale are reserved for the display of weak echo signals deriving from the parenchyma, while the small upper part is reserved for the signals derived from the major interfaces, the variations of which are almost solely dependent on the inclination of the interfaces themselves.

5.3.1 Digitized memory image converters

The shades of grey required are not provided by a conventional storage tube, so that two types of information backing systems have been developed, the mosaic memory of television image converters and electronic memories for discrete signals stored in digital form (Fig. 5.3.1.1).

The images can be formed on a television picture tube, maintaining the grey levels written in digital form by a memory that is read according to the standard television raster, which is generally different from that of the writing sequence which is dependent on the law of scanning of the ultrasonic beam, but maintaining the true relative position of the image dots.

It is interesting to consider the possibility of selecting different programmes to vary the law of assignment of the amplitude of echo signals at different levels of grey or colour (Fig. 5.3.1.2). The example in Fig. 5.3.1.2 illustrates how this type of preprocessing permits separation in programme A of two echo signals (c, d) which are assigned to the same grey level in programme B. The future applications offered by this innovation could increase the potential of identifying tissues for each particular study, selecting the assignment programme best suited to differentiating the echo signals scattered by the parenchyma of two different organs in the same patient.

An essential prerequisite for the clinical application of this potential is the accurate setting of the equipment and adequate operating stability.

The availability of images already in digitized form allows both manual and automatic scanning systems to transfer the data directly to a computer when complex processing such as quantification of ultrasonic data, image reconstruction and data extraction for tissue characterization are required, or images need to be stored for later comparison.

In automatic scanning systems it is important to be able to freeze single images, maintaining the display with its grey scale. In this case the memory is no longer updated at the rate of sequence of ultrasonic images, but stores the content of the chosen image, which is repeatedly read at the rate and with the raster of the television standard used.

When required by the system's characteristics or the conditions of use, with this digital storage system a flicker-free display can also be obtained of ultrasonic images formed at a low frame rate.
A further possibility provided by digitized storage devices for parallel line electronic scanning systems, is the formation by interpolation of extra lines of sight with respect to those physically obtained by the transducers. Finally, if digitized memories with an adequate capacity are available, potentially interesting real time processing can be developed such as: comparison between different images, display of different levels of the image using chromatic codes, computation of contours and areas or histograms, display of data on spectral changes of the signal due to selective absorption or Doppler effect, by using for these data chromatic codes superimposed on the grey scale image.

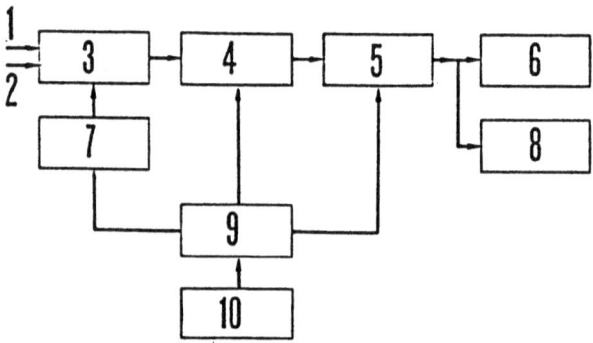

Fig. 5.3.1.1 - Block diagram of digitized memory and scan converter system. 1) Echo signals; 2) Ultrasonic beam position and direction signals; 3) Analog to digital signal converter; 4) Digital memory; 5) Digital to analog signal converter; 6) Display; 7) Preprocessing; 8) Video tape recorder; 9) Microprocessor; 10) Key board for patient data entering and processing control.

5.4 Radio frequency signal

As seen in Fig. 5.4.1, the echo signal received is amplified and detected, filtered, possibly differentiated and amplified yet again prior to formation of the image. Research is currently underway to extract information from the radio frequency (RF), i.e. the signal in the form it assumes prior to detection [46].

Fig. 5.3.1.2 - Characteristic preprocessing curve for the assignment of echo signal amplitudes to grey levels or chromatic scale. Two combinations between echo signal amplitudes and grey levels for two different programmes are shown on the lower part.

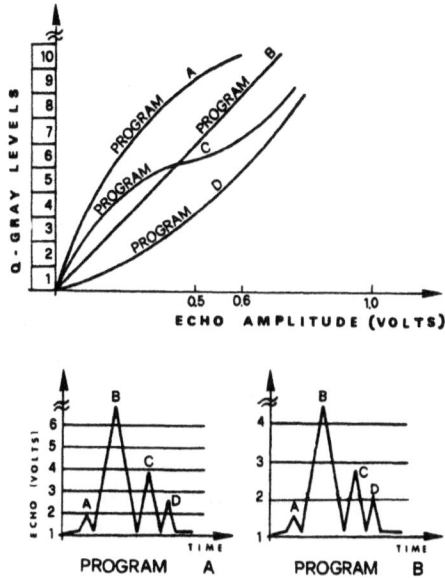

Fig. 5.4.1 - Analog processing operation performed on the received echo signal prior to display. a) Basic RF signal; b) Amplified RF signal; c) Rectified signal; d) Detected signal envelope; e) Detected signal leading edge.

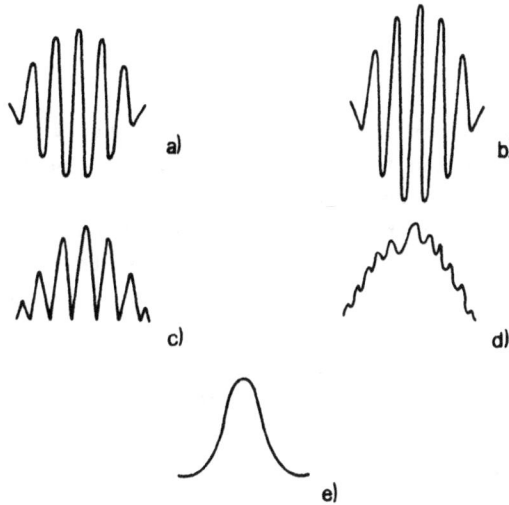

6. Recent developments

6.1 Basic characteristics of new echographic equipment

Ultrasound equipment for medical diagnosis is gradually becoming more sophisticated under the impetus of intense research activity that is underway on different technical and medical aspects. Several of the latest innovations have been incorporated in equipment already on sale; others are still at the experimental stage in laboratory prototypes.

Two research trends still characterize the work devoted to development of the diagnostic potential of ultrasound equipment. The first can be characterized as perfecting the ultrasonic field to be created within the human body in the region of interest and consists of:
a) Developing the "optics" of ultrasonic transducers as regards size, shape, static focussing law and dynamic focus programming;
b) Improving the modalities of exploration in the zone of interest such as scanning type and velocity;
c) Improving the ultrasonic signal emitted by the transducer.

The second aim of research can briefly be summarized as the development of the possibilities for extracting information supplied by the echo signals, that has been reinforced by the above mentioned developments in improving the spatial distribution of ultrasonic energy in the organ to be examined. This field can be divided into two wide branches:
1. Use of amplitude data contained in the echo signals, which has already led to the introduction of the grey scale, histograms and chromatic codes;
2. Use of not only the data linked to the arrival time of echo signals, and hence the position of the interface of origin, but also information on the form of the returning signal and hence its content in terms of frequency; linked on the one hand to the Doppler effect, i.e. the velocity of displacement, and on the other to the structure and nature of the reflection and scattering of biological tissues.

With equipment recently placed on the market, and some still at the prototype stage, it is possible to collect qualitative data on the spatial distribution of blood velocity in the heart and large vessels. Differentiation of tissues by means of the spectral content of radio frequency echo signals and spatial distribution of speckle are still at the initial experimental stage.

6.2 Several basic principles of new equipment

The principles behind several pieces of the latest equipment will be examined, although it is impossible to deal with all aspects of new developments in this field.

It should be emphasized that recent research has concentrated on perfecting the spatial distribution of ultrasonic energy in the organ under examination in order to collect greater information. Particular importance has been placed on the scanning law of the ultrasonic beam during exploration of the zone of interest. Automatic scanning systems of the ultrasonic beam have been developed alongside hand-held probes.

6.2.1 <u>Mechanical automatic or mixed mechanical electronic scanning</u>

Mechanical automatic or mixed mechanical electronic scanning is characterized by the use of electric motors to move the transducers and electronic switching to operate the transducing elements according to suitable laws when multiple transducers are used. Whilst the ultrasonic beam moved in this way explores the area of interest, the return signals are displayed as intensification - B (brightness) mode - of the illuminated dot on the screen, depending on the organization of the lines forming the display on the screen, according to the section under examination. An image is produced for each scan of the transducers. If a sequence of scans is performed at a sufficiently high frequency, a continuous *real time* display is supplied of sections of the organ, even though it is in motion.

There are various automatic scanning systems of the ultrasonic beam.

I - Sectorial oscillation of the transducer like the movement of a pendulum (Fig. 6.1(a)), (Fig. 6.1(b)), (Fig. 6.1(c)):
- In direct contact with the patient;
- By means of a coupling pouch full of liquid;
- By oscillation on a reflecting mirror placed in the path of the ultrasonic beam emitted by the fixed transducer (Fig. 6.2).

II - Rotation of a round multiple structure with transducers on the periphery, either directly coupled to the patient or, in the latest models, not directly in contact with the skin surface (Fig. 6.3);
- Rotation of a hollow round multiple structure carrying internal transducers with fixed mirrors to direct the beam inside the patient with scanning in the rotation plane, or according to a sector having as its axis the rotation axis (Fig. 6.4(a));
- Rotation of several round multiple structures with transducers on the periphery for sectorial or compound scanning (Fig. 6.4(b)).

III - Curved multiple structure with an intermediary water bath with electronically switched transducers oscillating to achieve sectorial or compound scanning (Octoson) (Fig. 6.5);

- Curved multiple structure oscillating with an intermediary water bath and electronically switched transducers for sectorial or compound scanning (Fig. 6.6).

IV - Rotating or oscillating structures fixed on endoprobes for examination of various organs through the gastro-intestinal tract, the prostate through the anus, the bladder through the urethra , the hear through the oesophagus [47] (Fig. 6.7).

V - Oscillating structures or sectorial electronic scanning arrays, fixed on the end of the arm of manual scanning devices to obtain simple or compound scans (Fig. 6.9.1).

Systems I and II supply sectorial images whilst system III provides curvilinear trapeziform images. System IV can supply sectorial or circular images depending on whether rotation is complete or is co fined to oscillation within a limited angle.

The latest types of linear array or electronic parallel line scan endoprobes, fitted into endoscopes, supply rectangular images.

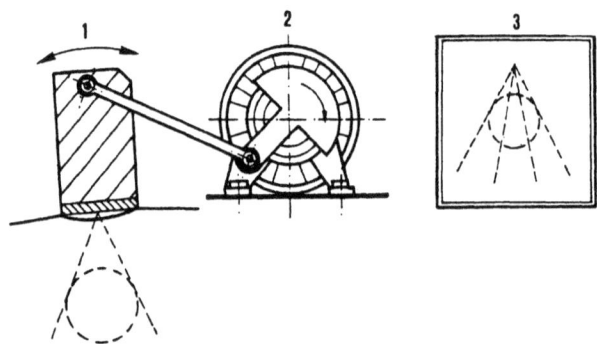

Fig. 6.1(a) - Diagram of a sectorial mechanical probe; 1) transducer; 2) electric motor; 3) oscilloscope screen.

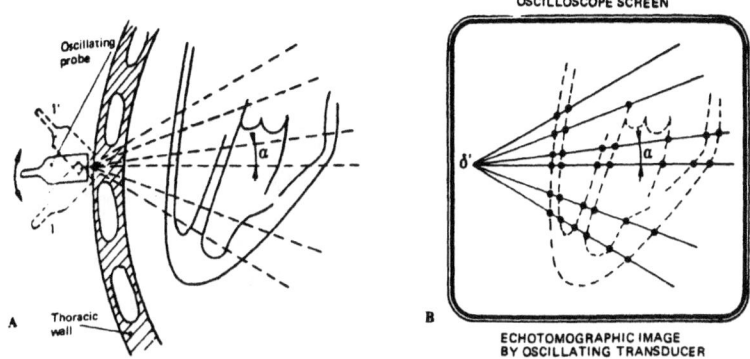

Fig. 6.1(b) - Diagram of a sectorial mechanical scanning probe; A) In contact with the thoracic wall; B) The diagram on the right illustrates a simplified echotomographic image.

Fig. 6.1(c) - Diagram of an oscillating mechanical scanning sectorial probe (Aloka, Siemens). 1) Crank; 2) Connecting rod; 3) Coupling membrane; 4) Transducer; 5) Position coding for lines of sight; 6) Holder containing starter motor.

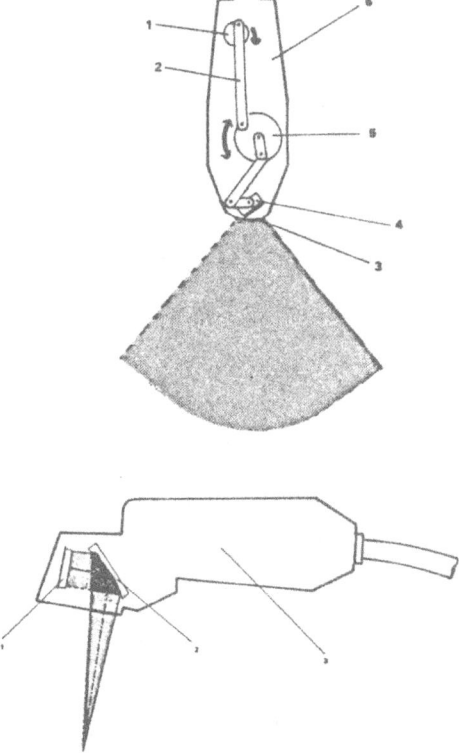

Fig. 6.2 - (a) Sectorial scanning probe with fixed transducer and oscillating mirror. 1) Transducer; 2) Oscillating mirror; 3) Housing for motor and angular position transduction to transmit data from the line of sight to the display system (Technicare, USA).

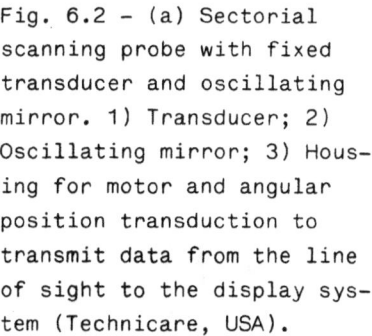

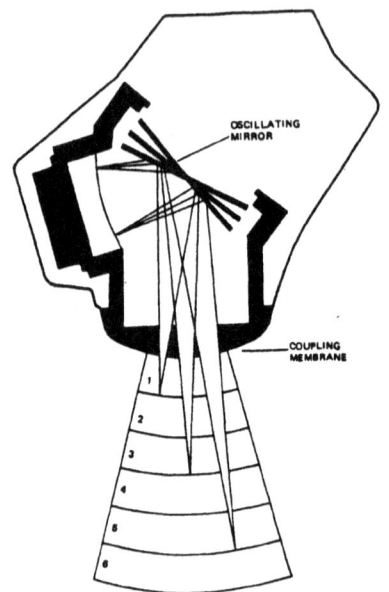

Fig. 6.2 - (b) Dynamically focussed concentric annular array probe (Fig. 3.2.1.2.1) with oscillating mirror, A, for beam scanning through an elastic membrane, B, (Smith and Kline).

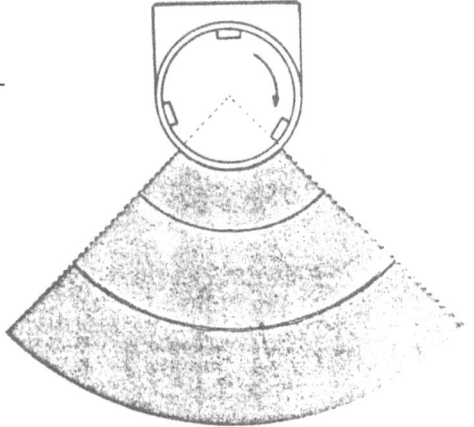

Fig. 6.3 - (a) Rotating probe with multiple transducers fixed on the periphery.

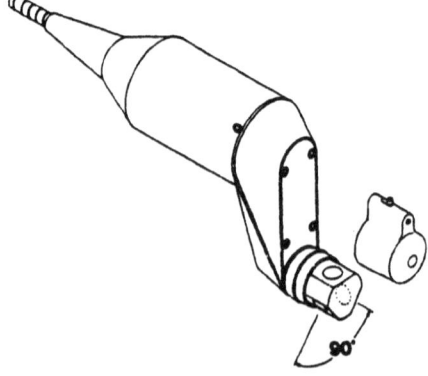

Fig. 6.3 - (b) Diagram of a rotating probe with several transducers. The transducers are fixed on a rotating wheel. Probe manufactured by ATL. Corp., Seattle, Washington.

Fig. 6.4 – (a) Rotating probe made up of a hollow circular structure bearing transducers; 2) On its internal surface, with fixed mirrors; 3) To direct the beam, as a sectorial scan in the rotation plane, through the lateral window; 4) Or scanning in a plane parallel to the rotation axis, through the axial window, 1, (G.E., USA).

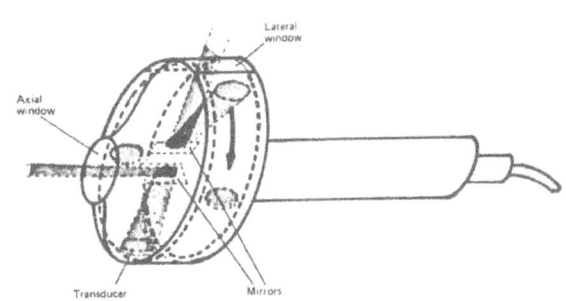

Fig. 6.4 (b) – Diagram of a multiple probe for sectorial and/or compound scanning. 1) Starter motor holder and coding device to obtain position data of lines of sight; 2) Coupling membrane; 3) Timing belt for motion transmission; 4) Transducer; 5) Gear wheel carrying transducer (Siemens).

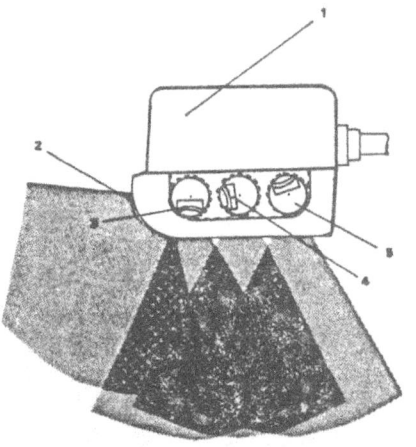

Fig. 6.5 – Scanning system with 8 transducers, fixed on an arc, each of which oscillates ±15°, electronically switched at a suitable sequence for simple or compound sectorial scanning (Octoson, Ausonics).

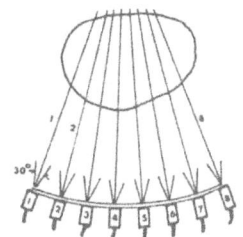

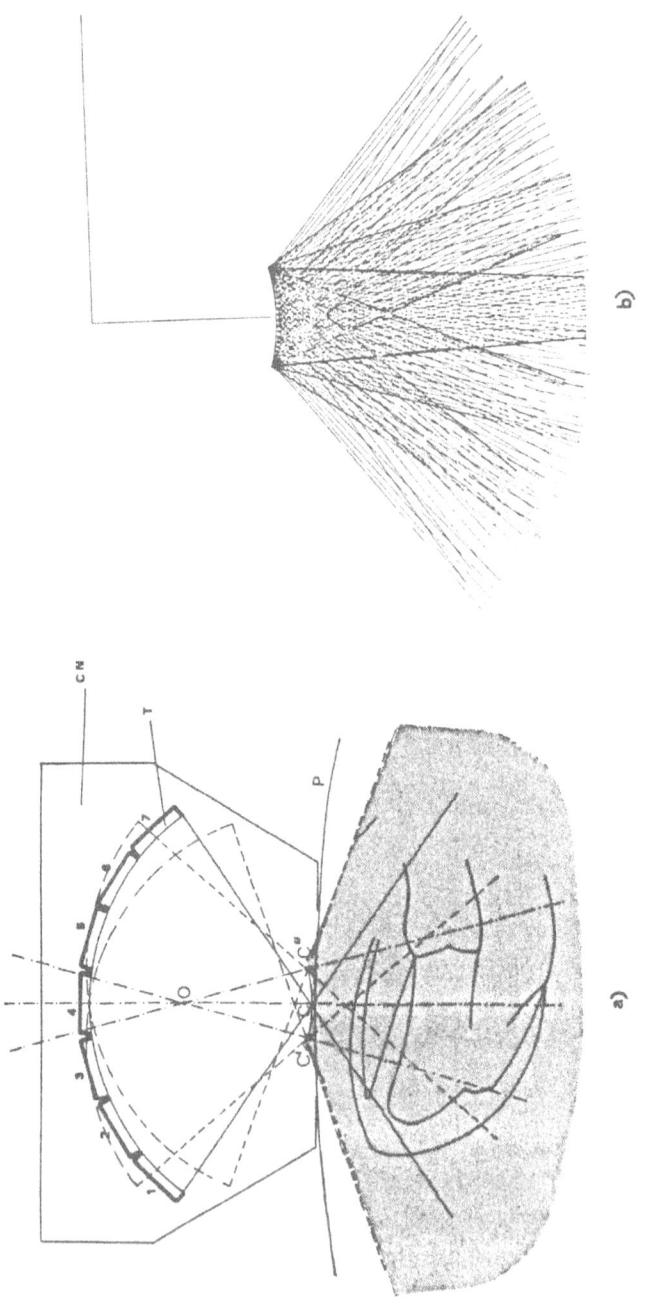

Fig. 6.6 - Diagram of a sectorial and/or compound scanning multiple probe, with a water bath between transducers and patient. T = Long focus double back transducer. The seven transducers are fixed on an arc which oscillates around point O with an angular swing of 30°. The transducers are electrically switched in a suitable sequence controlled by the operator (Eptacomp, prototype developed by L. Masotti, Institute of Electronics, University of Florence). CN = container; P = patient. a) Oscillating arc with transducers; b) Pattern of lines of sight for compound scanning in one of the possible switching sequences of the transducer.

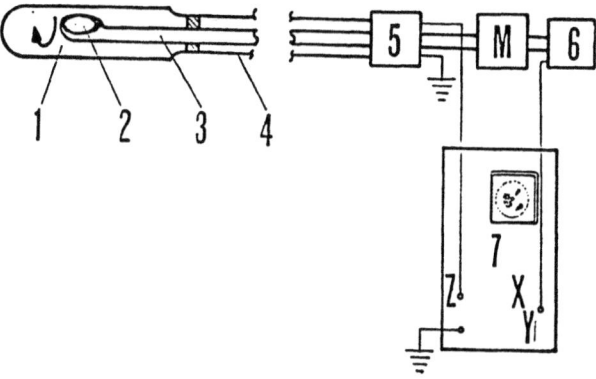

Fig. 6.7 - Endoprobe. 1) Head of the endoprobe, possibly inflatable with water or oil to contact the walls at the cavity in which it is inserted; 2) Transducer; 3) Rotating hollow internal sheath which transmits the rotatory or oscillatory motion to the transducer and contains the supply cable to the transducer; 4) External sheath which can be sterilized; 5) Structure to transfer the electrical signals to the cable of the rotating transducer; M) motion; 6) Transduction system to transmit data on the direction of the ultrasonic beam to the display system; 7) Display system (L. Masotti).

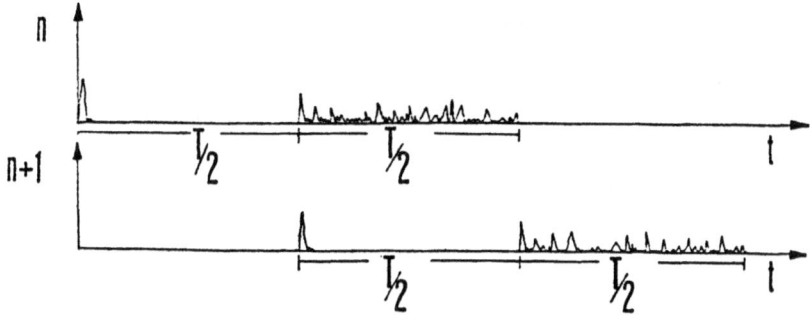

Fig. 6.8 - Diagram of multiple probes interleaving operation of two consecutive transducers. When the nth transducer starts to receive the signal from within the human body, the next transducer n + 1 begins transmitting and does not receive signals for the whole interval of the water bath, lasting T/2, between the transducer and the membrane coupled to the patient's skin.

6.2.1.1 Advantages of mechanical automatic or mixed electronic mechanical scanning systems

Mechanical scanning probes have several advantages and some of these are quite significant. Oscillating sectorial probes and some rotating devices have a small head which can be angled in a wide range of directions as long as no air enters between the probe and the skin surface. Furthermore, given the limited area of contact, it can be placed above an intercostal space for examinations of the hear eliminating the shadow effect of the ribs.

The mechanically moved transducer maintains its optical characteristics such as focalization and side-lobe level both in the scanning and perpendicular planes, as in any other plane passing through its longitudinal axis. This is extremely important for the quality of the images and the accuracy of measurements on TM tracings. As stated below, this advantage is not yet found in electronic scanning systems

Due to their greater simplicity, mechanical scanning probes often allow reliable real time echographic equipment to be produced at a limited cost, compared with electronic scanning probes.

There are several advantages in inserting a water bath:
- Use of wide diameter transducers with good focalization at the same frequency over all planes passing through the acoustic axis;
- Use of large concentric ring transducers to obtain dynamic focalization (Fig. 3.2.1.2.1);
- Use of the ultrasonic beam in the zone in which it is well focussed;
- No reduction in the number of images a second (provided that an appropriate scheme of interleaving between transmission and reception is used - see Fig. 6.8);
- When the bath is open, organs such as the breasts and testicles can be examined without a change in shape due to compression;
- Study of superficial organs without the problem of an extended blind zone in the image just under the skin surface.

6.2.2 Automatic electronic scanning

These probes allow the ultrasonic beam to explore the zone of interest without mechanical movement of the transducer. Basically there are two electronic scanning systems:
a) Electronic switching of one or more transducing elements of an array to change the line of vision by moving the beam parallel to itself (Fig. 6.10) or in a sectorial way (Fig. 6.9.1b).
b) Variation of the relative phase of the transducing elements of an array with the resulting variation of the direction of the ultrasonic

beam within a sector without moving the structure, but electronically creating the delay which could otherwise be physically introduced between the various transducing elements by physical rotation of the array (Fig. 6.11) (Fig. 6.13).

As the beam explores the zone of interest, the returning signals are applied to the intensification of the illuminated spot on the screen which is moved along lines which produce true images, i.e. with an accurate geometry, of the organ sections under examination.

Using type (a) scanning alone, the images formed are rectangular or sectorial. The number of transducing elements has been increased in the latest models (up to 380) and dynamic focalization has also been implemented in this type of parallel scanning array (Fig. 6.12). Using type (b) alone the images are sectorial, whilst a combination of both forms of scanning produces simple or compound rectangular, sectorial or trapezoidal images (Fig. 6.14).

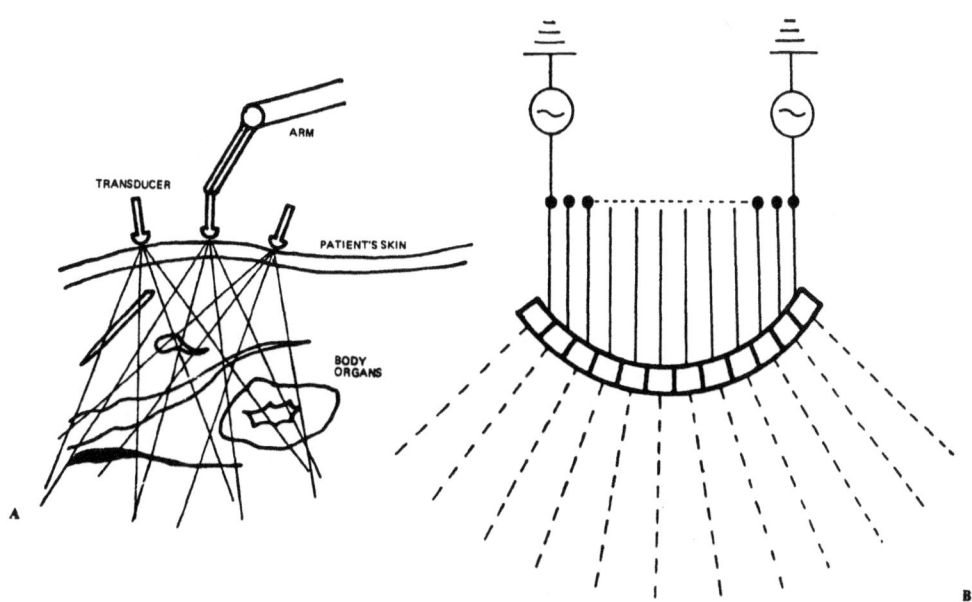

Fig. 6.9.1-Electronic switching sectorial scanning probe fitted onto the arm of a manual scanning device (Aloka, Japan).
a) Compound scanning with a manual scanner; b) Convex array transducer.

Fig. 6.9.2 - Mechanical sectorial scanning probe fitted into the arm of a manual scanning device (Technicare, USA).

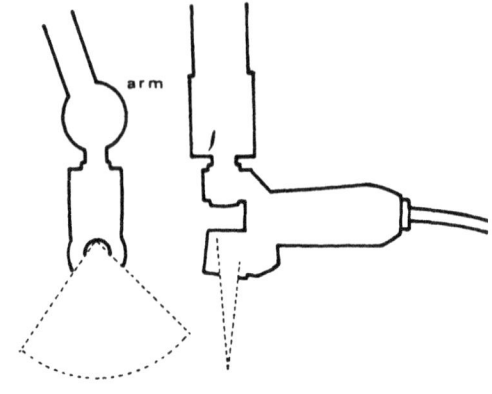

Fig. 6.10 - Electronic scanning probe using parallel lines beam obtained by means of a linear array transducer.

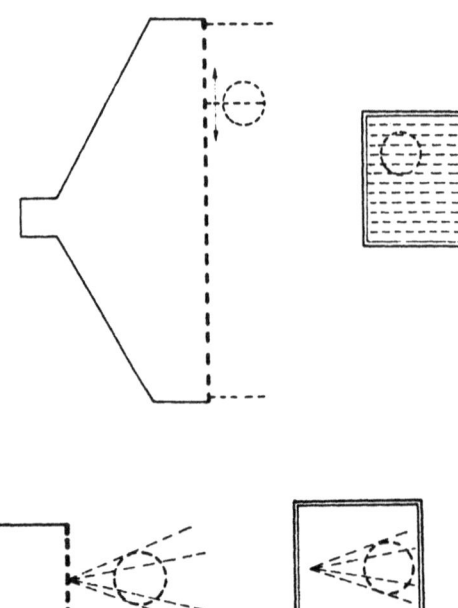

Fig. 6.11 - Sectorial electronic scanning probe using an array of transducers with variable delay between the signals of the various elements.

Fig. 6.12 - Linear array with parallel lines electronic scanning and dynamic focussing.
a) Qualitative behavior of the delays for the excitation of the various elements of a group.
b) Qualitative behavior of the focussed beam.

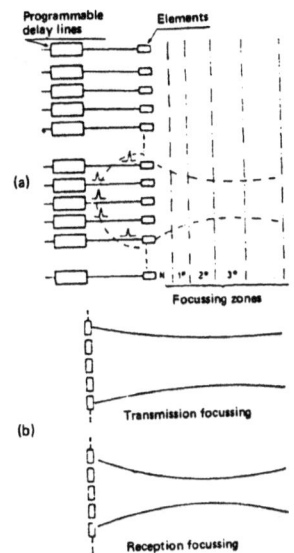

Fig. 6.13 - Phased array; beam scanning by varying electronically the delay $\tau_1, \tau_2, \tau_3, \ldots$ between the piezoelectric elements according to an appropriate law.

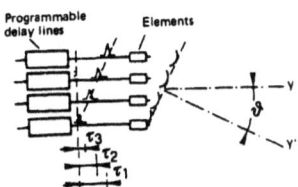

Fig. 6.14 - Electronic scanning probe for the following types of scanning: a) Parallel lines, b) Sectorial, c) Trapeziform, d) Compound.

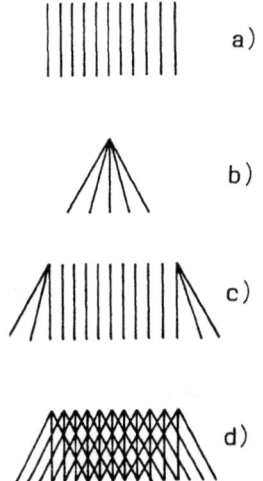

6.2.2.1 Phased transducer array

The probe is made up of a certain number of very narrow transducing elements (sixteen, twenty-one, thirty-two or sixty-four in current models) up to half a wavelength (in biological tissue at the working frequency) along the direction of alignment, each connected to a programmable delay line (Fig. 6.13) operating both in transmission and reception.

In practice, the lines are only used in reception, whilst simpler circuits are used in transmission to variously delay the excitation pulses of different elements. When the delays' supplied by the delay lines are null or equal to each other, the direction of maximum sensitivity, i.e. the direction of the major beam lobe, coincides with the axis y, normal to the emitting face of the structure, similarly to what occurs for the arrays described above and for the single transducers [49].

6.2.2.2 Advantages of the automatic electronic scanning systems

One advantage of the parallel beam scanning array is its easy application. In fact, this system displays real-time rectangular images which, due to only slight variations in degrees of freedom, make it possible to obtain very quickly sectional images of the zone of interest.

The rectangular image is clearly legible even in the portion covering the first few centimetres of tissue and displays a constant line density for the whole depth. Functional simplicity has the advantage over reliability and cost.

Equipment with this type of probe, if well made and fitted with transducers at different frequencies for various applications, appears very versatile. The limited lateral dimensions of the sectorial electronic scanning probe permit wide flexibility in viewing alignment and a good adaptability to the small pericardial window for applications in cardiology.

The TM tracing is of good quality, even though it is obtained at the same time as the two-dimensional real time image. In fact, the rate of the line of sight chosen for TM can be very high, comparable to that of the single probe as, unlike the mechanical sector scanner, it is possible for this device to be excited and receive a great number of times in the chosen direction, possibly with a slight reduction in the rate of two-dimensional images. Furthermore, the TM tracing for this type of probe can be perfected, thanks to the sighting possibilities available, unlike that of a parallel lines scanning device.

6.3 Characteristic parameters of automatic echographic systems

Brief mention should be made of the characteristics involved in the formation of automatic scanning two-dimensional images which are the basis of general and objective criteria of comparison for the various systems already available or at the experimental stage.

By assigning a certain maximum depth D to be visualized within the human body, the time required to receive the echo signals returning from the maximum depth is obtained from $T_L = 2D/v$ which corresponds to the time taken by the return journey of the ultrasound signal for the distance D at the velocity of propagation v. If the system supplies sectorial images in which d lines appear per degree which extend over θ degrees, we have d · θ lines per image. An image will be formed in a time $T_1 = d\theta T_L$, i.e. the time required for each line multiplied by the number of lines in an image. The number of images R in a second is given by: $R = 1/d\theta T_L = v/2Dd\theta$.

Fig. 6.15 illustrates the pattern of R as a function of the angle and depth D for sectorial systems. It is clear how the number of images a second R is reduced when the depth to be visualized D or the angle visualized θ increases, or the lines per angle unit become dense.

For high quality systems the number of lines per image must be large (several hundreds); the flicker effect that would be introduced by the reduction in the number of images a second, is avoided by using digital memory as for static or manual scanners.

In order not to lose the data from moving structures, such as the heart, i.e. for real time systems, the number of images a second must exceed 15 so that the depth D or the number of lines per image must be reduced.

Fig. 6.15 – Mechanical or electronic sectorial scanning probe; pattern of the number of images a second R as a function of the maximum depth displayed D and the scanning angle θ.

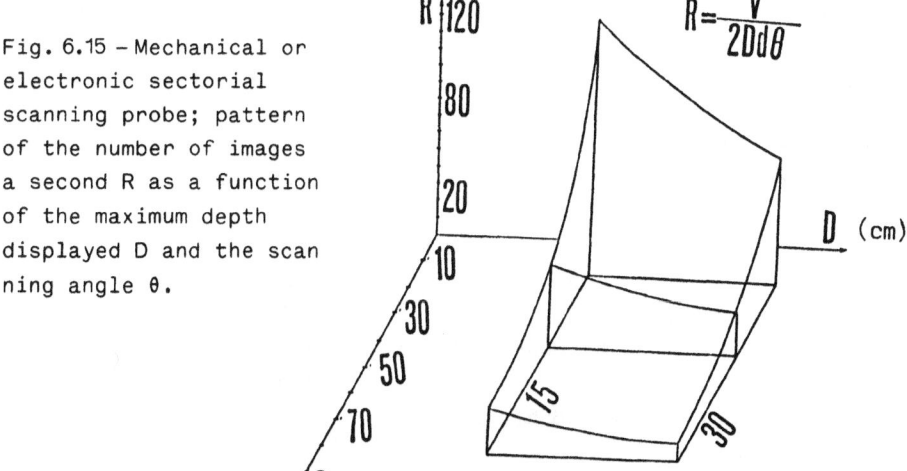

References

1. Hueter, T.F. and R.H. Bolt. Sonics. J. Wiley and Sons, New York, N.Y., 1965.
2. Diagnostic Ultrasound. Edited by C.C. Grossman, Plenum Press, New York, N.Y., 1966.
3. Biological Engineering. Edited by H.P. Schwan, McGraw-Hill, New York, N.Y., 1969.
4. Ultrasonics in Clinical Diagnosis. Edited by P.N.T. Wells, Churchi Livingstone, London, 1972.
5. Francini, G. and L. Masotti. Ultrasuoni. Apparecchiature di Diagnc si. Enciclopedia dell'Ingegneria. Aggiornamenti. Isedi. Mondadori, 1975.
6. Dunn, F., P. Edmonds and W. Fry. Absorption and Dispersion of Ultr sound in Biological Media, in Biological Engineering. Edited by H. P. Schwan, Mc-Graw-Hill (Inter-University Electronic Series, vol. 1969.
7. Wells, P.N.T. Physical Principles of Ultrasonics Diagnosis. Academ Press, London, 1969.
8. Beyer, R.T. and S.V. Letcher. Physical Ultrasonics. Academic Press New York, N.Y., 96, 1969.
9. Bhatia, A.B. Ultrasonic Absorption. Oxford Press, London, 174, 196
10. Pinkerton, J.M.M. The Absorption of Ultrasonic Waves in Liquids ar in Relation to Molecular Constitution. Proc. Phys. Soc. (London) E 129, 1949.
11. Carstensen, E.L. and H.P. Schwan. Acoustic Properties of Hemoglobi Solutions. J. Acoust. Soc. Amer. 31: 305, 1959.
12. Edmonds, P.D., T.J. Bauld et al. Ultrasonic Absorption of Aqueous Hemoglobin Solutions. Biochim. Biophys. Acta 200: 174, 1970.
13. Gramberg, H. Absorptionmessungen an biologischen Substanzen bei neidrigen und ihre Abhängigkeit von der Frequenz. Naturwissenschaf 39: 21, 1952.
14. Mayer, A. and H. Vogel. Ultraschallabsorption von Hamoglobinlosung im MHz-Bereich. Z Naturforsch 20b: 85, 1965.
15. Schneider, F., F. Muller-Landau and A. Mayer. Acoustical Propertie of Aqueous Solutions of Oxygenated and Deoxygenated Hemoglobin. Biopolymers 8: 537, 1969.
16. Goldman, G.E. and T.F. Hueter. Tabular Data of the Velocity and At sorption of High-Frequency Sound in Mammalian Tissues. J. Acoust. Soc. Amer. 28: 35, 1956.
17. Goldman, G.E. and T.F. Hueter. Errata: Tabular Data on the Velocit and Absorption of High-Frequency Sound in Mammalian Tissues. J. Acoust. Soc. Amer. 28: 655, 1957.

18. Chivers, R.C. and C.R. Hill. Ultrasonic Attenuation in Human Tissues. Ultrasound Med. Biol. 2: 25, 1975.
19. Colombati, S. and S. Petralia. Assorbimento di Ultrasuoni in Tessuti Animali. Ric. Sci. 20: 71, 1950.
20. Dankwerts, H.J. Discrete Relaxation Processes as a Model of the Absorption in Liver Homogenate. J. Acoust. Soc. Amer. 55: 1098, 1974.
21. Dunn, F. Temperature and Amplitude Dependence of Acoustic Absorption in Tissue. J. Acoust. Soc. Amer. 34: 1545, 1962.
22. Mountford, R.A. and P.N.T. Wells. Ultrasonic Liver Scanning: the A-Scan in the Normal and Cirrhosis. Phys. Med. Biol. 17: 261, 1972.
23. Pauly, H. and H.P. Schwan. Mechanism of Absorption of Ultrasound in Liver Tissue. J. Acoust. Soc. Amer. 50: 692, 1971.
24. Dunn, F. Attenuation and Speed of Ultrasound in Lung. J. Acoust. Soc. Amer. 56: 1638, 1974.
25. Dunn, F. and W.J. Fry. Ultrasonic Absorption and Reflection by Lung Tissue. Phys. Med. Biol. 5: 401, 1961.
26. Fry, F.J. and F. Dunn. Ultrasound: Analysis and Experimental Methods in Biological Research, in Nastuk (ed.). Physical Techniques in Biological Research, vol. 4, Special Methods. New York, Academic Press, 261, 1962.
27. Shung, K.K., R.A. Sigelmann and J.M. Reid. The Scattering of Ultrasound by Red Blood Cells. Appl. Radiol., 1976.
28. Bergmann, L. Der Ultraschall. Stuttgart, Hirzel, 1954.
29. Nicholas, D. and C.R. Hill. Acoustic Bragg Diffraction from Human Tissues. Nature (London) 257: 305, 1975.
30. Atzeni, C., G. Castellini, P.L. Emiliani, C. Lombardi, S. Manetti, L. Masotti, C. Raffini. L'Assorbimento Selettivo degli Ultrasuoni nell'Ecografia Clinica. Atti del 1° Congresso Società Italiana Studio Ultrasuoni in Medicina, Edizioni Centro Minerva Medica, 54, 1976.
31. Hueter, T.F. Messung der Ultraschallabsorption in menschlichen schadelkpoken und ihre Abhängigkeit von der Frequenz. Naturwissenschaften 39: 21, 1952.
32. Flynn, G.H. Cavitation Dynamics I. A Mathematical Formulation. J. Acoust. Soc. Amer. 57: 1379, 1975.
33. Flynn, G.H. Cavitation Dynamics II. Free Pulsation and Models for Cavitation Bubbles. J. Acoust. Soc. Amer. 58: 1160, 1975.
34. Fry, F.J., G. Kossoff, R.G. Eggleton et al. Threshold Ultrasonic Dosages for Structural Changes in the Mammalian Brain. J. Acoust. Soc. Amer. 48: 1413, 1970.

35. Dunn, F. and F.J. Fry. Ultrasonic Threshold Dosage for the Mammalian Central Nervous System. IEEE Trans. Biomed. Engin. BME 18: 253, 1971.
36. Clarke, P.R. and C.R. Hill. Physical and Chemical Aspects of Ultrasonic Disruption of Cells. J. Acoust. Soc. Amer. 47: 649, 1969.
37. Child, S.Z., E.L. Carstensen and M.W. Miller. Growth of Pea Roots Exposed to Pulsed Ultrasound. J. Acoust. Soc. Amer. 58: 1109, 1975.
38. Braeman, J. et al. Human Lymphocyte Chromosomes and Ultrasonic Cavitation. Br. J. Radiol., vol. 47, 158-161, 1974.
39. O' Brien jr., W.D. Safety of Ultrasound. Handbook of Clinical Ultrasound. Edited by M. de Vlieger, J. Wiley and Sons, New York, N.Y., 1978.
40. Fry, W.J., V.J. Wulff, D. Tucker et al. Physical Factors Involved in Ultrasonically Induced Changes in Living Systems: I. Identification of Nontemperature Effects. J. Acoust. Soc. Amer. 22: 867, 1950.
41. Taylor, K.J.W. and J.B. Pond. A Study of the Production of Haemorrhagic Injury and Paraplegia in Rat Spinal Cord by Pulsed Ultrasound by Low Megahertz Frequencies in the Context of the Safety for Clinical Usage. Brit. J. Radiol. 45: 343, 1972.
42. Stewart, H.F., G.R. Harris and H.M. Frost. Development of Principles and Concepts for Specification of Ultrasonic Diagnostic Equipment Performance. Ultrasound in Medicine.
Edited by D. White and R.E. Brown, Plenum Press, New York, N.Y., vol. 3B, 2115, 1977.
43. Rose, J.L. and B.B. Goldberg. Basic Physics in Diagnostic Ultrasound J. Wiley and Sons, New York, N.Y., 1979.
44. Kossoff, G. Balance Technique for the Measurement of Very Low Ultrasonic Power Outputs. Letter to the editor. J. Acoust. Soc. Amer. 38: 880, 1965.
45. Hertz, H., L. Masotti, C. Ligvoet, C.H. Eversdijk, J. Ridder, L.F. Van Der Wall, A.J. Berkhout, H. Hofmann and N. Bom. Report of the Workshop on New Diagnostic Ultrasound Techniques. International Congress Series No. 553 Recent Advances in Ultrasound Diagnosis 3. Proceedings of the 4th European Congress on Ultrasonics in Medicine, Editors A. Kurjak and A. Kratochwil. Excerpta Medica Amsterdam - Oxford - Princeton, 1981.
46. Bastogi, A., A. Casini, G. Castellini, A.G. Costantinides, F. Lotti, L. Masotti, S. Rocchi. Digital R.F. and Video Processing of Echographic Signals. Ultrasonic Tissue Characterization 3. Proc. of the Third EC Workshop, Stuttgart, Nov. 1983. Edited by J.M. Thijssen and K. Irion, Commission of the European Communities.
47. Bertini, A., L. Masotti, A. Zuppiroli, F. Cecchi. Rotating Probe for Trans-Oexophageal Cross-Sectional Echocardiography. J. of

Nuclear Medicine and Allied Sciences, 1984 (in press).
48. Masotti, L. Strumentazione per Tomografia con Ultrasuoni: Principi Fisici ed Apparecchiature. Ultrasuonodiagnostica Ed. M. Lenzi, B. Talia, G.C. Canossi; Edizioni C.E.L.I., Bologna, 1982.
49. Masotti, L. Introduction to Ultrasonography. Physical Principles and Equipment. Diagnostic Ultrasound in Gastroenterology, Ed. L. Bolondi, G. Labò, L. Gandolfi. Edizione Piccin/Butterworths, Padova/Borough Green, 1984.
50. Costa, P.L., L. Masotti, M. Dal Pane, S. Cappelli, C. Camporesi, G. Fontana. The 'Mirror-Image Effect': an Artifact of Hepatic Ultrasonography. Clinical Advances in Ultrasonology Ed. G. Labò, L. Bolondi, G. Rizzatto. Edizione Masson, Milano, 1983.
51. Masotti, L. and B. Talia. La Caratterizzazione dei Tessuti Mediante Ultrasuoni. Ultrasuonodiagnostica Ed. M. Lenzi, B. Talia, G.C. Canossi; Edizioni C.E.L.I., Bologna, 1982.
52. Nicholas, D. Ultrasonic Diffraction Analysis in the Investigation of Liver Disease. Br. J. Radiol., No. 52, 949-961, 1979.

PHASED ARRAY ACOUSTIC IMAGING SYSTEMS

H. Edward Karrer

Hewlett Packard Laboratories, Palo Alto, California

What is an ultrasound image? An image is a reproduction or imitation of the form of something. A major thrust of modern technology in the past century has been to enhance or complement the capability of the human sensory system with new imaging modalities. Examples that come to mind include the optical telescope, radar, sonar, infrared, and X-ray imaging systems.

The imaging process consists of two parts. First is the illumination of the objects to be imaged by some radiation. This radiation interacts with the object by means of reflection, absorption, or scattering. The second step is a reconstruction of the energy received from these interactions to form an image of the object.

The primary goal of medical imaging systems is to "see" inside the human body noninvasively. Our eyes are not useful for this since biological tissue is largely opaque to visible light. Fortunately, other forms of radiation like X-rays, some nuclear particles, and ultrasound readily pass through and interact with tissue.

Ultrasound brings several useful capabilities to medical imaging. An ultrasound image represents the mechanical properties of the tissue (i.e., parameters such as density and elasticity). Most people can immediately recognize common anatomical structures in an ultrasound image since the organ boundaries and fluid-to-tissue interfaces are easily discerned. This mechanical information complements the results of other imaging techniques, such as X-ray imaging, which displays X-ray absorption.

The ultrasound imaging process can be done in real time. This means that the viewer can follow rapidly moving structures such as the heart without motion distortion. Also, it allows the operator to move the small handheld transducer probe over the surface of the patient's body to select the proper view in an interactive way.

Ultrasound appears to be one of the safest diagnostic imaging techniques. It does not use ionizing radiation like X-ray and hence is used routinely for fetal and obstetrical imaging. There have been many studies done on the possible biological side effects of ultrasound on tissue and none has shown any harmful effects during clinical examination.

Areas where ultrasound imaging is particularly useful include cardiac structures, the vascular system, the fetus and uterus, abdominal organs such as the liver, kidneys, and gall bladder, and the eye. However, ultrasound cannot be used to image all portions of the body. Air pockets, for instance, are excellent reflectors of ultrasound and limit the penetration of sound into the lungs and bowels. Bone highly attenuates ultrasound, which makes imaging the adult brain through the skull difficult.

Physical Principles

Ultrasound generally refers to sound that has a frequency or pitch above the range of human hearing. Sound waves in human tissue are compressional (longitudinal) waves. These waves consist of repetitive or periodic regions of local compression and rarefaction which propagate through a medium at some velocity v. The spacing between successive regions of compression is called the acoustic wavelength . These parameters are related by the expression $v=f\lambda$, where v is the velocity in meters/second, f is the frequency in hertz, and λ is the wavelength in meters. Because it is not possible to resolve objects smaller than a wave length, it is desirable to image at the highest possible frequency (smallest wavelength) to get the best resolution.

The most common mode of ultrasound imaging is the reflection of pulse echo mode. The analogy to radar is valid. A short burst of acoustic energy is directed into the body and the reflected energy is received at a later time. Different tissues reflect acoustic energy depending on their characteristic acoustic impedance. This impedance is defined by the expression $Z=pv$, where Z is the acoustic impedance in rayls, p is the density of the tissue in kilograms/cubic meter, and v is the velocity in meters/second.

As the ultrasound pulse passes from one tissue type to another, a portion of it is reflected in a way analogous to reflection from a discontinuity on an electric transmission line.

For instance, when a pulse crosses the boundary between muscle tissue ($Z=1.7 \times 10^6$ rayls) and blood ($Z=1.6 \times 10^6$ rayls), about 0.1% of the acoustic energy is reflected. This echo is used to create the image of the blood-muscle interface. The rest of the pulse propagates across the interface and continues into the body to image deeper structures.

The ultrasound pulse is transmitted and received with a piezoelectric transducer. The piezoelectric material is a polycrystalline ceramic which converts an electrical signal into acoustic energy and vice versa. This transducer is the source and eye of the imaging system. It is usually placed directly on the skin surface.

As the ultrasound pulse propagates through the body, its acoustic intensity is attenuated with propagation distance. The acoustic attenuation also increases with frequency. A typical attenuation coefficient for soft tissue is 1 dB/cm/MHz. When imaging a structure that is 10 cm deep in the body at 3.5 MHz, the round-trip attenuation is 70 dB. This is an easily detectable signal when using clinically acceptable transmitter powers. Note that at 10 MHz the round-trip attenuation would be 200dB. This points out a basic tradeoff in ultrasound imaging; as the frequency is increased to resolve finer structures, only shallow structures can be imaged. Typically, 2.5 to 3.5 MHz is used for deep abdominal imaging, 5 MHz is used for organs near the surface and in pediatric work, and 5 to 15 MHz is reserved for "small parts" imaging such as the thyroid, testicles, peripheral vascular vessels, and the eye.

Other structures can also interact with ultrasound, giving different tissues different textures. Objects much smaller than a wavelength cause Rayleigh scattering. This diffuse scattering depends on the fourth power of the frequency and the ultrasound pulse tends to scatter uniformly in all directions. Images made at higher frequencies tend to appear more "filled in" because of this effect. If an object is much larger than a wavelength, it becomes a specular reflector and acts much like a mirror.

B or brightness mode scanning is the most common type of ultrasound imaging. A B scan is a view of a cross-sectional slice through the object. A narrow pencil beam of ultrasound is swept through a sector to define the scan plane. The beam is formed from bursts of ultrasound. The repetition rate of ultrasound pulse generation is selected so that the transmitted pulse has time to travel to the deepest target and back again before the next pulse is launched. The pulse is assumed to travel in a straight line at a constant velocity, a good assumption in soft tissue. As the pulse propagates into the body along any scan line, echoes are generated which travel back to the receiver. These echoes vary in intensity according to the type of tissue or body structure causing them. This data is presented on a cathode-ray-tube (CRT) display in which the brightness (hence the term B mode) depends on the echo strength. This image can be formed in real time since it takes only 260 us for ultrasound to travel 20 cm into the body and return. If the display frame rate is 30 frames per second, 125 lines can be displayed in the image.

Ultrasound imaging systems differ in the way that the sector scan is implemented. A single transducer can be mechanically rocked or pivoted to create a sector scan. The phased-array approach uses a stationary array of many small transducers which are electronically controlled to steer and focus the beam. This concept is shown in Fig. 1.

In effect, the phased array acts like an acoustic lens with electronically variable focal length. Let us assume that a region of tissue at location O has reflected a small amount of an incident short pulse of ultrasound. The echo reaches each transducer element (T_n) along the array at a different time depending on the position of O. Variable time delay elements (T_n) in series with each transducer element are rapidly varied under computer control to bring the electrical pulses generated by the echoes received at each transducer element into coincidence at the summing junction. For instance, if the object is on the axis of symmetry of the transducer array, but is far away, the returning echo wavefronts are essentially planar and the time delays are set equal. If the object is off-axis at some angle in the far field, the time delays must be linearly varied across the array aperture for coherent addition at the summing junction. When the object is close to the array, as shown in Fig. 1, the approaching wavefronts are more curved and the delay distribution across the array is more nearly parabolic. Changing the individual transducer delays to accomodate the curvature of the wavefronts is called dynamic focusing and is necessary to achieve maximum resolution in the near field of the array.

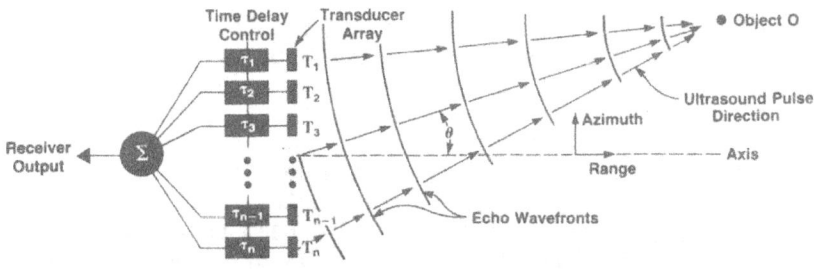

Fig. 1. Phased Array Principle

In a similar manner, the outgoing ultrasound pulse can be directed to a desired location. By varying the time at which each element of the transducer array is excited by the transmitter, the direction in which the ultrasound pulses generated by each element coherently add to form one pulse can be changed from one side of the axis to the other. This is called beam steering.

In practice, the transmit and receive functions are separate. Consider the events necessary to generate one line of the image. First, a set of ultrasound pulses is launched so as to provide a coherent wavefront along a given scan direction. This beam is focused at midrange. As the transmitted wavefront propagates into the body, it is scattered by objects along the scan line and echoes start returning to the array. In the receive mode, the array continuously changes its focus as echoes are received from successively deeper regions. This dynamic focusing process allows an array with an aperture of 2 cm to have a varying depth of focus from 2 to 20 cm.

Resolution is the ability to separate small objects in the scan plane visually. It has three components: range resolution (along a scan line), azimuth resolution (perpendicular to a scan line within the plane of the sector scan), and elevation resolution (the thickness of the sector scan slice). The range resolution is determined by the ultrasound pulse length. A shorter pulse gives higher resolution. The pulse length is primarily determined by the system bandwidth. Two targets 0.75 mm apart in range can be resolved with a 1us ultrasound pulse (3 cycles at 3.5 MHz).

The resolution in the azimuth direction depends on the array aperture (length of the array) and the acoustic wavelength . The principles are the same as for an optical telescope. High azimuth resolution is achieved with a large aperture and a short wavelength. Dynamic focusing optimizes the azimuth resolution of the imaging system.

A block diagram for a general ultrasound imaging system is shown in Fig. 2. The transmitter excites the transducer elements with short electric pulses so that a burst of ultrasound is generated. The returning echoes are applied to a variable-gain stage in the receiver called a time gain compensation (TGC) amplifier. This amplifier increases its gain with time, thus compensating for tissue attenuation as echoes come from deeper regions of the body. In a phased array system, each element of the transducer has its own TGC amplifier. The beam former combines the outputs of the individual receiver channels by using variable time delay and phase adjustment to bring the received signals into coincidence and hence bring an object into focus. Since the received echoes have a very wide dynamic range, the signal processing stage uses signal level compression. For instance, when imaging the heart, the strong echo from the posterior wall of the left ventricle can be 50 dB greater than the diffuse echoes from the endocardial tissue. This data must be compressed to be compatible with the 25-dB dynamic range of normal CRT displays. The compressed signal is then converted from analog to digital form so that an entire image frame can be stored in the memory of the digital scan converter. The digital scan converter changes the scan format from a sector display to a conventional television raster scan. It also permits digital postprocessing of the images. These various activities--the transmitter, TGC amplifier, beam former, scan converter, and display--are coordinated under microprocessor control. (1)

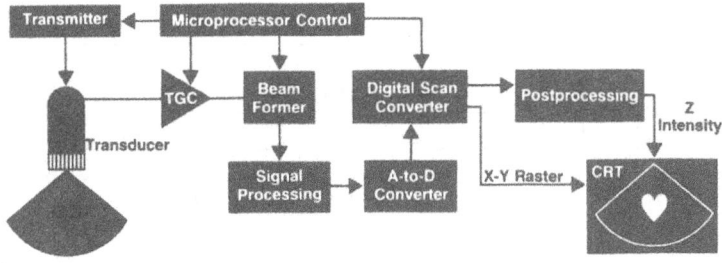

Fig. 2. Imaging System Block Diagram

Phased Array and Single Disc Mechanical Sector Scanners

Fig. 3 shows a general block diagram for a mechanical scanner (upper) and the phased array scanner (lower) (2). In the mechanical scanner the acoustic lens and mechanical scanner do the spatial processing and this is followed by the transduction process. In a phased array the spatial processing and transduction blocks are reversed. The transducer array preceeds the spatial processing which is done in a beamformer. This beam former is usually a series of electronically variable delay lines.

Other differences between a phased array and single transducer mechanical scanner are listed below:

1) Aperture - As mentioned before, the resolution of an acoustic imaging system increases with the number of wavelength across the aperture. In a mechanical sector scanner the effective aperture is usually less than the body contact aperture since the transducer must be recessed to accomodate the motion (Fig. 4). In a phased array the effective aperture and contact aperture are the same but the aperture falls off as $\cos\theta$ as the beam is steered.

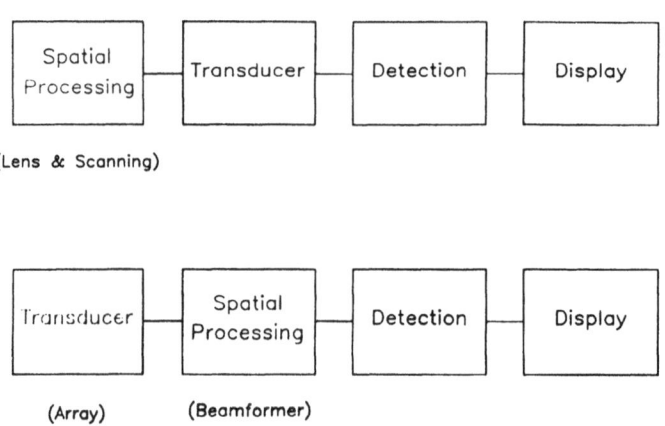

Fig. 3. Mechanical and Phased Array Block Diagrams.

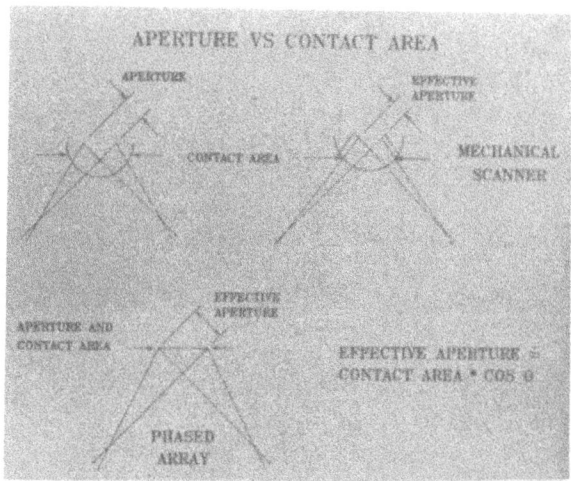

Fig. 4. Mechanical and Phased Array Apertures

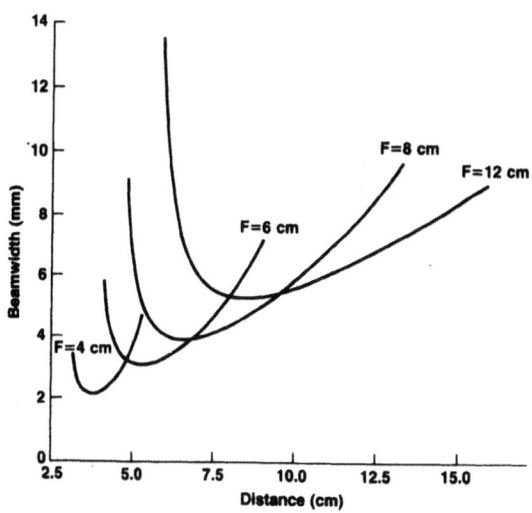

Fig. 5. Transmit beamwidth versus distance for equal aperture 5 MHz transducers with different focal lengths.

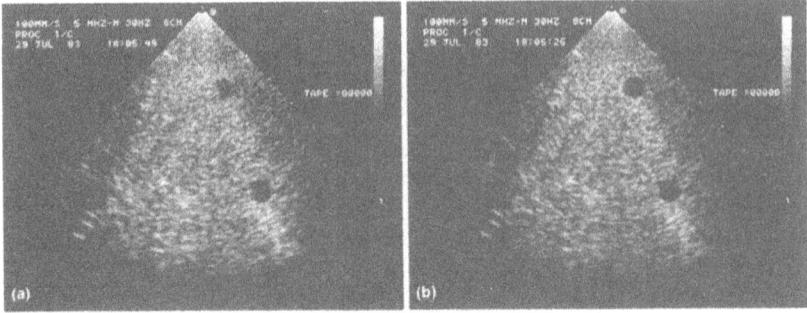

Fig. 6. Effect of Dynamic Focusing on Image Quality. (a) Image using a transducer with fixed receive focus at 8 cm. (b) Image using a transducer dynamically focused during reception.

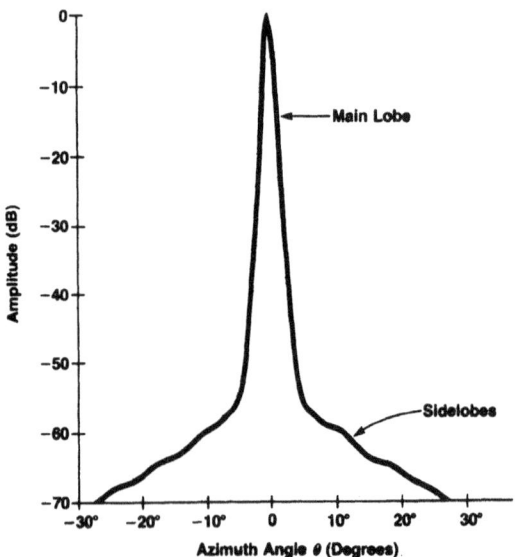

Fig. 7. Plot of Beam Intensity versus Azimuth Angle

2) Dynamic focus - A single disc transducer has a very narrow depth of focus as shown in Fig. 5. Historically this problem was the stimulus for the development of phased array systems which can achieve a diffraction limited focus at any range. The effect of dynamic focus on image quality is shown in Fig. 6.

3) Image clutter - A very important specification for any imaging system is the point spread function or beam plot. An example for a 3.5 MHz, 64 channel phased array system is shown in Fig. 7. The width of the peak near the maximum is the azimuthal resolution. Experience has shown that the sidelobe level and noise floor away from the main lobe must be in the -50 to -70 dB region to achieve clutter free images. In a phased array system this can be achieved by using a large number of elements (less than $\lambda/2$ spacing), proper apodization of the aperture, a fine time delay quantization and thermal noise limited electronics. In a mechanical scanner the reverberations in the fluid path between the transducer and the enclosure must be reduced to a similar level to avoid image clutter.

4) Doppler - The phased array has unique advantages for doppler. In a phased array multiple beams can be formed in real time so that the same transducer aperture can be used for 2D imaging and doppler. This is advantageous in cardiology where the physiological aperture is limited. Also the beam geometry can be varied electronically to change the doppler sample volume size and location.

Delay Line Technology

Many variable delay methods have been used in phased array imaging systems. These are listed in Figure 8 and several are discussed briefly below. The requirements for delay lines are delays of 10 us with 32 ns steps, video bandwidths and 60-80 dB of dynamic range.

1) Heterodyne - The mixing method was first developed simultaneously by Manes (3), Burchardt (4), and Maslak at Hewlett Packard (5, 6). It supposed that the return echo can be modeled in the form $r(t)=A(t) \cos(w_0 t + \phi(t))$, where the amplitudes and phase are varying slowly relative to the center frequency w_0. Coherent addition of the many channels can be achieved by using coarsly quantized delay lines to align the amplitude envelopes and phase shifters to align the phases. A practical way to implement the phase shifters is with mixers. Each return echo is mixed with a local oscillator whose phase is adjustable. This method has been implemented on 64 channel imaging systems.

2) Analog to a Digital Conversion - Currently most systems do an analog to digital conversion after the receive channels are summed and detected. It is possible to do that conversion earlier in the receive chain and do the time delay in digital

VARIABLE DELAY TECHNOLOGY

Electromagnetic (Lumped Element)

Charge Transfer Devices

Serial Analog Memories

Digital (A/D Converters)

Heterodyne Methods

Surface Wave Methods

Fig. 8. Variable Delay Technologies

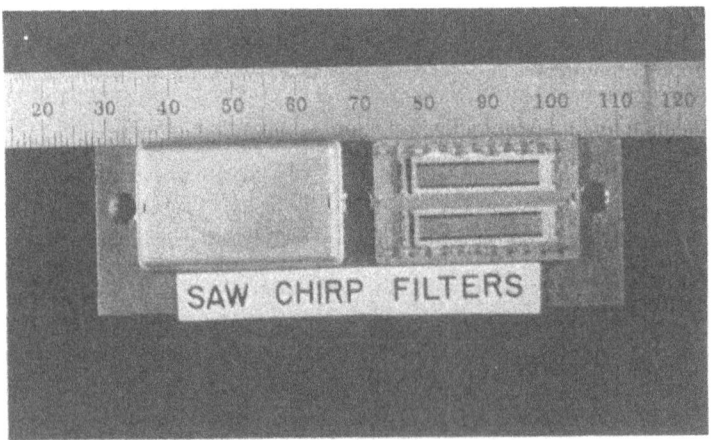

Fig. 9. Surface Acoustic Wave Delay Line

circuitry. This requires A to D converters that can convert 12 bits at 15 MHz rates and this is currently too expensive for systems with many channels.
3) Surface Wave Devices - Surface wave devices can be used for variable delay lines with wide bandwidths. The delay occurs as an acoustic surface wave propagates on the surface of a piezoelectric substrate. Dispersive delay elements must be used (7). An example of a variable delay line using this technology is shown in Fig. 9.

Transducer Arrays (8)

The acoustic transducer array is the analog front end of an ultrasound imaging system. It provides a large number of independent channels, transduces electric signals to acoustic pressure, and generates sufficient acoustic energy to illuminate the various structures in the human body. In turn, it converts the weak returning acoustic echoes to a set of electrical signals which can be processed into an image. The key transducer requirements are to:

Generate 10 to 100 mW/cm^2 of acoustic power from reasonable input voltages
Provide good signal-to-noise ratio
Have low cross-coupling between elements
Generate short acoustic pulses, 2 us in duration
Couple acoustic energy to the patient efficiently
Damp the acoustic backwave
Achieve broad angular coverage
Suppress undesired vibration modes
Be lightweight and handheld.

Although a variety of techniques for generating and detecting sound are available, piezoelectric transducers are preferable because they can both generate and receive acoustic waves, and they are several orders of magnitude more sensitive than other possible transducers.

The basic geometry of a phased array transducer is shown in Figure 10. An acoustically matched and absorbent backing is used to mount the transducer. The effective Q is lowered to ≈ 2 and the pulse length is reduced to 1 us. The acoustic energy propagated into the backing, or backwave, is lost by acoustic attenuation and no secondary resonances are set up. For example, for lead metaniobate ceramic material operating at 2.5 MHz and transmitting ultrasound into human tissue, the pulse duration is 1.3 us. The insertion loss, including transduction efficiency and the impedance mismatch of ceramic to tissue is -28 dB. This technique clearly optimizes the pulse response, although most of the power (>99%) is lost in the backing. It also has the disadvantage of minimizing the number of acoustic bonds and acoustic parts. One or more matching layers between the transducer and patient can be used to improve the transmission of acoustic energy into the body. For example, a typical PZT ceramic with two matching layers of appropriate acoustic impedances interposed between the ceramic and the patient has a -4dB insertion loss and a 2.1 us pulse duration. This represents a large improvement in transduction efficiency with some loss of pulse length.

A basic requirement of a phased-array transducer is that the elements be placed on half-wavelength ($\lambda/2$) centers to sample the aperture properly. Here λ is measured in the subject material. For the 1.5 to-2.5-cm apertures used for medical imaging, 60 to 80 elements are required. In turn, the ceramic transducer must be half-wavelength ($\lambda/2$) thick to operate properly. Here λ is measured in the ceramic. Thus, the elements have a width-to-thickness ratio directly proportional to the velocity of sound in the piezoelectric ceramic and inversely proportional to the velocity in tissue. This ratio is about 3:1, resulting in tall narrow elements. An insulator is placed between the backing and the ceramic. A metal foil is bonded over the elements to form the ground connection, protect the patient, and keep grease out of the kerfs between elements (the elements are cut apart to support cross-coupling). An important modification is to use a second layer of piezoelectric ceramic as the insulating layer. This gives suppression of the unwanted mass-spring mode and increases the acoustic energy radiated by the transducer.

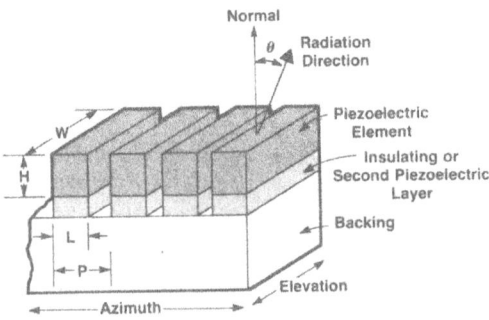

Fig. 10. Acoustic Transducer Array

Each array element appears electrically to be a frequency-dependent, lossy capacitor with capacitance $C = \varepsilon_o WL/H$ where ε_o is the clamped dielectric constant and W, H, and L are defined in Fig. 10. As will be seen later, these dimensions are constrained by the need to control spurious modes and grating lobes, and to obtain a narrow beam in the elevation direction. A compromise between high-frequency, shallow-penetration operation on one hand and low-frequency, deep-penetration operation on the other leads to choosing a center frequency of 2.5 MHz, a frequency which is assumed in the examples to follow. To satisfy the above conditions, the dimensions L=250u, period P=320u, W=10mm, and H=600u for PZT-5H ceramic material were chosen, and C =55 pF.

Exposure of mammalian tissue to average power densities of of 100 mW/cm^2 or less has been found to cause no significant biologial effects. Detailed calculations show that for PZT-5H, a single-layer array element can achieve 100mW/cm^2 for a 200:1 duty cycle with 216 volts peak-to-peak drive. A double layer element develops the same acoustic power output at 130 volts peak-to-peak. The use of acoustic matching layers can allow more efficient power generation. For example, a single matching layer used in conjunction with a single PZT layer could result in a transduction efficiency increase of 8 dB, or around 90 volts peak-to-peak to achieve 100 mW/cm^2.

Since the acoustic arrays are operated in a pulse mode to achieve good range resolution, wideband operation becomes a prime consideration. Factors influencing this include frequency-sensitive driving-point impedance, epoxy bond thickness, and frequency-dependent transduction efficiency. Other vibration modes can cause narrowband extended time duration response. The transducer response is quite dependent on the quality of the acoustic properties of the bonded array. Chief among these are the thicknesses of the epoxy-layers used to cement the PZT to the backing, the surface layers present on the backing, and the degree to which the backing impedance is the same as the PZT acoustic impedance. The epoxy bond has an acoustic impedance of 3.2×10^6 compared to 25×10^6 rayls for PZT-5H. This 8:1 mismatch dictates that the bond be very thin to prevent narrowing of the passband. To ensure good response, bond thicknesses less than 2 um are required.

In an acoustic imaging array the elements should have a single mode of vibration, namely a piston-like motion of the front surface. By making the elements sufficiently narrow, and reducing cross-coupling, the acoustic intensity should be uniform at various angles from the normal, that is, omnidirectional. With the element thickness H comparable to L, additional modes can be expected to exist at frequencies near the desired thickness mode frequency. Such vibrations include the dilatational or breathing mode, the mass-spring oscillation mode, Lamb wave on a foil, and the Rayleigh surface-wave mode. Of the modes discussed, the thickness mode is desired and all others are undesired. The dilatational mode is not suppressed, but by choosing narrow elements, the mode is moved to a higher frequency where it is conveniently filtered out. Of the remaining modes, the mass-spring mode is most troublesome. It is strongly excited and has high Q. Its occurrence around 1 MHz is inconveniently close to 2.5 MHz in terms of filtering. In one scheme, this mode is suppressed by using two oppositely poled pieces of PZT to cause a zero net center-of-mass motion. This results in an order of magnitude reduction of the mode as measured by the real part of the input impedance. Shorter ring-down times, less cross-coupling, and more uniform acoustic radiation patterns result.

The Lamb wave is suppressed by choosing a very thin foil. Since the asymmetric mode is largely responsible for Lamb-wave propagation, making the foil thin reduces the group velocity and prevents effective coupling from the array elements to the foil. Since the Rayleigh wave is bound to within a few wavelengths of the backing surface, making deep cuts extending well into the backing effectively suppresses it.

The acoustic beam generated by the one-dimensional phased array described here can only be electronically focused and steered in the azimuth plane. To improve the resolution and sensitivity further, a cylindrical acoustic lens is added to give a fixed focus in the orthogonal elevation plane.

The main properties of interest in a lens are the resolution at focus, radius of the curvature to achieve a given focus, the depth of field about that focus, and the intensity gain caused by focusing. The lens must be sufficiently strongly focusing to achieve better resolution than an unfocused beam, yet have enough depth of field to allow imaging over a useful range. This involves a compromise in the elevation aperture W. In addition, reverberations caused by poor lens impedance match to the patient are to be avoided. Finally, low attenuation in the lens and a convex outer surface are important considerations. Referring again to Fig. 10, the fabrication of an array probe involves the following processes, materials, or steps.

Synthesis of a highly attenuative backing material with close impedance match to PZT
Cutting, polishing, and plating the various ceramic materials and matching layers
Bonding the array together with sufficiently thin bonds
Dicing the elements

Providing electrical connections to the closely spaced elements
Applying a top ground foil electrode
Synthesizing and attaching a suitable lens
Packaging the array into a probe complete with cable and connectors.

The backing is required to match PZT acoustically and have sufficiently high acoustic loss to damp any backwave to a level below the system noise. Typically a 50 to 60 dB round-trip loss at any signal frequency above 1 MHz is required. If the loss is not large enough, multiple echos will return and cause bright lines or "range markers" in the image. The backing material chosen is a composite of tungsten for high impedance and polyvinyl chloride (PVC) plastic as a binder and dissipative medium. Typical parameters achieved are an acoustic impedance of 25×10^6 rayls, a density of 14.2×10^3 kg/m^3, and an attenuation of 20 dB/cm at 1 MHz. Typically the attenuation increases as frequency squared, so at 2 MHz the loss is 80 dB/cm.

The raw PZT-5H material used for each element is wafered to the appropriate dimensions, then ground and polished to a final thickness of 600 to 700 um. The thickness and the parallelism of the sides are carefully controlled. The parts are poled by a high electric field in a heated oil bath to make them piezoelectrically active.

The backing and ceramic parts are very carefully cleaned under dust-free conditions, then bonded together with low viscosity epoxy resin. Matching layers are also bonded at this stage, as is the electrical lead structure. To avoid the various cross-coupling problems outlined earlier, the 64 individual elements are separated by sawing. The array is thoroughly cleaned again and a thin metal foil is bonded on to complete the ground connection and isolate the array elements from infiltration by grease, coupling gel, or water.

A variety of acoustic lenses can be used. A convex single-element lens is an effective choice, but the selection of useful materials is limited to those in which the acoustic velocity is less than that in human tissue (1.54×10^3 m/s). The lens material used is a polyurethane rubber, Sylgard 170. It provides a good impedance match to human tissue and the acoustic velocity in Sylgard 170 is 1.02×10^3 m/s. This allows the design of a convex lens with a radius R=36 mm for a 7-cm elevation focal length. It is fabricated on a thin foil by casting and then is bonded to the array.

The final array is wired to a suitable coaxial cable containing 64 individual leads. It is then packaged in a waterproof plastic case.

Future Directions in Phased Array Imaging

The evolution of a new technology like phased array systems follows an "S" shaped curve (9) as shown in Fig. 11. Initially the invention and birth of the technology are achieved in a research lab with relatively little investment and initially low performance. If the technology looks promising, the investment rate is increased with dramatic improvements in performance. This is often accompanied by a technical breakthrough leading to rapid acceptance and market growth. As the technology matures, increased investment does not lead to improved performance and the practical limits of the technology are reached. A replacement technology often follows.

Fig. 12 shows the state of acoustic imaging on this curve today. Mature technologies include the conventional B scanner and mechanical scanners. Phased arrays are in a rapid state of development with substantial gains in image quality still occurring. Tissue characterization and annular arrays are emerging technologies.

Current phased array systems are used in cardiology, radiology and obstetrics. These systems operate in the frequency range 2.5-7.5 MHz. The coherent dynamically focused transducer apertures vary from 15-80 mm. The number of independent elements varies from 15 to 128. Image quality of the phased array system has steadily improved. A typical cardiac image is shown in Fig. 13.

The evolution of phased array systems will probably proceed through the 3 stages shown in Fig. 14. Image enhancement has occured due to reduction of image artifacts caused by under sampling the aperture (grating lobes), excessive side lobes (improper apodization), spurious vibration modes in transducer elements, and non-optimum scan conversion. The systems will also be enhanced by features such as doppler and automatic TCG.

Several recent techniques may have dramatic effects on phased array systems.
1) Parallel processing of the received information can increase the effective frame rate beyond 30 FPS (10). Several lines of data received can be processed for each transmitted pulse. This increased frame rate can be traded off for reduced dosage or to allow image averaging.
2) Systems for 2D flow mapping (11) are evolving. These systems will allow a simultaneous presentation of 2D morphology and 2D doppler flow maps showing quantity and direction of flow.

3) Quantitative backscatter images will provide the first step towards tissue characterization (12). When corrections are applied for speckle, propagation attenuation and beam variations, the image brightness can be calibrated quantitatively to indentify healthy and diseased tissue.
4) Aberrations caused by the false assumption that the speed of sound is constant in all tissues can be corrected for (13). This correction could cause significant improvement in image quality for systems with f numbers less than two.
5) Improvements in transducer materials such as PVF or newer materials may result in transducers that are more efficient and easier to fabricate at high frequencies.

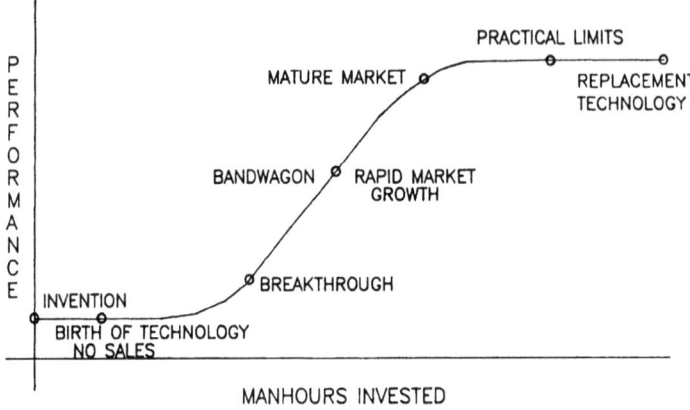

Fig. 11. Technology Evolution

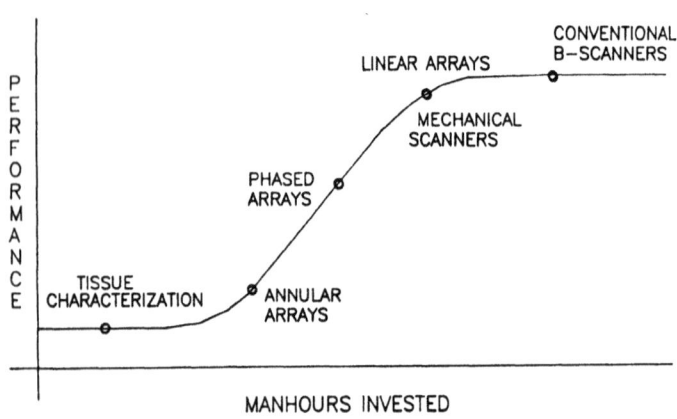

Fig. 12. Acoustic Imaging Evolution

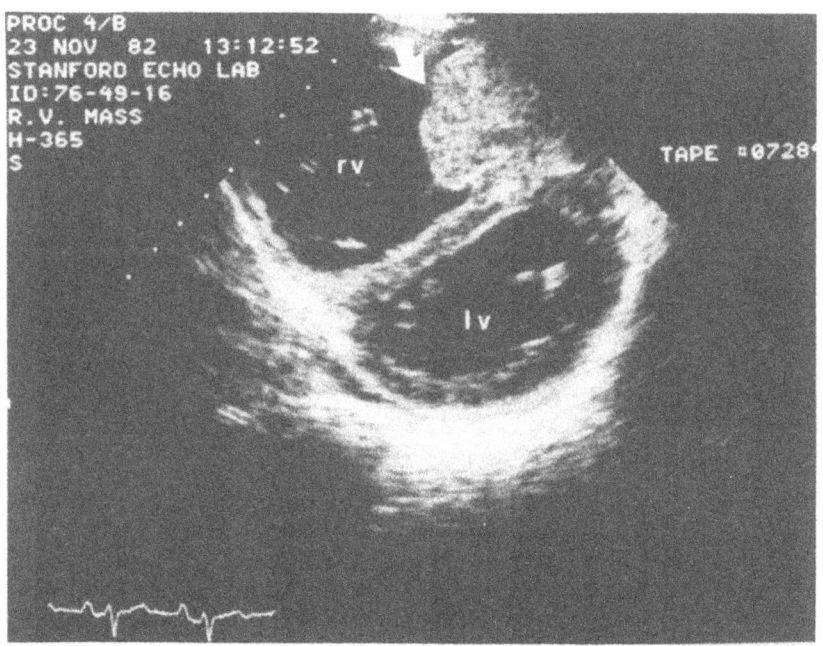

Fig. 13. Cardiac Image
(Section through right and left ventricles).

PHASED ARRAY SYSTEM EVOLUTION

Enhancement
Image Quality
Auto TGC
Doppler

Quantification
Tissue Characterization

Corrections
Adaptive Systems

Fig. 14. Stages of Phased Array Evolution.

REFERENCES

1) Hewlett Packard Journal, Oct 1983 and Dec 1983
2) J.L. Sutton. Proc. of IEEE, 67(4), Apr 1979, Pg. 557
3) G.F. Manes et al. Ultrasonics, Sept 1979, Pg. 225-228
4) C.B. Burkhardt et al. Echocardiography 1979, Pg. 385-393
5) S. Maslak. U.S. Patent #4,140,022
6) R. McKnight. Hewlett Packard Journal, Dec 1983, Pg. 16
7) V.S. Dolat et al. 1976 Ultrasonics Symposium Proceedings, Pg. 419-423
8) J.D. Larson. Hewlett Packard Journal, Oct 1983, Pg. 17-22
9) R.N. Foster. Business Week, May 24, 1982, Pg. 24-33
10) D.P. Shattuck et al. J. Acoust. Soc. Am., 75(4), Apr 1984, Pg. 1273
11) C. Kasai et al. Acoustic Imaging, vol. 13, Pg. 447
12) M. O'Donnell. IEEE Trans on Sonics & Ultrasonics, vol. 30, no. 1, Jan. 1983, Pg. 26
13) D. Wilson. SRI Report EDU 2333, 1984

ULTRASOUNDS IN CARDIOLOGY:
RECENT RESULTS, LIMITATIONS AND FUTURE NEEDS

Alessandro Distante, Eugenio Picano, Elena Moscarelli.

Institute of Clinical Physiology, C.N.R.
Institute of Medical Pathology
University of Pisa
PISA, ITALY.

INTRODUCTION

Ultrasonic techniques represent today such an unique combination of "information and safety" that, in some clinical settings, they are used for conclusive assessment before surgical procedures. After clinical evaluation, chest X-Ray and electrocardiogram, the safety factor makes echocardiography an attractive technique in situations where other existing procedures offer "competitive" information but involve either the invasive approach or the use of radiation doses that cannot be administered repeatedly, to the patient.

Diagnostic ultrasounds nowadays exploit mainly 2 tools:

1) M-Mode (T-M) and two-dimensional (2-D) echocardiography, which allow the study of anatomy and function of heart and vessels with a very high temporal and spatial resolution.

2) Doppler techniques which allow the study of intra and extracardiac blood flows.

Ultrasonic tissue characterization, though at a stage of experimental validation, can be considered a third emerging tool.

We will briefly summarize our experience in these 3 fields of application of ultrasounds attempting to extrapolate from current trends those which appear to be clues for future possibilities.

ECHOCARDIOGRAPHY IN TRANSIENT MYOCARDIAL ISCHEMIA

General background

Acute myocardial ischemia has been for a long time a "forbidden fruit" for echocardiography, due to its intrinsic features of phenomenon transient in time and regional in space. In recent years, the temporal restriction was overcome with a less "static" application of echocardiography.
This technique - as is the case with electrocardiography - gives much more information when just applied during the ischemic attack rather than during the intercritical periods. In fact, only a few seconds after the resolution of ischemia no mechanical "fingerprints" are left on myocardial contractility.
On the other hand, the "spatial" limitation, inherent to the M-Mode echocardiographic approach, was overcome with the availability of the two-dimensional technique which allows several regions of the left ventricle to be simultaneously explored. This is a crucial aspect when dealing with a strictly regional abnormal phenomenon in which the transient ischemic impairment of a myocardial segment occurs simultaneously with normal or even compensatory supernormal function of other non ischemic areas.
Our studies stem from these considerations and from the experimental evidence that ultrasounds are capable of detecting beat by beat changes in cardiac mechanics, caused by coronary occlusion, just a few seconds after the ligation of the coronary vessel (1). Clinical studies proved that episodes of variant angina are caused by a sudden vasospastic reduction in coronary blood supply, thus resembling the "stop flow" pattern of the experimental acute myocardial ischemia. The echocardiographic technique was therefore applied to the clinical model of angina at rest with ST segment elevation which, if compared to other clinical models of ischemia, appears to be more "echogenic" for several reasons:
1) no excessive tachicardia or hyperventilation are present during ischemic attacks, making it less difficult both to obtain good quality recordings and to properly interpret them (this is not the case, for instance, in exercise echocardiography);
2) The patient may lie quietly in the position most suitable for echocardiographic monitoring;
3) The site of ST elevation correlates fairly well with the site of ischemia (thereby varying from ST depression - by far the most common ECG pattern in demand induced ischemia - where the site of ischemia cannot be predicted on electrocardiographic ground). Our echocardiographic recordings were obtained in patients with variant angina in "warm" phase or during ergonovine testing performed for diagnostic purposes. In all cases the reliability of the findings was supported by two very important

conditions:
1) each patient acted as his own control (recordings were carried out "from basal to basal", going through ischemia, or "from ischemia to basal").
2) within each patient, the contractility of the ischemic wall could be compared to the simultaneous contractility of the other non ischemic walls.

Ultrasonic findings in acute transmural myocardial ischemia

Echocardiographic signs of transient myocardial ischemia with ST segment elevation follow a well defined time sequence (2,3), which is schematically summarized in table I, together with their relationship with the conventional markers of the ischemic event (ST elevation and pain).

	Pre ECG phase	ECG phase	Post ECG phase
1) Echocardiogram			
a) Wall signs:			
- Wall motion	↓	↓↓	↑
- End-diastolic thickness	↓	↓	=
- % systolic thickening	↓	↓↓	↑
b) Cavity signs:			
- End-diastolic diameter	=/↑	↑	=/↓
- % fractional shortening	↓	↓↓	↑
2) Electrocardiogram	ST =	ST↑	ST =
3) Anginal pain	NO	YES	NO

Table I: time sequence of clinical, ECGgraphic and mechanical events during acute transmural myocardial ischemia. The time sequence of echocardiographic signs of acute ischemia in ergonovine-induced attacks and their relationship to conventional markers of ischemia (pain and ST segment elevation) are schematically shown in this table. (↓) = marked decrease; (↑) = increase; (=) = unchanged relative to basal.

It is important to underline that such observations cannot be extended to angina at rest with ST depression where different alterations both in regional myocardial perfusion (non transmural but more extensive) and contractile function have been described by radioisotopic techniques (4). Most of these ultrasonic signs are the expression of regional impairment in contractility, an early consequence of ischemia (Fig. 1).

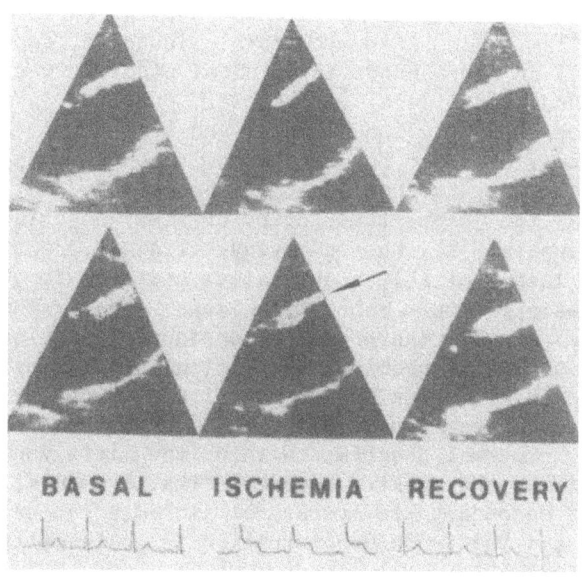

FIGURE 1:
Selected spots of a continuous two-dimensional echocardiographic monitoring during an episode of transient myocardial ischemia with ST segment elevation in man. From top to bottom end-diastolic frames (upper row), end-systolic frames (middle row) and ECG (lower row) are shown, while basal, ischemic and recovery findings are reported in columns.
During ST segment elevation (middle column), systolic thickening of the septum is impaired: in fact, a "step sign" (arrow) can be observed between the proximal and the distal part of the septum which, due to ischemia, has transiently lost its contractile function. Echocardiography is the only technique which permits a non invasive imaging, with high spatial and temporal resolution, of the mechanical changes which may occur in human hearts.

In particular, the mechanical impairment may be the only sign of the ischemic nature of attacks characterized only by minor T wave changes (Prinzmetal "abortive" attacks) (5).
The "post-electrocardiographic" contractile rebound is linked to reactive hyperemia, and, therefore, it is less evident when a severe organic stenosis limits reflow after spasm resolution (6).
This reported experience, performed during a rapidly changing phenomenon like transient myocardial ischemia, shows the marked potentialities of ultrasounds in clinical studies, where monitoring of regional and global left ventricular function is required with a high degree of resolution in space and time.
Being absolutely specific for the ischemic event, the mechanical marker is the only "stand alone" criterion. Such a statement - correct from the conceptual point of view - should, however, be cautiously applied to the everyday clinical practice, since at present "we lack reliable quantitative criteria for the detection of hypokinesia with echo techniques" (7). The risk of overdiagnosis should therefore be considered, particularly taking into account technical problems and biological variability (in time - in response to different environmental and psychological factors - and in space, since a physiological gradient of contractility exists, even in normal hearts, within the left ventricle, going from the base to the apex). However, "that segmental contraction abnormalities secondary to myocardial ischemia can be demonstrated with 2D-echo and that such demonstration is clinically useful is beyond question" (7).

DOPPLER TECHNIQUES

The use of Doppler in cardiology is a recent acquisition if compared to M-Mode and 2-D techniques. Nowadays, 15 years after its first applications, Doppler expansion in clinical practice seems to be in an exponential phase. This diffusion is based on the fact that Doppler techniques add to echocardiography quite new parameters which all stem from blood flow velocity measurements. These new parameters represent such a different type of information that a challenging effort is required to correctly understand their meaning. Cardiologists are, indeed, trained to think of cardiac hemodynamics in terms of pressure, pressure drop, stroke volume, cardiac output and volume of shunts, which are measurements derived from the use of intravenous or intraarterial catheters. No parameters of these, however, although collected in the catheterisation laboratory, provide measurements of blood flow velocity.
The early generation of Doppler velocimeters employed continuous wave ultrasonic probes which provided evaluation of blood flow velocities, without spatial definition of the site of sampling (8). The introduction of pulsed Doppler has overcome this limitation,

since it is possible to control both the depth and the dimensions of the sample volume on which flow velocity is detected (9). However, pulsed Doppler technique, even if combined with M-Mode or with 2-D echocardiography, can only partially overcome some crucial limitations in the accuracy of velocity measurements, since: a) it is unable to correctly display high blood flow velocity, due to the aliasing phenomenon (10); b) the recorded values of velocity are highly dependent on the angle between ultrasonic beam and flow direction.

The possibility of imaging the heart from different acoustic windows greatly helps as far as angle dependence of velocity measurements is concerned, whereas the aliasing phenomenon can only be overcome by the use of continuous wave Doppler which has, practically, no limits in velocity detection and display.

New perspective in Doppler imaging

Very recently, the potentialities of Cardiac Doppler in the analysis of blood flow velocity within the cardiac chambers and great vessels have been further increased by the commercial availability of the so-called "Color Doppler" technique. The flow information is given, in color and in real time, within the anatomical cross-section offered by the 2-D echocardiographic technique (Fig. 2). The information on blood flow, given in terms of mapping of velocity direction and intensity, added to real-time imaging of anatomy and function of structures, represents a major break-through in modern non invasive cardiology (11-12).

Clinical applications of Doppler techniques

Valves incompetence

Detection of regurgitant flow from an incompetent valve is the kind of information simple to obtain by pulsed Doppler techniques. While echocardiography allows only indirect signs of valve insufficiency, Doppler reveals not only the presence of a regurgitant flow but also the direction, the width and the length of the jet. Although several attempts have been made to quantitate the regurgitant volume, at the present time the semiquantitative approach seems to be the most accurate. Using a traditional Doppler system, a precise mapping of the jet in a cardiac chamber is a difficult target. However, this information can be easily and quickly obtained by a two-dimensional Color Doppler system; in fact, in each frame it displays the instantaneous mapping of flow velocities in cardiac chambers, even if at a rather low frame rate (Fig.3).

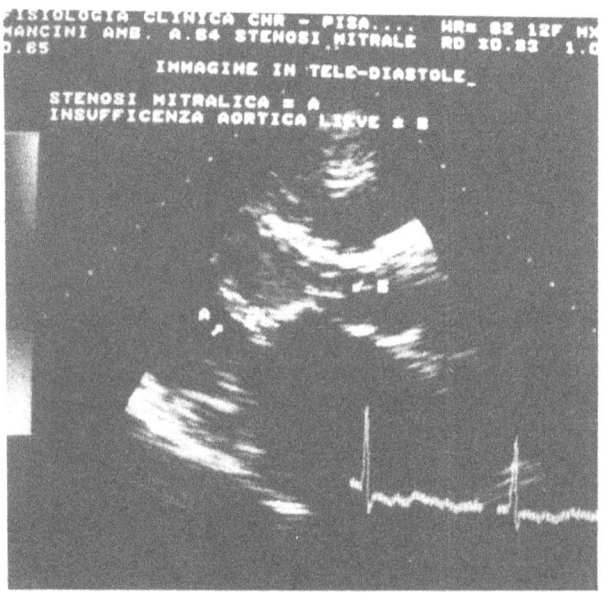

FIGURE 2:
Combined valvular disorder: mitral stenosis and aortic regurgitation. Non-invasive intracardiac blood flow mapping with two-dimensional Echo-Doppler imaging instrument (Toshiba SSH 65A). This image was recorded from the parasternal approach during diastole in a patient with acquired valvular disease. It is clearly evident that flow through the mitral valve (A) is limited to a small orifice (mitral stenosis) and it occurs contemporarily with regurgitant flow (B) from the incompetent aortic valve. The two diastolic jets (A = mitral and B = aortic) have different sites of origin but both are directed toward the left ventricle; only a two-dimensional Color Doppler system can allow a quick and clear evaluation of these combined lesions.

For colour reproduction see colour section at the end of the book

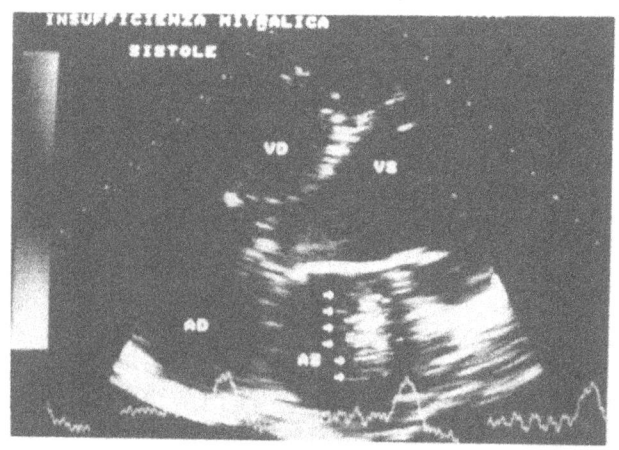

FIGURE 3A
Color Doppler flow imaging in a patient with mitral insufficiency. The image, obtained in mid-systole from the apical approach, clearly shows the geometric characteristics of the regurgitant volume in the left atrium.

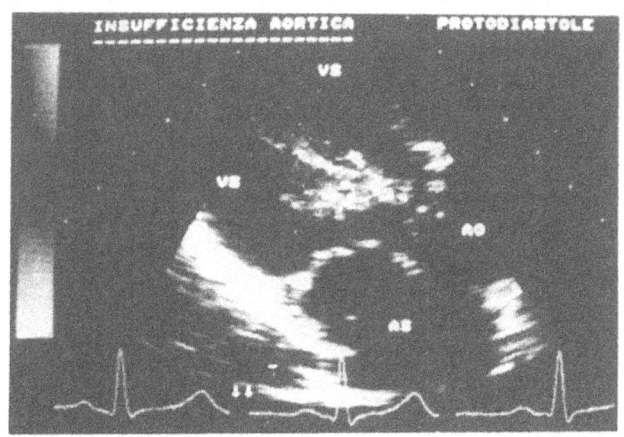

FIGURE 3B
Color Doppler flow imaging in a case of aortic insufficiency. The coloured "mosaic" appearance of the regurgitant jet is of the utmost evidence in this early diastolic still frame. Ao = aorta; VS = left ventricle; AS = left atrium.

A similar application of Doppler is performed when abnormal flows between the two ventricles, either congenital or acquired, or between the two atria or the large vessels (patent ductus arterious) are searched for.

Prosthetic valves

This promising field of Doppler application counteracts the known limits of echocardiography; in fact prosthetic valve dysfunction can be easily detected if a valve incompetence can be revealed by means of the Doppler examination. In the near future, a better knowledge of the normal flow through the different types of prosthetic valves will permit an early diagnosis of dysfunction and the results of surgical interventions will be easily followed up non invasively.

Pressure gradient across stenotic valves

The aim of this application is to derive non-invasively the pressure drop across a stenotic valve from absolute values of blood flow velocities measured by Doppler. The quantitative assessment of pressure drop has been validated in mitral stenosis by Hatle and co-workers (13) by means of a continuous wave Doppler, according to a simplified Bernoulli equation. In fact, blood flow velocity across a stenotic orifice is related to the pressure gradient across the stenosis by the simple relation $DP = 4V^2$, where DP is the pressure drop, V is the maximal peak blood flow velocity through the valve and 4 is a constant.
Moreover, the measurement of the time required by the pressure gradient to drop to one-half of its initial peak value allows an estimation of the valve area in those patients in whom valve leaflets are heavily calcified or the subvalvular apparatus is so thickened that the echocardiographic measurement of the valve area may not be accurate.

Cardiac output: monitoring of changes
and absolute measurements

Measurement of cardiac output can be useful in two main settings:
a) to monitor its changes with time;
b) to know its value at a specific moment (the first assessment of a patient).
The choice of a particular kind of Doppler technique depends on the final goal which must be reached: continuous wave Doppler can be satisfactorily used for monitoring changes in cardiac output (14) (Fig. 4), while a combination of echocardiography and Doppler instrumentation is necessary to measure absolute values of this parameter.
The principle on which the use of blood flow velocity for cardiac

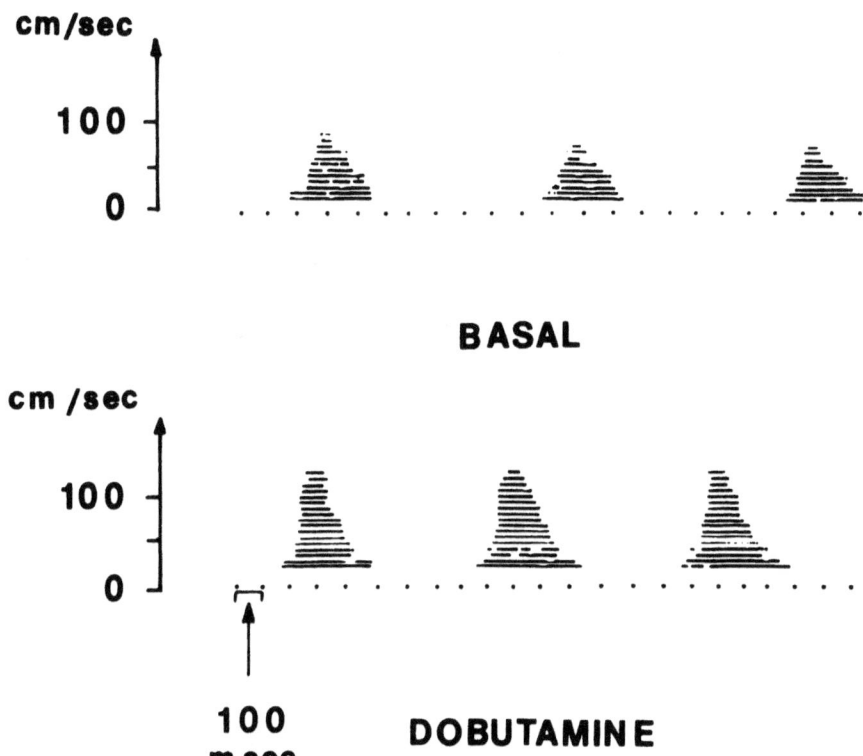

FIGURE 4:
Non-invasive blood flow velocity measurements obtained by insonating the descending part of the aortic arch by means of a continuous wave Doppler technique (Transcutaneous Aorto Velography, Muirhead Ltd).
Doppler tracings recorded in basal condition (on top) and during Dobutamine intravenous infusion of 5 ng/Kg/min (on bottom) are shown. A marked increase in the area of blood flow velocity complexes, expression of an increase in stroke volume, is clearly evident during Dobutamine administration, if compared to basal state (14). As the heart rate is almost equal in both conditions, it follows that cardiac output is also increased during the infusion of the drug.

output (CO) measurement is based is expressed by the following equation:
CO = $\bar{V}$ x A, where $\bar{V}$ is the time averaged blood flow velocity in the vessel and A is its cross sectional area normal to the direction of flow. If the value of A remains constant CO and $\bar{V}$ are directly proportional so that changes in CO are parallelled by proportional changes in $\bar{V}$.
An important assumption to be made is that blood flow should be nearly laminar in the site of measurement, so that the instantaneous blood flow velocity is roughly equivalent in each point of the cross sectional area of the vessel. If a continuous wave Doppler with a wide beam is used to insonate the vessel, the time averaged value of blood flow velocity shall be more accurate than that obtained with a pulsed Doppler instrument which has to be used with a small sample volume.

TISSUE CHARACTERIZATION

General background.

Ultrasonic tissue characterization consists of the use of ultrasounds to define the physical state of the tissue. The hypothesis underlying this application is that pathological changes alter the physical and mechanical properties of the tissue and that these changes can be detected and quantified by ultrasound. Such an hypothesis can be considered "proved" - in the experimental setting - for various pathologies of the heart (acute and chronic myocardial infarction, some cardiomyopathies, cardiac contusion) (15).
We will briefly summarize the results obtained in our laboratory on atherosclerotic aortic walls.

Findings in atherosclerotic disease

A major problem for quantitative ultrasonic diagnosis is the presence of a phase cancellation effect inherent to piezoelectric transducers. Phase cancellation at a receiving transducer occurs because tissue is inherently inhomogeneous. When a sound wave is launched, it has a well defined shape, but as it moves through the tissue, which has spatial variation in its composition and texture, parts of the wave front, or phase, move ahead or fall behind. Such a small shift in the wavefront may cause a distortion of the electrical signal received and, consequently, misinterpretation of the intrinsic structural properties of the tissue giving rise to the ultrasonic signal (16).

A first set of experiments was therefore performed in our laboratory in order to assess - by means of statistical indexes - the relevance of phase cancellation effects in the in vitro study of normal and diseased arterial specimens (17). It was shown that small diameter focused transducers may effectively minimize phase cancellation artifacts, which are however more relevant in atherosclerotic specimens (probably due to higher structural inhomogeneity as compared to normal walls).
In subsequent studies, we showed that backscatter (18) and attenuation (19) may discriminate normal from fibrofatty and calcific specimens (Fig. 5). By attenuation, even fibrous samples may be separated from fibrofatty samples.
The parameters of attenuation and backscatter are complementary; in fact, each of them provides information not present in the other. Therefore, it is likely that an approach based on the measurement of both will be most useful for clinical studies (16).
Further in vitro studies are needed anyway before an effective transfer of this information to an in vivo setting (20).

Perspectives of tissue characterization

With the use of technologically advanced transducers and exploiting the very sophisticated electronic features of instrumentation, it will be possible: a) to select a window within cardiac and/or vascular wall structures shown by two-dimensional echoes;
b) to analyze those structures according to radiofrequency parameters such as backscatter and attenuation.
c) to obtain speckle-free images and texture images.

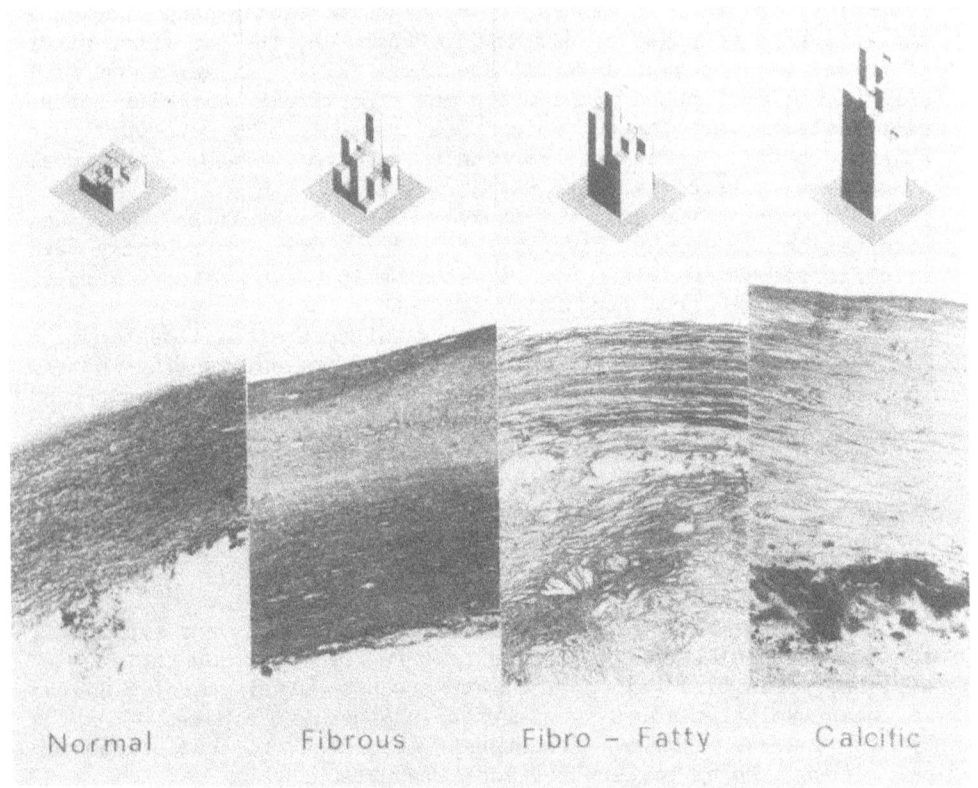

FIGURE 5:
Pictorial three-dimensional display (by 4 x 4 matrix) of four specimens of atherosclerotic plaques: normal, fibrous, fibrofatty and calcific.
For each specimen, 16 different values of ultrasonic attenuation were measured and displayed in three-dimensional histograms (upper part of the figure). In the lower panel, the histological slice shown (Weigert-Van Gieson, 32x) is a typical one out of the 16 slices, perpendicular to the tissue surface, performed for each specimen.
(Kind permission of Circulation Research: Picano E et al.: 56: 4, 1985).

CONCLUSIONS

The morpho-functional information provided by echocardiography has greatly questioned and often replaced the central role of cardiac catheterization which, until a few years ago, was almost invariably considered a "mandatory step" in the decision making process toward cardiac diagnosis. Nowadays, echocardiography is a solid cornerstone among the available diagnostic tools, providing prompt, easy-to-obtain, inexpensive and non invasive real time images of cardiac structures.
In order to remain the cornerstone of diagnosis, as in recent years of our "echocardiographic era in cardiology", increasing information with decreasing costs has to be offered by ultrasounds. Ultrasounds now appear to be in the same condition as Alice in Wonderland: "to remain in the place where you are, you must run with all your might. To go further, you must run twice faster".
It is reasonable to foresee that, within a few years, commercial instruments will have conventional M-Mode and 2-D imaging, Doppler flow imaging and quantitative imaging for tissue analysis, all built in the same basic hardware. Future needs and "leading edges" of echocardiography can be foreseen in the following schematic manner:
1) Small and inexpensive two-dimensional instruments for bedside use in the hospital and at home, in the out-patient clinics and in private offices, etc..
2) Computer assistance to analyse and quantitate ventricular function, to enhance ultrasonic images for automatic detection of internal borders and, memorizing anatomic cross sections from multiple viewpoints, to reconstruct in a three-dimensional display.
3) Radiofrequency analysis to explore the minute anatomical structure of the myocardium, valves and vessel walls (tissue characterization by means of new ultrasonic parameters such as quantitative backscatter, differential attenuation, etc.).
4) New and safe contrast agents to study myocardial perfusion in man with the help of digital substraction techniques.
5) Doppler imaging to map the type and the direction of flow within the cardiac chambers and in the great vessels, as well as to quantify transvalvular pressure gradients, shunts, etc.
6) Intraoperative use of high resolution echocardiography either to map blood flow velocities or to locate plaques in the stenotic vessels or to quickly control the surgical procedures performed (Fig. 6).

Paper partially supported by C.N.R. Progetto Finalizzato TBMS (Director: Prof. L.Donato) (Sottoprogetto ultrasuoni) and by Ministero Pubblica Istruzione (Fondi 60%).
Eugenio Picano M.D. is recipient of A.R.MED Research Fellowship.
Elena Moscarelli M.D. is recipient of "Assegno di formazione professionale" Legge 285, C.N.R.

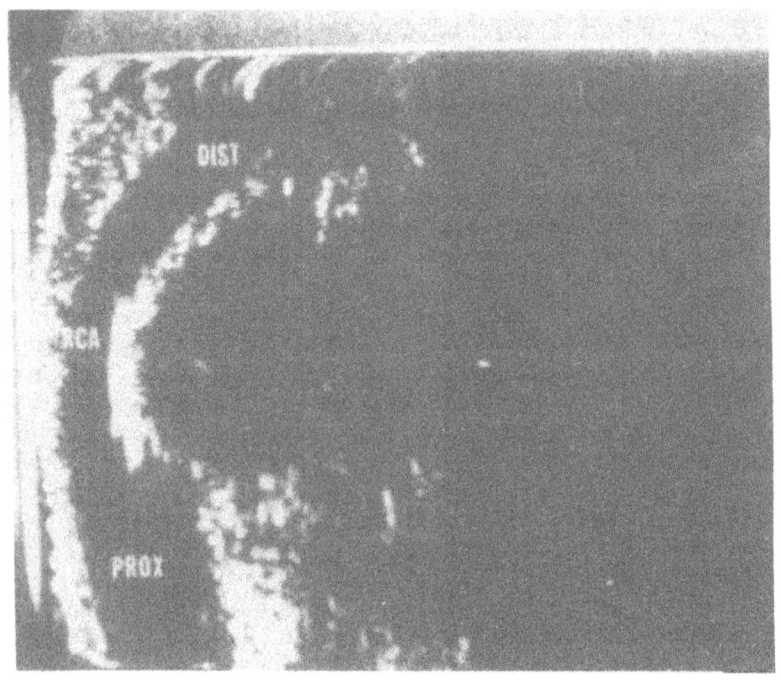

FIGURE 6:
Intraoperative application of high resolution 2-D echocardiography during open heart surgery.
A right coronary artery is visualized with an obstructive lesion between the proximal (PROX) and the distal (DIST) segment. Please note the marked reduction in lumen diameter due to the presence of an atherosclerotic plaque.
(Kind permission of Circulation: Sahn DJ et al.: 66: 1034, 1982).

REFERENCES

1) Kerber RE, Martins JB, Marcus ML: Effects of acute ischemia, nitroglycerin and nitroprusside on regional myocardial thickening, stress and perfusion. Experimental echocardiographic studies. Circulation 60: 12, 1979.
2) Distante A., Rovai D, Picano E, Moscarelli E, Palombo C, Morales MA, Michelassi C, L'Abbate A.: Transient changes in left ventricular mechanics during attacks of Prinzmetal angina: an M-Mode echocardographic study. Am Heart Journal, 107: 465, 1984.
3) Distante A, Rovai D, Picano E, Moscarelli E, Morales MA, Palombo C, L'Abbate A.: Transient changes in left ventricular mechanics during attacks of Prinzmetal's angina: a two-dimensional echocardiographic study. Am Heart Journal: 108, 440, 1984.
4) Parodi O, Bencivelli W, Camici P, Marzullo P, Davies JG, Maseri A, L'Abbate A: A new technique for the simultaneous assessment of myocardial perfusion and contractility in man. Am J Cardiol 47: 394, 1981.
5) Rovai D, Distante A, Moscarelli E, Morales MA, Picano E, Palombo C, L'Abbate A.: Transient myocardial ischemia with minimal electrocardiographic changes: an echocardiographic study in patients with Prinzmetal's angina. Am Heart Journal, 109: 78, 1985.
6) Distante A, Picano E, Rovai D, Moscarelli E, Morales MA, Palombo C, L'Abbate A: Post-ischemic contractility overshoot and degree of basal stenosis in coronary artery undergoing spasm. An echocardiographic and angiographic study in Prinzmetal angina. Circulation, 68 (Suppl. III): 256, 1983.
7) Falsetti HL, Marcus ML, Kerber RE, Skorton DJ: Quantification of myocardial ischemia and infarction by left ventricular imaging (editorial). Circulation 63: 747, 1981.
8) Light HL: Transcutaneous Aortovelography, a new window on the circulation. Br Heart Journal 38: 433, 1976.
9) Baker DW, Rubenstein SA, Lorch GS: Pulsed Doppler Echocardiography: principles and applications. Am J Med 63: 69, 1977.
10) Hatle L, Angelsen B: Doppler Ultrasound in Cardiology. Lea & Febiger Publishers. Philadelphia, 1985.
11) Omoto R: Real-time Two-dimensional Echocardiography. Lea & Febiger Publishers. Tokyo, 1984.
12) Namekawa K, Kasai C, Omoto R, Kondo Y, Katabami T, Hidai T, Yoshikawa Y, Tsukamoto M, Yokote Y, Takamoto S, Koyano A: Realtime two-dimensional bloodflow imaging using ultrasound Doppler. J of Ultrasound in Medicine and Biology 10 (Suppl. 2), 1983.
13) Hatle L, Brubbakk A, Tromsdal A, Angelsen B: Non invasive assessment of pressure drop in mitral stenosis by Doppler ultrasound. Br Heart J 40: 131, 1978.

14) Distante A, Moscarelli E, Rovai D, L'Abbate A: Monitoring of changes in cardiac output by Transcutaneous Aortovelography, a non-invasive Doppler technique: comparison with thermodilution. J Nucl Med All Sci 24: 171, 1980.
15) Miller JG, Perez JE, Mottley JG, Madaras EI, Johnston PH, Blodgett ED: Myocardial tissue characterization: an approach based on quantitative backscatter and attenuation. Proceedings of the 1983 IEEE Ultrasonics Symposium.
16) Miller JW, Sobel BE: Ultrasonic tissue characterization. Hospital Practice, 1: 143, 1982.
17) Landini L, Picano E, Sarnelli R: Attenuation measurements in atherosclerotic tissues: Problems with phase cancellation artifacts. Med & Biol Eng & Comput 23: 220, 1985.
18) Picano E, Landini L, Distante A, Sarnelli R, Benassi A, L'Abbate A: Different degree of atherosclerosis detected by backscattered ultrasounds; an in vitro study on fixed human aortic walls. J Clin Ultrasound, 11: 375, 1983.
19) Picano E, Landini L, Distante A, Benassi A, Sarnelli R, L'Abbbate A: Fibrosis, Lipids, and Calcium in Human Atherosclerotic Plaque. In Vitro Differentiation from Normal Aortic Walls by Ultrasonic Attenuation Circ. Res. 56: 4, 1985.
20) Landini L, Picano E, Sarnelli R: In vitro ultrasonic tissue characterization of atherosclerosis: state of the art, problems, and perspectives. In: Atherosclerosis Review, RJ Hegyeli Editor. Raven Press Publisher 12: 165. New York 1984.

ADVANCED APPLICATIONS OF ULTRASOUND IMAGING IN INTERNAL MEDICINE: RESULTS, LIMITATIONS AND FUTURE NEEDS

Licinio Angelini
IV Clinica Chirurgica
Universita di Roma
Rome, Italy

1   INTRODUCTION

Diagnostic ultrasound has experienced an extremely rapid and extensive development in general surgery in the last five years, in terms both of technological achievements and clinical applications. This development has been brought about by the impressive progress which has been made in ultrasound instrumenation for real time imaging.

In 1979, it was easy to predict that the future of ultrasound in surgery would depend upon the rapidity with which technological progress and industrial effort would make real time, high resolution, multi-probe portable equipment available. Nevertheless, at that time this view was not shared by all leading ultrasonologists and particularly by those from outside Italy. When the technology began to become available, there was a lag in the acceptance of real time scanning both in the diagnostic clinic (where the new instruments competed with static scanners) and in the operating theatre. Nowadays, the static scanner has largely been replaced by real time scanners of which the mechanical sector types are presently probably the most popular.

2   CLINICAL APPLICATIONS OF NEW TECHNOLOGY

The introduction of any new diagnostic procedure gives new hope and new enthusiasm in the otherwise discouraging management of patients with malignant disease. Thus, diagnostic ultrasound has widely proved to be a valuable tool for the diagnostician in the investigation of all neoplasms except for those arising within the lung parenchyma and in the skull. Sadly, however, there is no evidence that the introduction of diagnostic ultrasound has changed the mortality rates for cancer; the same applies to computed tomography and so this should not discourage investigators working on the technological and clinical areas of ultrasonography.

Opportunities for the improvements of ultrasonic diagnostic techniques are limited by physical considerations although in principle it should be possible to obtain more information by more complex techniques of retrieval and interpretation. In particular, the use of higher frequencies should lead to better resolution but higher frequencies have more limited penetrations. Another possibility is that of identifying tissues from their ultrasonic signatures thus leading to the realisation of "telehistology". This objective has attracted numerous investigators but it has to be admitted that progress so far has been generally frustrating and disappointing. Exceptions to this are that it may be possible to characterise tissues in terms of ultrasonic measurements of their attenuations and propagation speeds; computer reconstruction techniques using the transmission method are beginning to demonstrate this in the study of the breast. Nevertheless, no ultrasound tissue characterisation technique has yet become a routine clinical tool.

Despite the disappointing results from some laboratory work, clinicians have succeeded in expanding the usefulness of conventional ultrasonic diagnosis by developing guided needle aspiration and biopsy. Even when only bistable ultrasonic displays were available, ultrasound was shown to be an excellent means of guiding the direction of depth of a needle puncture in order to biopsy tissue or aspirate cells from suspected areas. The method was even used as a therapeutic manoeuvre for emptying fluid collections. Ultrasound guided needle aspiration and biopsy is becoming a common procedure now that real time equipment with good resolution is widely available. The procedure is now more easily performed, with less risk to the patient, especially when the region to be investigated is part of an anatomical structure that undergoes displacement during respiratory movements. Although only a few studies have reported the reliability of the method, there is no doubt that this interventional application of ultrasound does increase the diagnostic accuracy in many fields of pathology. In fact, ultrasound guidance is likely in the future to be the only technique capable of providing an accurate preoperative diagnosis in many types of neoplastic and diffuse parenchymal diseases.

3   INTRACAVITARY, ENDOSCOPIC AND INTRAOPERATIVE
    ULTRASOUND (IU)

Ultrasound frequencies greater than 5 MHz are capable of giving excellent resolution but generally they cannot be used transcutaneously because of the limitation in penetration which restricts access to intra-abdominal structures in most adult patients. One proposed solution to this problem, which incidentally also avoids the very annoying problem of intervening bowel gas, is to gain direct access to the organ under study. One approach is by intracavitary and endoscopic scanning.

The most widely investigated intracavitary scanning procedure is transrectal ultrasonography which in some countries (Japan, Italy etc) has become almost a routine diagnostic procedure for prostatic disorders. In fact with the transrectal probe the prostate gland is very nicely displayed and a lot of information can be obtained about its size, shape, contour and possible space occupying lesions. The contribution of this kind of information to differential diagnosis between benign and malignant disease is not negligible. At present transrectal ultrasonography is also used to stage rectal cancer more accurately. Work in progress in this particular area is very promising and if eventually clinically validated this diagnostic procedure would represent a major breakthrough in the treatment and follow-up of rectal cancer. As far as endoscopic scanning is concerned, the combined effort of endoscopy (Fuji, Olympus) and ultrasound (ATL, Aloka) equipment manufacturers has not yet resulted in appreciable progress in any clinical area. Nevertheless, this approach deserves further development and investigation because of its potential.

Another solution to the problem of limited penetration of high resolution probes is by direct application of the probe itself during surgical intervention. This has the great advantage that the surgeon can control the position of the probe and see directly the anatomical structure to which it is applied. The concept of using an ultrasonic probe during surgical operations is neither new nor recent. Since the early 1960s there have been reports about experience with the intraoperative localisation of kidney stones using A mode linear display equipment.

The introduction of high-frequency real-time B-scan equipment has remarkably extended the potential fields of application of intraoperative ultrasonography. Up to now hepatobiliary and pancreatic surgery have proven to be the areas where IU may give useful information. As for the biliary tract there is already sufficient evidence that intraoperative sonocholangiography and the traditional intraoperative X-ray cholangiography are competitive but sonocholangiography has the higher positive predictive value: therefore this examination could reduce the number of unnecessary choledocotomies. Regarding the rare but not exceptional cases of intrahepatic calculi, ultrasound examination is definitely more accurate than cholangiography.

At our own Institution we have investigated in particular the potential and ability of IU to detect occult neoplastic deposits in parenchymal organs such as the liver and pancreas. It is well known that in a not negligible percentage of cases liver metastases or endocrine tumours of the pancreas are localised deeply in the parenchyma and have a size (less than 1 cm) that prevents any preoperative investigation (by angiography, ultrasound or CT) to detect them and they also escape even the most accurate visual and palpatory examination at surgery. In both these conditions we have been able to demonstrate that using a 7.5 or 10 MHz probe, IU is far more accurate than any preoperative work-up resulting in the following advantages:
- more correct staging of the disease;
- reduction of expensive and invasive preoperative investigations; and
- reduction of unnecessary surgery.

There certainly are restrictions as indicated above since the technology for these applications is not yet perfected and there is difficulty in transferring echographic competence into the operating rooms.

In principle, endoscanning and intraoperative ultrasonography may eventually have the same indications and give images of similar quality. Assuming that the two procedures can achieve the same level of diagnostic accuracy, endoscanning will have the great advantage of providing the information before surgery.

4   EDUCATION AND TRAINING

The availability of new ultrasonic techniques will encourage many clinical specialists, such as those internal medicine, surgery and endoscopy, to begin to apply them in their practice. The availability of low cost equipment will encourage the use of ultrasound by the general practitioner.

The more widespread use of ultrasound is potentially of great benefit to the patients. This benefit will only be realised if appropriate education and training is provided beginning at the undergraduate level. This is already a demanding requirement and the provision of education and training facilities must not be delayed into the future.

FUTURE DIRECTIONS IN ULTRASOUND IMAGING: A CRITICAL EVALUATION

P.N.T. Wells

Department of Medical Physics
Bristol General Hospital
Bristol BS1 6SY, U.K.

1 INTRODUCTION

Ultrasonic imaging methods already have an established role in clinical diagnosis. Static and real-time scanning techniques, supplemented by A-scan and M-mode studies and by Doppler data concerning structure motion and blood flow, are vital to the modern practice of internal medicine, obstetrics, urology, cardiology and ophthalmology.

The future of ultrasound imaging depends mainly on the development of new technical methods, new clinical applications, complementary and competitive technologies and safety considerations. Some aspects of these factors are considered in the following sections.

2 THE DEVELOPMENT OF NEW TECHNICAL METHODS

2.1 Transducer Materials

Nowadays, lead zirconate titanate transducers [1] are by far the most commonly used in medical ultrasonics. For diagnostic applications, PZT-5H is a good pulse-echo transmitter receiver for transducers with diameters up to a few centimetres operating in the low megahertz frequency range; it has reasonably high transmitting and receiving constants, an adequate coupling constant and a fairly low mechanical Q factor. Lead metaniobate may be better than PZT5-H when the transducer has a large area, because of its relatively low dielectric constant.

The ferroelectric polymer polyvinylidene difluoride [2] has recently attracted much interest because of its potential advantages in ultrasonic diagnostic applications. These arise mainly because the material has low characteristic impedance (providing a good match to water and soft tissues) and low Q (giving good pulse response). The main difficulty is the low sensitivity of the material. It is likely that the problem may be solved by the development of blends of PVF2 and, for example, polyethylmethacrylate or copolymers with trifluoroethylene [3].

The available PVF2 film typically has a thickness of 30 µm and is electroded on each surface. It can be used as a single layer on a low impedance backing, as a single layer on a high impedance backing, or as a stack of transducer plates arranged to reinforce each other [4].

Pulsed Doppler transducer materials are chosen to optimise the same factors as exist in comparable pulse-echo situations, although a narrower frequency bandwidth may be acceptable and this can allow a greater sensitivity. For continuous wave Doppler applications, the probe usually has separate transducers for transmitting and receiving.

2.2 Transducer Array Construction and Associated Signal Processing

Transducer arrays are used to steer and focus ultrasonic beams by the introduction of electronically-controlled time delays which modify the velocity potential of the transducer surface to produce the desired diffraction pattern. At the moment, three types of array are in common use [3]: annular arrays, which are used to control the axial position of the focus of the circularly symmetrical beam [5] and to tailor the beam profile [6]; linear arrays, which allow the use of element groups to produce a rectangular format real-time scan and also to control the axial position of the focus in azimuth [8]. The array elements may be coplanar, but, in the case of annular arrays, some degree of curvature may be used to provide mechanical focusing so that the required time delay variation to control the axial position of the focus can be more easily provided.

The discrete nature of the array gives rise to grating lobes which have the effect of producing "ghost" images [9]. Grating lobes can be reduced by increasing the element density of the array. Small elements may be electrically connected in parallel to produce any required aperture. Another problem is that, particularly with phased arrays, the array is required to be sensitive to ultrasonic disturbances approaching at other than normal incidence.

A typical phased array transducer [8] for operation at 2.5 MHz consists of 64 PZT elements 0.24 mm wide, 14 mm long and 0.48 mm high, bonded to a 30 mm long alumina substrate attached to a tungsten-vinyl backing. The front faces of the elements are bonded to a brass foil, with an acoustic lens focused at a distance of 70 mm. The spaces between the elements are occupied by air.

The delay circuits associated with transmission and reception are usually separate. Transmission delays can be generated by voltage-controlled multivibrators or by digital timing pulses. Reception delays can be introduced either at the ultrasonic frequency or after the signal has been mixed with a local oscillator to shift it to the baseband frequency. The delay circuits have to be able to accommodate the full dynamic range of the ultrasonic signal (usually after compression by time gain control) and passive, lumped-constant delay lines have the advantage of having low inherent noise. The main difficulty with this approach is that the channel corresponding to each element in the array has to have its own separate delay circuit, so the expense and size are both rather large. Each delay line must typically provide hundreds of delay steps to cover the necessary overall delay range. A system which greatly reduces the component requirements [10] is based on separate and independent processing of the carrier and envelope of the echo pulses. Carrier phasing is accomplished by electronic phase-shifters, while envelope delay is provided by delay lines. The increments in delay line timings are much greater than would be required without the continuously-variable phase shifts.

2.3 Improved Resolution

As a result of progress in the design of ultrasonic transducers and electronic amplifiers, the ultrasonic frequencies used for clinical investigations have steadily increased over the past few years. For example, 3.5 MHz (and sometimes even 5 MHz) is now often used for abdominal studies, where 2.5 MHz would previously have been the limit. Together with the provision for choosing the transducer with the optimal aperture and focal length, or even swept focusing, image resolution has enjoyed a corresponding improvement.

Fortunately, there is still scope for further improvement. Firstly, it should be possible to optimise the transducer aperture so that the effects of inhomogeneities in the distributions of tissues with different speeds and attenuations [11] (which tend to distort the ultrasonic beam) are minimised in any given situation. Secondly, it should be possible to correct for inhomogeneities in speed distribution by the application of adaptive delays in one-dimensional or, better, in two-dimensional arrays to compensate for phase degradation [12]. Finally, the application of a fully-compensated synthetic aperture may result in diffraction-limited resolution throughout the entire scan plane [13], but there are several difficult problems to solve before this could be implemented.

2.4 Image Texture Analysis and Tissue Characterisation

The resolution of an ultrasonic pulse-echo imaging system is determined by the dimensions of the resolution cell. The image is characterised by a granular pattern, or "speckle", which varies from place to place in the tissue and which fluctuates in time as a result of motion. This speckle can be explained in terms of the coherent formation of the echo from the many small scatterers within the resolution cell [14]. Thus, the texture in the image does not bear a one-to-one relationship to the scatterers in the tissue, but it is an artifact which reflects the properties of the imaging system in addition to being characteristic of the geometrical distribution and strength of the scatterers.

Despite the fact that clinicians infer some properties of the examined tissues from the corresponding textures in the ultrasonic image, it can be argued that an ideal image should not contain any speckle since speckle is an artifact [1]. Speckle can be smoothed by combining images which are uncorrelated, apart from echoes directly related to actual targets. Images with uncorrelated speckle can be obtained by scanning from different directions, or by scanning at different ultrasonic frequencies [15].

There is great interest in the possibility that ultrasonic signals may contain clues about the histology and, more importantly, about the pathology of the examined tissues. For example, liquid-filled structures such as cysts are generally more anechoic and more transonic than solid tissues. Cirrhotic liver tends to be more echogenic than normal liver [16]. The dependence of attenuation on frequency, which can be estimated from backscattered signals analysed in terms of zero-crossing frequency [17] or frequency spectra [18], may be characteristic for different tissues. Other approaches to tissue characterisation are based on estimates of speed [19], nonlinearity [20] and the frequency or angular dependence of the scattered echo signals [21].

2.5 Phantoms and Methods of Standardisation

The establishment and definition of appropriate methods of measuring and reporting the performance of ultrasonic pulse-echo diagnostic equipments is the subject of a paper published in 1976 by a Working Group of the International Electrotechnical

Commission [22]. This document deals with acoustic frequency, echo detection capability, gain characteristics, display characteristics, geometrical resolution and geometrical alignment accuracy.

As a substitute for some of the rigorous tests specified by the IEC Working Group, it is often satisfactory, at least on a day-to-day basis, to make do with checks involving the use of phantoms. The simplest phantoms consist of water tanks containing fine wires stretched between plates and with geometries allowing the rapid evaluation of registration and resolution when scanned by the instrument under test [23]. More complicated phantoms are constructed from "tissue-equivalent" materials which mimic real tissues, at least over limited frequency ranges, in terms of speed, attenuation and scattering [24]. Phantoms of this kind can be used for grey scale assessment [25], texture evaluation [26] and resolution checks [27].

2.6 Computed Tomography

Ultrasonic computed tomography involves the acquisition of a complete set of transmission profiles (time-of-flight or amplitude) through the plane of interest and the subsequent reconstruction of the two-dimensional cross-sectional image (representing propagation speed or attenuation) [28].

The assumption that the ultrasonic beam remains straight in tissue greatly simplifies the mathematics of the reconstruction process, but neglects the beam distortion due to reflection, refraction, inhomogeneous attenuation and diffraction. For this reason, some of the early results of ultrasound computed tomography were rather disappointing. Beam distortion is less of a problem with time-of-flight reconstruction than with amplitude reconstruction, since the signal which is first to be detected is likely to have travelled along the shortest path, although its amplitude may be quite unrepresentative of that of the main beam. One method of taking the effect into account is to backproject the received waves to the centre of the object [29].

Although only a few structures, such as the female breast, are accessible to this method (because through transmission in every direction is ideally required), encouraging results are being obtained [30].

2.7 Analysis and Display of Doppler Data

Ultrasonic Doppler techniques depend on the change in frequency which occurs when a wave is reflected by a moving target [31]. Simple Doppler systems merely detect the amplitudes of the Doppler-shifted signals. They cannot distinguish between approaching and receding targets, nor can they measure the positions of the targets along the ultrasonic beam. Directional information can be obtained by phase quadrature detection or by upper and lower sideband filtering. Range information can be derived from time-of-flight pulse-echo techniques, although only with resolution which depends on the bandwidth of the transmitted pulse; a compromise is necessary, because wide band pulses also result in undesirable Doppler spectral broadening [32].

The simplest method of presenting the Doppler information is for the operator to listen to the frequency-difference signals. This is all that is needed in some clinical applications, such as for confirming that the fetal heart is beating or that a blood vessel is patent. The acquisition of quantitative data, however, requires quantitative analysis of the Doppler signals. Although zero-crossing frequency meters are still used in many commercially available instruments, they can be misleading with complicated signals [33]. Frequency spectrum analysis is preferable and this can be achieved either off-line using a slow-speed swept filter or by fast Fourier transform or other techniques [34].

For the assessment of arterial disease, the information in the frequency spectrum can be interpreted by several methods [31]. The degree of damping and transit time of the arterial pulse can be judged by inspection of the recordings. An appropriate index of pulsatility of the waveform of maximum velocity against time can be calculated and its variation along the arterial segment can be assessed. The waveform can also be described by its Laplace transform [35], giving numerical indices of arterial stiffness, proximal lumen size and distal peripheral impedance.

The Doppler signals derived from the region of a malignant tumour generally seem to have distinctive characteristics. The phenomenon has been studied mainly in connexion with breast cancer [36]. The advancing edge of the tumour is associated with neovascularisation and the Doppler signals have increased power and frequency. It seems likely that the observed spectra are partly due to arterio-venous shunting.

In studies of the vascular system, it is often useful to have two-dimensional maps showing the positions and shapes of blood flow patterns. With blood vessels, these maps can be obtained with a Doppler system linked to a two-dimensional position measuring scanner [31]. Continuous wave Doppler systems are limited to the production of plan views because they lack range resolution; cross-sectional imaging can be obtained by using multigated pulsed Doppler systems.

The combination of two-dimensional pulse-echo real-time imaging with a limited amount of pulsed Doppler information (so-called "duplex" scanning) [37] results in a powerful diagnostic approach. Although originally developed for short-range applications, the value of deep Doppler studies is beginning to emerge. At the moment, the results are usually based on subjective assessment of the frequency spectra of the Doppler blood flow signals and so there is scope for the development of quantitative techniques for analysis of such characteristics as the frequency spread function (which is affected by blood flow turbulence).

Although the data acquisition time for Doppler information is inherently much slower than that for pulse-echo imaging, it is possible to produce two-dimensional blood flow maps in real time. One method uses a scanned linear array [38] and is suitable for studies of peripheral blood vessels; another method is based on autocorrelation [39] and has produced spectacular colour-coded images of blood flow superimposed on real-time two-dimensional cardiac scans.

There are three different approaches to the ultrasonic measurement of blood-flow-volume rate. The first is based on a multigated Doppler imaging system, arranged to determine the vessel orientation (to allow correction for the velocity vector) and the blood-flow velocity profile [40], which is assumed to have circular symmetry. In the second method, the blood-vessel diameter is measured by pulse-echo ultrasound and the average blood velocity is estimated from Doppler signals collected at known angles [41]. In the last method [42], the total backscattered power and the spectral distribution of the Doppler signals from all the blood moving in the vessel are measured and the volume flow rate is obtained by correcting for attenuation in the intervening tissue. This attenuation is estimated from a measurement of the backscattered power from a small sample volume positioned entirely within the blood in the vessel. This method, which avoids difficulties due to errors in angulation and vessel diameter measurements, should give good results in vessels of intermediate to large sizes.

3   THE DEVELOPMENT OF NEW CLINICAL APPLICATIONS

3.1   Intraoperative Imaging and Flow Studies

The idea of using ultrasonic imaging and flow studies during surgical procedures is not new but it is only recently that the potential importance of the approach has been widely appreciated [43]. One of the main problems has been the need to develop suitable real-time scanning and Doppler probes to satisfy the requirements of easy access and surgical sterility. The main applications are likely to be in vascular surgery, surgery of the biliary tree and the pancreas, renal surgery and neurosurgery.

3.2 Screening

There are a very few diseases in which screening the asymptomatic population is emerging as being clinically worthwhile. Examples include the detection of carcinoma of the cervix and fetal neural tube defects. So far, ultrasound has not demonstrated its value in screening. The development of high-resolution imaging might change the pattern of neural tube screening, cost-effective carotid screening might reduce stroke incidence and a successful scheme for breast cancer screening might include ultrasound. Advances of this kind would have significant effects on the future of ultrasound imaging.

3.3 Contrast Agents

An important advance in diagnostic ultrasound occurred with the discovery that indocyanine green completely opacifies the intraluminal areas of blood vessels and heart chambers on ultrasonic echograms [44]. The effect is mainly due to the production of microbubbles by cavitation at the tip of the injection catheter. Almost any liquid produces ultrasonic contrast in this way and, in one study [45], ether was found to be the most effective.

In practice, the use of microbubbles as an ultrasonic contrast agent is limited to studies of the right side of the heart, since transmission through the capillary bed is potentially dangerous [46].

Recently, there has been growing interest in the possibility of developing ultrasonic contrast agents with specific affinities. Gelatin encapsulated microbubbles, being relatively stable, are trapped in the vascular rims of malignant tumours [47] and result in echo enhancement. Contrast without the need for gas can also be obtained in suitable circumstances; perfluoroctylbromide, which concentrates in the reticuloendothelial system in the liver and spleen, increases echogenicity [48] but has the disadvantage of being rather toxic.

3.4 Inexpensive Scanners

As the medical community has become more familiar with the role of ultrasound in diagnosis and as improvements have taken place in the technology, it has begun to seem possible that appropriate ultrasonic instruments could have a significant impact on the practice of medicine in primary health care and in the developing countries. In primary health care, it should be possible for non-specialists in ultrasound to use simple purpose-designed instruments to carry out specific tests, particularly in obstetrics and cardiology, reducing the need for expensive referral to specialist centres. In the developing countries, where apart from some X-radiography there are virtually no facilities for noninvasive imaging studies, the availability of suitable scanners designed for obstetrics and for the detection of some of the endemic diseases such as abdominal cysts and abscesses, could revolutionise some aspects of the quality of health care.

3.5 Veterinary Applications

Although it has long been recognised that ultrasonic scanning might be of great value in the study of animals in health and disease [49], it is only recently that the subject has begun to be taken seriously. In animal production, the measurement of fat thickness is quite useful. In both large and small animals, other areas of importance include pregnancy detection and investigation of diseases of kidney, ovary and heart, besides the detection of pleural effusion. In large animals in particular, scanning from the rectum or the vagina is often used to avoid the need for substantial tissue penetration.

4 COMPLEMENTARY AND COMPETITIVE TECHNOLOGIES

In parallel with the development of ultrasonic diagnostic techniques, advances have been made in other methods of medical imaging [50]. The most important of these methods are X-radiography, digital radiography, computed tomography, radionuclide imaging and nuclear magnetic resonance imaging; other methods include infrared and microwave thermography, light and infrared transmission imaging, microwave imaging, body surface potential mapping and electrical impedance imaging [51]. Innovations in imaging technology can be judged to be successful if they reduce the invasiveness or discomfort of the examination, reduce the dose of ionising radiation or obtain more information with the same dose, increase the flexibility or convenience, give increased accuracy or reliability, or improve cost-effectiveness. When evaluated on the basis on these criteria, it is clear that contemporary ultrasonic techniques have many advantages. Moreover, the expenditure of resources on ultrasonic research and development is well justified in view of the many opportunities for innovation and improvement.

5 SAFETY OF ULTRASONIC DIAGNOSIS

Ultrasound can modify biological systems by at least two different mechanisms. These are due to thermal effects and to the effects of streaming or relative motion often associated with the presence of gas bubbles or cavitation. Such effects are generally considered to be undesirable in diagnostic applications, although some of them, even if they do occur, have not been shown to be hazardous.

Whether or not biological effects occur in any particular circumstances is determined by the exposure conditions and the characteristics of the irradiated tissues [52]. Since, other things being equal, the amount of obtainable information increases with the amount of ultrasonic energy directed into the patient [53], it is tempting to instrument designers to use high ultrasonic intensities. To give positive guidance on this point, the American Institute of Ultrasound in Medicine has stated [54] that ultrasonic intensities below 100 mW cm^{-2} (spatial peak temporal average) are not known to have caused independently confirmed significant biological effects. Most contemporary instruments operate with lower intensities.

This remains the scientific situation. Changes in public opinion and sometimes even the requirements of regulatory bodies are not predictable, however, and there is no doubt that response to the occasional and happily so far always unfounded concerns of pressure groups could have an adverse effect on the health care which patients presently enjoy as a result of the benefits of ultrasonic diagnosis. Nevertheless, it is prudent for research into bioeffects to be encouraged so that benefits can be balanced against scientific estimates of risk.

REFERENCES

1   Hunt, J.W., M. Arditi and F.S. Foster. Ultrasound Transducers for Pulse-Echo Medical Imaging. IEEE Transactions on Biomedical Engineering BME-30 (1983) 453-481.

2   Ohigashi, H. Electromechanical Properties of Polarized Polyvinylidene Fluoride Films as Studied by the Piezoelectric Resonance Method. Journal of Applied Physics 47 (1976) 949-955.

3   Hadjicostis, A.N., C.F. Hottinger, J.J. Rosen and P.N.T. Wells. Ultrasonic Transducer Materials for Medical Applications. Ferroelectrics (1984) in press.

4   Swartz, R.G. and J.D. Plummer. On the Generation of High-Frequency Acoustic Energy with Polyvinylidene Fluoride. IEEE Transactions on Sonics and Ultrasonics SU-27 (1980) 295-303.

5   Dietz, D.R., S.I. Parks and M. Linzer. Expanding-Aperture Annular Array. Ultrasonic Imaging 1 (1979) 56-75.

6   Fu, C-C. and L. Gerzberg. Annular Arrays for Quantitative Pulsed Doppler Ultrasonic Flowmeters. Ultrasonic Imaging 5 (1983) 1-16.

7   Whittingham, T.A. and J.A. Evans. Ultrasonic Visualisation of the Heart. Ultrasonics International 1975, pp. 182-189 (Guildford, International Publishing, 1975).

8   Dias, J.F. Construction and Performance of an Experimental Phased Array Acoustic Imaging Transducer. Ultrasonic Imaging 3 (1981) 352-368.

9   Bardsley, B.G., D.A. Christensen and T.A. Pryor. Multi-frequency and Nonuniformly-Spaced Arrays: Effects on Grating Lobe Amplitude. Ultrasonic Imaging 4 (1982) 351-354.

10   Manes, G.F., C. Atzeni and C. Susini. Design of a Simplified Delay System for Ultrasound Phased Array Imaging. IEEE Transactions on Sonics and Ultrasonics SU-30 (1983) 350-354.

11   Halliwell, M. and R.A. Mountford. Physical Sources of Registration Errors in Pulse-Echo Ultrasonic Systems. Part I - Velocity and Attenuation. Medical and Biological Engineering 11 (1973) 27-32.

12   Smith, S.W., G.E. Trahey and O.T. von Ramm. Refraction Correction for Ultrasonic Imaging Through Tissue Layers. Ultrasonic Imaging 6 (1984) 210.

13   Berkhout, A.J., J. Ridder and M.P. de Graaff. New Possibilities in Data Measurement, Signal Processing and Information Extraction: Philosophy and Results. E.A. Ash and C.R. Hill (eds.) Acoustical Imaging, vol. 12, pp. 269-279 (New York, Plenum, 1982).

14   Wells, P.N.T. and M. Halliwell. Speckle in Ultrasonic Imaging. Ultrasonics 19 (1981) 225-229.

15   Foster, D.R., M. Arditi, F.S. Foster, M.S. Patterson and J.W. Hunt. Computer Simulations of Speckle in B-scan Images. Ultrasonic Imaging 5 (1983) 308-330.

16   Mountford, R.A. and P.N.T. Wells. Ultrasonic Liver Scanning: the A-scan in the Normal and Cirrhosis. Physics in Medicine and Biology 17 (1972) 261-269.

17 Flax, S.W., N.J. Pelc, G.H. Glover, F.D. Gutmann and M. McLachlan. Spectral Characterization and Attenuation Measurements in Ultrasound. Ultrasonic Imaging 5 (1983) 95-116.

18 Kuc, R. Estimating Acoustic Attenuation from Reflected Ultrasound Signals: Comparison of Spectral-Shift and Spectral-Difference Approaches. IEEE Transactions on Acoustics, Speech and Signal Processing ASSP-32 (1984) 1-6.

19 Robinson, D.E., C.F. Chen and L.S. Wilson. Image Matching for Pulse Echo Measurement of Ultrasonic Velocity. Image and Vision Computing 1 (1983) 145-151.

20 Law, W.K., L.A. Frizzell and F. Dunn. Comparison of Thermodynamic and Finite Amplitude Methods of B/A Measurement in Biological Materials. Journal of the Acoustical Society of America 74 (1983) 1295-1297.

21 Cosgrove, D.O. Tissue Characterization by Ultrasound. L. Angelini, G. Fegiz and P.N.T. Wells (eds.). Emerging Technologies in Surgery, pp. 49-59 (Milan, Masson, 1984).

22 Brendel, K., L.S. Filipczynski, R. Gerstner, C.R. Hill, G. Kossoff, G. Quentin, J.M. Reid, J. Saneyoshi, J.C. Somer, A.A. Tchevnenko and P.N.T. Wells. Methods of Measuring the Performance of Ultrasonic Pulse-Echo Diagnostic Equipment. Ultrasound in Medicine and Biology 2 (1976) 343-350.

23 Trimmer, W.S.N. and D. Vilkomerson. A New Wire Phantom for Accurate Measurement of Acoustical Resolution. Ultrasonic Imaging 5 (1983) 87-93.

24 Madsen, E.L. Ultrasonically Soft-Tissue-Mimicking Materials. G.D. Fullerton and J.A. Zagzebski (eds.). Medical Physics of CT and Ultrasound, pp. 531-550 (New York, American Institute of Physics, 1980).

25 McCarty, K. and W. Stewart. A Simple Calibration and Evaluation Phantom for Ultrasound Scanners. Ultrasound in Medicine and Biology 8 (1982) 393-401.

26 Madsen, E.L., J.A. Zagzebski, M.F. Insana, T.M. Burke and G. Frank. Ultrasonically Tissue-Mimicking Liver Including the Frequency Dependence of Backscatter. Medical Physics 9 (1982) 703-710.

27 Burlew, M.M., E.L. Madsen, J.A. Zagzebski, R.A. Banjavic and S.W. Sum. A New Ultrasound Tissue-Equivalent Material. Radiology 134 (1980) 517-520.

28 Greenleaf, J.F., J.J. Gisvold and R.C. Bahn. A Clinical Prototype Ultrasonic Transmission Tomographic Scanner. E.A. Ash and C.R. Hill (eds.) Acoustical Imaging, vol. 12, pp. 579-597 (New York, Plenum, 1982).

29 Greenleaf, J.F., P.J. Thomas and B. Rajagopalan. Effects of Diffraction on Ultrasonic Computer-Assisted Tomography. J.P. Powers (ed.). Acoustical Imaging, vol. 11, pp. 351-363 (New York, Plenum, 1982).

30 Schreiman, J.S., J.J. Gisvold, J.F. Greenleaf and R.C. Bahn. Ultrasound Transmission Computed Tomography of the Breast. Radiology 150 (1984) 523-530.

31 Atkinson, P. and J.P. Woodcock. Doppler Ultrasound and its Use in Clinical Measurement (London, Academic, 1982).

32 Wells, P.N.T. A Range-Gated Ultrasonic Doppler System. Medical and Biological Engineering 7 (1969) 641-652.

33 Lunt, M.J. Accuracy and Limitations of the Ultrasonic Doppler Blood Velocimeter and Zero Crossing Detector. Ultrasound in Medicine and Biology 2 (1975) 1-10.

34 Wille, S. A Computer System for On-Line Decoding of Ultrasonic Doppler Signals from Blood Flow Measurement. Ultrasonics 15 (1977) 226-230.

35 Skidmore, R. and J.P. Woodcock. Physiological Interpretation of Doppler Shift Waveforms - I. Theoretical Considerations. Ultrasound in Medicine and Biology 6 (1980) 7-10.

36 Burns, P.N., M. Halliwell, P.N.T. Wells and A.J. Webb. Ultrasonic Doppler studies of the Breast. Ultrasound in Medicine and Biology 8 (1982) 127-143.

37 Daigle, R.E., S.A. Rubenstein and D.W. Baker. A Duplex Scanning System for Pediatric Cardiology. D. White and R.E. Brown (eds.). Ultrasound in Medicine, vol. 3B, pp. 1209-1211 (New York, Plenum, 1977).

38 Arensen, J.W., R.S.C. Cobbold and K.W. Johnston. Real-Time Two-Dimensional Blood Flow Imaging Using a Doppler Ultrasound Array. E.A. Ash and C.R. Hill (eds.). Acoustical Imaging, vol. 12, pp. 529-538 (New York, Plenum, 1982).

39 Namekawa, K., C. Kasai, R. Omoto, Y. Kondo, T. Katabami, T. Hidai, Y. Yoshikawa, M. Tsukamoto, Y. Yokote, S. Takamoto and A. Koyano. Realtime Two-Dimensional Bloodflow Imaging Using Ultrasound Doppler. Journal of Ultrasound in Medicine 2, suppl. to no. 10 (1983) 65.

40 Fish, P.J. Recent Progress in the Field of Doppler Devices. A. Kurjak (ed.). Recent Advances in Ultrasound Diagnosis, pp. 54-63 (Amsterdam, Excerpta Medica, 1978).

41 Gill, R.W. Accuracy Calculations for Ultrasonic Pulsed Doppler Blood Flow Measurements. Australasian Physical and Engineering Sciences in Medicine 5 (1982) 51-57.

42 Hottinger, C.F. and J.D. Meindl. Blood Flow Measurement Using the Attenuation-Compensated Volume Flowmeter. Ultrasonic Imaging 1 (1979) 1-15.

43 Lane, R.J. Intraoperative B-Mode Scanning. Journal of Clinical Ultrasound 8 (1980) 427-434.

44 Gramiak, R. and P.M. Shah. Echocardiography of the Aortic Root. Investigative Radiology 3 (1968) 356-366.

45 Ziskin, M.C., A. Bonakdarpour, D.P. Weinstein and P.R. Lynch. Contrast Agents for Diagnostic Ultrasound. Investigative Radiology 7 (1972) 500-505.

46 Meltzer, R.S., O.E.H. Sartorius, C.T. Lancee, P.W. Serruys, P.D. Verdouw, C.E. Essed and J. Roelandt. Transmission of Ultrasonic Contrast Agent Through the Lungs. Ultrasound in Medicine and Biology 7 (1981) 377-384.

47 Carroll, B.A., R.J. Turner, E.G. Tickner, D.B. Boyle and S.W. Young. Gelatin Encapsulated Nitrogen Microbubbles as Ultrasonic Contrast Agents. Investigative Radiology 15 (1980) 260-266.

48 Mattrey, R.F., F.W. Scheible, B.B. Gosink, G.R. Leopold, D.M. Long and C.B. Higgins. Perfluoroctylbromide: a Liver/Spleen-Specific and Tumor-Imaging Ultrasound Contrast Material. Radiology 145 (1982) 759-762.

49 Stouffer, J.R. and R.G. Westervelt. A Review of Ultrasonic Applications in Animal Science. Journal of Clinical Ultrasound 5 (1977) 124-128.

50 Wells, P.N.T. Scientific Basis of Medical Imaging (Edinburgh, Churchill Livingstone, 1982).

51 Wells, P.N.T. Possible Directions of Alternative Imaging Modalities: a Critical Overview. (Published in these Proceedings.)

52 Hill, C.R. Biological Effects of Ultrasound. B.B. Goldberg and P.N.T. Wells (eds.). Ultrasonics in Clinical Diagnosis, 3rd. edn., pp. 228-236 (Edinburgh, Churchill Livingstone, 1983).

53 Hill, C.R. and C.R. ter Haar. Ultrasound. M.J. Suess (ed.). Nonionizing Radiation Protection (Geneva, World Health Organisation, 1982).

54 American Institute of Ultrasound in Medicine. Report of Committee on Bioeffects. Ultrasound in Medicine and Biology 2 (1976) 351.

DISCUSSION SUMMARY

PANEL ON ULTRASOUND IMAGING: CURRENT TRENDS AND CLINICAL APPLICATIONS

In reply to a question from Wells, Masotti confirmed that the speckle texture pattern in two-dimensional images does not bear a one-to-one relationship to tissue structure. Payne asked what developments in transducer design would lead to a closer match between the image and the anatomy and Masotti agreed that an increase in frequency bandwidth was required. Waller mentioned that the phase information, besides the amplitude information, seems to carry diagnostic data.

Dealing with Wells' point about resolution improvement, Karrer stated that increasing the aperture of the transducer should be an advantage. This led to a discussion of optimal aperture size and the effect of speed inhomogeneities in the examined tissues. It was concluded that the development of adaptive compensation for speed differences along the different ray paths of the array could in principle correct for this but that full correction would require a two-dimensional array. Payne introduced the subject of the safety of diagnostic ultrasound and it was agreed that contemporary operating intensities might be set lower than necessary; increase in intensity would allow higher frequency to be used for a given penetration, with consequent improvement in resolution. Heintzen mentioned that it is difficult to identify the cardiac borders in two-dimensional scans when the image scanning and TV frames are not synchronised and Karrer confirmed that electronic phased array scanning in principle could solve this problem.

Wells asked Distante whether blood flow in the coronary arteries could be detected by Doppler techniques and the reply was that spatial movement of the heart during the cardiac cycle made this virtually impossible with current methods; the development of a tracking system might solve the problem. Heintzen commented that digital processing of echographic image series has several significant applications especially in echocardiography. Thus, it can help to discriminate between the images of the structure and the equally echogenic contrast bolus, by digital subtraction of e.c.g.-gated pictures. Moreover, the information can be made clearer by various filtering procedures. Payne asked about the need for noninvasive pressure measurement, particularly in the heart, and Heintzen stated that this would be a highly significant advance for the paediatric cardiologist especially in the diagnosis and management of congenital and acquired heart diseases. Todd-Pokropek said that he was under the impression that the unsatisfactory cardiac images were obtained in 20-30 per cent of patients but Distante confirmed that it is nowadays possible to achieve successful studies in more than 90 per cent of cases.

Angelini, in response to a question from Wells, agreed that intraoperative ultrasonic imaging is generally both faster and more convenient than X-radiography during biliary surgery. Angelini also confirmed that the presence of hepatic metastases undetectable by any technique before surgery could be established by high-resolution intraoperative ultrasonic imaging and that it is often clinically worthwhile to remove such lesions.

Todd-Pokropek asked Wells to enlarge on the debate concerning the use of ultrasound for screening in obstetrics. Wells said that the N.I.H. Consensus Development Conference had wisely concluded that ultrasonic scanning should only be used when there is a medical requirement for diagnostic data. He went on to say that the efficacy of effectiveness of diagnostic ultrasound in obstetrics and, indeed, in most other applications has not yet properly been demonstrated scientifically and that, although practitioners are convinced of the value of the method, there is growing demand for randomised controlled trials to test this opinion. Allemand enquired whether the ultrasonic C.T. scanner could not be considered to be a clinical tool and Wells said that developments were still needed in image reconstruction techniques and that the instrument would in any event remain limited to the study of accessible organs such as the breast. Waller asked whether two-dimensional arrays would suffer from insuperable problems due to superficial obstructions such as the ribs. Wells replied that, on the contrary, such arrays could be used with adaptive control which would recognise and correct for the presence of such structures.

Poster Session

HIGH RESOLUTION MEDICAL ULTRASOUND: APPLICATIONS IN RHEUMATOLOGY AND DERMATOLOGY

P.A. Payne, MSc, PhD, MIERE, CEng

Department of Instrumentation and Analytical Science
The University of Manchester Institute of Science and
Technology, P.O. Box 88, Manchester M60 1QD, UK

INTRODUCTION

Medical ultrasound techniques have largely concentrated on the use of transducers resonant at frequencies between 1 and 15 MHz. Increasingly, there has been a realisation that considerable diagnostic information can be obtained by the use of higher frequencies, although applications are clearly limited to peripheral structures.

The use of transducers with resonant frequencies of 20 MHz and above, but additionally with broad band characteristics so that considerable energy is produced up to 40 MHz, enables higher axial resolution to be obtained in A- and B-scan applications. Transducer materials based on polyvinylidene fluoride (PVDF) have been employed in this context and show great promise (1). Polymer film transducers are readily constructed as either focused or unfocused devices, and both types have found application in dermatology. More recently, applications in rheumatology have emerged and these transducers have also been used as the basis for a single-channel pulsed Doppler system for the measurement of skin blood flow (2).

DERMATOLOGY APPLICATIONS

Clinical dermatology has for many years been concerned with determination of the thickness of skin which changes with diseased states and also with the topical application of steroids used in the treatment of diseases such as psoriasis. One traditional method for measuring skin thickness is to use a 'skin pinch' and a caliper or micrometer device to measure the thickness of the pinch which is itself assumed to be twice the skin thickness. This assumes that the skin is easily separated from the subcutaneous fat and is not compressed unduly during the measurement. An alternative method is to use xeroradiography. In the case of caliper measurements there is a danger of considerable operator variability and the measurement cannot be made on an area of skin lesion. Xeroradiography suffers from the obvious drawbacks of ionising radiation techniques and successive measurements on the same area of skin to follow the dynamics of treatment may not be possible. Ultrasound A-scan techniques have been widely used recently and their place in dermatology seems now to be assured.

A problem associated with A-scan measurements on skin occurs when the extent, for example of malignant melanoma, is to be assessed. When the skin is abnormal it is less easy to interpret than A-scan data and B-scans have shown their usefulness here. Again the role of B-scans at high resolution seems also to be assured in the area of dermatology.

Polymer film transducers have been used for both these modalities. In the case of A-scans a focused transducer can be useful where a very small area of skin is to be assessed dimensionally. However, unfocused transducers also prove of use in that the data obtained is averaged over a larger known area of skin For B-scan applications a focused polymer film transducer is preferred and work such as reported in reference (1) was performed with a transducer focused at about 4 cm with a beam width of less than 0.25 mm. Measurements have shown that the axial resolution of this type of transducer can be better than 50 μm.

RHEUMATOLOGY APPLICATIONS

A-scan and B-scan techniques at high resolution have also been applied to the study of soft tissue and blood vessels of human digits. A range of normal volunteers has been examined with the aim of establishing normal dimensions for important digital veins and arteries so that these may be compared and contrasted with the dimensions found in patients suffering from rheumatological disorders.

Of particular interest is the assessment of digital artery dimension changes resulting from hot and cold challenges in patients suffering from Raynaud's Disease. The high resolution B-scan system using a polymer transducer has proved valuable in this work and has also enabled us to begin to examine the dynamics of lumen dimension changes due to certain drug treatment regimes.

In Figure 1 a normal digit has been imaged from the side and the figure identifies a digital artery and places dimensions on this together with dimensions for various other structures. In Figure 2 a normal digital vein has been imaged and again the various structures have been measured and the dimensions are shown. Figure 3 shows the result of scanning the side of a digit on a patient with systemic sclerosis. Once again the various structures have been measured and the dimensions are presented. It is clear, looking at these three figures, that in systemic sclerosis much thicker soft tissue is present and that the lumen area of the artery identified is considerably smaller than that of a normal.

SKIN BLOOD FLOW MEASUREMENTS

A single-channel pulsed Doppler system has been used in conjunction with polymer film transducers, either focused or flat, and the system has been operated at frequencies ranging from 15 up to 30 MHz. The vasculature of the skin is extremely complex, but the blood vessels that feed the skin cell renewal process are largely those looping vessels that are adjacent to the papillary layer. These lie just below the basal layer of the epidermis and loop up from the dermal plexus.

Alternative techniques exist for the measurement of blood flow in the skin and some of these have been recently reviewed in reference (2). Thermal conductance methods are unable to separate the flow of blood in the papillary capillary loops from the blood flow in subcutaneous and subdermal vessels. Thus the blood flow which provides nutrition for skin renewal cannot be measured in this way. The laser Doppler technique is also not able to control the depth from which the light scattering occurs and is therefore also susceptible to measurement of flow from vessels at deeper layers. By using a range gated Doppler technique with gate pulses on the transmitter of 1 μs duration or less, it is possible to localise the measurement onto the papillary loops and so gain insight into the important data concerning flow in these blood vessels.

CONCLUSIONS

Ultrasound at higher frequencies giving rise to higher resolution has found a number of applications in medicine. No doubt there are others to follow, for example, in the area of ophthalmics.

The development of transducers for these applications is largely based on the use of PVDF material, however, copolymers of vinylidene fluoride and trifluoroethylene may well prove to be advantageous in this context. Much work remains to be done in this area, but there is no reason why an in vivo acoustic microscope cannot be devised capable of looking at the dimensions of such structures as the stratum corneum where an axial resolution of the order of a few micrometres may be required.

REFERENCES

1. Payne, P.A., Grove, G.L., Alexander, H., Quilliam, R.M. and Miller, D.L. Cross-sectional ultrasonic scanning of skin using plastic film transducers. Bioengineering and the Skin 3 (1981) 234-240
2. Payne, P.A. Measurement of skin blood flow. Electronics and Power 30 (1984) 219-221

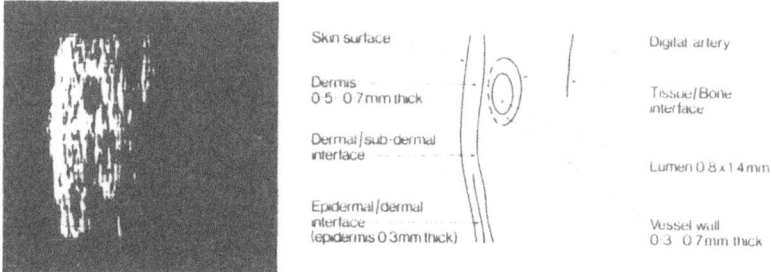

Figure 1 Ultrasound B-scan showing a normal digital artery

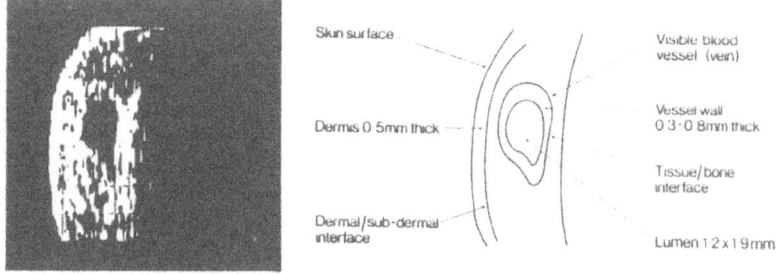

Figure 2 Normal digital vein

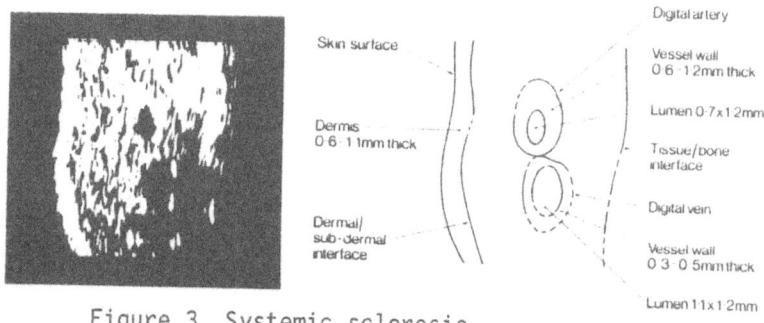

Figure 3 Systemic sclerosis

PART V GENERAL PROBLEMS I

Chairman: Robert Kruger (U.S.A.)

DIGITAL ARCHIVING OF MEDICAL IMAGES

D. KAPLAN

THOMSON-CGR, Direction des Etudes
48, rue Camille Desmoulins, 92130 Issy-les-Moulineaux FRANCE

This chapter presents an overview of the problems involved in archiving medical images on digital media and focuses on their solutions using optical disk technology. The context is a Medical Imaging Department in which there exist several digital imaging modalities, such as CT scanner, Magnetic Resonance Imaging or Digital Angiography. The emphasis is on these currently digital systems, rather than on an all-digital situation in which every modality, including conventional radiography would have been transformed to a digital format. To begin with we will discuss some of the issues involved and the technologies that may be applicable. Next, various elements on the solutions offered by Digital Optical Disks will be given. Finally, some of the alternatives are discussed briefly.

1 ISSUES

The general organisation of a Medical Imaging Department is presented in fig. 1. Several imaging machines corresponding to various digital imaging modalities comprise the activities of this department. Digital archiving is possible at each machine location. We shall call such an archiving a local archiving. Its main functions are :
. Extension of the length of time during which images can be consulted on-line on the imaging machine
. Constitution of a logging of all the images taken, thus permitting the constitution of a legal archive
. Collection of special images for teaching and research purposes
The second possible level of archiving is the constitution of a central archive. It is preferable for this archive to be connected to the modalities by a digital image network,

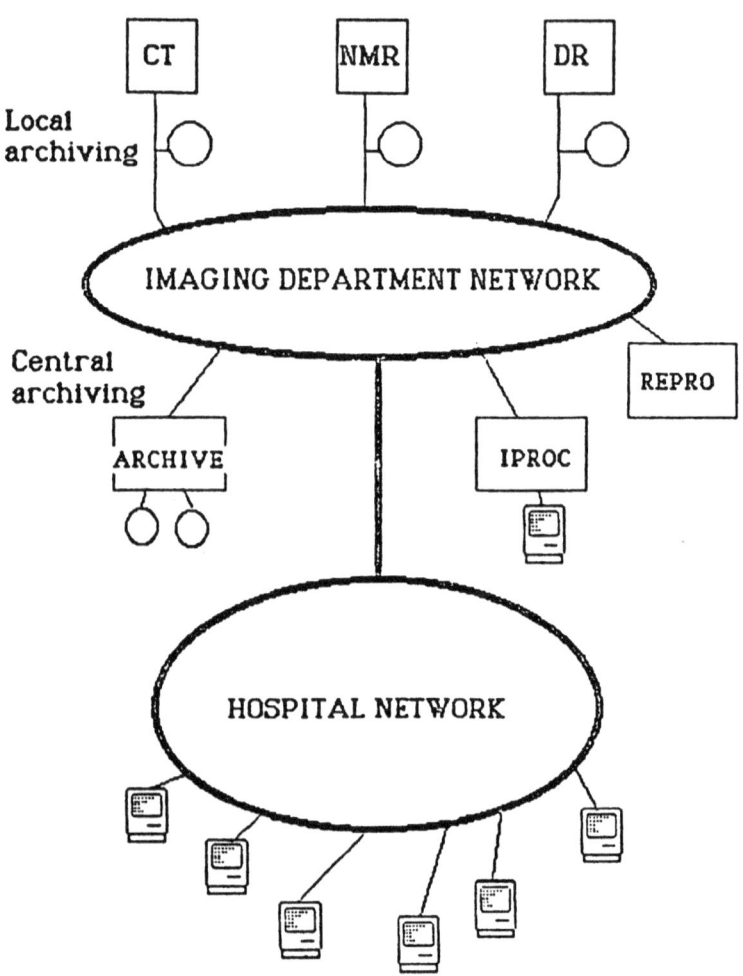

to allow for automatic transfers. The central archive is organized differently, e.g., instead of logging images in time succession, images corresponding to a single patient are bunched together to allow for rapid retrieval of a single patient data. The functions of this central archiving are thus:

. Diagnosis involving several modalities on a single patient

. Patient disease and therapy monitoring.

Consultation of these images may be envisaged within the department only, or outside the department extending to the hospital as a whole or even the referring physician. The technical and economic demands involved in large scale consultation are important and it is not clear when they can be met. For the purpose of this presentation we shall remain within the framework of the imaging department only.

2 TECHNOLOGIES

Digital archiving implies writing on and reading off an archiving medium. For these two functions, there exist mainly two approaches : magnetic and optical.

Magnetic storage techniques use magnetic heads to write patterns of magnetization orientation in the medium. Reading is performed by detecting voltages induced in the reading head by the pattern moving close to it.

Optical storage usually relies on burning holes or blowing bubbles in suitable materials to store the data. Optical reading is performed by observing the changes of diffusion or reflectivity produced by these patterns. Recently new hybrid systems have appeared (1) in which storage is performed using a laser beam to induce a magnetization pattern in a magneto-optical material. Reading is made optically, and these systems combine the spatial resolution of optical storage with the ability to erase the digital data.

The storage density is determined by the minimum size needed to store or retrieve a bit. For optical approaches, this size is constrained by the wavelength of the light of the order of 1 micron. If we assume that a high reliability will impose the order of three wavelengths on every spatial direction for each bit, the storage density turns out to be 10 Mbits per square centimeter, which is a fair estimate of current densities in commercial systems. This implies that it is unlikely that optical disks storage densities will be enhanced by several orders of magnitude in the forthcoming years. In the case of magnetic storage, the limitation is of a more practical nature. New developments such as vertical recordings are expected to yield densities approaching those of optical storage. Today techniques to significantly exceed this are not apparent.

In summary of this rapid overview, we expect that, over the next few years, different technologies will make available storage densities of the order of one million characters per square centimeter. These will exist in both erasable (magnetic) and non-erasable (optical) form.

3 OPTICAL DISK SOLUTIONS

Currently, digital optical disk systems are offered by several companies (e.g. Philips, Alcatel-Thomson, Shugart...). They are in general non-erasable disks.

As an example a typical 30 cm diameter disk will offer 1000

million characters (Gigabyte) storage capacity on each face of the disk. Access time is of the order of 100 ms. Transfer rates are several Mbits/s. The error rate is in the 10^{-12} range, making this disk suitable for numeric data storage. Shelf lifetime is considered to be over 10 years. Systems with somewhat improved performance in terms of capacity or access time have been proposed, but with higher costs that make them difficult to envisage in the present applications.

To see how the above type of disks can be used in the medical imaging department, we have listed below estimates of the disk capacity in terms of weeks of activity of different imaging modalities. It is assumed that all images are stored. Two cases are considered depending on whether a compression algorithm without information losses (i.e. reversible) is used or not.

	IMAGE SIZE (MBITS)	NUMBER PER HOUR	SINGLE SIZE CAPACITY (WEEKS)
DSA	2	100	.7 (1.4)
CT	4	20	1.7 (3.4)
MRI	1	60	2.2 (4.4)

Assumptions : 60 Hours per Week
No Image Selection

( ) : Compression factor = 2

From this data, we see that the introduction of optical disk storage allows for on-line access to the image data for periods ranging from several days to several weeks. In terms of the size of the archive, given the disk thickness of 2 cm, the shelf space needed per modality per year is less than one meter in length in all cases. The large storage rooms that were necessary to store the data on magnetic tape can be eliminated together with much of the inconvenience in retrieving the data.

Although the introduction of optical disks is a big improvement in the functioning of a local archive, the question of how to organize a central archive remains still unsettled. The number of disks necessary to handle the output of five digital modalities for five years is still of the order of several hundred. Juke-box systems are currently offered with access times of the order of 20s. However, they have typical capacities of only 50 to a 100 disks, so that using a battery of them is an expensive proposition. At least three approaches to this problem can be envisaged:

. Development of automatic disk library systems able to handle 1000 disks or more, albeit with longer access times than the current juke-box.

. Use of compression algorithms involving loss of data, but increasing the compression factor by an order of magnitude. This is possible, provided one accepts that no sophisticated mathematical treatments are to be made on the archived data, which are meant to be pictures of already processed data.

. Systematic selection of meaningful images. This is a debated issue since, although many agree that a large fraction of the images will not be retrieved at all, some physicians insist that the effort needed to perform this selection is not compatible with a heavily overworked imaging department.

A possible strategy, for the near future, is data compression of most images, with uncompressed data being stored for specially identified cases.

4 ALTERNATIVE SOLUTIONS

Other technological solutions may challenge Digital Optical Disks in the longer term. Optical tape (2) for instance has the capacity of storing larger volumes of data, thus making the design of the archive a simpler proposition. Alternatively, we may cease to archive most images in the hospital and give the patient himself an optical card (2) to contain his image data. Improvement in storage capacity should make magnetic storage an active contender at the level of local archiving. However, cost considerations make it unlikely that it is to be used in a general central archive. In the short term however, the Digital Optical Disk appears to be the most realistic answer to archiving medical images.

REFERENCES
1. R.M. WHITE   IEEE SPECTRUM p.32, August 1983
2. J. DREXLER   SPIE VOL 418 Picture Archiving & Communication Systels p.30 (1983)

PART VI GENERAL PROBLEMS II

Chairman: Vito Cappellini (Italy)

3-D DISPLAY

A Todd-Pokropek

Dept. of Medical Physics
University College London, U.K.

ABSTRACT

The sampling of data in Medical Imaging is, of its essence, 3-dimensional. 3-D displays can be classified into groups as follows: the use of colour as a depth cue, 2-D representations of 3-D objects using shaded surfaces, stereo pairs, holograms, time coding and depth cueing, the varifocal (vibrating) mirrors and other mechanical systems, and, finally, true 3-D displays. Brief descriptions of some algorithms for the production of stereo pairs, the use of the kinetic depth effect, and shaded graphics are presented. A fundamental problem is that of the perception of interior structures, which implies the use of interaction, for example, by selective high-lighting and elimination of concealing structures. The volume of data generated by current systems is so large, that a fast powerful 3-D display is essential. Some suitable architectures are presented.

1. INTRODUCTION

Medical images are produced by sampling a 3-D volume- the patient. The nature of most systems is that the data collected must be reduced to two dimensions. Typical methods are by working with 'line-integrals' e.g. Radiology and Nuclear Medicine, defining slice planes, CT, NMR (MRI!) and conventional ultrasound, or by using some other coding, such as ultrasound M-scanning and Doppler. However, many systems are capable, at least in principle, of producing true 3-D information, albeit after solution of an appropriate inverse equation relating a set

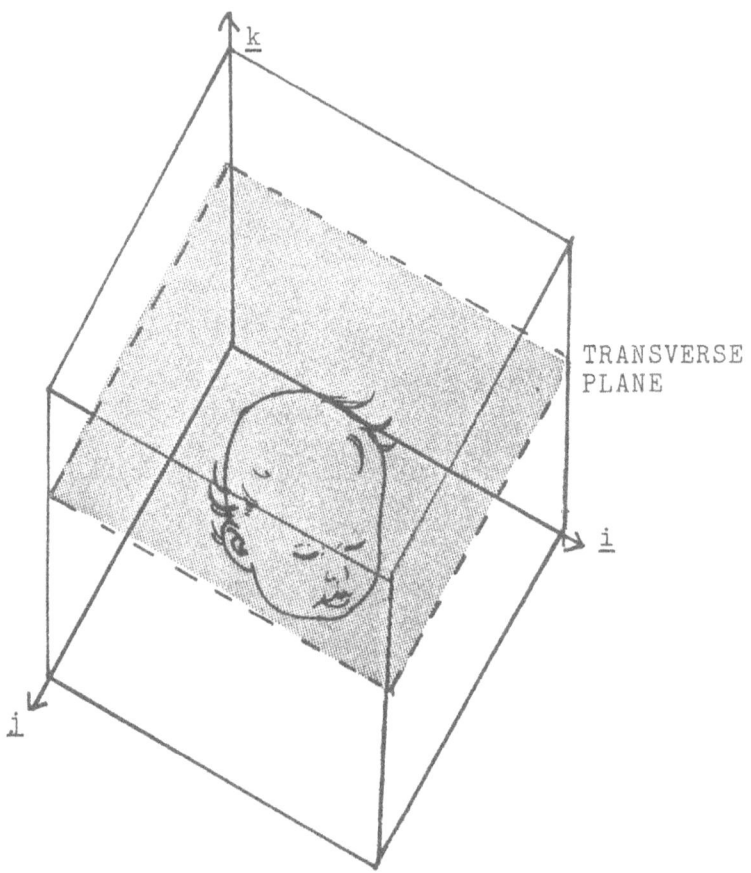

Fig 1. Diagram to illustrate the three orthogonal vectors $\underline{i}$ $\underline{j}$ and $\underline{k}$, and the corresponding plane selected for $\underline{k}$ = k'.

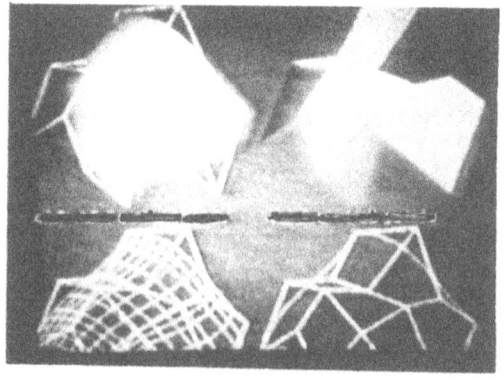

Fig 2. Illustration of some bicubic splines as wire diagrams and as shaded objects.

of 'measurements' **M** to the 3-D sample estimates of some parameter **P**. Let us suppose that a series of observations **M** are made, and that the system may be completely determined by a set of coefficients **A**. In general, if it is desired to find the values **P** of the clinical parameter in the patient, since

$$M = A \cdot P$$

then

$$P = A^{-1} \cdot M$$

where **A** must be known and hence A^{-1} must be found. Thus **P** is a set of data in 3-D, found from the solution of the above inverse equation. The aim of this paper is to present some of the ways in which such data sets may be handled, and to discuss some associated problems.

2. SORTING

The matrix **P** in 3-D may be expressed as P(i,j,k) where **I**, **J**, **K** are the three orthogonal unit vectors. Conventional tomography generally implies the formation of an image $I_{k'}(i,j)$ assumed to be identical to a slice though the 3-D data set, P(i,j,k') where k' is a constant indicating the corresponding transverse slice plane. This is illustrated in Fig 1. Clearly, orthogonal planes P(i',j,k) and P(i,j',k) may also be defined being images of slices conventionally termed 'sagittal' and 'coronal'. The collection of a series of transverse planes $I_k(i,j)$ for $k_1 < k < k_2$ permit the definition of a three dimensional array P(i,j,k) between the limits k_1 and k_2, from which the other orthogonal planes can be determined by fixing either i or j, or in other words, by sorting. Thus simply by reading the data from a set of transverse axial slices in different orders, images can be generated with various alternative 3-D orientations.

However, in many cases the sampling of the data matrix **P** may not be identical in all three axes. This is notable in the case of X-ray CT. The voxel (3-D volume element) is not a cube; space is filled with abutting parallelepipeds. Typical values of a voxel in X-ray CT are 0.5mm by 0.5mm by 2mm, where 2mm is the slice thickness. A second problem is that we may desire to create slices at other angles than the three orthogonal planes defined so far, e.g. oblique slices. Both these problems require suitable interpolation. The value of P(x,y,z) is desired at some arbitrary point x,y,z in continuous space, determined from a set of values known at points (i,j,k) sampled in discrete space. A general solution is given by the matrix multiplication

$$P(x,y,z) = P \cdot W$$

where **W** is an appropriate set of weights, for example formed from two dimensional sinc functions. Thus one aim in handling 3-D display is the determination of a suitable compact form for **W**, in particular one where the weights do not vary as a function of x,y or z. Note also that this has implications in terms of the hardware used in a display, in that it is likely that the display of the data will require a fast matrix multiplier. Although a general rotation (with translation and perspective) is just a multiplication by a 4x4 matrix, such an operation is not sufficient for the general interpolation problem.

It must be noted that, while inverse problems in 3-D can be stated in general, almost all practical systems are implemented by measuring **M** for some predefined slice and then estimating **P** from that restricted set of values. If the full 3-D problem is posed, the size of **A** may be of the order of $(512^3) \times (512^3)$ and beyond the capacity of present systems to manipulate. The matrix **A** does however tend to be very sparse. Solutions of such inverse problems, while of considerable interest, are beyond the scope of this paper. However, it is likely that within the near future such true 3-D inverse problems may become manageable, and that as a result, a considerably improvement in 3-D image quality may become available, together with an increased need to work with 3-D displays.

3. THE REPRESENTATION

One of the most important issues in 3-D displays is that of the internal representation of the data being displayed, dependent on which the form of the hardware used may be quite different. It has been suggested in Section 2 that the most natural representation of a 3-D medical image is in the form of a matrix **P** of size NxN by n slice planes. Dependent on the technique used for sampling, N is then likely to have values of the order of 512, and n will tend to N, such that the complete data set will approach $\sim 512^3$ or 128M data points. The method of storing such images in an array of voxels has been recommended by Gabor Herman and co-workers [1,2,3]. An implementation has been described by Herman's group working with a set of $\sim 0.6M$ voxels in CT, presumably corresponding to an array of size 84^3. Note that N=n=512 is equivalent to a resolution in 3-D of $\sim$1mm for a chest. With the notable exception of conventional (plane film) radiography which is not a 3-D imaging method, this is probably adequate for all current techniques for the next few years.

Various alternative forms have been suggested as methods for reducing the total amount of data. If one can determine

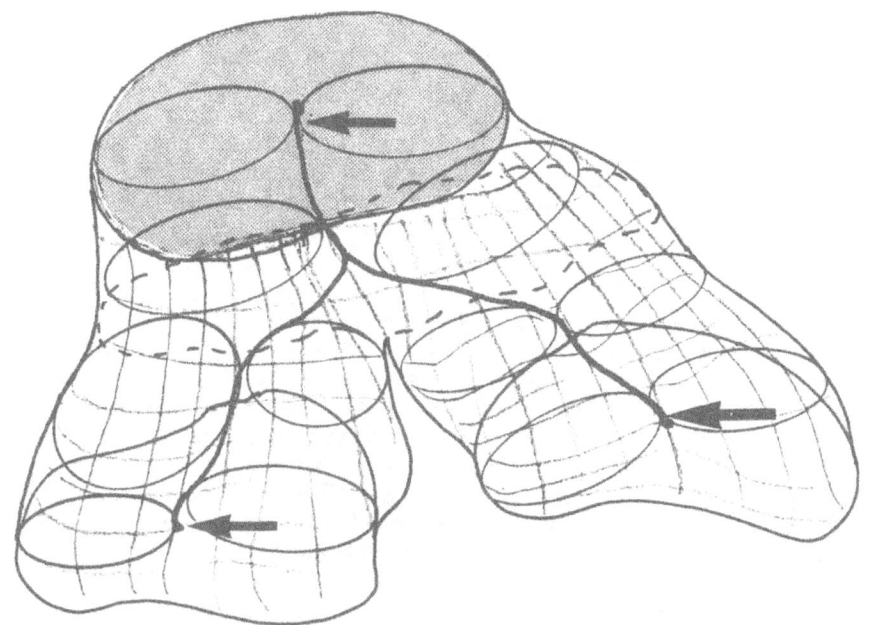

Fig 3. An artificial 3-D object, as shown in this diagram may have its skeleton (arrowed) extracted by filling the object with spheres (shown as ellipses).

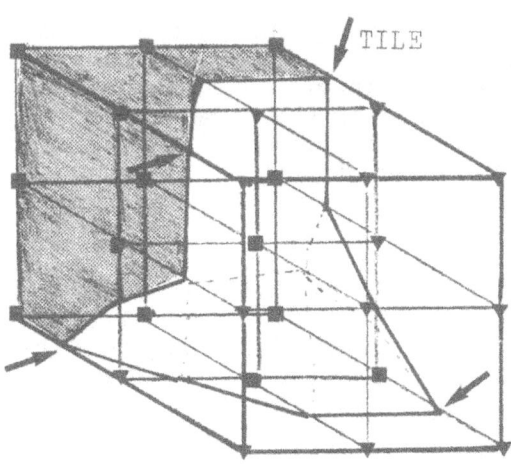

Fig 4. A 2x2x2 domain where nodes can take either the value■ or the value▼ A tile is defined in 3-D seperating these two domains.

boundaries between different portions of the image, then surfaces are defined (e.g. [4,5,6] and many others). This is a technique almost always employed for natural scenes, images of runways, in robotics etc, but is far less obviously viable than for medical images. However, if such surfaces can be defined, then a coding scheme for storing these surface may be constructed, for example by using 'tiles' or 'patches'. A tile (patch) is defined as a polygonal segment of a surface in 3-D, located by the values of its apices, and with some 'shape' well-defined by some mathematical function, for example bi-cubic splines, as illustrated in Fig 2. Since a complete surface comprises a set of contiguous tiles, the number of tiles will tend to approach the number of apices. Reasonable estimates for the number of apices can be found from sampling theory, e.g. an apex needs to be defined whenever a 'significant' change in slope has occurred. Typical values for a single surface defined with a 3-D array of size 512^3 are of the order of 10->50K. Thus considerable data reduction can be achieved, at a considerable increase in the complexity of the form of storage of the data.

These two representational forms are by no means the only types that can imagined. The use of 3-D skeletons, as illustrated in Fig 3 has also been proposed [7]. Alternative (related) systems are to describe the object by that minimal set of spheres which can be closely packed within the object, and the symmetric axis transform [8]. However, in order to generate an image which can be perceived, the internal representation of the object must be converted into an external representation, normally a set of display intensities within some display hardware. Typically, the display hardware will have a set of controllable display positions. The total number of positions might be of the order of 1024x1024 or 1M altogether, while the number of values to be displayed in the raw data P was estimated as being of the order of 128M. This is therefore a problem of coding. Many different schemes have been proposed.

4. A CLASSIFICATION OF 3-D DISPLAY SYSTEM CODING SCHEMES.

Basically, it is suggested in this paper that 3-D display coding schemes can be classified as shown in the following list. Several of these may be combined.
1. The use of colour as a depth cue.
2. 2-D representations of 3-D objects using shaded surfaces etc, i.e. 'art'.
3. Stereo pairs, i.e. 'binary' coding.
4. Holograms, or other systems compressing 3-D into 2-D, i.e. coding at the microscopic level.
5. 2-D display devices using time to code the 3rd dimension, such as rotating images, the use of depth cueing etc.

6. Varifocal (vibrating) mirrors and other mechanical systems using time to code the 3rd dimension so as to generate 3-D images by visual integration.
7. True 3-D images, such as computer generated (wax!) models, laser/frequency coding etc.

In general most of these are essentially 2-D systems designed to give the human observer the impression of some 3-D object. Some form of coding is employed. It is suggested that the distinction between 2-D and 'true' 3-D displays is artificial in that, if the observer can 'perceive' the 3-D object with sufficient accuracy via the 2-D display, then it is no different from a 'true' 3-D display. Effectively, all that is required is to match the output of the display system to the input of the human observer, the two eyes!

This classification of 3-D display will now be considered in more detail.

5. THE USE OF COLOUR

One of the most obvious coding schemes that can be employed is the use of colour. In section 3, it was estimated that the difference between the number of display positions (on a 2-D display device) and the number of voxels in the matrix P was of the order of 100. Thus, if at each position, the number of display intensities is much greater than the number of values that any voxel can take, a coding scheme can be employed, for example representing the voxel value by the brightness of the display, and coding one axis of the data, for example z, by hue. Thus 'near' could be indicated by red, and 'far' by blue, and voxel value by intensity [9]. This could be reversed, using colour for voxel value, and intensity for distance.

An immediate problem is that this mapping is not unique. Many voxels have to be encoded simultaneously at each given display position. Thus it may be desired to mix one intensity at one hue together with other intensities at other hues. The human visual perception mechanism cannot distinguish such combinations. The eye appears only to be able to make sense of the resultant 'contaminated' data for very simple objects. One simplification which may be employed is not to map all voxels within the complete data set, but only those lying on 'nearest' surfaces.

6. SHADED SURFACES

Most 3-D display systems have been concerned with shaded surfaces (e.g. [5,6,10] and others). Defining a surface may be considered in several steps [11,12]. Firstly some rule must be established for detecting a surface. Let a voxel be defined as a box where each apex has some value. One rule for detecting an 'iso-value' surface is that the surface is said to pass through the voxel if and only if not all the apices have values greater than, or less than, the corresponding 'iso-value'. A a 'patch' or 'tile' in then generated within the voxel. All voxels satisfying this condition for a given value may be flagged and indicate in a general way the position of the surface. The complete surface associated with the value used for testing is formed by linking such tiles in some structure, and is the equivalent in 3-D of an iso-value contour. Herman [1] has stated that this linking process can be represented as traversal of a directed graph, where each flagged voxel is one node of the graph. Herman has also stated that, in a total space of 85^3 voxels, for CT data, the number of flagged voxels is over 66K. It should be noted that, when considering individual voxels in this way, Herman suggests that a binary tree may be created and the search considerably simplified. An alternative representation is as on oct-tree, as suggested by Meagher [13,14,15].

An oct-tree (a 3-D form of the well known quad-tree) is defined as follows. The root is the complete 3-D image (the universe) and is a cube of side L. This can be subdivided into 8 cubes each of side L/2. These children are linked in standard order to the parent, and flagged as being: empty, partially full, or completely full (i.e. containing an object). This process is repeated recursively down to the final (smallest) size of voxel desired. The order of the linkages, each parent having 8 children, permits obscuration of any element at a given level to be determined. Any such node which is obscured need not be followed to lower levels, since all the elements at any lower level are by definition also obscured. This permits fast searches to be made of the 3-D structure.

An alternative technique [11,16] is to locate the surface by the fitting of tiles, not within each individual voxel, but, as illustrated in Fig 4, by defining rules for the curvature of the tile, and fitting it over a much larger volume than a single voxel. This can considerably reduce the number of tiles. Various functions, such as oblate spheroids, have been used. However, formation of what is effectively a linked list still needs to be performed.

A more common, but less exact, technique is to start by defining contours in 2-D in each slice plane [16]. Tiles may then be established by linking the contour in one such plane with contours in adjacent planes. This is illustrated in Fig 5. Ambiguities often exist which normally can only be resolved by heuristic methods.

It is also possible, and may be desirable, to define surfaces not with respect to some 'iso-value' but with respect some other parameter of the image for example the 3-D gradient of the voxel values [10,17,18], the surface being defined at that surface passing through all points of steepest gradient. This same operation can be carried out starting from 2-D planes, and then cross-linking the data. In all cases, the final result is a list of tiles, identified by the location of their vertices, with some defined 3-D curvature. These are only some examples of the many different techniques that have been used in the 3-D segmentation of an image.

Satisfactory display of such a display list normally implies the removal of hidden surfaces [9,19]. The rule is that an observation angle is defined. This observation angle is normally variable, allowing us to 'rotate' the display. A tile which is behind another tile with respect to this angle is (at least partly) obscured, and therefore not displayed. This rule may be extended to cover 'transparent' tiles, where the 'hidden' tile is 'modified' by some mapping function, rather than merely eliminated. The problem of partial obscuration may be solved by dynamically subdividing the 'hidden' tile into sub-tiles, each of which is either visible, or obscured. An alternative, when using small tiles, is to suppose that all partially obscured tiles are in fact completely obscured, and that any 'significant' exceptions are eliminated by subdivision prior to display. The hidden surface problem then becomes a sorting algorithm, and many possible solutions have been proposed in the literature [19]. Essentially a tree structure may be defined as a linked list where the tile obscuring other tiles are linked with them. Only the first tile is such a linked list needs to be displayed. The power of such algorithms resides in making the linked list essentially independent of the angle of observation.

Finally, the tiles must be displayed with shading, and, in certain applications, texture. The two basic shading algorithms are by interpolation using apex values only [20], and continuously [21].

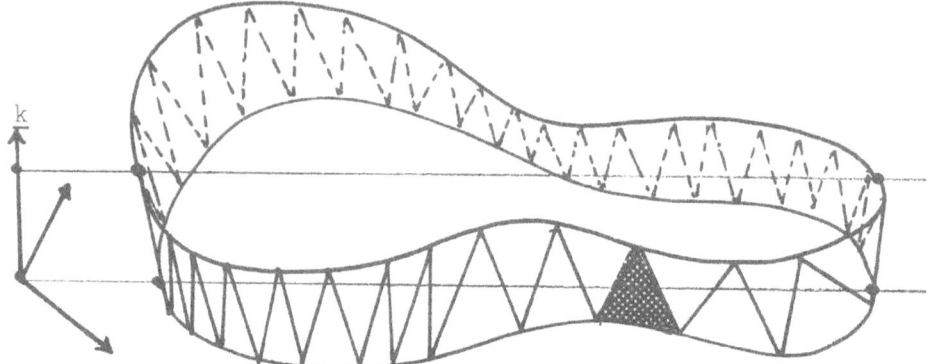

Fig 5. Two contours defines in two tranverse slices may be linked together by a series of triangular tiles.

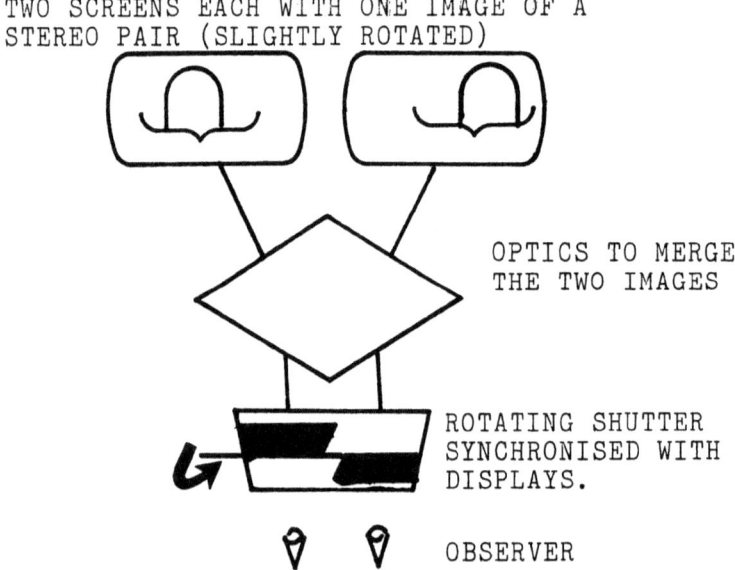

Fig 6. One of many schemes to enable a stereo pair of images to be observed independently by each eye. The system may also perform other manipulations, such as simultaneously rotating the two images.

7. STEREO PAIRS

Matching of the display to a human observer with two eyes suggests the idea of creating 'stereo pairs' of an image. It is well known that the perception of distance for an object in 3-D is facilitated by the use of the differences in the object for the angles of observation corresponding to each eye. It is not so well known that this is not a very powerful depth clue. The technique suggested in section 6 could then be modified by generating two slightly different images for the two angles corresponding to right and left eyes, which are then viewed by an observer [22]. The rotation is a simple matrix multiplication.

There are many methods of displaying such stereo pairs, of which the worst must surely be the use of a pair of images in red and green viewed by the observer with corresponding filters over each eye. A much simpler technique, as illustrated in Fig 6, is to use two separate display screens and appropriate mirrors so that the observer sees them at the same virtual position. A third technique is to use a single display switching between the two stereo pairs at high speed (e.g. video frame rates) synchronised with a mask, obscuring either the right or left eye of the observer. The stereo separation of the images (i.e. the angular difference in viewing angle) needs to be continuously adjustable to match individual observers.

The problems associated with the use of stereo pairs are, firstly, the power of the 3-D clue is not very great, secondly, it does not help with complex objects, and thirdly, it can normally only be used by one single observer at any one time.

8. HOLOGRAMS

A very good optical technique for coding a 3-D image on to a 2-D surface exists: the hologram [23]. The image is formed by the interference patterns of the object when illuminated from more than one direction with a coherent light source, for example a laser. Holograms have in the past been of relatively poor quality, but, recently, the technology of producing such images has improved dramatically, and good 3-D images of medical data can be produced.

There are, however, some limitations which severly restrict the value of this technique. The density of data in a hologram is much greater than the density of data, or to be precise, the sampling requirements, for a conventional display. The sampling density of the hologram needs to be greater by a factor of about 1000 then for the raw image, and there are also increased requirements for the dynamic range needed. Although computer driven implementations exist, such a display is not very convenient in that conventional display devices such as CRTs are quite inadequate. The total amount of data to be transferred is also great, normally many times the original volume of data in P. Thus, with present technology, it is difficult to see how interactive displays which use such techniques can be devised. However, some preliminary (but very pretty) results have been obtained, for example in CT [24].

9. ROTATING IMAGES

As mentioned in section 6, it is common to display 3-D images from different view points by rotating the image and viewing it from a different angle. A powerful 3-D clue, much more powerful than the stereo pair, is generated by the so-called kinetic depth effect, e.g. the way in which the image changes as the view point of the observer is modified as a function of time. This may be achieved by an observer moving the head from side to side, or it may be achieved by moving the object, for example by rotating it continuously. Both of these can give very powerful impressions of 3-D depth. Thus, time can be used as an alternative coding method to reduce the data from 3-D to 2-D. Simple rotation about one axis can be achieved with little effort. Rotation about an arbitrary axis requires matrix multiplication (by a 4x4 matrix), voxel by voxel, in real time. In certain cases, for example in SPECT, the raw data itself, when displayed as a movie, permits this with no computation.

10. THE VARIFOCAL (AND OTHER MOVING) MIRROR SYSTEMS.

An alternative time coding system has been implemented by combining a changing display with some mechanical system synchronised to the display, such that, by visual integration, an impression of a genuine 3-D image is obtained. Typical of such systems is the varifocal mirror [25]. As illustrated in Fig 7, a display is placed above such a mirror. The mirror, made out of some flexible reflective material, is made to change its radius of curvature, and therefore its focal distance, as a function of time. The reflected image of the display then appears at a different **virtual** depth. Synchronising the display with the different virtual distances permits the display to write to different positions in perceived (virtual) 3-D. However, it is important to examine the data rates involved.

If it is assumed that the mirror is driven with a sine wave at some frequency of the order of 50-60Hz, then it is likely that one would want to define say 100 different positions in depth. The minimum time between two successive positions, under these conditions, is of the order of 50usec. Thus the complete image of a slice must be changed in a time of <~50usecs. Note that any

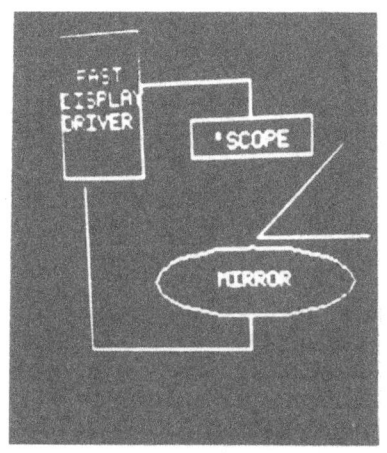 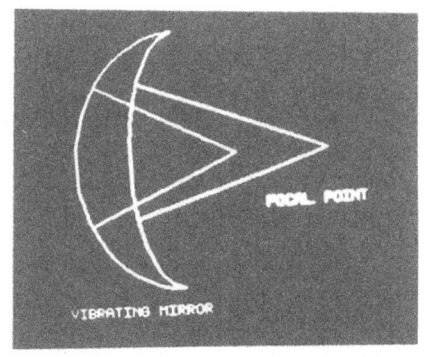

Fig 7. Above, a diagram of how the varifocal mirror system functions, left, a block diagram, and right, a diagram showing how the focal length changes as a function of the radius of curvature of the mirror. Below, a photograph of an image is shown being the letters UNC, being a reflection of an apparently straight line in the display (Courtesy of S.M. Pizer).

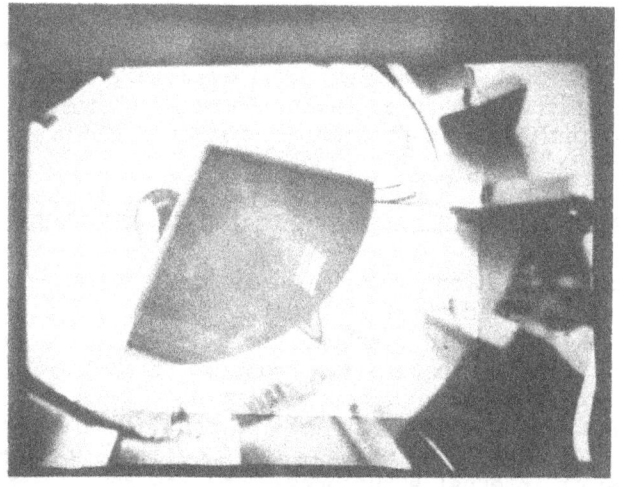

persistence of the display phosphor will create a blurring in depth. Thus, a very fast display and display generator is required.

The data may be structured as a list of x,y,z coordinates, or elements, where x,y indicates the position, and z is directly used as time. Thus, for convenience, the data should be sorted in z order, after which displaying and refreshing the data may be achieved at the desired data rates, provided that the length of the display list is not too long.

Other systems have been devised, for example using a rotating spiral mirror [26]. An alternative suggestion for handling the data rate problem is to use multiple displays, and then optically to switch between displays (for example with a Kerr cell), synchronised with the mechanical system.

11. TRUE 3-D IMAGES

Some efforts have been made to generate true 3-D image under computer control, for example, by computer controlled machine cutting. Such systems are of little (other than pioneering) interest. However, the stacking of sets of (normally transparent) displays can achieve true 3-D displays in a less 'invasive' manner. Any transparent sheet where an element within can be controlled by a change in state controlled by input from the edge, could be used in this manner. High definition controllable liquid crystal displays are now available and used in flat screen televisions. These could be stacked to give some kind of 3-D display. An extension of this technology (or some variation of it) should permit within the near future a true 3-D high definition addressable volume display. In such a display a one-to-one mapping would exist between voxel elements in the 3-D image data, and 3-D points in the volume display. However, the existence of such a mapping, while probably reducing the data rate requirements of such a system, do not in themselves solve all display problems, in particular that of translucence.

12. INTERACTION AND THE DISPLAY OF INTERNAL STRUCTURES.

The major problem with 3-D display systems in medical imaging, is the display of internal structures. If something is in front of, for example, lesion, it is desirable to see BOTH the lesion, and the structure in front of it [26]. This is quite different to the use of such display systems in other applications. Thus the use of shaded graphics is often not appropriate, in that, as such, it specifically prevents the observation of internal structures. The raw data is the complete set of values in 3-D, all of which need to be displayed, or at least, displayable. Rotating the image does not solve this problem either. One solution is to imagine a 'translucent' object, which can be compared to that obtained when pouring ink into a swimming pool. Voxels are treated as been partly transparent. An alternative approach is to use highly interactive procedures. Herman has shown [1], with CT images of dogs hearts, how surfaces can be defined, and then the object manipulated, for example by splitting into two sections, and then rotating each half such that the 'inside' becomes visible. This system has been implemented to give high quality 3-D CT images [27], and forms an important part of so-called computerized surgery systems [5,6]. Masking, and the use of inverse intensity can also help. Here, everything outside an object, for example an organ, is removed. Objects inside the organ are displayed inversely with respect to their voxel values. This process may be repeated to find objects within objects within objects. This same method can also be used for stereo pairs, and rotating (kinetic depth effect) images. However, interactive control of the process, for example by using a continuously variable surface detection under user control, needs to be implemented. Thus the observer, for example, might interactively selects a point in the 3-D image and the set of surfaces passing though this point are displayed. The hardware implications of this are very significant, and tend to exclude non-interactive devices such as holograms.

13. A DESIGN FOR A FUTURE 3-D DISPLAY SYSTEM

In suggesting a design requirement for a suitable 3-D display system, the usual convention of assuming a considerable improvement of technology has been assumed. See also [28,29]. Thus, it is suggested that the most appropriate form for storing the data from the 3-D medical images is to do so directly in a memory of size ~512^3 by 32bits or about 0.5Gbytes. This memory needs to be rapidly accessible along any line in 3-D. The 'depth' of the memory is required to place information associated with flags, the linked lists, and indications of surface orientation etc.

A simple form of read out, then, is to extract display intensities plane by plane (where a plane is described arbitrarily) during which time simple algorithms manipulating individual voxels may be employed. The read out time of a complete image must be of the order of a second, giving a read/write time per voxel of the order of 8nsecs. This implies that the image must be visually integrated by some external device. This fast cycle time is primarily required to permit interactive operations to be achieved within reasonable operator response times (e.g. <2secs). Dedicated hardware would be required to manipulate the raw data matrix at the necessary speed, but is within the range of current technology. Likewise, special purpose hardware will be required for writing to the display, handling appropriate structures, octrees, tiles etc, rather than directly manipulating primitives of the form WRITE-INTENSITY at 3-D position (x,y,z). A multilayer optical storage device is required for visual integration of the image.

14 SUMMARY AND CONCLUSIONS

The need for 3-D display systems is of increasing urgency, Some good clinical examples of the use of prototypes have been shown in CT [2,27,30] and in NMR [31,32] and for craniofacial surgery [5,6]. The technology needed to implement more advanced systems, with sufficient power and flexibility to perform operations as described in the last section, is just beyond current capabilities. The volume of data is very substantial. Although a true 3-D display is desirable, alternative approaches using suitable coding, for example the varifocal mirror might prove adequate. Work on devising suitable methods for interaction with the data seems to be essential, in order to resolve the problem of internal concealed objects. The development of suitable hardware, and in particular, data structures and algorithms needs to be pursued.

Acknowledgements

The author would like to thank many colleagues, notably Drs Pizer and Fuchs of UNC Chapel Hill, Drs Herman and Bajcsy of Philadelphia, Dr Barrett of Tucson, Dr Baxter of Salt Lake City, Dr Francoise Soussaline of Paris, and co-workers Drs Linney, Arridge and Grindrod at UCH London.

Bibliography
1. Herman, G.T. and D. Webster. Surfaces of organs in discrete three-dimensional space. In 'Mathematical Aspects of Computerized Tomography' Eds Herman G.T. and Natterer F., (Springer Verlag, Berlin, 1981) pp204-224.
2. Herman, G.T. and H.K. Liu. Three-dimensional display of human organs from computed tomograms. Comp. Graph. and Image Processing 9 (1979) 1-21.
3. Frieder, G., Faux, I.D., Ostowski, M.C. and K.G. Pasquill. Back-to-front display of voxel-based objects. IEEE Comp. Graph. and Applications 5 (1985) 52-60.
4. Sunguroff, A. and D. Greenberg. Computer generated images for medical applications. Computer Graphics, Proc Siggraph 78, 12 (1978) 196-202.

5. Vannier M.W., Marsh J.L. and J.O. Warren. Three dimensional CT reconstruction images for craniofacial surgical planning and evaluation. Radiology 150 (1983) 179-184.
6. Vannier M.W., Marsh J.L. and J.O. Warren. Three dimensional computer graphics for craniofacial surgical planning and evaluation. Computer Graphics 17 (1983) Proc. Siggraph '83 263-273.
7. Bookstein, F.L. The line skeleton. Comp. Graph. and Image Processing 11 (1979) 123-137
8. Nackman, L.R. and S.M. Pizer. Three-dimensional shape description using the symmetric axis transform. In Medical Image Processing, ed Goris, M.L., (Stanford University, Div. Nucl. Med. Stanford, 1981) 363-396.
9. Di Paola, R. Personal communication
10. Fuchs, H., Abram, G.D. and E.D. Grant. Near real-time shaded display of rigid objects. Computer Graphics 17 (1983) 65-72.
11. Artzy E. Frieder G. and G.T. Herman. The theory, design, implementation and evaluation of a three-dimensional surface detection algorithm. Comput. Graph. and Image. Proc. 15 (1981) 1-24.
12. Rhodes M.L. Towards fast edge detection for clinical 3-D applications of computer tomography. IEEE CH1404 (1979) 321-327.
13. Meagher D. High speed display of 3-D medical images using octree encoding. IPL-TR-021 Image Processing Lab. Ressenlaer Polytechnique Inst. (1981).
14. Meagher D.J. Interactive solids processing for medical analysis and planning. Proc. Natl. Computer Graphics Assoc. (1984)
15. Meagher, D. Geometric modeling using octree encoding. Comp. Graph. and Image Processing 19 129-147 1982.
16. Fuchs H., Kedem Z.M. and S.P. Uselton. Optimal surface reconstruction from planar contours. Comm. A.C.M. 20 (1977) 56-58.
17. Zucker, S.W. and R.A. Hummel. A three-dimensional edge operator. IEEE Trans. Pat. Anal. and Mach. Intel. PAMI-3 (1981) 324-331.
18. Akima H. A new method of interpolation and smooth surface fitting based on local procedures. J.A.C.M. 13 (1970) 589-602.
19. Sutherland, I.E., Sproull, R.F. and R.A. Schumacker. A characterization of ten hidden surface algorithms. Computing Surveys 6 1974.
20. Gourand H. Computer display of curved surfaces. IEEE Trans. Computers C-20 (1971) 623-629.
21. Phong B.T. Illumination for computer generated pictures. Comm. A.C.M. 18 (1975) 311-317.
22. Barber, D.C. and I. Skellas. Three-dimensional display of tomographic data. Clin. Phys. Physiol. Meas. 2 (1981) 153-155.

23. Greguss P. Holographic displays from computer assisted tomography. J. Comp. Ass. Tomography. $\underline{1}$ (1977) 184-186.
24. Exhibition and Symposium on 3-D Imaging, 3rd World Congress of Nuclear Medicine and Biology, August 1982, Paris, France.
25. Pizer, S.M., Fuchs, H., Heinz, E.R., Staab E.V., et al, Interactive 3D display of medical images. In Information Processing in Medical Imaging, ed Deconinck F., (Nijhoff, Boston, 1984) 513-526.
26. Bradley-Moore P.R. and E.A. Woloshuk. Time as depth. Handout and exhibit 27th Soc. Nucl. Med. meeting Detroit 1980.
27. Real-time solid modeling system: Insight. Phoenix data systems Inc.Albany N.Y., USA.
28. Flynn M., Matteson R., Dickie D., Keyes J.W. and F. Bookstein. Requirements for the display and analysis of three-dimensional image data. SPIE $\underline{418}$ Picture Archiving and Communication systems (1983) 213-224.
29. Goldwasser, S.M. A generalized object display processor architecture. IEEE Comp. Graph. and Applications. $\underline{4}$ (1984) 43-55.
30. Artzy E. Display of three-dimensional information in computed tomography. Comp. Graph. and Image Processing $\underline{9}$ (1979) 196-198.
31. Kramer D.M. Schneider J.S., Rudin A.M. et al. True three dimensional nuclear magnetic resonance images of a brain. Neuroradiology $\underline{21}$ (1981) 239-244.
32. Schlusselberg, D.S., Smith W.K., Lewis, M.H., Culter, B.G. and D.J. Woodward. A general system for computer based acquisition analysis and display of medical image data. Proc. ACM Ann. Meeting Oct 1982, 18-25.

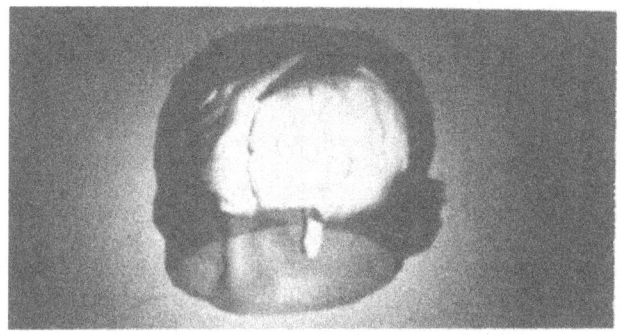

Additional Figure. Two 3-D shaded graphics images from the literature. Above is the image of a brain inside the surface of the head, obtained from a set of NMR (MRI) slices (Courtesy of D.S. Schlusselberg). Below, the 3-D image of a section through the orbits is shown, obtained from CT data (Courtesy of G.T. Herman and Phoenix Data Systems).

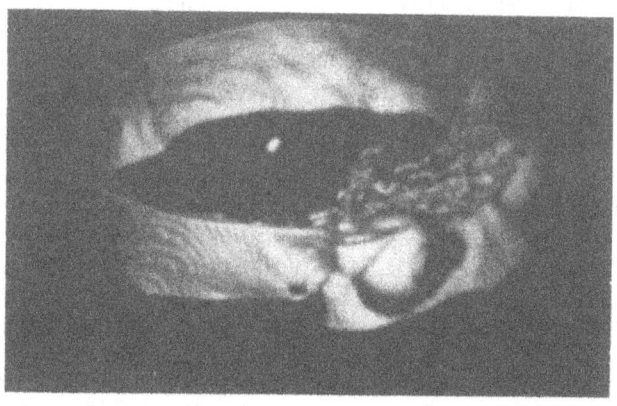

QUALITY ASSURANCE IN MEDICAL IMAGING

C. Leon Partain, M.D., Ph.D.
Jon J. Erickson, Ph.D.
James A. Patton, Ph.D.
Ronald R. Price, Ph.D.
David R. Pickens, Ph.D.
A. Everette James, Jr., J.D., M.D.

Department of Radiology & Radiological Sciences
Vanderbilt University School of Medicine
Nashville, Tennessee, 37232 USA

ABSTRACT

The philosophy and general test methods that can be used on a routine basis to assure the quality of medical imaging systems are summarized in this article. Quality assurance must be observed throughout the entire imaging process from the initial order for a particular procedure to the generation, interpretation, and reporting of results. Key areas of concern include the optimization of the decision process (selection of the proper imaging procedure or sequence of procedures); the utilization of contrast agents, pharmaceuticals (including radiopharmaceuticals), and pharmacologically enhanced imaging procedures; the biodistribution and dosimetry; and the possible side effects of external agents.

INTRODUCTION

Quality control of the medical imaging process is a topic which is receiving increased attention as the complexity and cost of medical instrumentation rises to unprecedented levels. Most professional organizations have at least one committee that is charged with the responsibility of recommending quality assurance procedures appropriate to their respective specialities. In spite of this widespread increase in interest, there has not been a unified approach to the problem of quality assurance in the general field of diagnostic imaging equipment. This is not surprising in light of the disagreement that is evident among individuals involved in promolgating the protocols for the various imaging modalities. For example, it is possible to become embroiled in long arguments over tests intended to examine such relatively simple concepts as the uniformity of the scintillation camera image. Furthermore, the increased use of computers and the attendant software makes absolute quality assurance testing an exceedingly difficult task. The need for a universal quality assurance program for medical imaging is obvious. The implementation of this concept, however, is not yet realized and the problems present complex challenges.

Although it may be possible to suggest some unifying concepts such as spatial resolution, measuring times, density or chemical sensitivity, it is unlikely that there is much to be gained by attempting to coordinate actual testing protocols across modalities. In fact, it may be argued that the lack of consensus concerning the detailed protocols are of less value than are the mental attitudes which their use creates. Thus, which protocol is used for daily evaluation of the scintillation camera or the CT scanner is probably of less significance than the fact that the operator is doing something and thereby being reminded that image quality is important and must be monitored.

The clinical importance of quality assurance in medical imaging is well recognized in diagnostic medicine (1-4). Discussed below are objectives and components of a quality assurance program followed by comments on appropriate implementation.

OBJECTIVES

Quality assurance programs are designed to provide maximal diagnostic information at the minimum possible risk to the patient. They include an analysis of both efficacy and benefit/risk ratio of each medical imaging procedure.

The quality control of the use or external agents include assurance that the agent is 1) administered to the patient in the form and amount prescribed; 2) pure and safe for in vivo use; and 3) sterile and pyrogen free. Instrumentation utilized to establish the above must be evaluated routinely for optimal and stable performance.

Quality control in the operation of any medical imaging instrument seeks to ensure that the image represents actual variation in intensity, transmission, or activity distribution within a patient and not variations in instrument performance. Hence, imaging system performance must be continually evaluated.

Similarly, data storage, retrieval, processing, and interpretation should ensure the detection of subtle changes in biodistribution of activity, intensity, or differential transmission. Beyond that, the subtle differences should be attributable to pathophysiological conditions with maximal sensitivity and specificity.

COMPONENTS OF QUALITY ASSURANCE

Decision: Which Procedure Should be Used?

Usually the referring physician determines the need for a particular procedure in consultation with the medical imaging physician. Key considerations include 1) benefit; 2) possible alternative tests with less risk and/or more diagnostic data; and 3) minimal risk. The need for medical judgment may at times be incorporated with the logical desire to maximize benefit/risk ratios.

Utilization of External Agents

Monitoring for sterility, apyrogenicity, purity, and safety should accompany preparation and administration. An accurate record keeping system for the *in vivo* utilization of all external agents is essential.

Measurement of Spatial Distribution of Information in Patients

Quality assurance measurements may be characterized by four types of tests: 1) confidence tests; 2) performance tests; 3) parameter determination; and 4) hardware diagnostic procedures.

Confidence tests are simple, quick, and easy tests which require no special equipment and may be performed several times a day. They provide confidence in correct system operation by providing an estimate of "go/no-go" operation but do not establish correct system operation.

Performance tests require more time and material than confidence tests. They may be performed as seldom as once a day or week. They provide a check of correct system operation, monitor system parameter stability and may indicate impending failure. These tests are performed in the event of suggested system failure. Examples include measures of image uniformity, spatial linearity, and evaluation of possible artifacts.

Tests of parameter determination are performed after installation and following major repair. They may require significant time and effort and are used to characterize system performance. Examples include measures of imager/computer deadtime and measures of the relationship of detector surface with pixel separation in the image.

Hardware diagnostic tests are used to isolate hardware failures. These do not guarantee successful and accurate execution of new software. They are usually performed by a system

Perception of Results and Interpretation

Factors which influence perception and observed performance in medical imaging include intensity, contrast, and the size of abnormalities. These factors have recently been applied to the interpretation of scintigraphic abnormalities (5).

IMPLEMENTATION OF QUALITY ASSURANCE PROGRAM

The quality assurance program should be established as an integral part of the operation of every medical imaging department. The initiation and maintenence requires the commitment of time and trained personnel. The process has been described as involving education and regulation (6). The concepts and philosophy of quality assurance and phantom design have been recently proposed for nuclear magnetic resonance imaging systems (7).

In conclusion, it is obvious that a functioning quality assurance program is essential on a medical, legal, ethical, financial and technical basis.

Acknowledgments

The author gratefully acknowedges the editorial assistance of Mrs. Margaret Moore.

REFERENCES

1. Quality Assurance in Nuclear Medicine, Proceedings of an International Symposium and Workshop, Washington, D.C., April, 1981. HHS Publication FDS 84-8224.

2. Erickson JJ and Rollo FD, eds: Digital Nuclear Medicine. Philadelphia, J. B. Lippincott, 1983.

3. Waggener RF and Wilson CR, eds: Quality Assurance in Diagnostic Radiology. New York, American Association of Physicists in Medicine, 1980.

4. Gray JE, Winkler NT, Stears J, and Frank ED: Quality Control in Diagnostic Imaging. Baltimore, University Park Press, 1982.

5. Schultz AG, Kohlenstein LD, Knowles LG: Factors affecting recognition of scintigraphic abnormalities. Seminars in Nuclear Medicine 3:327, 1973.

6. Hendee WR: How to achieve quality assurance in nuclear medicine. In Rhodes BA (ed): Quality Control in Nuclear Medicine, Chapter 15. St. Louis, C.V. Mosby, Inc., 1977.

7. Price RR, Patton JA, Erickson JJ, Pickens DR, Partain CL and James AE: Concepts of quality assurance and phantom design of NMR systems. Transactions of American Association of Physicists in Medicine, Portland, OR, August 1985.

MEDICAL AND NON-MEDICAL IMAGING: CROSS-FERTILIZATION

Vito Cappellini

Dipartimento di Ingegneria Elettronica, University of Florence and
IROE - C.N.R., Florence, Italy

1. INTRODUCTION

The area of image acquisition, analysis and processing ("Imaging") has increased greatly in importance over the last few years, particularly as a result of the impressive advances and innovations in digital methods and technology. The following aspects, in particular, are to be outlined: definition of new and efficient algorithms; new image acquisition and digitizing systems; construction of special digital microelectronic devices with high complexity (such as LSI-VLSI, microcomputers, array processors) at a decreasing cost; production of fast computers and microcomputers.

Imaging methods and techniques, in particular of the digital type, have already found many applications in different fields such as communications, radar-sonar systems, remote sensing, manufacturing automation, robotics, office automation, telematics and biomedicine.

In this paper we consider the cross-fertilization which has already occurred, and that which will occur in the near future, between medical and non medical imaging, particularly in relation to the advancement of biomedical image processing, (not neglecting, however, the additional possibility of transferring efficient techniques from biomedicine to other fields).

First the different image processing methods and techniques are reviewed, such as digital transformations, digital filtering, local space operators, data compression and image storage, geometrical transformations and pattern recognition. The different implementation systems for image acquisition, analysis, processing and transmission are also presented, both as hardware and software solutions, outlining the real-time and off-line configurations. Hence some digital techniques and systems, which were already developed for the fields indicated above and which can be of interest and utility for medical imaging are described, as they increase the efficiency and open new trends in this field. In particular, techniques are presented, which use special multi-dimensional digital filters, data compression and pattern recognition and some typical examples are given. Finally some considerations are developed to transfer interesting results obtained in medical imaging (special sensing and acquisition systems and tomography techniques) to other fields (such as remote sensing and robotics).

2. IMAGE PROCESSING METHODS AND TECHNIQUES

Some important image processing methods and techniques, mainly of the digital type, are briefly reviewed in the following pages, with special reference to digital transformations, digital filtering, local space operators, data compression, geometrical transformations and pattern recognition.

2.1. DIGITAL TRANSFORMATIONS

An invertible digital transformation of the two-dimensional (2-D) type can be defined by the following relation (1):

$$F(k_1, k_2) = \sum_{n_1=1}^{N_1} \sum_{n_2=1}^{N_2} f(n_1, n_2) A(n_1, n_2; k_1, k_2) \qquad (1)$$

where $f(n_1, n_2)$ are the input data (samples of the analog image) and $A(n_1, n_2; k_1, k_2)$ represents the forward transform kernel, N_1 and N_2 being two positive integers. The inverse transformation provides a mapping from the transform domain to the image space as given by

$$f(n_1, n_2) = \sum_{k_1=1}^{N_1} \sum_{k_2=2}^{N_2} F(k_1, k_2) B(n_1, n_2; k_1, k_2) \qquad (2)$$

where $B(n_1, n_2; k_1, k_2)$ denotes the inverse transform kernel.

The most important 2-D digital transformations are represented by Fourier transform (in particular cosine and sine transforms), Hadamard transform and Walsh transform, Haar transform, slant transform, SVD (Singular Value Decomposition) transform and Karhunen-Loeve transform. Fast computational algorithms have been discovered for the above transforms, excluding only the Karhunen-Loeve transform. Of special interest for digital image processing are 2-D FFT (Fast Fourier Transform) and FWT (Fast Walsh Transform).

2.2 DIGITAL FILTERING

A 2-D linear digital filter can be defined by the following relation (2):

$$g(n_1,n_2) = \sum_{k_1=0}^{N_1-1} \sum_{k_2=0}^{N_2-1} a(k_1,k_2) f(n_1-k_1, n_2-k_2)$$

$$- \sum_{k_1=0}^{M_1-1} \sum_{k_2=0}^{M_2-1} b(k_1,k_2) g(n_1-k_1, n_2-k_2) \qquad (3)$$

$$k_1+k_2 \neq 0$$

where $f(n_1, n_2)$ are the image data, $g(n_1, n_2)$ are the output filtered data (samples of the analog output image), $a(k_1, k_2)$ and $b(k_1, k_2)$ are the digital filter coefficients (specifying the 2-D space frequency response), $N_1 N_2 M_1$ and M_2 being suitable positive integers.

If all the $b(k, k)$ coefficients are zero, the 2-D digital filter is called FIR (Finite Impulse Response) type: in this case the difference equation (3) is a convolution between the input image matrix and the coefficient matrix and no feedback of previous outputs is present. Otherwise the 2-D digital filter is of causal IIR (Infinite Impulse Response) type. FIR digital filters have a non-recursive structure, while IIR filters have a recursive structure. Furthermore FIR digital filters can easily give frequency responses with linear phase (which must have no phase distortion), while this is difficult to obtain with IIR digital filters. Moreover IIR digital filters have stability problems. However, with regard to the implementation cost, IIR digital filters require, in general, a lower number of coefficients than FIR digital filters.

Due to the above properties, 2-D FIR digital filters are in general used for digital image processing, because, in particular, they have no phase distortion and stability problem. But when higher speed or lower cost processing is required, IIR filters are preferred.

2.3 LOCAL SPACE OPERATORS

Local space operators correspond in general to low complexity 2-D digital processing systems: small blocks of data (image samples) are processed in the space domain (3). By evaluating, for instance, the mean value of the block data, a "smoothing" is obtained, while by performing the difference of data along lines or columns "enhancement" effects are the result.

A very important class of 2-D local space operators is

represented by "edge detectors", which extract boundaries or edges in the processed image. The most part of these operators are based on the evaluation of the gradient through a test on a given image point (pixel) and its close points. In fact if the magnitude and the direction of the gradient in a point are know and if the magnitude is greater than a given threshold, it is assumed that in the point there is an edge or contour, whose direction is orthogonal to the gradient direction. The techniques used for this purpose can be divided in two groups: to the first group belong the operators which evaluate two orthogonal components of the gradient; the second group is based on gradient detection by means of a set of "templates" or "masks" of different orientation. Well known operators are: Roberts operator, smoothed gradient operator, Sobel operator, Prewitt operator, isotropic operator, Robinson operator, Chen-Frei operator.

Recently a special edge operator was introduced (4) for extracting edges in noisy images. This operator considers a block of 3x3 data: to each one of the 8 pixels surrounding the central one a binary value is given, according to the difference among the pixel value and the central value. In this way, 256 configurations result: they are divided in 5 classes, there being a decreasing probability that the central pixel is a part of an edge or contour. Adaptive criteria can be used to estimate if the central pixel pertains to an edge, depending on the noise characteristics in the processed image. Another advantage of this operator is represented by its speed of implementation: practically, to estimate whether or not a pixel is a part of an edge, after the binary values have been obtained, it is sufficient to compare the actual binary configuration to a memorized "decision table".

Of increasing interest are 2-D local space operators performing non-linear filtering operations, assuring very fast image processing. An interesting example is represented by the following non-linear smoother of noisy images. If we consider a block of 3x3 data and we denote with P_0 the value of the central pixel, while P_1, P_2, ..., P_8 are the values of the surrounding pixels, the smoother is defined by the following relation (5):

$$P'_0 = \frac{1}{n} \sum_{P_i \in S} P_i \qquad (4)$$

where $S = \{P_i : |P_i - P_0| \leq K\}$ and i $= 0,1,2,.....8$.

By means of this smoother the value of each pixel is replaced by the average of itself and its neighbouring values, except those which have level differences greater than a fixed threshold in absolute value. In this way, small amplitude noise is removed, while no degradation is resulting for edges present in the processed image regions. Therefore, the use of this operator is recommended before the edge extraction through a usual edge operator, especially in noisy image processing.

2.4. DATA COMPRESSION

Data compression is a transformation performed to reduce the amount of redundant data ("redundancy reduction") and is particularly useful for image processing, due to the large number of sampled data representing each image. Several data compression methods and techniques have been introduced of either the "reversible" or "irreverseble" type: "reversible" means that the inverse transformation or "decompression" can recover all the original data.

Some important data compression methods include the following: adaptive sampling, prediction, interpolation, filtering, encoding and the use of transforms (Fourier, Hadamard, Walsh, Haar, Karhunen-Loeve ...). All one-dimensional (1-D) data compression methods can also be applied to image processing if the image is processed line by line (6).

Two particular techniques of appreciable interest are: 2-D digital filtering and the use of 2-D digital transformation as described above. 2-D digital filtering of low-pass or band-pass type, by itself represents a sort of data compression because a limited part of the space frequency spectrum is extracted, requiring a lower number of data to be represented. Further 2-D low-pass digital filtering can be used for pre-processing before the application of other compression algorithms because the smoothed data can be more efficiently compressed.

2-D digital transforms are, in general, followed by simple procedures such as thresholding, variable word-length encoding, prediction-interpolation. A method of using 2-D FFT or FWT (6) consists of dividing the transformed image data into several squares of small size (4x4, 8x8, 16x16) and in employing, for each of them, a minimum word-length (a bit number sufficient to represent the maximum absolute value in the square plus one bit for the sign). An additional fixed-length word is inserted before the square amplitude values in order to specify the number of bits used to represent these square values. In a modified method, no value is maintained for those sub-areas or squares, in which the addition of the absolute value of the transformed date lies below a given threshold.

2.5. GEOMETRICAL TRANSFORMATIONS

In many practical applications the available images are to be geometrically transformed for their final utilization. This happens for instance when there are several images taken by different equipment or sensing devices, corresponding to the same observed "scene". A typical example is represented by images obtained from different remote sensing equipment and instruments, in particular, at different heights or with different ground space resolutions.

In the above cases geometrical transformations such as "rotation", changes of the "point of view", geometrical scale variation, etc. are to be performed. Suitable geometrical relations are available for this purpose.

An interesting practical situation is represented by the need (more often emerging, for instance, in remote sensing) to compare and correlate images obtained from different equipment and having different space resolutions. A special processing technique has been defined (7) to solve this problem. First geometrical transformations are performed, in such a way as to "register" the different images on specific "reference points". Then a 2-D low-pass digital filter is applied to the image with higher space resolution (to limit its spectrum to the same extent as that of the lower resolution image): a "decimation" (data reduction) is then performed on the filtered image to reduce its space sampling interval to the same value as the lower resolution image.

2.6. PATTERN RECOGNITION

In the most part of image processing applications, a very important processing step is represented by "pattern recognition" in which useful patterns or configurations are extracted, recognized and classified for final utilization and decision.

A first relatively simple approach to pattern recognition is represented by comparison with "prototypes". In this approach each pattern to be recognized has a prototype in the memory of the processing system. The incoming pattern or configuration is compared with each one of the prototypes and the decision is taken to recognize the incoming pattern by the prototype nearest or most similar to it (or more precisely the prototype having a minimum "distance" or "error").

More generally, pattern recognition methods can be classified in two main groups: "statistical decision" methods and "syntactical" or "structural" methods. In the methods of the first type, each pattern is characterized by one or more "features", significant measurements which are considered invariant properties of the patterns; the pattern recognizer thus consists of two main parts: a "feature extractor" and a following "classifier", which makes the final decision on the incoming pattern depending on the extracted features. In the methods of the second type, each pattern is decomposed in a large number of elementary "sub-patterns" with a syntactic or structural description (for instance a "tree" structure); the pattern recognizer thus consists of a sub-patterns extractor, a classifier of obtained sub-patterns and a final decision (suitable languages are also used to describe the useful patterns as a "composition" of elementary sub-patterns) (8).

3. IMPLEMENTATION SYSTEMS

Implementation systems are indeed very important for the practical use of the image processing methods described above and techniques in the different fields such as communications, radar-sonar systems, remote sensing, manufacturing automation, robotics, office automation, telematics and biomedicine. In the following pages, different implementation aspects are briefly reviewed with special reference to hardware implementation, software implementation and some image acquisition, processing and transmission systems. Both the state of the art and the near future evolution are considered.

3.1. HARDWARE IMPLEMENTATION

The technology of integrated digital circuits has a very fast development, in terms of working frequencies and complexity, with large scale integration (LSI) and very large scale integration (VLSI) implementations. With regard to the evolution trend, we can outline that, whereas now silicon devices are available with delays of one elementary circuit (as a logical gate) in the order of nanoseconds, in a decade from now they are expected to have delays in the order of 100 picoseconds or less. By means of Josephson effect or Ga-As devices, delays of 10-30 picoseconds are expected. With regard to the number of elementary circuits in a chip (in particular a microprocessor), it is expected that over the next decade this will rise from about 10^5 elementary circuits presently implemented to 10^6 and more.

Arithmetic circuits are now produced, which have multiplication times (16-24 bits) of the order of about 100 nanoseconds or less, allowing the implementation of fast processing units. At the same time memories are available with capacities which range from thousands of bits to thousands of bytes, with access times which range from a few nanoseconds to some hundreds of nanoseconds. At lower clock frequencies, MOS technologies (e.g. CMOS) allow the integration (using VLSI implementation) of very complex signal processing primitives, which can then be used in "pipeline" or parallel organizations as building blocks of complex image processing facilities, where the complexity of the control is traded off for the use of a less expensive technology (9)(10).

These advances in technology have their impact even in the peripherals, which are necessary to implement efficient image processing facilities. A typical example is the storage problem both in the implementation of fast buffers to be used during the process and of very large storage systems. The impact of the new memory chips in the production of buffer memories is obvious, but very interesting developments are under way in other directions too. For instance digital tape recorders are under development (HDDT - high density digital tape) with capacities ten times higher than those now available (greater than 10^{11} bits).

By using optical technologies, optical records ("optical disk"), obtained by means of laser beams, are available with capacities of up to 10^{10} bits/record and with transfer rates of about 10 Mbits/s, while higher capacity records (up to 10^{11}) are under development. With regard to the processing, "integrated optics" are very promising for performing different operations such as spectral estimation, convolution, correlation (11).

Correspondingly, good quality systems for image presentation are produced. High resolution TV monitors (up to 1000x1000 pixels and more) are now available and, generally, they are incorporated in microcomputer based presentation facilities, which allow the storage of one or more images with simple local processing on a single or small sequences of images.

Some interesting developments are also under way in the implementation of specialized processors for image processing applications, in two different directions. The first approach is the study of very high-speed processing units, which, in the typical arrangement, make use of efficient memory structures and multiple data buses, obtaining very high throughputs (essentially in structured operations such as the ones employed in image processing applications). The second approach is the development of parallel structures, with distributed processing units and memories. These allow the use of simpler logic and the identification of processing sub-structures, suitable for VLSI implementation. This, in turn, requires the development of very efficient architectures where the above-defined building blocks are suitably interconnected to implement complex operations. Bus structures have to be defined in order to transfer the data among the different parts of the processor and to use them in an efficient way together with efficient control structures and algorithms.

With reference to the above point, it is important to outline that most activities in the development of digital signal processing techniques have been in the reduction of the number of multiplications, which in conventional implementations (as on a general purpose computer) is the "limiting factor" in the processing speed (the use of integer coefficients in digital filters is for instance an example of processing speed increase). Now this is not the only problem to be taken care of because several other factors such as the "segmentability" of the algorithms and the simplicity of the control are indeed very important.

Improvements are also in progress in the use of general purpose computers, due essentially to the increase in the computation speed, to the availability of large central memories even in small computers or microcomputers and to the increased capacity of the transfer-rate of disks.

3.2 SOFTWARE IMPLEMENTATION

In the software implementation, general purpose computers or microcomputers are used to perform digital image processing through suitable "programs". In general, computers having fast CPU ("central processing unit") and high data transfer-rates with disks and other peripheral units, are preferred, due to the large amount of data to be processed, often in a short time, in image applications. The evolution trend, also for large computer systems, is to have several fast computing units interconnected among them and with large capacity memories by means of fast multiple data buses; in particular for matrix operations, as required in image processing, fast "array processors" are more frequently utilized. With regard to speed indication, while we now have systems working at 10-100 MIPS (millions of instructions per second), it is predicted that in a decade these will reach 1000 MIPS and more.

With regard to the programs for image processing, we can distinguish among three types of programs (in addition to the internal programs assuring the basic working of the computer system): design programs, simulation programs and processing programs. Design programs are used to design digital operations (digital filtering, data compression, pattern recognition, ...) with the purpose of determining the digital operation "parameters" best suited for the desired application. Simulation programs are used to evaluate the performance of a given digital operation, in general by varying the operation parameters and obtaining the corresponding performance results. Processing programs are indeed used to actually perform the desired digital operation and processing application by means of the parameters defined through the design programs and tested through the simulation programs.

Some general criteria used to define good computer programs are: modularity (that is to decompose the program in suitable "sub-routines" to be used in several different programs), flexibility and transportability (possibility of using the same program in different computer systems).

Many computer languages are known. Some specific languages have been defined for processing applications regarding signals and images, such as SPL/1 defined at the Naval Research Laboratory in Washington, ADA used for defence problems but also extended to other applications, LISP defined at MIT for artificial intelligence problems. High level languages are studied for the future computer systems (and in particular for the "fifth generation computers") with the aim of obtaining the highest processing efficiency and speed.

3.3 IMAGE ACQUISITION, PROCESSING AND TRANSMISSION SYSTEMS.

An image processing system can consist as outlined above of special harware processors, microprocessors, array processors or of a standard computer (often interconnected with some of the above processors). In any case, two important parts of the overall image processing system are represented by the image acquisition unit and by the transmission unit.

With regard to the input acquisition unit, several solutions are available: opto-electronics scanners, laser systems, special TV cameras (in particular using CCD devices). These units are available for acquisition of 1000x1000 pixels and more for black-white and colour input images; high resolution TV monitors are also available, as already observed, for the visual presentation of these acquired images. The trend is to implement "integrated" units, where acquisition, image storage and presentation are performed together under the control of suitable fast microprocessors, eventually devoted also to pre-processing operations. With this last purpose, optical processors, as already observed, are also carefully considered, for future systems.

Regarding the transmission unit, it is important to outline that the image data exchange with other computer systems or input-output devices (in particular remote acquisition or utilization units) is presently of great relevance to the overall performance of the computer systems and will be of even greater relevance in the future. Indeed in several application areas (remote sensing, office automation, telematics), in addition to standard TV systems or teleconference systems, images are to be efficiently transferred from one place to another with the lowest possible distortion. In addition to cables and microwave ground links, satellite communication systems and fiber optics are becoming very important, due to the high transmission rates (1 Gbit/s and more). While satellite systems are seen as the best solution for long and medium distance communications, optical fibers systems appear to be the best solution for lower distance communications (presently distances in the order of 50 Km and more can be covered without the use of repeaters). Optical fibers systems represent in particular a very attractive solution for the interconnection of different image processing systems in the same building or in different buildings in a town: local communication networks can be implemented.

In the above communication systems, it is very useful to have image data which are already compressed , due to the bandwidth reduction that, in this way, can easily be obtained (a lower amount of data can be transmitted in a lower time with the same bandwidth or in the same time with lower bandwith) (6). Furthermore, if noise or distortion problems arise in the communication link, suitable error control coding techniques (for simple error detection and also for error correction), can be applied, using, for instance, block coding or convolutional coding (12).

4. DIGITAL PROCESSING TECHNIQUES AND SYSTEMS DEVELOPED IN OTHER FIELDS OF INTEREST FOR MEDICAL IMAGING

Some of the digital image processing techniques and implementation systems presented above have been already applied in the biomedical area. In the following pages we mainly consider those processing techniques and systems which have been only partially utilized for biomedical image processing up to now or have not been applied at all. Acquisition, processing and transmission aspects are outlined.

With regard to image acquisition, some sensing devices and equipment already developed in other fields can enter biomedicine in a more consistent form. An interesting example is represented by the "microwave radiometry", widely used in remote sensing. This sensing technique is useful for giving more information inside the tissues, in comparison to the more standard "infrared radiometry", which offers more space resolution on or near to the surface. Some prototypes are appearing such as Bruker TMO 3000, that work in the microwave S band (3 GHz) and are also available in the X band (10 GHz) such as the TMO 10000 model (13). The innovation trend on this line does indeed correspond to the integration of the microwave with the infrared radiometry in order to combine, in the best possible way, the two different sensing capabilities, outlined above. In these new systems for non-invasive clinical analysis (in particular of cancerous tumours) the main processing problems are represented by the need of performing an efficient integration of the two types of images: 2-D digital filtering techniques in combination with geometrical transformation, as described above, can be very useful in solving these problems. Interesting experiments on this new implementation line have been performed recently in Florence in cooperation with S.M.A. S.p.A. and Dipartimento di Ingegneria Elettronica of Florence University (14).

Further digital image acquisition systems, converting each black-white or colour image in 1024x1024 pixels, can be more commonly employed in the biomedical area, due to their availability in different structures and configurations at a decreasing cost. In particular CCD TV cameras can be used in connection with digitizing units and memory buffers together with some processing capability offered by fast microprocessors, as outlined above. Different solutions are available on the market (for instance CCD cameras by Hamamatsu and digitizing-storage-processing units by IBM or VDS in Florence). These systems can be useful for acquisition and digitizing of different types of bioimages, such as those obtained in thermography, ultrasonics, X-radiography etc.

With regard to the digital image processing, efficient digital filtering, data compression and pattern recognition techniques can be more extensively applied in the biomedical area. Concerning digital filtering, 2-D digital filters can be used for biomedical image enhancement and restoration to obtain higher quality images for a better diagnosis: an example of the application of a special 2-D FIR digital filter of "parabolic" type to a part of a computer tomography image is shown in Fig. 1 (different results: b, c, d). Further 3-D digital interpolations or digital filters are very useful for 3-D reconstruction of body parts starting from single 2-D images: an example of the application of 3-D digital interpolation to computer tomography images is shown in Fig. 2 (a complete lower image is at the left and 30 interpolated images of a small sub-part are at the right) (15) (16). Concerning data compression, the different techniques developed first in space telemetry and remote sensing fields are indeed also very useful for biomedical image processing, due to the increasing amount of bioimages taken every day to be not only analysed but also stored in data banks or transferred from one place to another. Some experimental results obtained by applying digital transformation techniques (2-D FFT and FWT) to nuclear medicine images, pre-filtered through 2-D low-pass digital filters of FIR type, are shown in Table 1: the values of the obtained compression ratios (data reduction from the original to compressed images) and of the errors (peak and r.m.s.) are given (12).

Table 1 - Results obtained by applying 2-D digital transformations to pre-filtered nuclear medicine images

	compression ratio = 6		compression ratio = 8	
	peak er.	r.m.s. er.	peak er.	r.m.s. er.
2D-FFT	0.1322	0.0134	0.1581	0.0164
2D-FWT	0.0483	0.0074	0.1088	0.0160

With further regard to pattern recognition, high efficiency techniques have been developed for automatic recognition of patterns and configurations, also in connection with artificial intelligence principles, in different fields such as character recognition, remote sensing and in particular robotics. Also if some pattern recognition techniques have already entered the biomedical area, much greater impact is expected due to the advantages of separating different tissues and especially of extracting ill or altered parts from the overall analysed bioimages. Two pattern recognition situations are also of particular interest for biomedical images: recognition and tracking of moving objects (moving parts of the body such as the heart); decomposition of complex objects into their elementary parts (complex organs into their different tissues and structural elements). Just as an indication of the actual capabilities, Fig.

3 shows an example of automatic recognition and tracking of moving objects (each one identified by a different colour, appearing here as different gray levels), while Fig. 4 shows an example of complex object decomposition (a circuit board decomposed in the different components with identification of the position of each component through its centroid and elongation axis) (17) (18).

With regard to the transmission of biomedical images, advanced digital communication techniques can be utilized: data compression and error control coding techniques with communication systems such as optical fibers or communication satellites. Indeed telemedicine systems have been developed, which transmit biomedical data and bioimages through different communication channels (from the telephone lines to special data transmission lines and also to optical fibers). A trend for the future is represented by the set-up of large data banks containing biomedical data and, in particular, bioimages with easy access to these banks from remote regional places and fast exchange of data and bioimages among the different data banks in a region.

5. CONCLUSIONS

The evolution of imaging techniques, image acquisition, processing and transmission is very fast, with innovations appearing in the different fields such as communications, radar-sonar systems, remote sensing, robotics, telematics and biomedicine. We have reviewed the state of the art and the evolution trends in the imaging area, pointing out some aspects which can be transferred through the other fields to biomedicine e.g. bioimages, and have illustrated some typical examples.

From another point of view, it is also to be observed that some interesting results obtained in medical imaging, can be transferred to the other fields. This is the case with special sensing and acquisition systems such as those developed in medical ultrasonics, X-radiography and computer tomography. In particular, ultrasonics and X-radiography equipment can be extensively applied to the analysis, monitoring and testing of mechanical components and machines and of other composite structures. Ultrasonic equipment developed in biomedicine with high sensitivity can be useful in manufacturing automation and robotics, to give data and images related to the mechanical parts position and internal structure. Furthermore, new tomographic techniques can also been applied to manufacturing automation and robotics: y-ray techniques, in particular, are very promising at this advanced level (19).

In conclusion, the cross-fertilization among medical and non medical imaging appears to be very important in order to exchange innovations and new implemented systems with the advantages of efficiency increase and cost reductions.

ACKNOWLEDGEMENTS

We are very grateful to Drs. A. Del Bimbo, A. Mecocci and R. Carla' for their useful cooperation in image processing experiments. Furthermore this work was developed with the support of Ministero Pubblica Istruzione (Special 40% Project in cooperation with Prof. F. Rocca, Politecnico di Milano).

REFERENCES

(1) Pratt, W.K. Digital Image Processing (New York, John Wiley & Sons, 1978).
(2) Cappellini, V., Constantinides, AG. and P. Emiliani. Digital Filters and Their Applications (London-New York, Academic Press, 1981).
(3) Cappellini, V. and P.L. Emiliani. 2-D Digital Systems and Applications the State of the Art, in Tzafestas, S.G. Ed., Multidimensional Systems (New York, Marcel Dekker, 1984).
(4) Cappellini, V. and L. Odorico. A New Operator for Edge Detection. Proceedings of IEEE Intern. Conference on Acoustic, Speech and Signal Processing (Atlanta, IEEE Press, 1981).
(5) Cappellini, V. Non-Linear Digital Filtering Techniques for Fast Image Processing. Proceedings of IEEE Intern. Symposium on Circuits and Systems (Newport Beach - California, IEEE Press, 1983).
(6) Benelli, G., Cappellini, V. and F. Lotti. Data Compression Techniques and Applications. The Radio and Electronic Engineer, vol. 50, n. 1/2 (1980) 29-53.
(7) Cappellini, V., Carla', R., Conese, C., Maracchi, G.P. and F. Miglietta. Digital Comparison and Correlation Techniques of Remote Sensing Images with Different Space Resolution. EARSeL/ESA Symposium on Integrative Approach in Remote Sensing, Guilford - England (1984).
(8) Fu, K.S. Digital Pattern Recognition (Berlin-New York, Springer-Verlag, 1976).
(9) Cappellini, V. Elaborazione numerica delle immagini (Torino, Boringhieri, 1984).
(10) Clementi, E. Lo sviluppo tecnologico negli Stati Uniti nel prossimo decennio. Note di Informatica - IBM Italia n. 7 (1984) 21-44.
(11) Sottini, S., Russo, V. and G.C. Righini. Integrated Optical Devices for Signal Processing. Proceedings of Intern. Conference on Digital Signal Processing, 333-340 (Firenze, Tipografia Giuntina, 1981).
(12) Cappellini, V. Ed. Data Compression and Error Control Techniques with Applications (London-New York, Academic Press, 1984).
(13) Robert, J., Edrich, J., Leroy, Y., Mamouni, A., Escanye, J.M. and P. Thouvenot. Clinical Applications of Microwave

Thermography. Journal of Optics and Photonics Applied to Medicine, vol. 211 (1980) 149-153.

(14) Prosperi, E. Esperienze di radiometria infrarosso e a microonde. Thesis, Ingegneria Elettronica, Universita' di Firenze (1983).

(15) Cappellini, V., Carla', R. and M. Melani. Implementation of a 2-D FIR Digital Filter of Parabolic Type for Biomedical Applications. Proceedings of Intern. Conference on Digital Signal Processing, 691-695 (Amsterdam, North-Holland, 1984).

(16) Pazzaglini, G. Elaborazione di immagini tomografiche: analisi spettrale e interpolazione a tre dimensioni. Thesis, Ingegneria Elettronica, Universita' di Firenze (1983).

(17) Cappellini, V. and A. Del Bimbo. Digital Processing of Time Varying Images, in Chen, C.H. Ed., Issues in Acoustic Signal/Image Processing and Recognition (Berlin-Heidelberg, Springer-Verlag, 1983).

(18) Cappellini, V., Del Bimbo, A. and A. Mecocci. Image and Vision Computing, vol. 2, n. 2, (1984) 109-113.

(19) Guzzardi R. Private Communication (1984).

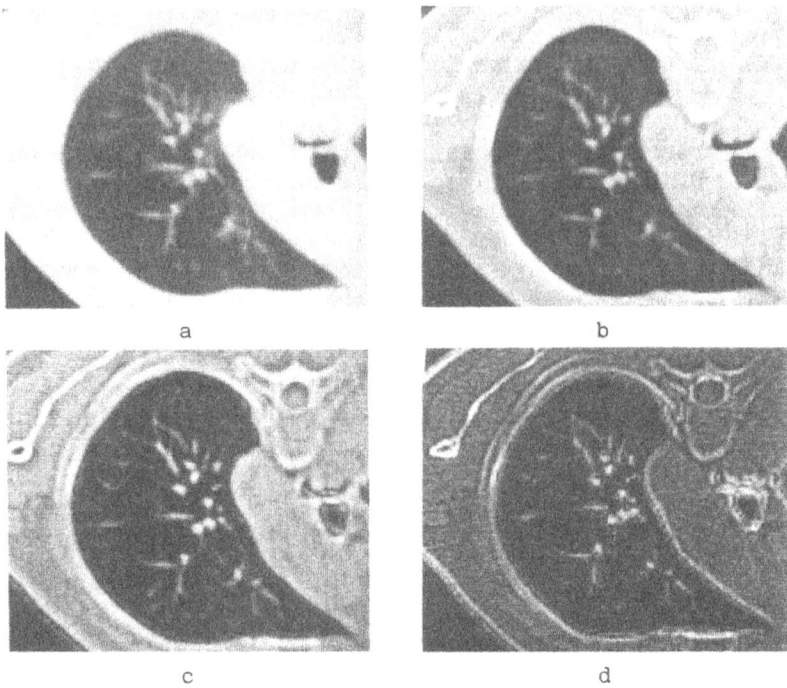

Fig. 1 - Original image (a) and processing results (b,c,d).

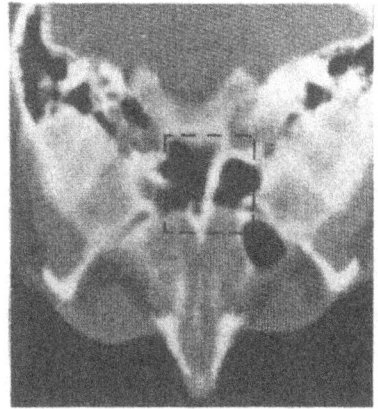 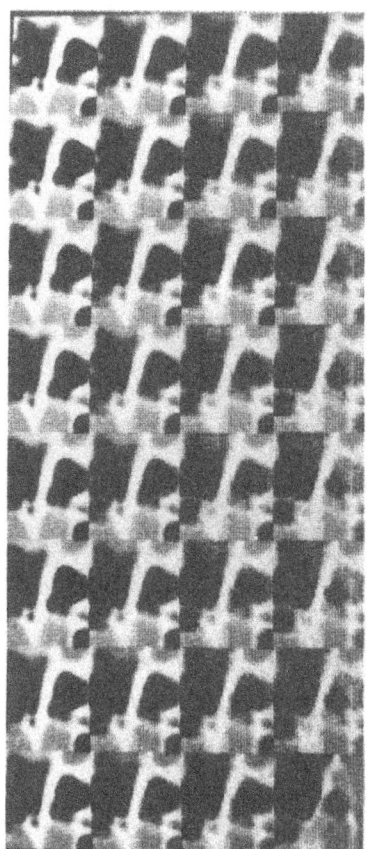

Fig. 2 - 3-D digital interpolation on a tomographic image.

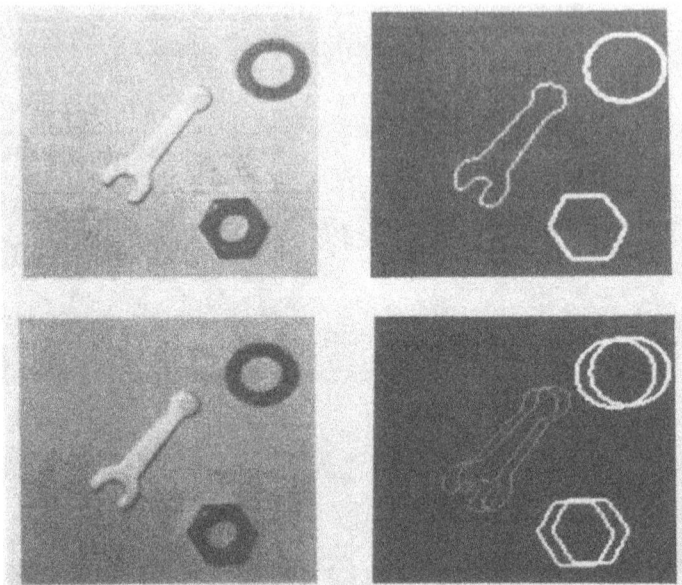

Fig. 3 - Example of the recognition-tracking of moving objects.

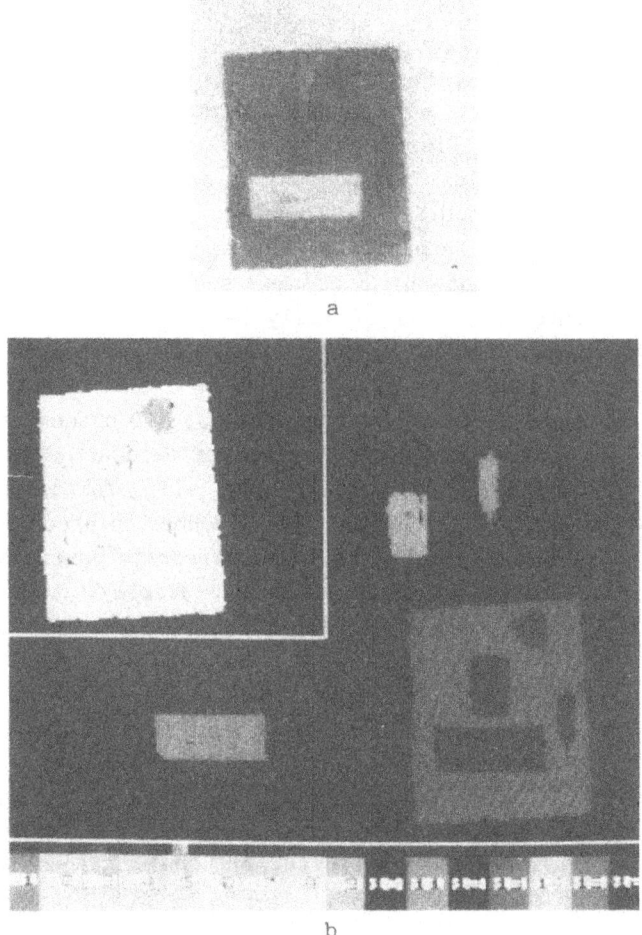

Fig. 4 - Example of the recognition-decomposition procedure on a circuit board (a): four components are recognized and three are already extracted from the board, identifying their exact geometrical position (b).

DISCUSSION SUMMARY

SESSION OF GENERAL PROBLEMS II

Four lectures were presented in the session on General Problems such as 3-D Display, Pictorial Information Systems, Quality Control of Medical Imaging Devices and Cross-Fertilization aspects of Medical and non Medical Imaging.

Several speeches were given and many questions raised. Philippe Garderet pointed out that the "segmentation" is the key point of data interpretation of fully 3-D medical data and that the segmentation procedure must be the central part of an "interactive" 3-D display. Leon Partain observed that, by continuing to increase the amount of images, 3-D presentation can become very useful in summarizing available data and in relating abnormal to adjacent structures, while also following their response to a specific therapy. Karl Höhne pointed out that presenting a 3-D image with a varifocal mirror is practically the same as rotating a shaded image in a 2-D display. On the other hand, Andrew Todd Pokropek observed that the biomedical data are quite complex, due to internal structures and are more difficult to represent than other 3-D data (such as, for instance, data regarding an aircraft). During the discussion it was also observed how holography can be a good way of "archiving" 3-D data.

In conclusion, besides focussing on general problems in biomedical and non medical image processing, it was also outlined that Cross-Fertilization can represent an attractive and inexpensive solution for the future.

PART VII OTHER IMAGING MODALITIES

Chairman: Carlo Corsi (Italy)

CURRENT STATE, LIMITATIONS AND NEW PERSPECTIVES IN FUNCTIONAL
PATTERNS OBTAINED BY INFRARED AND MICROWAVE RADIOMETRY

Carlo Corsi

Elettronica S.p.A. - Rome - Italy
Present Address: RSE Selenia S.p.A. - Rome - Italy

1   INTRODUCTION

The ever growing medical interest in functional information besides morphological structure analysis is encouraging the development of new techniques suitable for supplying pattern distributions of physiological states in the human body.

One of the most promising techniques is based on the measurement of thermodynamic properties and, in particular, on the measurement of thermodynamic activities of the human body: in particular the macroscopic information, detectable as pattern distributions of the temperature of the fundamental organs or vital parts of the body, are generating a growing interest for future clinical horizons. Moreover, the potential use of radio-frequency electromagnetic waves to produce local hyperthermia for cancer therapy has generated the necessary close development of the understanding of how electromagnetic waves interact with the human body, with an accurate prediction and control of subsequent electromagnetic power dissipation and heat distribution in the various body tissues and organs.

Infrared radiometry, generally called telethermography, has been recently growing in technical performances and system philosophy use, allowing to get reliable and significant information on health status to be obtained in different applications although limited to epidermic pattern emission due to the specific blackbody emission of the human skin in the infrared region. New radiometric developments in the microwave field, due to the partial transparency of the human body to microwaves, are nowadays allowing internally generated thermal radiation to be detected from an outer measurement.

The results reported above outline the possibility of

developing a system capable of radiometric measurements which, by correlating surface infrared images with internal microwave patterns, can supply a thermodynamic pseudo-image inside the human body.

This completely passive system, capable of tomographic reconstruction, has to be designed on the basis of the functional requirements derived from the emerging fields of IR thermography, microwave radiometry and e.m. radiation induced hyperthermia.

2 HUMAN BODY TEMPERATURE DISTRIBUTION

The diagnostic information acquired by thermography, is to be correlated to a "normal" body temperature distribution, to be evaluated in the right terms.

This is not a simple and monotonic correlation because, although the homeostatic mechanism involved in the regulation of body temperature tends to stabilize the temperature within narrow limits, the mechanism cannot prevent small fluctuations in temperature due to external and internal variations. Therefore, it is implicit in any concept of a "normal body" temperature that the specific conditions under which the temperature is measured must be stated accurately, especially if considering absolute measurements. Even more important is the control of the major factors which contribute to the generation of the heat within the body, like:

a) Exergonic reactions, that is the exergonic chemical reactions that contribute to heat production by the body and their relationship to the basal metabolic rate in conjunction with overall energy balance. These oxidative reactions liberate the heat energy as a by-product of the various specific metabolic processes.

b) Ingestion of food stuffs, which increases basal heat production that varies in accordance with the type and quantity consumed.

c) Endocrine factors can greatly modify heat production within the body.

d) Contraction of skeletal muscles. The principal source of heat in the human body is derived from muscular work; i.e., by the contraction of skeletal muscles that accompanies various types of bodily activity. (Shivering is an involuntary rhythmic contraction of the skeletal muscles that serves as a physiological mechanism to increase heat production in very cold environments).

In addition to these four major factors, the body's thermal loads may be increased somewhat by the ingestion of large quantities of very warm foods and/or beverages, although in general this is a physiological factor of minor importance.

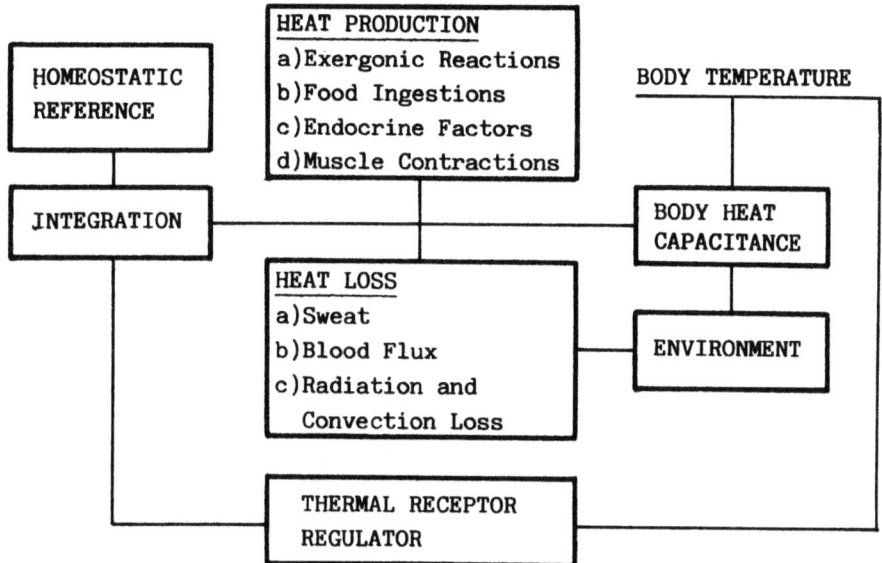

Fig. 1 - Block Diagram of Human Thermoregulating System.

Thus, the total heat produced by the body at any particular time is the sum of the individual thermal contributions that are made by the several factors mentioned above. Moreover, due to the fact that the human body is not a closed system, there is also a balanced exchange of materials and energy between an organism and its environment. (Fig. 1).

Although the body temperatures are normally stabilized within narrow limits due to the homeostatic mechanism, the complexity of the interactions can cause some variations due to internal or external conditions. Some of these variations may be normal either for the widely varying environmental temperature (also associated with some physical exercise) or for regular diurnal variation (circadian cycles) or for longer monthly variations due to the sexual cycle in women. (Figs. 2-3).

All the previous considerations underlie the complexity and the statistical meaning of the temperature distribution in the human body. Then, when considering the temperature distribution for a diagnostic interpretation it is convenient to assume some tissue structure model based on the bio-heat equations for the heat transfer taking care of the metabolic heat processes and of the heat exchange, especially by the blood system flux.

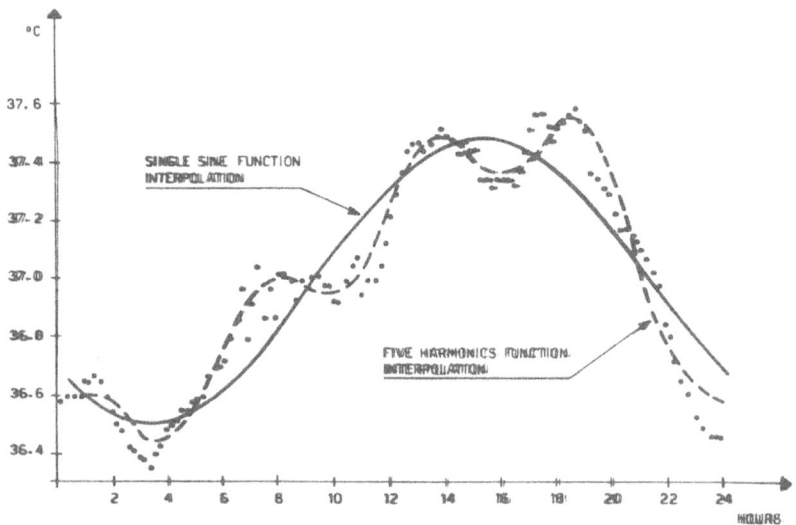

Fig. 2 - Data on 1-Day Measurement of Rectal Temperature
(from ref. 1)

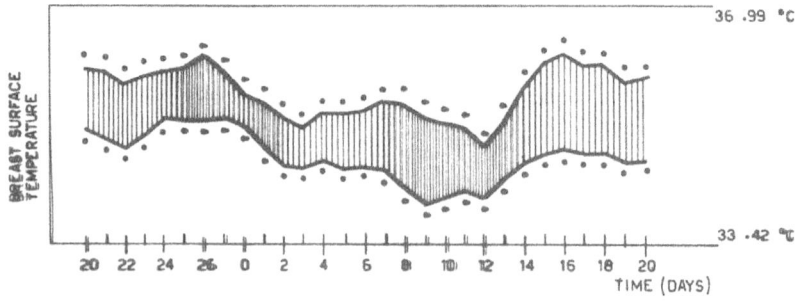

Fig. 3 - Data on Menstrual Cycle Breast Temperature Changes
(from ref. 1)

In general, we can assume for biophysical systems the following mathematical expressions for the bio-heat transfer phenomena (3):

(1)
$$\rho(r)Q(r)\frac{\delta T(r,t)}{\delta t} = \nabla[C(r,T)\nabla T(r,t)] - B_S(r)[T(r,t) - T_S(r,t)] + M(r) + A(r,t)$$

where: $C(r,t)$ = thermal conductivity $T(r,t)$ = local temperature
       $\rho(r)$ = density $T_S(r,t)$ = blood temperature
       $Q(r)$ = specific heat $B_S(r)$ = exchange coefficient
       $M(r)$ = metabolic heat
       $A(r,t)$ = external applied heat

In equation (1) we have assumed several simplifying hypotheses, such as the biological tissues being isotropic, linearly non homogeneous, and with time independent physical characteristics, and that the metabolic heat produced by unit volume $M(r)$ is time independent.

Moreover, the above expression for the bio-heat transfer equation is based on the assumption that heat exchange between blood and tissue is rescricted to the "capillary" part of the vascular system; microvascular contributions which can strongly influence temperature variations on small scale spatial distributions, are not included in the heat transfer model. So in addition to the perfusion terms there are two other contributions to be considered in heat transfer due to the microvascularization: one proportional to local blood perfusion velocity and the other due to the effective thermal conductivity (4) (5).

3 PRINCIPLES OF INFRARED AND MICROWAVE THERMOGRAPHY

Information on functional activities of the human body have assumed increasing importance in the last years especially if correlated with clinical information based on morphological structures. So besides structural imaging techniques, related to the reflecting and transparency of tissues, such as X-rays and more recently ultrasounds, new functional imaging techniques are supplying biological and physiological information; the best known examples of these techniques are nuclear magnetic resonance, which supplies an image mapping of the relaxation time of molecular resonance, microwave and infrared radiometry, which supply the temperature distribution of the internal and external human body, respectively, and recently biomagnetism, which supplies a pattern distribution of magnetic activity collateral to the electrical activity of the body.

Confining our discussion to radiometry, normally it is classified as infrared thermography and microwave radiometry, depending on the spectral band of the electromagnetic spectrum in which the radiometric systems are operating. Both measure the energy emitted by the body, at proper bands (infrared, microwaves) and their signals can be associated to the temperature values corresponding to the intensity of emitted energy by the Planck's law or Blackbody's radiation law.

(2) $I(T,\nu) = \varepsilon(\nu) \dfrac{2h\nu^3}{c^2}$

where: $I(T,\nu)$ = intensity of emitted energy
$\varepsilon(\nu)$ = emissivity
ν = frequency
T = absolute temperature
c = light speed
h = Planck's constant

This law can be approximated by the Raileigh-Jeans expression in the microwave region (where $h\nu \ll kT$):

(3) $I(T,\nu) = \varepsilon(\nu) 2kT\nu^2/c^2$

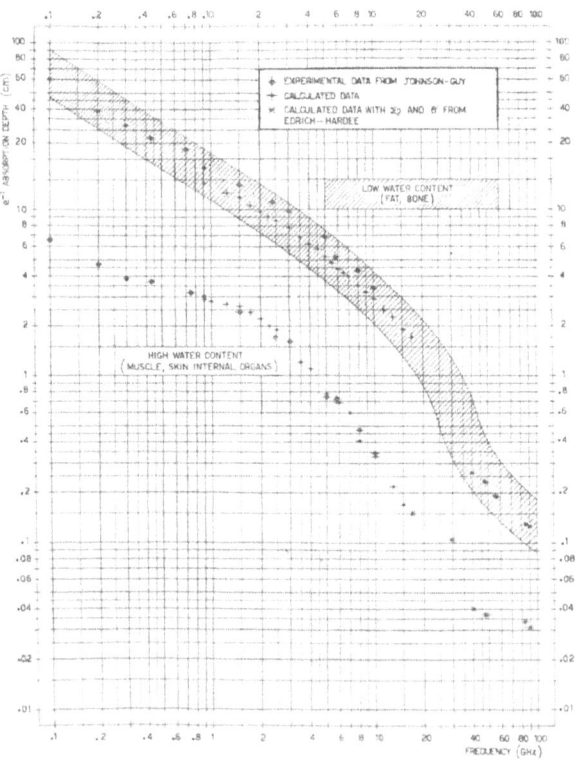

Fig. 4 - Penetration Depth vs Frequency of e.m. Radiation in the Human Body

The main difference in the content of information between infrared and microwave radiometry is strongly dependent on the transparency of the tissues which, being almost zero in the infrared region, allows a precise mapping of only the cutaneous temperature distribution of the human body to be obtained. Although some information on deeper layers inside the body due to thermal conductivity of tissues might also be derived in the infrared region, this limitation can be overcome by shifting toward lower spectral frequency, such as microwave frequencies, where the opacity of tissues is strongly reduced allowing deeper penetration for investigating deep physical-biological process provoking thermal pathologies (Fig. 4) (6÷10).

3.1 Computerized Radiometric Systems

The complexity of a diagnostic system is almost proportional to the amount of data to be interpreted. It is therefore obvious how important computerized systems are in the case of diagnostic techniques based both on acquisition of an enormous mass of data (such as in the acquisition of images or more generally of "patterns") and on the use of complex algorithms for reconstruction of tomographic images.

An example of such a new generation of systems is the development of integrated computerized systems based on radiometric techniques and therefore totally passive. Such a system will be initially directed towards applications for breast cancer screening (naturally an extension to vascular disease etc. will be immediate).

The social importance of such equipment capable of mass screening for the precocious diagnosis of breast cancer is widely accepted: today there is still controversy over the validity of purely passive diagnostic techniques in obtaining an efficient and reliable diagnostic capability. On the other hand the enormous increase in diagnostic capabilities of radiometric techniques is nowadays evident. This is a result of a strong lowering in false positives and, mainly, in the minimization of false negatives, as it has been recently shown (11-12).

These improvements are evident in the development of elaboration of IR images by computer systems.

The new generation of integrated computerized systems, from the experience of most advanced diagnostic laboratories for thermographic systems interfaced to a computer, will show some characteristics particularly important in operational technology:
- "A priori" knowledge in system acquisition
- Space signature analysis

- "Pattern Recognition" and topologic representative decision
- Quantized and intercorrelated decision levels
- Data bank for controlling physiological evolution and improvement in diagnostic capability.

3.2 <u>Computerized Infrared Systems</u>

In present thermographic equipment the IR image is acquired by a complex optical-mechanical scanning system which provides interlacing of the image points, normally obtained by one or more detectors, with a low precision in the real resolving power and strongly limited in achieving a real time processing.

The most advanced development in the field of IR systems today allows IR multisensor array structures with many elements well defined in geometrical patterns to be obtained. The advantage of a solid state approach for electronic scanning is quite important even if limited to one axis, because the perfectly defined geometry and quantized spatial characteristics of IR detector arrays allow simple and accurate geometrical laws to be obtained for the acquired patterns or image, and it is therefore possible to obtain a strong improvement in the information content by an on-line digital computer processing (13).

One of the most advanced developments provides, in particular, a 512 sensor linear array which by a simple one-axis scanning supplies a real television image, already pre-processed in real time during acquisition phase (14). Such development using a resolution structure perfectly "matched" to the requirements in space resolution of IR pattern, allows one to take advantage of the "a priori" knowledge in system acquisition using:

A completely integrated structure capable of utilizing the analysis of spatial signature previously developed by the pre-processor so as to optimize the specific information content by using an automatic adaption capability.

A "pattern recognition" and a topological representation based on "almost real time" elaboration techniques.

A data bank which allows the updating and development of diagnostic algorithms, and moreover the control of physiological evolution capability in prognostic applications.

4 ELECTROMAGNETIC FUNCTIONAL MORPHOLOGICAL IMAGING

The importance of obtaining a functional imaging of internal body sectors without interference from other regions has recently become an important goal of biomedicine. Hence, very recently, attention has been focused on developing e.m. imaging techniques.

Two main classes of imaging have recently been under

development: a) imaging based on emission of radiation and reconstruction of the pattern derived by different absorption of tissues, b) imaging derived from natural e.m. emission of the body such as is derived by infrared and microwave radiometry. The last one is particularly important for the higher content of functional information and the absolute innocuity due to its completely passive technique.

4.1 <u>Microwave Computerized Active Tomography</u>
The importance of computerized tomography (CT) in X-ray diagnostics has given a great stimulation to the development of the CT method by using different types of rays, e.g. ultrasonic (15) and particularly microwave (16) rays, active tomography has been developed by reconstructing images as a cross sectional distribution from transmission measurements or by reconstructing the distribution of reflectivity using the CT concepts (17-18).

In both cases microwave imaging has shown good results in diagnostic medicine, as this technique allows information to be obtained on several parameters which are not available in either X-rays or ultrasonic diagnostic because of the different absorption and interaction phenomena with the tissue for detecting, locating and representing the organs and their malformations.

In contrast to X-ray imaging, complex algorithms are involved in developing an image basically because the path of radiative exchange in the microwave regions is dependent on the spatial distribution of conduction within the body.

As a result, while, for example, the X-ray imaging problem is usually reduced to find a solution of a linear system of equations in the form:

$$[C][A]=[P]$$

where $[C]$ is a coefficient matrix, $[A]$ is a vector representing the unknown densities at the mathematical cells and $[P]$ consists of the values of the line integrals measured for discrete rays, for e.m. imaging the resulting system of equations will be of the form: form

$$[C(A)][A]=[P]$$

where the coefficient metric $[C(A)]$ depends on the solution A, and hence the problem is non-linear. To take into account non-linearities a simple extension of the well-know algebraic reconstruction techniques is to be developed assuming a given set of boundary conditions and then performing the finite difference method (19).

4.2 Computer Aided Tomographic Radiometry

Two main approaches to the solution of a computer-aided tomographic thermography have been proposed: both methods, although in some ways similar to computer-aided X-ray tomography, are much more complex due to the essentially diffusive, non-linear nature of governing equations and the as yet unfamiliar characteristics of human modelling in this region of e.m. spectrum.

a) Tomographic radiometry based on incoherent propagation of the thermal noise power emitted by internal tissues (20-21-22). In this case a numerical modelling has been developed by taking advantage of the antenna reciprocity principle by using either an active transmission process or a passive detection process (22).
This technique is aimed at obtaining a microwave thermal pattern by assuming some specific signatures for the thermal structure of the tissue under consideration. In this case the thermal power emitted in the dissipative medium from a source, at a unit form temperature T can be assumed equal to:

(4) $$P(\nu, \Delta \nu) = A \sum_{i=0}^{\infty} |E_i(\nu)|^2 T$$

where : $E(\nu)$ = Amplitude of the electrical field associated to the elementary volume under consideration for a monocromatic frequency
T = Temperature of medium.

Moreover:

(5) $$P(\nu, \Delta \nu) = K T \varepsilon(\nu) \Delta \nu$$

where : $\varepsilon(\nu)$ = emissivity.

In the case of considering a source embedded in a diffusing medium with thermal distribution $T_i(x,y,z)$ we can write:

(6) $$P(\nu, \Delta \nu) = A \sum_{i=0}^{\infty} |E_i(\nu)|^2 T_i(x,y,z)$$

This equation allows thermal signatures to be computed by scanning the probe in front of the source and by integrating the relation in the frequency domain.

b) A different approach is based on the radiative heat transfer equation for governing the coherent propagation of e.m. radiation in a diffusing and inhomogeneous medium (23-24).

In this case the temperature profile of biological tissues is derived by assuming a planar stratified model for the tissues and determining the emitted e.m. power by a suitable process of inversion of the multispectral microwave radiative value.

Generally a simplified model is assumed for the tissues which are modelled as a stratified medium of planar layers (normally thin layer: skin, fat and muscle).

The region of thermal anomaly can be considered as a generator of thermal power which transversing the intermediate layers emerges across the skin to be collected by the antenna receiver.

Assuming a transmission line model it is possible to describe the energy transmission in terms of temperature profile T(z) (where z is the coordinate perpendicular to the three planar layers).

Assuming a temperature T(z) roughly constant and equal to T_j, for each layer in a certain frequency interval $\Delta \nu$, it is possible to relate the antenna temperature T_a to the individual temperature T_j of the internal layers by the linear combination (24).

(7)
$$T_A(\nu_i) = \sum_{y=1}^{i} a_i(\nu_i) T_j$$

The coefficient $A_{ij} = \alpha(\nu_i)$ depends on geometry assumed for tissue models on the propagation coefficients and receiver characteristics. Similar to computer tomography and remote sensing an inversion procedure can be used for a numerical reconstruction of the temperature profile of the biological tissues under measurement.

Indeed several aspects of the problem deserve some discussion as thermal emission in the microwave region from various parts of the human body are affected by the local layered character of the tissues. In fact, the surface layers of a body consist in general of skin-fat-muscle, typical thickness of the three layers are in the millimeter and centimeter range, so that interference effects leading to partially coherent emission processes might significantly affect the apparent brightness of the structure at microwave frequency. In this case the problem of retrieving the temperature profile from a set of radiometric data by solving the resulting Fredholm integral equation has been brightly afforded by means of Kalman filtering.

This solution is quite valid because the Kalman filtering besides its good retrieving characteristics, exhibits the additional advantage of recursivity which is useful whenever the temporal evolution of the thermal profile is of interest, as in the case of hyperthermical treatments.

In particular starting from the assumption that a transmittance $\tilde{\tau}(z)$ can be defined so that the brightness temperature T_B can be written

(8)
$$T_B = \int_0^{1-R} T(z)\, d\,\tilde{\tau}(z)$$

where R is the reflectivity of biological structure and $\tau(-\infty)=0$
T(z) = thermodynamic temperature within the tissues.

The highest temperature of the body can also be written in the alternative form of a Fredholm integral equation of the first kind:

$$T_{BP}(\alpha) = \int_{-L}^{0} W_P(\alpha, z) T(z) \, dz \tag{9}$$

where the weighting function $W(z) = d\tau/dz$ is derived from the second order moment of the field, where α has the meaning either of angle of observation or of frequency, P is indicating the polarization, and L is the depth within the tissues beyond which the contribution to the brightness becomes negligible.

Equation (9) is supplying the relation between the measurable function T_B (the brightness temperature which is given by the radiometric receiver) and the internal unknown temperature profile $T(z)$: a suitable inversion technique has therefore to be applied to extract the unknown function $T(z)$ from the measured values of T_B at different frequencies.

The Kalman filtering estimation algorithm has been proven to be quite an effective technique both from the point of view of accuracy in retrievals and attainable spatial resolution (25).

With this approach, the emitting structure has been regarded as a linear stochastic dynamic system and the brightness temperature T_B, which is supplying the information content about the thermal state, is related to the thermal state vector $\vec{T}$, by means of the Kalman linear estimation procedure, which yields a minimum variance estimate of $\vec{T}$ from the data $\vec{T_B}$.

Naturally, an a priori expected thermal profile is to be assumed to initiate the filter and considering the big difficulty in obtaining sufficiently wide statistics from in vivo measurements, a thermal model of human living tissues has to be assumed. Taking into account the metabolic heat generation and the heat exchange by convection due to the effect of the heat flow and by conduction due to the heat exchange with the environment, the obtained results based on three layers model for different frequencies are reported in fig. 5.

These results show the interference effect quite clearly: a more suitable model taking into account the complex morphology of the human body and the different thicknesses in layers of different tissues is to be assumed for a more realistic tomographic representation.

Undoubtedly the results obtained can be assumed as starting

temperature profile while a better matching to the real temperature profile can be derived by assuming as boundary conditions of the Fredholm integral equation the surface temperature measured by infrared radiometry.

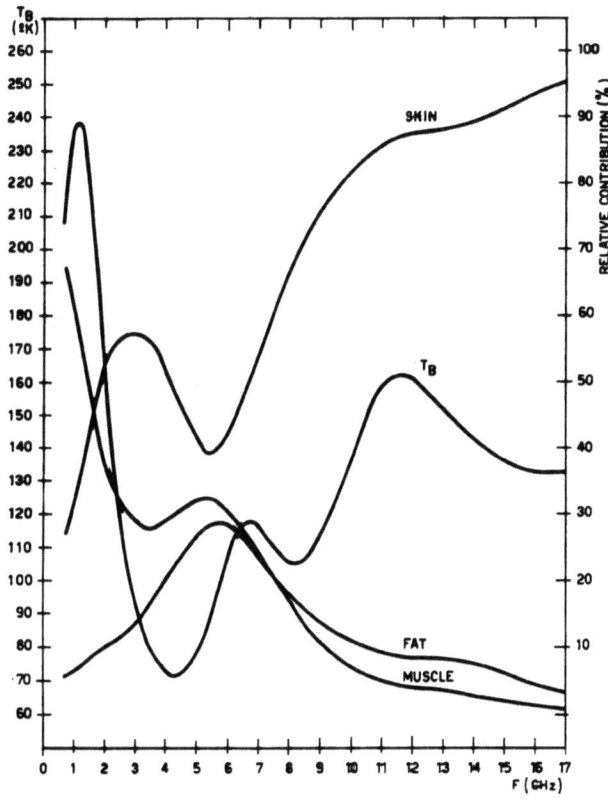

Fig. 5 - Brightness Temperature T_B vs Frequency with Relative Contributions from Skin, Fat and Muscle (from ref. 24).

5 CONCLUSION

The complexity of the equation to be assumed for deterministic information on the clinical status from the temperature measurements underlie two main general assumptions:

a) Deep correlations of temperature measurements of different layers of the human body (from the infrared surface imaging through the inner layer of temperature patterns acquired by microwave radiometry) are to be developed to extract complete and reliable information on functional thermo-dynamic activities.

b) A statistical approach has to be developed and used in any diagnostic evaluation of thermal pattern analysis.

IR thermography is supplying the surface thermal pattern of the body in relation to metabolism and vascularization of the underlying tissues; therefore it is strongly affected either from normal phenomena (e.g. in the breasts thermophysiology, menstrual cycle or pregnancy important conditions are to be taken account of) and/or pathological processes. While the bio-heat transfer equation appears to give adequate results in several applications, a precise description of the heat transfer in tissues remains a tedious but a challenging problem. Moreover, models and data on thermal properties, intratumour blood flow rates, and metabolism of tumour are limited. Therefore, it is important to have and provide accurate measurements of infratissue temperature distributions during normothermia and hyperthermia.

Anyway, a statistical approach based on symmetry of data patterns/hystograms shows the possibility of correlating the radiometric data obtained in the μW regions with those detected in the IR region, allowing an integrated system to be developed.

An integrated infrared microwave radiometric system is actually one of the most advanced diagnostic techniques under development: this integrated system will be particularly dedicated to monitoring inner temperatures in hypertermic therapy.

In fact, the combined use of infrared imaging together with microwave tomography can increase the resolution of inner spatial distribution and control the evolution of temperature profile as the dynamical response to the electromagnetic heating in hyperthermia.

Acknowledgments:
The author wishes to express his recognition to Professor F. Bardati and D. Solimini for the useful discussions on radiometric sensing techniques

References
1. J. De Prins and W. Malbey "Statistical Analysis of Thermal Biorhythms". Biomedical Thermology pp. 123÷132, Ed. Michel Gautherie and Ernest Albert, Alan Liss Inc. New York, 150 Fifth Avenue, N.Y. 1982.

2. H.W. Simpson, D. Wilson, K. Griffiths, F. Mutch, F. Halberg, M. Gautherie, pp. 133÷154, ibid. Ref. 1.

3. H.F. Bowman, E.G. Cravalho, M. Woods "Theory, Measurements and Applications of Thermal Properties of Biomaterials". Ann. Rev.

Byoophys., Byoeng. pp. 43+80 Vol. A, 1975.

4. M.M. Chen, K.R. Holmes "Microvascular Contributions in Tissue Heat Transfer" pp. 137+150 in Thermal Characteristics of Tumours: Application in Detection and Treatment". Ed. R. K. Jain and P.M. Gullino. The New Academy of Sciences, New York, N.Y. 1980.

5. E.G. Cravalaho, L.R. Fox, C. Kan "The Application of the Bioheat Equation to the Design of Thermal Protocols for Local Hyperthermia" pp. 86+97. Ibid. Ref. 4.

6. A.M. Barret, P.C. Myers, N.L. Sadowsky "Detection of Breast Cancer by Microwave Radiometry", pp. 167+171, Vol. 12 Radioscience, 1977.

7. J. Edrich "Centimeter and Millimeter Wave Thermography: a Survey of Tumor Detection", pp. 95+104 J. Microwave Power, Vol. 14, 1979.

8. J. Edrich, W.E. Jobe, R.H. Cacak, W.R. Hendce, C.J. Smith, M. Gautherie, C. Gros, R. Zimmer, J. Robert, P. Theouvenot, J.M. Escanye, C. Itty "Imaging Thermograms at Centimeter and Millimeter Wavelenghts" pp. 456+474. Ibid. Ref. 4.

9. J. Bigu del Balnco, C. Romero-Sierra, G. Watts "Microwave Radiometry and its Potential Applications in Biology and Medicine: Ecperimental Studies" pp. 298+316 Biotelemetry Vol. 2, 1975.

10. P.C. Meyers, A.M. Barret "Microwave Thermography of Normal and Cancerous Breast Tissue" pp. 443+455 Annals of the N.Y. Academy of Sciences, Vol. 335, 1980.

11. M. Gautherie, C. Gros, M.A. Meged, B. Keith, P.L. Wendel "Computer Processing of IR Thermograms of Breast Cancers Applied to the Recognition of Thermologic Classifications" Proc. Biosigma, April 1979, Paris.

12. A. Amalric, D. Giraud, C. Altschuler, F. Amalric, J.M. Spitalier, H. Brandone, Y. Ayme, A. Alvarez Gardiol "Does Infrared Thermography Truly Have a Role in Present Day Areas Cancer Management" pp. 269+276, Ibid. Ref. 1

13. C. Corsi "Computerized Radiometric Systems for Diagnostic Applications", proc. Ist International Conference on Applications of Physics to Medicine and Biology pp. 141+163, Trieste 1982.

14. C. Corsi "Computerized System for Diagnostic Applications"

ACTA Thermographica Int. Journal of ART, pp. 95÷100 Vol. 7 n.2 1984.

15. R.K. Mueller, M. Kaveh, G. Wade "Reconstructive Tomography and Application to Ultrasonic" Proc. IEEE pp. 567÷587 Vol. 64, 1979.

16. Maydy, F. Iskander, Karldurney "Electromagnetic Techniques for Medical Diagnosis a Review", Proc. IEEE pp. 126÷132 Vol. 68, 1980.

17. H. Hermet, F. Fulle, D. Miller "Microwave Computized Tomography" pp. 424÷426, Proc. 11th Euro Conf. (Amsterdam), 1981.

18. J. CH. Bolomey, A. Izadnegahdar, L. Jofre, CH. Pichot, G. Peronnet, M. Solaimani "Microwave Diffraction Tomography for Biomedical Applications", IEEE trans. MTT, Vol. 30 n. 11, 1982.

19. R. Maini, T.F. Iskander, C.H. Durney "On the Electromagnetic Imaging Using Linear Reconstruction Techniques" Proc. IEEE, pp. 1550÷1552 Vol. 68, 1980.

20. P. Edenhofer "Electromagnetic Remote Sensing of the Temperature Profile in a Stratified Medium of Biological Tissues by Stochastics Inversion of Radiometric Data", pp. 1065÷1069, Radio Science, Vol. 16, n. 6, 1981.

21. P. Pantazatos, M.M. Chen "Computer Aided Tomographic Thermography: a Numerical Simulation", Journal of Bio-Engineering, Vol. 2, pp. 397÷410, Pergamon Press. Inc. 1978.

22. D.D. Nguyes, M. Robillard, M. Clive, Y. Leroy, Y. Audet, C.H. Pichot, J.C.H. Bolomey "Microwave Thermography, the Modelling of Probes: an Approach Toward Thermal Pattern Recognition" pp. 232÷236 Proc. 11th Euro Conf. (Amsterdam), 1981.

23. F. Bardati, U. Conventi, D. Solimini "Determination of Temperature Profiles in Biological Layered Media" pp. 681÷683 International URSI Symposium, Santiago de Compostela, August 1983.

24. F. Bardati, D. Solimini "Radiometric Sensing of Biological Layered Media", pp. 1393÷1401 Vol. 18, Radio Science, Nov. Dec. 1983.

BIOMAGNETISM: A NON-INVASIVE NEW APPROACH FOR IMAGING OF BIOELECTRICAL SOURCES IN THE HUMAN BODY[°]

Gian Luca Romani and Roberto Leoni

Istituto di Elettronica dello Stato Solido - CNR
Via Cineto Romano 42, 00156 Roma, ITALY

ABSTRACT

Biomagnetic investigation is proving to be a powerful tool for the study of physiological and pathological activity in the human heart, and particularly in the brain, and shows promise of providing a new means for functional imaging of the human body. Measurements of magnetic fields at the body surface can provide new information directly related to the bioelectric source under investigation, with minor effects due to the interposed medium. The appropriate use of mathematical models achieved impressive results in the three-dimensional localization of active areas in zones of the cerebral cortex devoted to handling primary or higher levels of brain functions. The most promising results in the clinical situation regard the possibility of identifying the equivalent sources of epileptic foci.

1 INTRODUCTION

The impressive ability of SQUID systems to detect the extremely weak magnetic fields associated with physiological

---

[°] Work partially supported by Progetto Finalizzato "Tecnologie Biomediche e Sanitarie" - CNR.

and pathological activity in the human body has started a new field of research which is raising interest from a variety of scientists, including laboratory researchers and clinicians.

The first magnetic signals generated by biochemical current flow in the human heart were measured more than twenty years ago (1). In 1970 the use of a superconducting magnetometer provided the first magnetocardiogram featuring a signal to noise ratio comparable with that of a standard electrocardiogram (2). This measurement was performed inside a magnetically shielded room which, at that time, represented the only means of eliminating ambient magnetic noise. After about a decade, during which the greatest efforts were devoted to improving instrumentation performance in order to also achieve operation in unshielded environments, significant results were also collected in the clinical situation. During the last three years the refinement of data analysis procedures and the use of appropriate mathematical models permitted the three-dimensional localization of sources of physiological and pathological activity in various organs, thus showing promise of becoming a new, nonivasive tool for "functional" imaging of the human body.

2 INSTRUMENTATION AND MEASUREMENT PROCEDURES

A measurement of biomagnetic fields is characterized by two fundamental problems: i) the extreme weakness of fields to be measured and, ii) the huge ambient noise, which more correctly we should define as unwanted signals. Indeed any experimental environment is filled with various spurious signals which are of orders of magnitude higher than fields emanating from the human body. Fig. 1 shows the amplitudes of representative fields and the frequency range within which they are commonly studied. But for the strong signals associated with the presence of magnetic contaminants in the lungs of people exposed to occupational pollution, we note that the typical amplitudes of fields produced by bioelectric events in the human body span over about three orders of magnitude. Signals as weak as a few tens of femtoTesla (1 fT=10^{-15} T) have been observed and this limit is actually set by instrumental sensitivity. By contrast, the earth's magnetic field has a typical value of 10^{-5} T. Its "micropulsations", due to the interaction between the solar wind and the ionosphere,

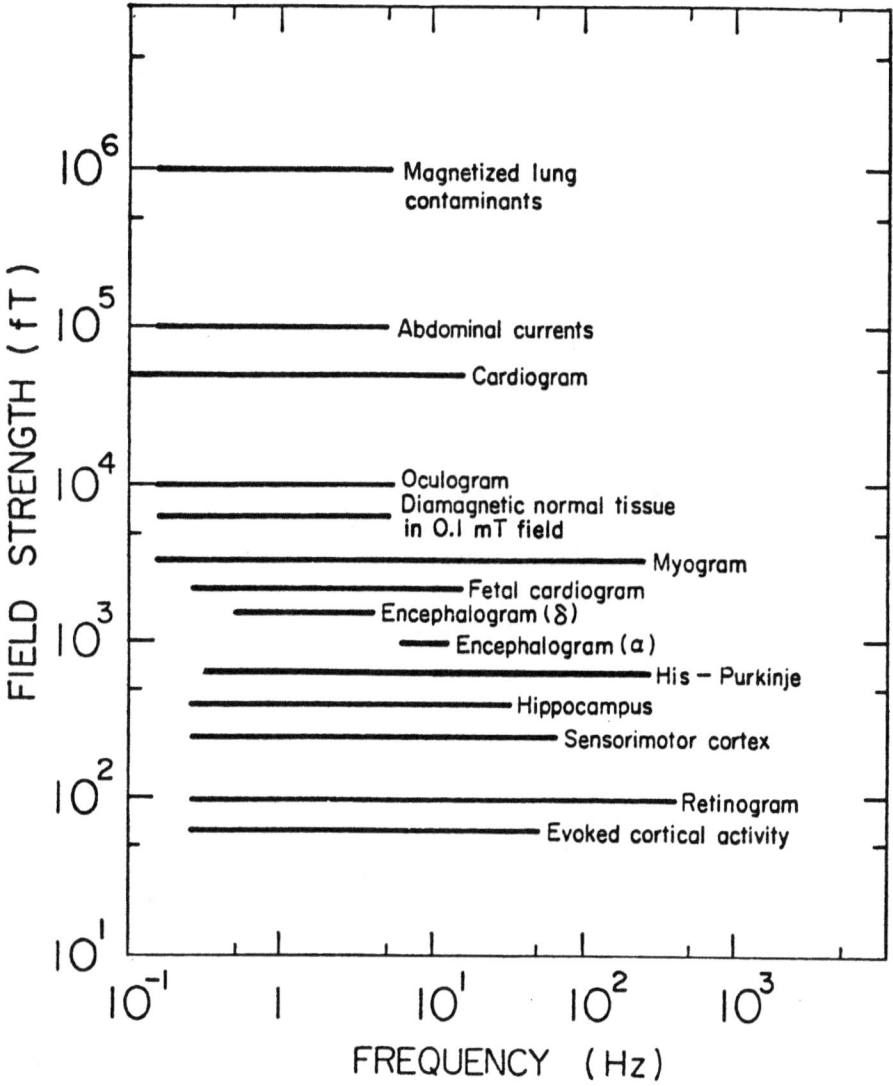

Fig.1 Typical amplitudes and frequency ranges for the most studied biomagnetic fields. Field strength is expressed in femtotesla, or 10^{-15} T. The amplitudes of disturbing fields and 'urban noise' are well above the upper limit of the scale.

show a 1/f behavior and can be as strong as 10^{-9} T at 1 Hz. Finally, the power line magnetic noise, at the line frequency and harmonics, plus additional contributions at specific frequencies due to the unavoidable presence in urban ambients of big instrumentations, fans, pump elevators, etc. constitute a serious drawback. The use of large magnetically shielded rooms - multiple layers of high permeability metals and pure copper or aluminum - permits strong reduction of dc fields and an even higher attenuation of ac fields (3). Nevertheless, these rooms have high costs and sometimes pose serious psychological problems with specific patients. This forced investigators to develop alternative techniques of eliminating ambient fields which will be described in the following pages.

The fundamental configuration of a biomagnetic instrumentation consists of a superinsulated fiberglass dewar inside which a superconducting circuitry is located and kept cold at liquid helium temperature (4.2 K) for about a week without refilling. The SQUID, which actually senses the magnetic flux and

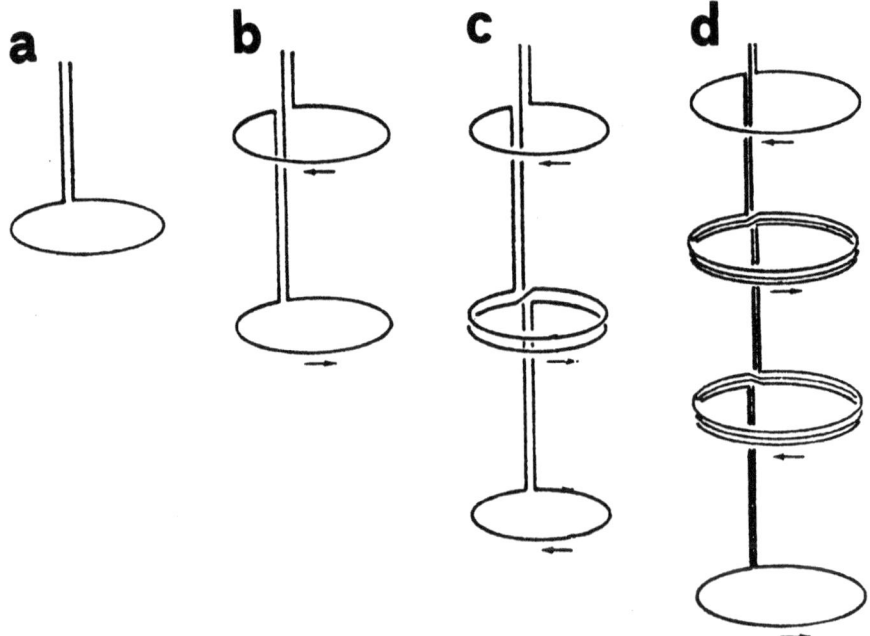

Fig.2 Some of the possible configurations for detection coils used with a SQUID to achieve spatial discrimination.

provides a voltage output linearly proportional to it (3), is located inside a superconducting shield and coupled to the external world by means of a superconducting flux transformer. The use of such a closed loop, consisting of a primary coil, the "detection" coil, to pick up the external field and an "input" coil tightly coupled to the SQUID, permits a significant portion of the applied signal to be transferred to the magnetometer whereas the geometry of the detection coil can be suitably modified.

Some of the configurations typically used for the detection coil are depicted in Fig.2. A single coil - generally referred to as a magnetometer - is shown in (a); this geometry works properly inside magnetically shielded rooms. A first-order gradiometer (b) is insensitive to fields uniform in space and is generally used in low-shielding environments or in rural environments. More complex geometries, such as second- c) or third-order (d) gradiometers are needed to operate in urban laboratories and in hospitals. These configurations are sensitive only to the second- (c) or third-order (d) spatial derivative of the ambient fields plus, obviously, higher order derivatives. Indeed, far fields can be satisfactorily assumed as having a constant gradient. This assumption is verified in experimental practice and the measurement is performed with the lowest coil of the gradiometer as close as possible to the source under investigation. In fact, the rejection due to the other coils is strongly reduced and a field measurement is actually performed in the case of "local" fields. By contrast, a progressive reduction in sensitivity occurs when using higher orders of "spatial discrimination". Nowadays systems operating inside magnetically shielded rooms' feature sensitivity of the order of a few femtoTesla in unit bandwidth, whereas the best instrumentations based on dcSQUID devices provide sensitivities of 15-20 $fT/\sqrt{Hz}$ in unshielded environments.

Practical measurements are performed by positioning the tail of the dewar over the appropriate region of the body surface and detecting the signal at that location. The measurement is successively repeated at different sites in order to obtain the spatial distribution of the magnetic field which is needed for further analysis. Fig.3 shows an overall view of one of the instrumentations operating at the Istituto di Elettronica dello

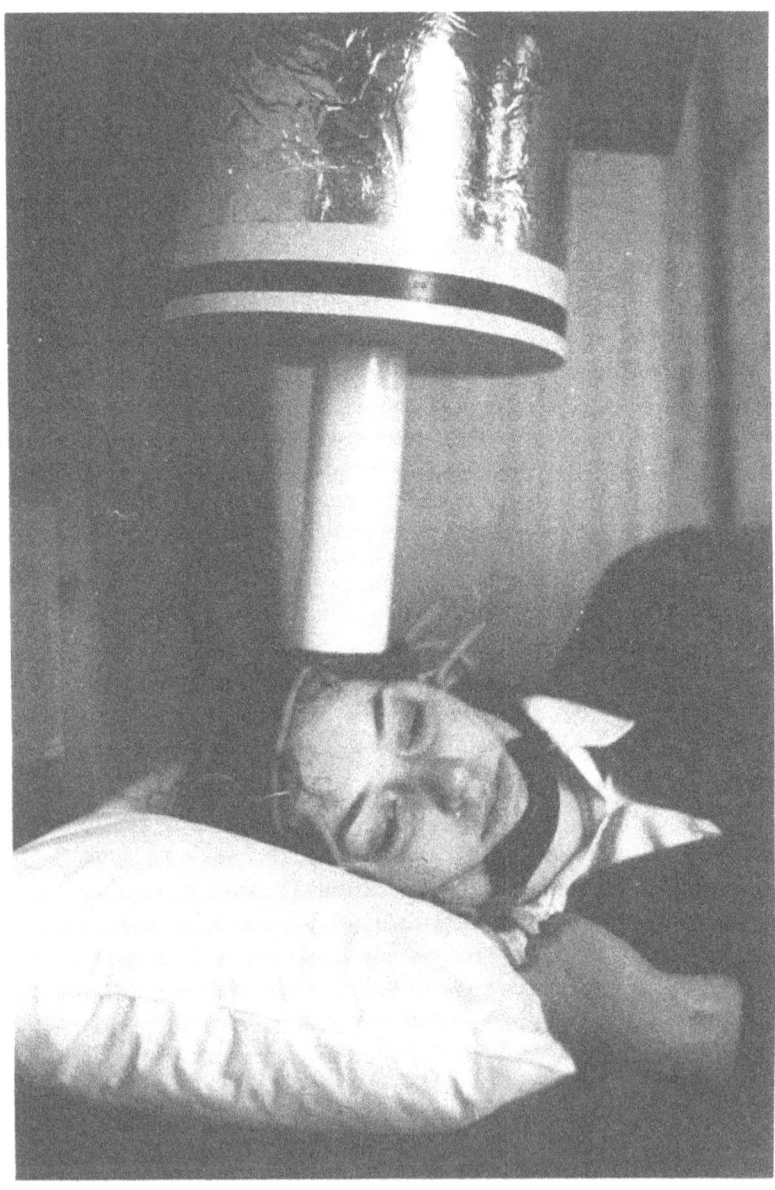

Fig.3 View of one of the biomagnetic instrumentations developed at the Istituto di Elettronica dello Stato Solido in Rome and used for neuromagnetic studies.

Stato Solido in Rome, during investigation of brain activity. One
of the most serious drawbacks experimentalists have to face,
particularly when dealing with clinical measurements, lies in
this non-simultaneity of magnetic measurements. In fact,
significant information can be lost due to variability in the
actual activity of the investigated source. Furthermore, the
very lengthy duration of the recording session is often
unbearable for some patients. Consequently, great efforts are
being devoted to the development of multi-channel systems for
achieving simultaneous detection of fields in 3 or 4 sites of the
body surface. Presently only two multi-SQUID instrumentations are
operating in unshielded environments (4): a five-channel system
based on dcSQUIDs and electronic noise cancellation by four
additional rfSQUIDs, operating at the Neuromagnetism laboratory of

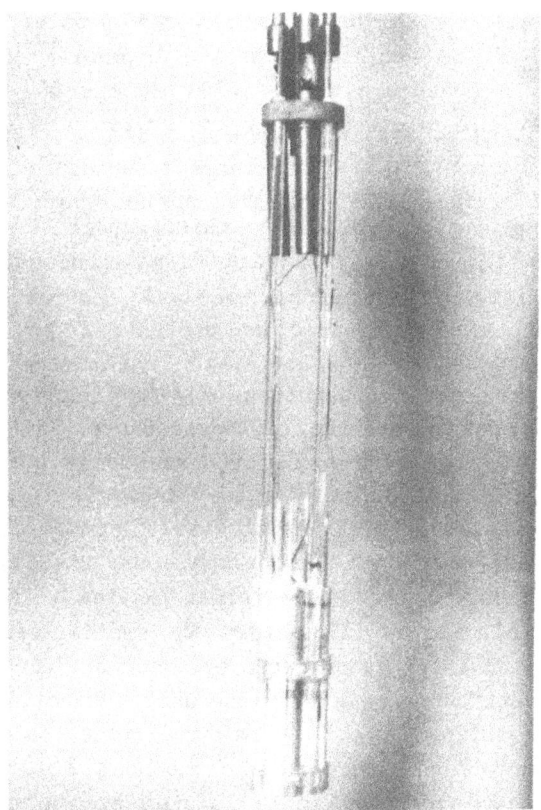

Fig.4 Close-up view of the four channel system under test at the
Istituto di Elettronica dello Stato Solido in Rome.

the New York University, and a four-channel system based on rf-SQUIDs, coupled to second-order gradiometers permanently adjusted, operating at the Istituto di Elettronica dello Stato Solido in Rome. Fig.4 shows a close up view of the four gradiometers of the Rome instrument. The sensitivity of the system should improve significantly by coupling the gradiometers to micro-fabricated dcSQUIDs and reach a level of about 10 $fT/\sqrt{Hz}$. This value is particularly satisfying as an intrinsic subject noise of approximately the same amplitude has often been observed. It seems to be a threshold to instrumental sensitivity and also to studies performed inside magnetically shielded rooms.

3 SOURCE LOCALIZATION

It is well known that the inverse problem, i.e. the determination of the configuration and intensity of sources in the body from a measurement of fields at the body surface has infinite equivalent solutions. Only the choice of a simple source model allows the problem to be challenged and source localization to be achieved. One of the simplest and consequently most used models is the current dipole: this source, schematically represented in Fig.5a as immersed in a homogeneously conducting medium, consists of a current flow J_p concentrated in an elementary volume dv and of volume currents J_v which close the loop. J_p represents the intracellular ionic currents which are responsible for the propagation of the activation inside excitable cells. The magnetic field associated with this source is represented by the transverse circles and is due only to the primary current J_p, according to the Biot-Savart law (5). This fortunate circumstance is still valid if the medium is bounded by an infinite flat surface or by a spherical one, provided that only the component of the field normal to the surface is taken into account (5). Fig.5b illustrates the spatial distribution of this normal component B_n as produced by a current dipole located 2 cm below the surface of a homogeneously conducting sphere and oriented tangentially to it. Two important points must be made: i) only the tangential component of the dipole contributes to B_n and ii) a dipole located at the centre of the sphere produces no external field. These drawbacks are partially compensated for by the consideration that the overall symmetry of the pattern of fig. 5b is maintained when the orientation of the

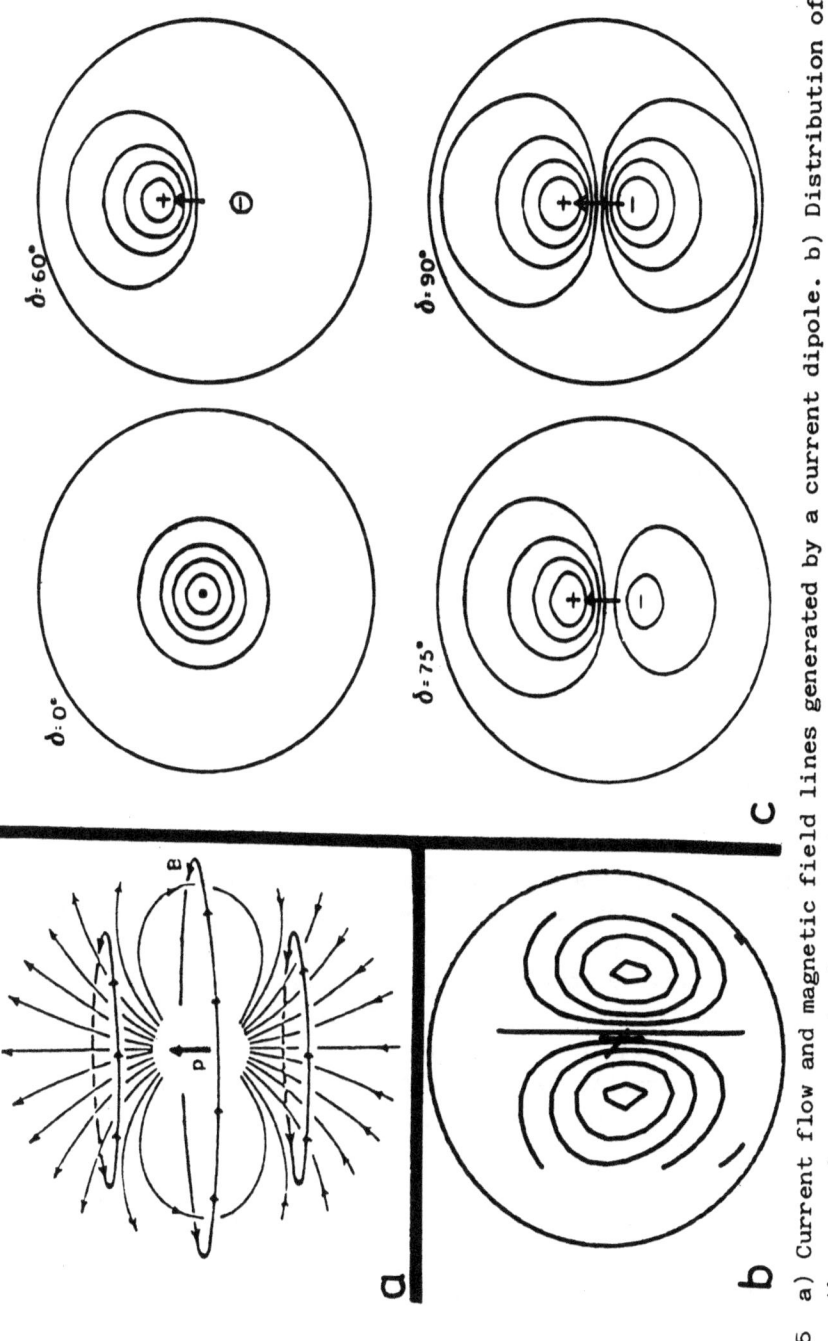

Fig.5 a) Current flow and magnetic field lines generated by a current dipole. b) Distribution of the normal component of the field over the surface of a sphere as generated by a dipole located 2 cm below the surface and oriented parallel to it. c) Distribution of the electric potentials as produced by the same dipole for four different orientations.

dipole is changed from a tangential direction to a radial one. Only the relative amplitude will decrease towards zero. As the relationship between the spatial distribution and the depth of the generator is unique, it is always possible to localize the generator if it has a tangential component, provided that the instrumentation has sufficient sensitivity. Fig.5c shows the electric potentials pattern for a radial dipole $\delta=0$, tangential dipole $\delta=90$ and two in intermediate positions. For $\delta=90$ the pattern presents the same symmetry as Fig. 5b, but 90 degree rotation whereas the symmetry is lost in all the other cases. This complicates the localization of the source.

The interpretation of experimental magnetic patterns in terms of a simple model like the one described above - provided that the basic hypotheses concerning the model are satisfied and substantial similarities between the measured and the theoretical distributions are observed, yields three-dimensional localization of the equivalent generator. Generally the procedure consists in a five-parameter fit (three for the coordinates of the dipole and two for the intensity of its tangential component) performed inside the best sphere, fitting the appropriate portion of the head, by means of interative numerical procedures. As a result, the dipole position is provided, together with the appropriate uncertainty region and a level of significance, which indicates the reliability of the localization.

A crucial point is the inadequacy of the spherical geometry for representing particular regions of the head. Furthermore, more complicated source configurations should be studied, as they will probably prove essential for interpreting signals related to complex phenomena, such as higher brain functions. Nevertheless, the present state-of-the-art is satisfactory for many investigators, and has permitted significant progress to be made in the study of human physiology and pathology.

4 IDENTIFICATION OF ACTIVE SOURCES IN THE HUMAN BRAIN

The procedure illustrated in the previous paragraph has been successfully applied to the identification of equivalent generators for sources of bioelectrical activity both in the

human heart and brain. One important point concerning the choice of the dipole model must be "a priori" made: it was sometimes questioned that such a simple model could not appropriately account for the activity of large bundles of excitable cells, and in particular for the extremely high number of neurons originating the scalp's electric and magnetic fields. The basic idea underlying this choice is that the dipole model is the only mathematically tractable and sufficiently realistic tool.
Consequently, the identification of an equivalent generator means essentially to localize the center of gravity of the active area in the investigated organ. Variations in source location according to time evolution or to modifications of physiologically significant parameters can provide information on the functional structure of the source and, in clinical cases, eventually yield the localization of the pathological area.

Many of the most important results achieved so far by the biomagnetic approach concern the investigation of brain activity. Although cerebral magnetic fields are extremely weak, the interpretation of scalp distributions is probably favored by the particular geometry of the skull, which can be satisfactorily represented by a sphere, at least in its posterior and central portion. The cerebral cortex covers all the basic structures of the brain and develops into an incredible number of folds - namely, convolutions and fissures. The cortical width is approximately constant and within this 5 mm of grey matter at least one population of neurons - the so-called pyramidal cells - is preferentially aligned in a direction normal to the cortex surface. As a consequence, it is expected that the most active areas from a magnetic point of view are those located inside fissures, rather than those distributed along convolutions. This is fortunately the case for many of the "primary" areas, which are devoted to the first analysis of input signals from peripheral sensory systems. A typical procedure for investigating these areas consists in repetitively stimulating the chosen system and detecting fields which are time-locked to the stimulus over the appropriate region of the scalp. The neuromagnetic study of cerebral activity evoked by sensory stimuli has marked several milestones in the understanding of brain organization and functioning (6). Other important achievements are being collected in the investigation of higher levels of brain functions (6,7,8). In order to illustrate which kind of functional imaging can be achieved by the neuromagnetic approach, we will place our accent on the study of magnetic fields related to spontaneous brain activity which is proving to be one of the most interesting research areas also from a clinical point of view.

4.1 Normal spontaneous activity

The alpha rhythm, which represents the strongest bioelectrical activity spontaneously arising in the human brain, has long been investigated, since the first recording of an electroencephalogram (EEG) in 1929 (9). A quasi-periodic electric signal - approximately 10 Hz frequency - is detectable over the occipital region of the scalp of almost everybody. The alpha waves are stronger when the subject keeps the eyes closed and are generally significantly reduced by visual input or by execution of simple mental tasks. At present, however, experimentalists are still uncertain about the possible structure and location of their source(s).

The neuromagnetic approach to the study of this phenomenon is particularly difficult, in which the non-simultaneity of magnetic recordings prevents information on the relative phase of the measured signals from being obtained. A possible solution to the problem consists in simultaneously recording the EEG and the MEG and in studying the correlation between these signals. In effect this procedure, which has been referred to as the Relative Covariance (RC) method (10), calculates the covariance between the magnetic and electric channels after filtering around the frequency of interest (~ 10 Hz). The covariance is divided by the variance of the electric signal to compensate for possible variations in source intensity. A similar analysis, repeated for all the recording positions with respect to the same reference lead, provides a spatial distribution of the RC coefficient which reflects that of the magnetic field. Negative or positive RC values correspond to out-of-phase or in-phase magnetic and electric signals, provided that they come from the same source. Fig.6a shows the iso-RC pattern from a normal subject by the described procedure. The distribution was interpreted as due either to a quite deep, single dipole, or to two sinchronously acting, shallower sources. The latter hypothesis was preferred on the basis of several arguments (10). In particular, the amounts of magnetic alpha on the two sides of the occipital scalp were

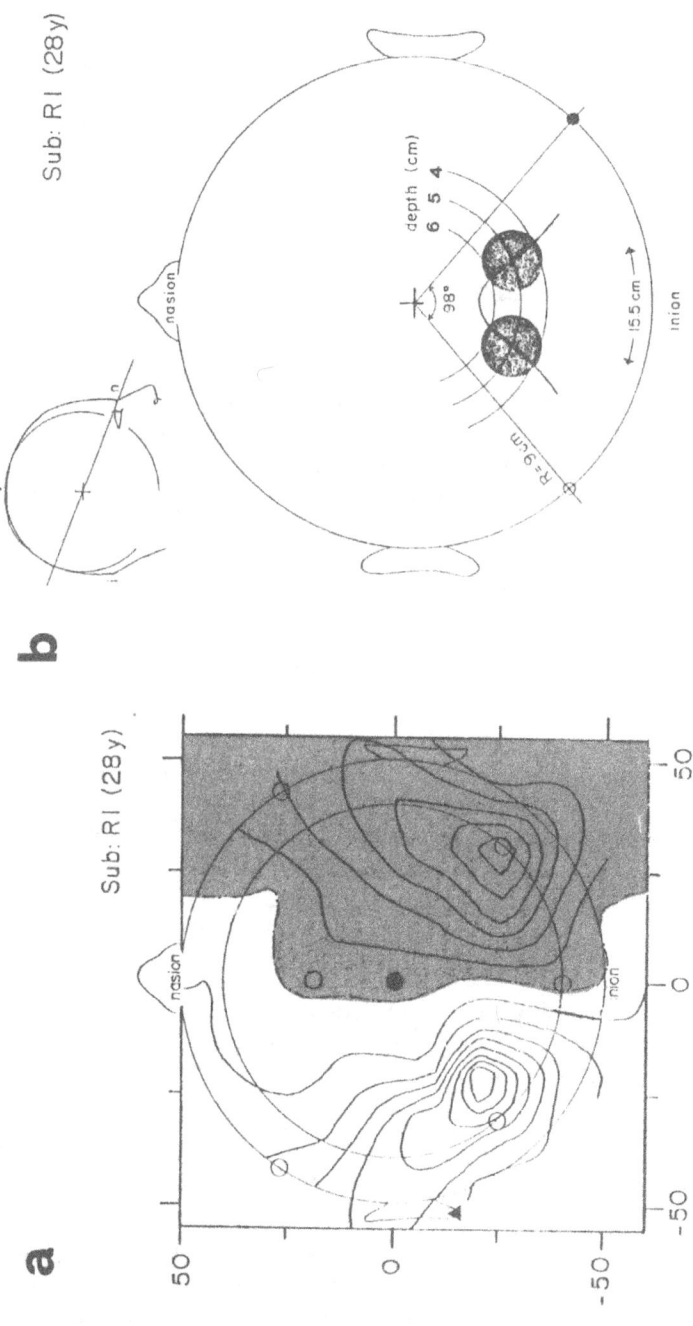

Fig.6 a) Relative Covariance pattern over the scalp of a normal subject reflecting the measured distribution of the magnetic alpha rhythm. The shaded area represents negative RC values. b) localization of the equivalent generators: the shaded circles represent the equivalent cortical area possibly involved.

selectively suppressed by stimulating both visual fields separately. Furthermore, the strength of a single deep dipole would be too large as compared with typical values of neural currents. The χ^2 fit provided further support to the hypothesis that the major portion of the occipital alpha rhythm could be accounted for as produced by two equivalent generators approximately located as shown in Fig. 6b, and involving the equivalent area of cortex indicated by the circles.

4.2 Localization of epileptic foci

The investigation of pathological spontaneous activity by the neuromagnetic method represents one of the most promising areas of research, particularly from the clinical point of view. During the last few years several studies (11-13) have shown that the magnetic signals measured over the scalp of patients affected by focal epilepsies - during interictal intervals - often display a dipolar-like distribution. This finding suggests that the neural source underlying the measured activity is relatively concentrated: consequently, great efforts have been devoted to refining the procedures of localization and confronting the results obtained with those available from other techniques.

It should be emphasized that we are still far from achieving localization of the pathological source in all focal epilepsies. On the basis of the results so far achieved we can classify the clinical cases successfully investigated according to two main categories, depending on whether or not there is presence in the EEGs of repetitive spike-like signals of large amplitude: i) those for which an averaging procedure can be applied to obtain magnetic field distribution over the scalp, and ii) those which can be studied only by the Relative Covariance method described in the previous paragraph.

Fig.7 and Fig.8 illustrate the results of the procedures mentioned above. Subject (SC) is affected by left parietal lobe epilepsy which should be related to the abnormality in that lobe clearly shown by the CT scan. The measurable pathological activity featured clearcut spikes both in the MEG and in the EEG. The "anatomical" localization and that provided by the averaging procedure show excellent correspondence.

469

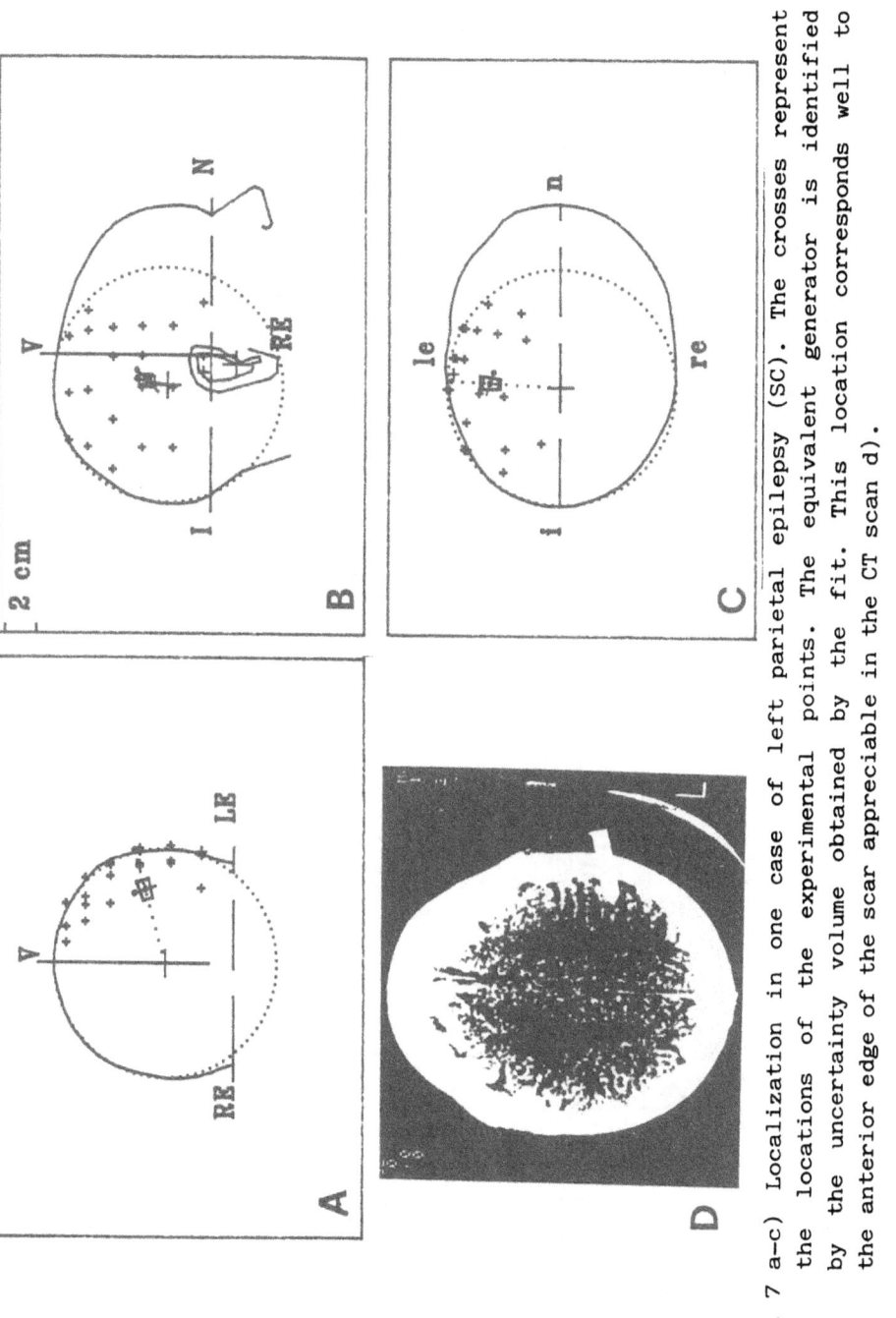

Fig. 7 a-c) Localization in one case of left parietal epilepsy (SC). The crosses represent the locations of the experimental points. The equivalent generator is identified by the uncertainty volume obtained by the fit. This location corresponds well to the anterior edge of the scar appreciable in the CT scan d).

The same encouraging result is achieved for the second patient (EI). In this case the validity of the neuromagnetic localization can be checked on the basis of the clinical history of the patient, who shows sensory-motor seizures involving the right hand as a consequence of surgical removal of a parasitical cyst in the rolandic area. The localization of the equivalent source shown in Fig.8a-c) is based on the iso-RC map reported in d) and well matches the appropriate region in the sensory cortex.

More than a dozen cases have so far been investigated by our own group (14) and for all but one the neuromagnetic approach has proved to be successful in localizing the source of pathological activity. To these results we should add several others investigated by the UCLA group (11,15). The overall experience is therefore particularly encouraging and gives promise of further important achievements.

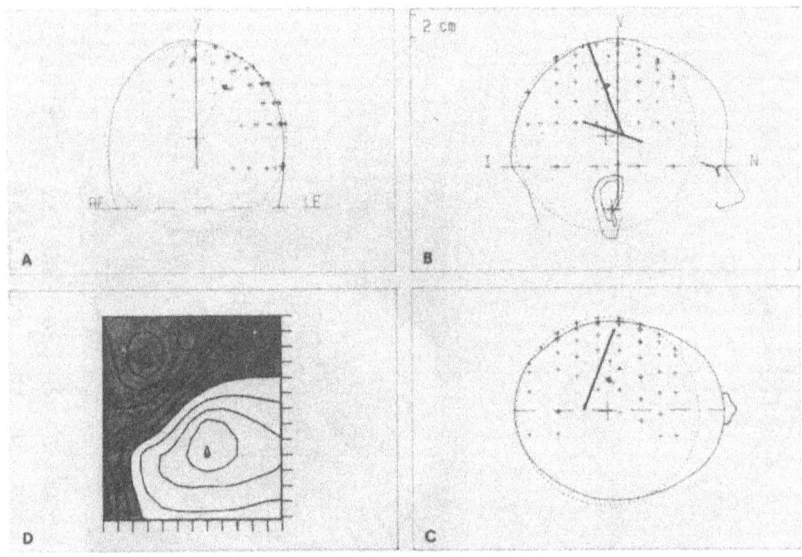

Fig.8 a-c) Localization in a case of right motor epilepsy (EI). Details as in Fig.7. d) Constant contour map illustrating the RC values distribution. Distance between tics, 1 cm. The iso-RC lines are spaced 4 pT/mV.

5   CONCLUSIONS

The purpose of this article has been to provide a brief overview of what is likely to be achieved in functional imaging by means of the biomagnetic approach. The survey of results has been unavoidably limited by lack of space. We have not dwelt on the important achievements which are being collected in the study of higher levels of brain functions. Had we space enough to just touch upon cardiomagnetic measurements, we should at least mention the fundamental progress achieved in the study of the conduction system of the heart and of the abnormal conduction pathways typical of the Wolf-Parkinson-White disease (16).

We remark that recording and mapping field patterns over the appropriate region of the scalp or the torso requires very lengthy sessions. For instance, a complete magnetic map in an epileptic patient is typically recorded in three hours. This is a serious drawback which can prove to be insurmountable with specific patients. The development of multichannel systems is therefore a decisive step thanks to which fundamental advances are likely to be gained. We are just now entering a new era, the final target being the set up of systems with a number of channels at least comparable with that of standard electro-encephalography, say 20 sensors distributed inside adequate dewars in order to cover a large portion of, or possibly all the scalp. These large systems should be coupled to appropriate computer facilities for data analysis and reconstruction of "functional images". If things proceed as fast as in the last few years it is expected that these goals are not far away.

ACKOWLEDGEMENTS

The authors are indebted to all the other members and collaborators of the Rome biomagnetic group and in particular to Prof. I.Modena for helpful discussions and suggestions. Special thanks are due to Prof. A. Paoletti for continuous encouragement and guidance.

REFERENCES

1. Baule, G.M. and R. Mc Fee. Detection of the magnetic field of the heart. Am. Heart J., 66 (1963) 95.
2. Cohen, D., E.Edelsack and J.E.Zimmerman. Magnetocardiograms taken inside a shielded room with a superconducting point-contact magnetometer. Appl. Phys. Lett. 16 (1970) 278.
3. Romani, G.L., S.J.Williamson and L.Kaufman. Biomagnetic instrumentation. Rev. Sci. Instrum. 53 (1982) 1815.
4. Romani, G.L. Biomagnetism: an application of SQUID sensors to medicine and physiology. Physica, 126B (1984) 70.
5. Williamson, S.J. and L.Kaufman. Magnetic fields of the cerebral cortex, in: Biomagnetism, Eds. S.N.Ernè, H.D.Hahlbohm and H.Lubbig (Walter de Gruyter, Berlin, New York, 1981) 353.
6. Williamson, S.J. and L.Kaufman. Application of SQUID sensors to the investigation of neural activity in the human brain. IEEE Trans. Magn. MAG-19 (1983) 835.
7. Weinberg, H., P.A.Brickett, J.Vrba, A.A.Fife and M.B.Burbank. The use of a SQUID third order spatial gradiometer to measure magnetic fields of the brain. Annals of New York Academy of Sciences (1984) in press.
8. Fiumara, R., F.Campitelli, G.L.Romani, R.Leoni, M.Caporali, M.Zanasi, A.Cappiello, G.Fioriti and I.Modena. Neuromagnetic study of endogenous fields related to the contingent negative variation. Proc. 5th World Conference on Biomagnetism, Vancouver 1984, in press.
9. Berger, H. On the electroencephalogram of man. Arch. Psychiat. 87 (1929) 527.
10. Chapman, R.M., R.Ilmoniemi, S.Barbanera and G.L.Romani, Selective localization of alpha brain activity with neuromagnetic measurements. Electroencephalogr. Clin. Neurophysiol. (1984), in press.
11. Barth, D.S., W.H.Sutherling, J.Engel and J.Beatty. Neuromagnetic localization of epileptiform spike activity in the human brain. Science 218 (1982) 891.
12. Ricci, G.B., I.Modena, S.Barbanera, F.Campitelli and G.L.Romani. Tridimensional biomagnetic localization of epileptic foci. Acta Neurochirurgica, Suppl.33 (1984) 85.
13. Chapman, R.M., G.L.Romani, S.Barbanera, R.Leoni, I.Modena, G.B.Ricci and F.Campitelli. SQUID instrumentation and the

relative covariance method for magnetic 3-D localization of pathological cerebral sources. Lett. Nuovo Cimento 38 (1983) 549.
14. Ricci, G.B., R.Leoni, G.L.Romani, F.Campitelli, S.Buonomo and I.Modena. 3-D neuromagnetic localization of sources of interictal activity in cases of focal epilepsy. Proc. 5th World Conference on Biomagnetism, Vancouver 1984, in press.
15. Barth, D.S., W.Sutherling, J.Engel and J.Beatty. Neuromagnetic evidence of spatially distributed sources underlying epileptiform spikes in the human brain. Science 223 (1984) 293.
16. Ernè, S.N., personal communication.

POSSIBLE DIRECTIONS OF ALTERNATIVE IMAGING MODALITIES:
A CRITICAL OVERVIEW

P.N.T. Wells

Department of Medical Physics
Bristol General Hospital
Bristol BS1 6SY, U.K.

1　INTRODUCTION

This paper touches on aspects of imaging techniques not discussed elsewhere in the present NATO ASI. Advances in X-radiography, interventional radiography, light and infrared transmission imaging, microwave imaging, electrical impedance methods and body surface potential mapping are considered. These techniques expand and complement the capabilities of the conventional imaging methods.

2　ADVANCES IN X-RADIOGRAPHY

2.1　Contrast Media

The use of contrast agents, usually containing compounds of either barium or iodine, has an established role in the enhancement of X-radiographic images. Contrast media are currently or potentially capable of delineating vascular anatomy, excretory pathways, organ anatomy, cerebral spinal fluid pathways, bronchial structure, body cavities, haemorrhagic foci and the reticuloendothelial system.

A new generation of contrast media for intravascular use has recently been developed. These substances either have low osmolarity or are nonionic [1] and so they generally are free from the systemic toxicity associated with ionic contrast media.

Other new X-ray contrast agents include perfluoroctylbromide emulsions [2], particulate media [3] and radio-opaque liposomes [4], all of which have been used in imaging the reticuloendothelial system in the liver and the spleen.

2.2 Raster Scanned Equalisation Radiography

Significant improvement in X-radiograph quality can be obtained by the use of a scanned collimated X-ray beam which is more effective for scatter reduction than conventional radiographic grids. Scanning slot [5] and rotating wheel [6] collimators have been used. The reduction in scatter results in improved soft-tissue contrast. The wide dynamic range of X-ray images of certain structures (particularly the chest) remains a problem, however, since there may be negligible contrast over the thicker body parts. Thus, for example, it may be very difficult or impossible to examine lung tissue in the shadows of the heart, diaphragm and mediastinal regions when the exposure has been optimised for the lung fields.

The problem of nonuniform exposure can be largely solved by scanned equalisation radiography [7]. In a typical system, a beam of radiation (35 x 35 mm) is swept over the patient's chest in a raster fashion to expose a conventional radiographic film. As the beam is swept, it is rapidly pulsed and measurements of the transmitted beam intensity are made by a large detector placed behind the film cassette. Thus, it is possible to control the regional X-ray exposure so that the film exposure uniformity is greatly improved.

This type of exposure control can lead to image artifacts [8], which may offset the advantages of the method if they are not suppressed. The potential artifacts are due to nonuniform filling of the image field and consist of sharp lines and ripple patterns. They can only be avoided when the beamwidth is an integral multiple of the interpulse spacing and when a variable frequency X-ray source is used.

2.3 Dose Reduction

X-radiography is a multiple step process and most steps are capable of improvement which would result in a reduction in the dose of radiation received by the patient without an unacceptable deterioration in image quality.

An analysis of possible improvements [9] is set out in the following table:

Area of improvement	Potential dose reduction factor
Detector efficiency	<2 (beyond rare earth phosphors)
Scatter rejection	2
Optimal spectra	2-3
Resolution	1.5-2 (small objects)
Image display	>2 (large objects)
Low attenuation materials	1.3

If the best of all these improvements were simultaneously realisable, the dose reduction could be rather more than a factor of 60. It is reasonable to conclude that an improvement by a factor of 20-40 should be achievable. Moreover, the widespread use of image storage techniques during screening procedures could well lead to a further significant reduction in dose.

2.4 Image Trapping

As an alternative to the conventional screen-film combination for X-radiography, it is possible to use photo-stimulable phosphor crystals set in an organic binder. A 1 mm thick imaging plate can store, or "trap", X-ray energy in quasistable states. Once the image has been trapped, the plate is scanned with a 633 nm helium-neon laser beam. This causes the plate to emit visible or infrared radiation that corresponds to the absorbed X-ray energies. The luminescence is detected by a photomultiplier and digitised for processing, analysis and display. The display can be on photographic film directly exposed to a scanned modulated laser light beam. With the present prototype system [10], the entire process takes 3 minutes. Sampling resolution is 10 points per millimetre. The dynamic range is 100:1, which is better than many types of film-screen combinations. The patient radiation dose averages 20-50 µGy. The imaging plate can be reused after the residual trapped energy has been erased by a flood of light. Thus, the advantages of the method are: low but variable dose; wide dynamic range; flexibility of digital system; and conventional kind of display.

3   INTERVENTIONAL RADIOLOGY

Since the mid-1970s, interventional radiology - the performance of therapeutic procedures guided by imaging techniques - has emerged as a cost effective and relatively atraumatic substitute for several traditional surgical operations [11]. The main applications are as follows:

- Percutaneous transluminal angioplasty of arterial obstructions;
- Selective embolisation of vascular neoplasms and bleeding sites;
- Drainage of obstructed biliary tracts;
- Guided biopsies;
- Drainage of obstructed urinary tracts;
- Drainage of abdominal abscesses;
- Selective infusion for chemotherapy of tumours; and
- Removal of stones and retained foreign bodies.

4   LIGHT AND INFRARED TRANSMISSION IMAGING

It is more than forty years since the first descripton of the application of a light torch to the underside of a pendulous female breast (diaphanography) providing a simple and safe method of visualising lesions [12]. The skin and the tissues act as an optical filter, so that illumination with white light gives a yellow or red appearance depending on the amounts of fat and fibroglandular materials. Malignant lesions are strongly absorbing and cast brown or black shadows with illdefined margins. This seems to be due to the concentration of blood in vessels associated with malignant tumours, especially at their advancing edges [13].

When the transilluminated breast is viewed by the unaided eye of the investigator, the results are unreliable. A substantial improvement is obtained by photographing the image by means of film sensitive to infrared radiation. The disadvantage of this is that special processing facilities are required for this type of film. This problem can be avoided by the use of a suitable television camera.

Although white light, covering the spectrum from 400 nm to 1200 nm (which is in the infrared), is commonly used for diaphanography, it has been argued that better results can be obtained by removing those wavelengths from the light which do not differentiate between lesions and normal tissues [14].

Diaphanography alone is still not a reliable method for breast cancer screening but, used in conjunction with other methods, such as palpation, fine needle aspiration cytology, X-ray mammography, ultrasound and thermography, it can be expected to have a useful role. Diaphanography may also prove to be helpful for examining other small and superficial structures such as the neonatal head, the scrotum and the sinuses.

5 MICROWAVE IMAGING

Electromagnetic waves of frequencies 1-10 GHz in the microwave region of the spectrum (300 MHz to 300 GHz) have adequate penetration to allow images to be made of the dielectric properties of the soft tissues of the body [15]. At 4 GHz, the loss is about 135 dB over a 20 cm path length in the thorax or abdomen; this is about the highest loss which can be measured by a state-of-the-art S-band receiver with a noise floor of around -140 dBm. Higher frequencies can be used for smaller structures. The wavelength at 4 GHz is 75 mm in free space and it is obvious that such a long wavelength would be capable of giving only very poor resolution. One solution to this problem is to use a material with a high dielectric constant to fill the waveguide-based antennae and to provide the coupling medium with the target. Relative to that in air, water contracts the wavelength by a factor of 9, to just over 8 mm. Quite promising results have been obtained by in vitro orthogonal transmission raster scanning of excised canine kidney, with both copolarised and crosspolarised detection. The main problems with the method are that arrays of antennae are necessary to acquire images in reasonable scan times and that multiple paths degrade the data.

Even with the best possible wavelength contraction, the application of ray optics to microwave imaging is bound to have rather poor resolution. Attempts to produce more rigorous and accurate solutions to the structure of an object from its scattered radiation may be grouped under the comprehensive title "inverse scattering". The application of a multiview/single frequency approach to microwave imaging by the convolution/back projection method promises to realise diffraction limited resolution [16].

6   ELECTRICAL IMPEDANCE METHODS

6.1 Electrical Impedance Imaging

The resistivities of typical biological materials range from around 0.5 Ωm for saline, CSF and plasma, through 2 Ωm for muscle, 6 Ωm for liver, 20 Ωm for lung, to 45 Ωm for bone [17]. The first attempt [18] to image the distribution of electrical impedance within the intact human body resulted in disappointing results. A matrix of 144 mutually guarding electrodes was used to make 100 spatially specific measurements across the thorax from a common plate electrode; the main problem was that the guarding technique was apparently not very effective in maintaining parallel straight-line current paths within the tissue.

Following the failure of the orthogonal imaging approach, it was natural that computed tomography by reconstruction from impedance profiles in a two-dimensional plane should be tried. A linear array of electrodes with an opposing common electrode were rotated around the object to be imaged [19]. The fact that the current paths were not straight was recognised. An initial guess of the object was made and for this guess the current paths and the resistances along the current paths were compared with the measured resistance projections. The guessed object was then corrected by back projecting the differences along the calculated, generally curved, paths. The same procedure was repeated for all other orientations of the object, each time using the corrected object from the previous step. Usually, sufficient convergence was not obtained with one revolution and so several revolutions had to be made. Although quite encouraging results were obtained, problems of anisotropy and nonlinearity were identified and the need to extend the analysis into three dimensions was recognised.

In an attempt to solve the problem of the curved current paths, all the inter-electrode potentials for every possible current injection electrode pair around an annulus containing the structure to be imaged has been tried [20]. An important feature of this approach was that voltages were not measured at the current-injecting electrodes, but only at the other electrodes where high impedance connexions were possible. For an annulus of N electrodes,

Number of independent current pairs = $N(N-1)/2$
Number of independent voltage measurements per current pair = $N-3$
Therefore, total number of independent voltage measurements = $N(N-1)(N-3)/2$

For example, for 16 electrodes there are 1560 independent voltage measurements. An iterative reconstruction process was used, with the initial assumption that the resistivity distribution was uniform. Back projection was followed by recalculation of the isopotentials and expected peripheral potentials for the back projected image. This forward projection involved solving Laplace's equation for the given spatial distribution of resistivity. An image of a human arm in cross-section was produced, using 50 kHz current and 16 electrodes applied directly to the skin. It was recognised that three dimensional reconstruction should result in significant improvement. Moreover, it has been suggested [21] that a modified algorithm may lead further improvement by adjusting the impedance profile.

Although the published work on electrical impedance imaging shows that much development needs to be done before the clinical value of the method can be assessed, the potential advantages of safety, high speed and tissue differentiation are well worth pursuing.

6.2 Dielectric Scanning

The dielectric constant of biological soft tissue generally decreases with increasing frequency. Softer tissue tends to have lower conductivity and dielectric constant than harder tissue [22]. An image of the dielectric constant of the tissue close to the skin can be obtained by applying an array of electrodes to the skin and measuring the impedance associated with the paths between each electrode and a common electrode applied to a distant part of the body. An instrument based on this principle, with an 8 x 8 array of 7 x 7 mm electrodes in a 10 x 10 cm square matrix surrounded by a guard electrode has been constructed for breast cancer studies [23]. The applied signal had an amplitude of 1 V peak-to-peak and a frequency of 1 kHz. The impedances associated with the 64 elements were measured in a total scan time of 1 s and displayed with up to 16 gray levels. In the preliminary studies, the four quadrants of the breast were examined in sequence. Although it was not possible to distinguish between benign and malignant lesions, abnormal images were obtained in all 57 patients examined with palpable masses [24].

It is worth noting that the so-called dielectric scanning method is really a variant of the original impedance imaging technique [18]. The reason that it offers some chance of success is that it aims only to detect quite large discontinuities in dielectric constant in tissue situated close to the detection electrode array.

7 BODY SURFACE POTENTIAL MAPPING

Electrocardiographic and electroencephelographic signals are traditionally displayed as strip chart recordings or as vector maps.

These physiological signals can alternatively be displayed on direct spatial maps corresponding to particular times during their acquisition. For example, one system for body surface potential mapping of the thorax used 180 active dry electrodes attached to an inflatable vest [25]. The electrodes were nominally equally spaced on the front and back of the torso. The e.c.g. signal from each electrode was amplified, sampled at 1 kHz rate and time multiplexed into groups of 15 onto one of 12 tracks of an f.m. tape recorder. The signals were played back with a time expansion of 32 to facilitate synchronous analogue-to-digital conversion under external clock control. The signals associated with each electrode were adjusted for baseline drift, low pass filtered to reduce noise, scaled and partly replaced by interpolated signals if this resulted in further improvement. Finally, the digitised data were converted into body surface potential colour maps.

REFERENCES

1   Almen, T. Experience from Ten Years of Development of Water-Soluble Nonionic Contrast Media. Investigative Radiology 15 (1980) S283-S288.

2   Mattrey, R.F., D.M. Long, F. Mutter, R. Mitten and C.B. Higgins. Perfluoroctylbromide: a Reticuloendothelial-Specific and Tumor-Imaging Agent for Computed Tomography. Radiology 145 (1982) 755-758.

3   Violante, M.R., P.B. Dean, H.W. Fischer and J.A. Mahoney. Particulate Contrast Media for Computed Tomographic Scanning of the Liver. Investigative Radiology 15 (1980) S171-S175.

4   Harron, A., S.E. Seltzer, M.A. Davis and P. Shulkin. Radiopaque Liposomes: a Promising New Contrast Material for Computed Tomography of the Spleen. Radiology 140 (1981) 507-511.

5   Barnes, G.T. and I.A. Brezovich. The Intensity of Scattered Radiation in Mammography. Radiology 126 (1978) 243-247.

6   Rudin, S., P. Bednarek and R. Wong. Design of Rotating Aperture Cones for Radiographic Scatter Reduction. Medical Physics 9 (1982) 385-393.

7   Plewes, D.B. and E. Vogelstein. A Scanning System for Chest Radiography with Regional Exposure Control: Practical Implementation. Medical Physics 10 (1983) 655-663.

8   Plewes, D.B. and E. Vogelstein. Exposure Artifacts in Raster Scanned Equalization Radiography. Medical Physics 11 (1984) 158-165.

9   Wagner, R.F. and R.J. Jennings. The Bottom Line in Radiologic Dose Reduction. Society of Photo-Optical Instrumentation Engineers 206 (1979) 60-66.

10 Fuji Computed Radiography. Ref No XM1-69E (Tokyo, Fuji Photo Film, 1982).

11 Wilkins, R.A. and M. Viamonte. Interventional Radiology (Oxford, Blackwell, 1982).

12 Cutler, M. Transillumination as an Aid to Diagnosis of Breast Lesions. Surgery, Gynecology and Obstetrics 48 (1929) 721-727.

13 Watmough, D.J. Diaphanography. Acta Radiologica Oncology 21 (1982) 11-15.

14 Carlsen, E. Transillumination Light Scanning. Diagnostic Imaging 4 (1982) 28-33&60.

15 Larsen, L.E. and J.H. Jacobi. Methods of Microwave Imaging for Diagnostic Applications. Reba, R.C., Goodenough, D.J., and Davidson, H.F. (eds.) Diagnostic Imaging in Medicine, pp. 68-123 (Boston, Nijhoff, 1983).

16 Adams, M.F. and A.P. Anderson. Synthetic Aperture Tomographic (SAT) Imaging for Microwave Diagnostics. Proceedings IEE (pt.H) 129 (1982) 83-88.

17 Geddes, L.A. and L.E. Baker. The Specific Resistance of Biological Material. Medical and Biological Engineering 5 (1967) 271-293.

18 Henderson, R.P. and J.G. Webster. An Impedance Camera for Spatially Specific Measurements of the Thorax. IEEE Transactions on Biomedical Engineering BME-25 (1978) 250-254.

19 Tasto, M. and H. Schomberg. Object Reconstruction from Projections and Some Non-Linear Extensions. Chen, C.H. (ed.) Pattern Recognition and Signal Processing, pp. 485-503 (Alphen aan den Rijn, Sijthoff and Noordhoff, 1978).

20 Brown, B.H. Tissue Impedance Methods. Jackson, D.F. (ed.) Imaging with Non-Ionizing Radiations, pp. 85-110 (Glasgow, Surrey University Press, 1983).

21 Kim, Y., J.G. Webster and W.J. Tomkins. Electrical Impedance Imaging of the Thorax. Journal of Microwave Power 18 (1983) 245-257.

22 Pethig, R. Dielectric and Electronic Properties of Biological Materials (Chichester, Wiley, 1979).

23 Sollish, B.D., E.H. Frei, E. Hammerman, S.B. Lang and M. Moshitzky. Microprocessor-Assisted Screening Techniques. Israel Journal of Medical Science 17 (1981) 859-864.

24 Man, B., B.D. Sollish, M. Moshitzky, Y. Choukron and E.H. Frei. Results of Preclinical Tests for Breast Cancer by Dielectric Measurements. XII International Conference on Medical and Biological Engineering, abstr. 30.4 (Jerusalem, 1979).

25 Ko, W.H., B.P. Bergmann and R. Plonsey. Data Acquisition System for Body Surface Potential Mapping. Journal of Bioengineering 2 (1978) 33-46.

DISCUSSION SUMMARY

PANEL ON OTHER IMAGING MODALITIES

The main questions on C. Corsi's paper Infrared and Microwave Radiometry have been on the capability of detecting deep temperature variations and on the reliability of the human body modelling. In particular E. Karrer asked if the described methods might be used to measure body hyperthermia temperature as deep as 10-15 cm. The answer pointed out that the method can supply real temperature data with good resolution for depth of some centimeters, while at 10-15 cm good resolution data can be provided but with a real spatial resolution of no more than a few centimeters.
P. Payne asked if the thickness changes around the body were not altering the validity of the modelling. The answer specified that the different layer thicknesses (skin, fat and muscle) have to be assumed just as a parametric value, to be changed according to the boundary conditions, derived by the measurements of the surface temperature in the infrared region and at high microwave frequency.
Finally Peter Wells asked about the possibility of detecting deep tumors by infrared techniques. A positive answer can be ascribed to the possibility of good thermal conduction by the vascular network, which can transfer part of the high metabolic heat activity of tumors to the breast surface. G. Romani and M. Viergever raised questions on G. Romani's paper respectively on the clinical use of the technique and on the difficulties of finding good solutions in the inverse problem. To the first question, Romani answered that improvements are expected by the use of a multisensor head (down to a few minutes, to carry out a complete diagnosis); the answer to the second question emphasized the importance of accuracy in the modelling, describing the phenomena and the careful calibration of the measuring devices.
The paper on Alternative Imaging Modalities by P. Wells raised questions mainly on the importance assumed by the algorithms on image reconstruction (Todd Pokropek) and more specifically on the main difficulties of the inverse problem: computation or modelling (M. Waller). P. Wells answered highlighting both aspects: software and hardware and more specifically computation algorithms as well as number and complexity of probes. A comment to the question on the inverse problem has been given by M. Viergever, who stated that the main difficulty is normally due to the critical

dependence of the results on the data and on the model underlying the inversion process, often underestimated in the context of medical imaging. To the last question of V. Cappellini on the possible use of the microwave computer tomography, P. Wells answered that it depends mostly on the level of the equipment which will be developed in the near future and on the acceptance of classical radiology for a widespread use.

PART VIII PRINCIPLES AND APPLICATIONS OF NUCLEAR MAGNETIC RESONANCE IMAGING

Chairman: Bruno Maraviglia (Italy)

BASIC PRINCIPLES OF NMR IMAGING

R. Campanella, C. Casieri, F. De Luca, B.C. De Simone,
B. Maraviglia
Dipartimento di Fisica
Universita' di Roma "La Sapienza"
00185 Roma, Italy

1 INTRODUCTION

NMR spectroscopy has been used since 1946 in the study of condensed matter. In recent years it has also been applied to research in fields related to medicine. The main applications are NMR Imaging and NMR High Resolution "in vivo" spectroscopy. In this paper we will be concerned only with the first topic. An immediate comparison with traditional radiography allows one to see the initial difference between the two techniques: whilst X-ray images are simply absorption maps of the system under examination, so that they can show only the electron density of the sample, an NMR image includes, besides the morphology of the body, chemical and physiological information. A second difference is the fact that the two techniques use frequencies which lie in ranges very far from each other: in fact NMR makes use of radiofrequencies (r.f.), so that it is non-ionizing; moreover, at the present moment, no harm was found to be produced by NMR imaging. Before analyzing the bases that have allowed the study of heterogeneous systems, it is necessary to give a brief description of the NMR spectroscopy principles.

2 NMR SPECTROSCOPY

Nuclear Magnetic Resonance is based on the principle that all the nuclei with non zero spin also have a magnetic moment μ. If we restrict ourselves to the case of nuclei with spin one half, when they are placed in a static magnetic field H_o, usually directed along the z axis of the reference frame, they will align along the direction of the field, in a parallel or antiparallel state, following a Boltzmann distribution. The energy difference between these two levels is $\Delta E = \hbar \omega_o$, where ω_o is the classical Larmor angular frequency given by $\omega_o = \gamma H_o$, with γ the gyromagnetic ratio. The population of nuclei oriented in the parallel state will be greater than the other because this state corresponds to a lower energy. The difference between populations results in a net macroscopic magnetization M_o aligned along H_o. The equilibrium situation can be modified by applying an r.f. electromagnetic wave, with energy equal to the separation between the two levels. The effect of this perturbation is to change the distribution of the populations. When the perturbation ends, the return to equilibrium of the system will be characterized by two relaxation times: the spin-lattice relaxation time T_1 and the spin-spin relaxation time T_2. The last one is the time constant with which the spins loose their phase coherence, while the realignment along the direction of the main magnetic field is characterized by the time constant T_1. These relaxation times can be measured using suitable sequences of pulses. The return to equilibrium can be detected with a coil that surrounds the sample; the variation of the component of the magnetization in a plane perpendicular to the z axis, called Free Induction Decay (FID), induces in the coil an efm signal. The Fourier Transform (FT) of this signal is the frequency spectrum of the system.

The spin-spin relaxation time gives information on the local fields experienced by the nuclei: these fields are related to the environment which surrounds the nuclei under examination. On the other hand, the spin-lattice relaxation time gives information about the energetic exchanges between the spin system and the lattice. This relaxation process is due, in fact, to the fluctuations of the local magnetic fields; the molecular motions tend to reestablish the thermodynamic equilibrium and to reorientate the spins in the direction of the static magnetic field.

From a classical point of view, the effect of the r.f. pulse is to rotate the magnetization of a flip angle around an axis, that will be denominated as x', of a reference frame rotating at the same frequency as the r.f. pulse.

P.C. Lauterbur (1) was the first to suggest a way

to obtain spatial images of the NMR parameters. His original idea was to correlate the resonance frequency of the spins in different parts of the sample and their spatial positions, by means of the induced interaction between them and a linear magnetic field gradient, superposed on the homogeneus field. The effect of the gradient is to change the Larmor frequency of the spins linearly with the position, so that it becomes possible to assign each frequency of the spectrum to a given coordinate.

3 GENERAL PRINCIPLES OF NMR IMAGING

When the magnetization is a function of the coordinates, as in the heterogeneous systems, the Bloch equation can be written (2):

$$\frac{\partial \vec{m}(\vec{r},t)}{\partial t} = \gamma \vec{m}(\vec{r},t) \times \vec{H}(\vec{r},t) - \{m_x(\vec{r},t)\hat{i} + m_y(\vec{r},t)\hat{j}\} / T_2(\vec{r}) - \{m_z(\vec{r},t) - m_o(\vec{r})\hat{k}\} / T_1(\vec{r}) \quad (1)$$

where $m_o(\vec{r})$ is the local equilibrium magnetization, T_1 and T_2 are functions of the spatial coordinates, and

$$\vec{H}(\vec{r},t) = H_{1x}(t)\hat{i} + H_{1y}(t)\hat{j} + [H_o + \vec{r}\cdot\vec{G}(t)]\hat{k} \quad (2)$$

In eq. (1) and (2) $\hat{i}$, $\hat{j}$ and $\hat{k}$ are unit vectors of the lab. reference frame, $H_{1x}(t)$ and $H_{1y}(t)$ are the components of the r.f. magnetic field, H_o is the static field and $\vec{G}(t)$ is the magnetic field gradient, defined by

$$\vec{G}(t) = \frac{\partial H_z(t)}{\partial x}\hat{i} + \frac{\partial H_z(t)}{\partial y}\hat{j} + \frac{\partial H_z(t)}{\partial z}\hat{k} \quad (3)$$

After the r.f. pulse, the magnetic field will be given by

$$\vec{H}(\vec{r},t) = [H_o + (\vec{r}\cdot\vec{G})]\hat{k} \quad (4)$$

and the solution of the Bloch equation for the transverse component of the magnetization $m_\perp(\vec{r},t)$, defined as

$$m_\perp(\vec{r},t) = m_x(\vec{r},t) + im_y(\vec{r},t) \qquad i = \sqrt{-1}$$

is given by

$$m_\perp(\vec{r},t) = m_o(r_G) \exp\{i\omega t - i\gamma\int_{t_1}^{t_1+t} \vec{r}\cdot\vec{G}(\tau)d\tau + \\ - t/T_2(r_G)\} \qquad (5)$$

where t=0 corresponds to the end of the excitation pulse and t_1 is the time when the gradient is turned on. Equation (5) is referred to a set of monochromatic spins for which

$$m_o(r_G) = \int_r \rho(x,y,z) dx\, dy\, dz \qquad (6)$$

is the equilibrium magnetization in the plane specified by $\vec{r}$ in the direction of the gradient $\vec{G}$, where $\rho(x,y,z)$ is the density of the resonant spins.

The total equilibrium magnetization M_o is given by the sum of the various $m_o(r_G)$ carried over all the isochromats

$$M_o = \int_{L_G} m_o(r_G) dr_G \qquad (7)$$

where L_G is the maximum extension of the sample in the direction of the gradient. In the same way the FID produced by the whole sample will be given by:

$$S(t) = \int_{L_G} m_\perp(r_G,t) dr_G \qquad (8)$$

From the expression (8) it is possible to obtain, with a suitable choice of the parameters that characterize a measure process, all the information from a heterogeneous sample. An imaging experiment will be defined by the sequence of excitation and by the temporal behaviour of the gradient vector because they both strongly affect the whole measure process and the information available. In particular, the use of the gradients distinguishes many different imaging methods among them. We now discuss the techniques applied in almost all the practical cases.

4 NMR IMAGING METHODS

4.1 Projection - Reconstruction (PR)

The Projection - Reconstruction technique is the first NMR imaging method that has been realized (1,3). In 1973, P.C. Lauterbur proposed the application of a linear, time independent magnetic field gradient over the homogeneous magnetic field. In this case the expression for the gradient G is:

$$\vec{G} = \frac{\partial H_x}{\partial x}\hat{i} + \frac{\partial H_z}{\partial y}\hat{j} + \frac{\partial H_z}{\partial z}\hat{k}$$

with

$$\frac{\partial H_x}{\partial x} = G_x = const; \quad \frac{\partial H_z}{\partial y} = G_y = const; \quad \frac{\partial H_z}{\partial z} = G_z = const$$

and the integral which appears in the expression (8) can be easily solved in the following way:

$$\int_{t_1}^{t_1+t} \vec{r}\cdot\vec{G}(\tau)d\tau = \int_0^t \vec{r}\cdot\vec{G}d\tau = (\vec{r}\cdot\vec{G})t \qquad (9)$$

From expressions (5) and (9) it can be shown that all the spins with

$$xG_x + yG_y + zG_z = const \qquad (10)$$

generate a single frequency of the spectrum; hence the relation (10) represents a plane, normal to the direction of $\vec{G}$, which contains the monochromatic spins. The FT of eq. (5) will give the amplitude of the spectral component associated to the plane which satisfies the condition (10). The real part of the FT is:

$$m_\perp(r_G,\omega) = 2m_0(r_G)\cdot T_2(r_G)$$
$$\{1 + T_2^2(r_G)[\omega - (\omega_0 + \gamma\vec{r}\cdot\vec{G})]^2\}^{-1} \qquad (11)$$

To obtain the whole spectrum, it is necessary to sum the expression (11) over all the planes orthogonal to $\vec{G}$, each resonating to a single frequency. Hence:

$$S(\omega) = \int_{L_G} m_\perp(r_G,\omega)dr_G \qquad (12)$$

Equation (11) represents a Lorentzian line produced by the plane defined by the relation (10), centered at the frequency

$$\omega = \omega_0 + \gamma\vec{r}\cdot\vec{G} \qquad (13)$$

with half height width given by $1/\pi T_2$ and amplitude

$$2m_o(\vec{r_G}) \cdot T_2(\vec{r_G}) \tag{14}$$

Equation (12) represents the whole spectrum; it is a superposition of Lorentzian lines, and if the strength of the gradient $|\vec{G}|$ is sufficiently high, so

$$\gamma |\vec{G}| L_G / N > 1/\pi T_{2min} \tag{15}$$

where T_{2min} is the minimum T_2 exhibited by the sample, eq. (15) becomes the spin density projection along the direction of $\vec{G}$. In the expression (15), $\gamma |\vec{G}| L$ is the spectral width of the sample in the direction of the gradient, and N an integer which defines the dimension of the reconstructed image, so that L_G/N is the achievable spatial resolution,.

The PR method consists of obtaining a set of projections, each one in a different direction. The procedure which allows one to reconstruct the image is called "back-projection", and it is similar to that used in the Computerized Tomography (CT). The NMR images, although called "density images", represent a spatial distribution of the product $m_o \cdot T_2$, as it is evident from eq. (11).

The simpler excitation technique makes use of an r.f. pulse which turns the magnetization by 90° around the x' axis of the rotating reference frame. The most commonly used sequences are generally based on a 90° pulse followed by a 180° pulse. This forces the spins that have dephased with the characteristic time T_2 to refocalize after a time 2τ from the beginning of the sequence. This procedure is called "spin-echo". The time delay τ between the pulses is much shorter than T_2, if one wants to reduce the dependence of the image on this parameter.

If a contrast in T_1 and T_2 is desired, the parameters that define the sequence must be changed or other pulse sequences must be obtained. A T_2 contrast can be obtained with a longer time delay between the 90° and the 180° pulses. A sequence that was given the name of "inversion-recovery" allows one to obtain a contrast depending mainly on T_1. It is made of a 180° pulse, followed after a time t_i by a spin-echo sequence. The time interval t_i should be comparable with T_1. Additionally a variation of the repetition time of the sequence influences the dependence of the image on T_1 and T_2.

The acquisition of data from a whole 3D sample

would require a very large memory and a long time to reconstruct the whole image, although in many cases the region of interest represents only a part of the body. For these reasons a reduction of the sample to a chosen slice is desired. This is operated in the following way: the sample is excited with a pulse whose shape in the frequency domain is a square of width $\Delta\omega/2\pi$, centered around the Larmor frequency, i.e. a sinc function. If the sample is irradiated in the presence of a gradient, let us say in the z direction, only the spins belonging to planes with z satisfying the relation

$$-\frac{\Delta\omega}{2\pi G_z} < z < \frac{\Delta\omega}{2\pi G_z}$$

will contribute to the signal.

4.2 Fourier Zeugmatography

This technique has been proposed by R.R. Ernst et al.(4), and is derived from a general class of experiments, that is referred to as 2D NMR spectroscopy. It makes use of pulsed field gradients after the excitation pulses, in the following way: immediately after the 90° pulse, a magnetic field gradient G_x is applied along the x direction for a time t_x, followed by a gradient G_y applied for a time t_y along y. The FID is finally recorded during a time interval t_z, under the influence of a gradient G_z. Mathematically, the behaviour of the z component of the magnetic field is described by

$$H_z(\vec{r}) = \begin{cases} H_o + G_x x & \text{for} \quad 0 < t < t_x \\ H_o + G_y y & \text{"} \quad t_x < t < t_x+t_y \\ H_o + G_z z & \text{"} \quad t_x+t_y < t \end{cases} \quad (16)$$

Obviously the phase of the FID at a time $t > t_x+t_y$ is a function of the previous time intervals t_x and t_y, hence we shall define it as $S(\underline{t}) = S(t_x,t_y,t_z)$. The tridimensional FT of the NMR signal $S(\underline{t})$ is a measure of the spin density function $\rho(\vec{r})$, and can be interpreted as a tridimensional image of the sample.

The observed signal $S(\underline{t})$ is formed by the contribution from the various sample parts, and can be written as

$$S(\underline{t}) = \iiint \rho(\vec{r}) \, s(\vec{r},\underline{t}) dv \quad (17)$$

where $s(\vec{r},\underline{t})dv$ represents the contribution of the volume element $dv = dx \cdot dy \cdot dz$ identified by the vector $\vec{r}$. The function $s(\vec{r},\underline{t})$ can be easily found as a solution of the Bloch equation. After a phase sensitive detection at a frequency ω_o, the cosine component of the signal will be given by:

$$s(\vec{r},\underline{t}) = \cos\{-\gamma G_x x t_x - \gamma G_y y t_y - \gamma G_z z t_z\} \qquad (18)$$
$$\exp\{-(t_x+t_y+t_z)/T_2\}$$

The tridimensional FT of $S(\underline{t})$, that will be written as $S(\underline{\omega}) = S(\omega_x,\omega_y,\omega_z)$, will be given by:

$$S(\underline{\omega}) = \iiint S(\underline{t}) \exp(-i\underline{\omega}\cdot\underline{t}) dt_x dt_y dt_z \qquad (19)$$

and can be expressed as a sum of the contribution from the various volume elements:

$$S(\underline{\omega}) = \iiint \rho(\vec{r}) \, s(\vec{r},\underline{\omega}) dv \qquad (20)$$

where $s(\vec{r},\underline{\omega})$ is the FT of $s(\vec{r},\underline{t})$, and is given by:

$$s(\vec{r},\underline{\omega}) \simeq 1/2 \; L(-\gamma G_x x - \omega_x) \cdot \qquad (21)$$
$$\cdot L(-\gamma G_y y - \omega_y) \cdot L(-\gamma G_z z - \omega_z)$$

where

$$L(\omega) = A(\omega) + iD(\omega) = \frac{1}{1+\omega^2 T_2^2} + i\frac{\omega T_2}{1+\omega^2 T_2^2} \qquad (22)$$

From eq. (21) we can demonstrate the validity of the following identity:

$$S(\vec{r},\underline{\omega}) = S(0,\underline{\omega}+\gamma\vec{G}\cdot\vec{r}) \qquad (23)$$

Substitution of eq. (23) into eq. (20) gives:

$$S(\underline{\omega}) = \iiint \rho(\vec{r}) \, S(0,\underline{\omega}+\gamma\vec{G}\cdot\vec{r}) dv \qquad (24)$$

If at this point we rewrite the frequency variable $\underline{\omega}$ in terms of a spatial variable $\vec{r}\,'$, i.e.:

$$\underline{\omega} = -\gamma\vec{G}\cdot\vec{r}\,'$$

eq. (24) becomes:

$$S(\underline{\omega}) = S(-\gamma\vec{G}\cdot\vec{r}\,') = \tilde{\rho}(\vec{r}\,') =$$
$$= \iiint \rho(\vec{r}) \, S(0,-\gamma\vec{G}\cdot(\vec{r}-\vec{r}\,')) dv \qquad (25)$$

This integral represents the tridimensional convolution between the "true" spin density $\rho(\vec{r})$ and the natural lineshape $L(\omega)$ through the function $s(\vec{r},\omega)$. Writing it explicitly:

$$S(\omega) = \tilde{\rho}(\vec{r}') = 1/2 \iiint \rho(\vec{r}) \, L[-\gamma G_x(x-x')] \cdot L[-\gamma G_y(y-y')] \cdot L[-\gamma G_z(z-z')] dv$$

The function $\tilde{\rho}(\vec{r}')$, which we could define as "filtered density", is a complex function. Its real and imaginary parts both contain the functions absorption and dispersion, which can hardly be distinguished. Hence it is better to calculate its absolute value $|\tilde{\rho}(\vec{r}')|$ which, under the assumption that the line shape is sufficiently narrow and the intensity of the gradients is strong enough, is a good measure of the density $\rho(\vec{r})$.

The advantages of this method rather than the backprojection technique can be found in the fact that no reconstruction process is needed to obtain the image, the 3D FT of the FIDs being itself a map of the sample. As in the case for the PR method, the need for too large a memory makes it necessary for the technique to be reduced to two dimensions.

In practice, the NMR imaging method most commonly used today is a derivative of the Fourier Zeugmatography, which was named "spin-warp" (5). The difference between the two techniques can be explained in the following way: the effect of the first gradient, for example G_y, is to change the phase of the spins in a plane characterized by a value y_0 of the y coordinate of an amount

$$\gamma \, y_0 \int_0^{t_y} G_y(t) dt$$

as can be easily seen from eq. (18). The value of such an integral can be modified either by varying the time interval t_y while keeping $|G_y|$ constant, or by varying the amplitude of the gradient $|G_y|$ with t_y fixed. This second way is usually preferred for practical reasons: it is simpler to maintain fixed the timing of the sequence and to gradually change the amplitude of the gradient than to change the length of the encoding gradient. The sequence we use on our machine is a spin echo, in which both pulses are selective.

In fig.1 the sequence for a transverse section of the body is shown. G_z is the selection gradient, and is

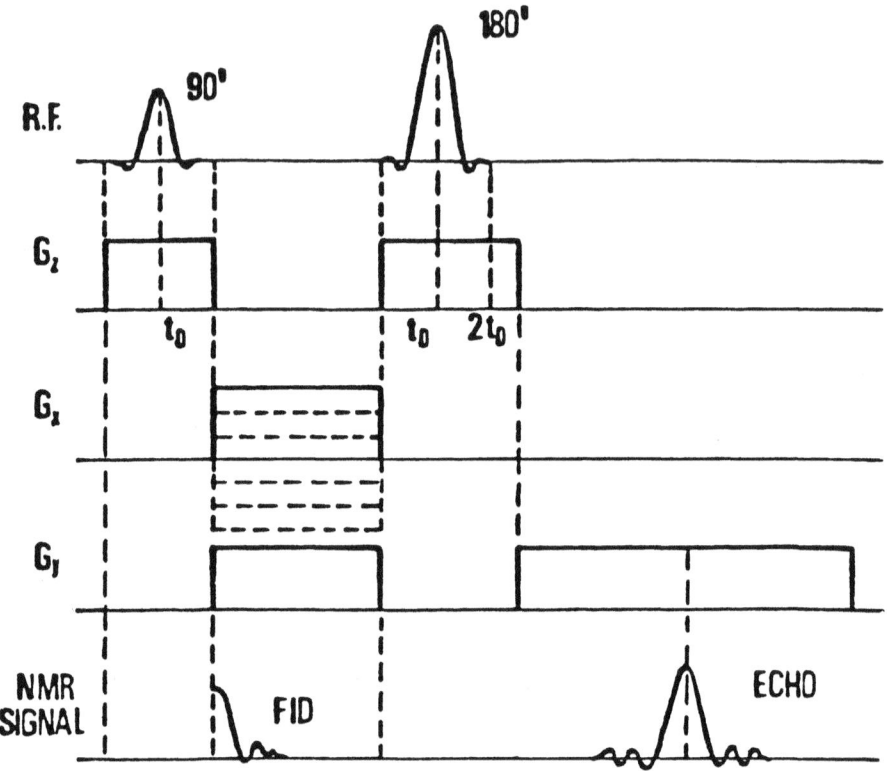

Figure 1.

Typical 2DFT sequence. It is a spin echo with both selective pulses. The gradient G_z is switched on to select an x,y slice during r.f. irradiation. The G_x gradient is the reading gradient, which is on while the echo is recorded. G_x introduces the frequency spread along the x axis. The phase encoding gradient G_y is applied with a whole set of amplitudes and for each one the echo is sampled. The 2DFT of the recorded signal gives the spin density map. T_1 contrast can be generated by applying an extra selective 180° pulse before the spin echo sequence (IR).

only turned on during the selective pulses.

G_y is the gradient which operates a phase encoding in the y direction. Its intensity is varied following the integral relation:

$$\gamma L_y \int_T G_y \, dt = 2\pi n$$

where L_y is the maximum sample length in the y direction, T is the duration of the gradient pulse and n is an integer which takes on the values:

$$-N/2 \, , \, -N/2-1 \, , \, \ldots \, , \, -1 \, , \, 0 \, , \, +1 \, , \, \ldots \, , \, N/2-1$$

if it has been assumed that each echo in the N points is to be sampled. The bidimensional FT of N echoes will give an NxN image of the object.

REFERENCES

1. Lauterbur, P.C. 'Image formation by induced local interaction: examples employing nuclear magnetic resonance' Nature, 242, 190 (1973)
2. Abragam, A. The principles of nuclear magnetism. Oxford Press, 1961.
3. Holland, G.N.; Hawkes, R.C.; Moore, W.S. 'Nuclear Magnetic Resonance (NMR) Tomography of the brain: coronal and sagittal sections' J. of Comp. Ass. Tomography 4, 429 (1980).
4. Kumar, A.; Welti, D.; Ernst, R.R. 'NMR Fourier zeugmatography' J. of Magn. Res. 18, 69 (1975).
5. Hutchison, J.M.S.; Edelstein, W.W.; Johnson, G. A whole body NMR imaging machine' J. Phys. E. Sci. Instrum. 13, 947 (1980).

COMPARATIVE EVALUATION OF NMR IMAGING TECHNIQUES

P. Mansfield

Department of Physics, University of Nottingham, England.

1.   INTRODUCTION

Nuclear magnetic resonance (NMR) imaging has rapidly developed over the last twelve years to the point where machines are being evaluated in clinical trials. The NMR principles on which these and other machines are based are discussed and reviewed elsewhere (1). Although much of the early clinical work was done in Britain, principally at Aberdeen, the Hammersmith Hospital, London, and at Nottingham University, many commercial machines have now been installed in hospitals, universities and institutions throughout the U.S.A., Europe and Japan for intensive clinical and technical evaluation. However, many of the potential users of such machines are not completely sure exactly what NMR has new to offer from a diagnostic point of view. Various research groups have different approaches to NMR imaging which can be confusing to both users and equipment manufacturers alike. In different circumstances, one might well argue that initially each idea is as good as the next and eventually the market place will sort out the clinically useful systems. But the fact is that all NMR imaging schemes are costly to produce, though there are varying scales within this high cost technology. In this case, especially when there are so many imaging methods to choose from, and when there is so much written about all the schemes, it behoves any manufacturer and indeed any potential user, to look carefully at what is on offer. The many choices of technique could well result in a costly imaging machine becoming obsolescent if not obsolete within a year or so of installation.

NMR imaging presents an unusual opportunity to the manufacturers and users in the following sense. After eight or nine years of invention and innovation, we are in a position to say with

certainty what the optimum performance for an ideal imaging machine
is. Such a machine, if possible to make, can never be exceeded in
performance and so may never be superceded by newer models, except
in trivial matters such as style and colour, etc.

However, we shall also see that such an optimum machine,
though approachable in practice, may, for reasons of cost, be
unattractive as a general purpose imaging machine. In such
circumstances, we may have to accept a lesser machine out of
economic necessity.

2. IMAGING METHODS

All methods of imaging fall into one of four categories:
(a) point scanning; (b) line scanning; (c) planar imaging and
(d) three dimensional imaging. The modes of imaging are
represented schematically in Figure 1 in which Figure 1(a)
represents sequential scanning of an isolated point or volume
element; (b) sequential scanning of an isolated column of volume
elements to form a line; (c) sequential scanning of an isolated
plane of magnetization and finally (d) simultaneous signal
reception from the whole volume. All methods and categories of
imaging are fully described elsewhere (1), only a brief discussion
of the various techniques is given in this presentation.

2.1 Point Scanning

Two different methods of imaging have evolved based on
magnetically localizing a small volume of material within a larger
object. In the first method (2) the point of interest is isolated
by placing the specimen in two orthogonal and roughly linear
gradients both of which are modulated at different frequencies.
The imposed time dependence of the gradients has the effect when
used with a suitable receiver filter, of washing out all signals
from the specimen except the slowly time dependent and time

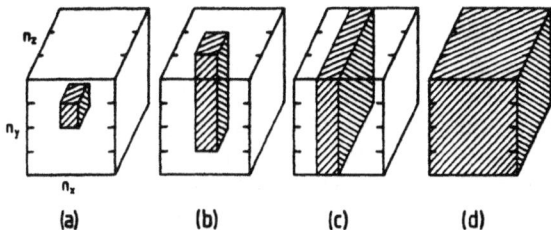

Figure 1. Diagrams of a rhombohedral object field of $n_x n_y n_z$ volume elements illustrating the classification of the various imaging methods:
(a) sequential point scanning
(b) sequential line scanning
(c) planar imaging
(d) simultaneous or true three dimensional imaging

independent signals from the selected sensitive point. Since information is required at only one point the magnetic field gradients can be quite non-linear compared with the other imaging modes we shall describe.

The sensitive point signal is read out point by point by a continuous spin interrogation method known as steady-state free precession (SSFP). This utilizes a continuous stream of high power RF pulses of short duration, typically 20 μsec. The object may be scanned to produce images in a single plane or a volume as required.

A second point scanning method (3) relies upon degrading the static magnetic field everywhere except at a point or aperture from which signal is read again by a repetitive pulse method. In this case the repetition period of the RF pulses is usually longer than that required for SSFP. The spot is swept by moving the specimen line and row-wise, to produce an image.

A further variant on this method (4) specializes to a single point of interest using very high homogeneity over the sensitive spot. In this case, analysable chemically shifted spectra are obtained from, for example, phosphorus resonances, enabling the phosphorus metabolites in the breakdown and synthesis of ATP to be followed in vivo.

2.2 Line Scanning

In line scanning, a whole line or column of material is examined simultaneously, thereby giving a degree of multiplexing in the received signal. The line of material may be defined by gradient modulation (5) or by combinations of switched gradients and a selective RF pulse (6). Selective pulses are shaped or tailored to excite specified range of spin magnetization in a given gradient. The RF pulses are of much lower power but usually last longer, typically a few milliseconds.

2.3 Planar Imaging

Three main methods exist for studying the spin magnetization in a plane of interest within an extended specimen. These are (i) Projection Reconstruction (PR) Imaging (7); (ii) Two Dimensional Fourier Transformation (2DFT) Imaging (8) and (iii) Echo-Planar (EP) Imaging (9). Initial slice selection may be achieved in all three methods by selective irradiation (10). In one form of projection reconstruction imaging slice selection utilizes gradient modulations as in the previously described point and line scanning methods, together with SSFP for the signal read-out. However, it is found from theoretical considerations that this form of slice selection is not precise and is sample dependent through T_1 and T_2. Moreover, SSFP as a signal read-out mode, though efficient, weights the observed signals with a sample dependent parameter $T_2/(T_1 + T_2)$. This has the effect of losing signal contrast in the images formed using this method.

A variant of the two dimensional FT method (11) is also in use. So far as can be seen at the present, initial slice definition using selective excitation is to be preferred together with a simple slowly repeated pulse read-out, avoiding the SSFP regime. Pictures obtained in this manner show a remarkable degree of image contrast, especially in the brain (12).

2.4 Three Dimensional Imaging

All three planar imaging methods may be extended to three dimensional imaging where the signal from the total volume of interest within the specimen is received and unravelled to produce a three dimensional image of the object. However, from a technical standpoint, it appears that 3D imaging from a series of projections is the easiest to achieve while 3D echo-planar imaging is probably the hardest.

A disadvantage of 3D projection reconstruction seems to be that one is forced to deal with a cubic array even when a few imaging planes may suffice. However, several variants both of projection imaging (13) and selective excitation imaging (14) combined with any of the planar imaging methods can overcome this problem, which, as we shall see later, relates to the imaging time.

3. PICTURE QUALITY

A full theoretical account of the factors affecting picture quality are given elsewhere (1). In this presentation we wish to bring out the salient general parameters affecting picture quality, namely, imaging time T, pixel signal-to-noise ratio R and picture element volume $\Delta v = \Delta x \Delta y \Delta z$, where Δx, Δy and Δz are the dimensions of the rhombohedral voxel.

For an ideal imaging system, the imaging time is given by (see also Reference 1):

$$T = KR^2/\Delta v^2 \qquad (1)$$

where K embodies all other factors relating to magnet field strength, receiver coil and sample parameters. Equation (1) as it stands gives the time T to image one voxel to the required signal-to-noise ratio. Clearly from our previous discussion of imaging modes, in a completely multiplexed, decodeable imaging technique, the time to image the whole volume of $n_x n_y n_z$ elements is the same as that required to image one. (In our sketch of Figure 1, we have taken $n_x = n_y$ where n_x is the number of voxels along one edge of the cubic array in the object field). Thus Equation (1) represents the optimum 3D imaging time. The total time to image the same rhombohedral object array by planar imaging is

$$T_{planar} = n_z T \qquad (2)$$

The corresponding time by line scan imaging is

$$T_{line} = n_y n_z T \qquad (3)$$

and by point imaging, the scan time is

$$T_{point} = n_x n_y n_z T \qquad (4)$$

Although T is thought of here as a continuous data accumulation time, in many experiments, T is in fact broken up into a series of m data accumulation windows of period T_o, i.e. $T = mT_o$. In this class of imaging experiment, the actual imaging time is clearly much longer since there are m-1 delay periods T_d between the sampling windows T_o to add in to the total imaging time. This latter consideration is the factor which limits the imaging speed of two of the three efficient imaging methods, namely; reconstruction from projections and 3D or 2D Fourier transform imaging. In echo-planar imaging, where it is in principle possible to obtain an image in a single shot experiment, Equation (1) is directly applicable.

As we have already indicated, single plane imaging, particularly combined with the possibility of looking at a few adjacent planes, is faster than 3D imaging and in my view is therefore likely to be more useful clinically. In this case, Equation (2) is the relevant imaging time with $n_z = 1$.

Another factor affecting imaging time is the resolution reflected through the pixel size. For equal resolution in the x-y plane, and with constant slice thickness Δz, the imaging time varies as $1/\Delta x^4$, whereas for cubic voxels the imaging time varies as $1/\Delta x^6$.

At the present time, most NMR images have been produced with a ratio of $\Delta z/\Delta x$ in the range 3 - 5 and this seems an adequate compromise on imaging time and spatial resolution.

From Equations (3) and (4) and our previous comment, it is clear that line and point scanning as imaging modalities are basically inefficient methods compared with planar and 3D methods, simply by virtue of the data multiplexing exploited in the latter techniques. On the other hand, 3D imaging by PR or FT takes so long to accumulate the data that it becomes impractical as a clinical imaging modality. Three dimensional EP imaging, though possible in principle to yield single shot images, will have immense technical problems which I do not minimize. It would seem that true 3D imaging, by any means, is not a profitable route to follow.

In this paper, I wish to concentrate on planar methods. In this case, we examine Equations (1) and (2) with $n_z = 1$ and plot R versus T with resolution as parameter for three values of Larmor

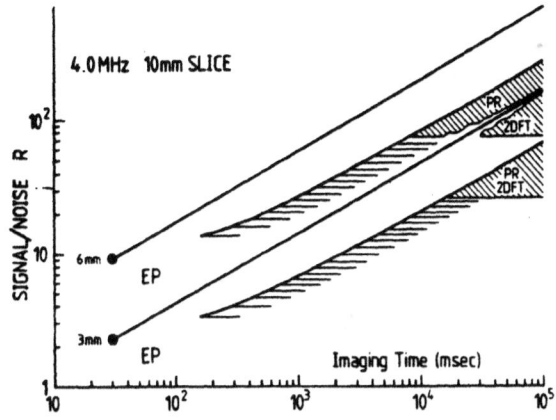

Figure 2. Signal/noise ratio R versus imaging time T for three planar imaging methods calculated for a 10 mm slice at 4.0 MHz. PR: projection reconstruction imaging; 2DFT: two dimensional Fourier transform imaging and EP: echo-planar imaging. Solid lines are Equations (1) and (2) for 3 and 6 mm resolution. Shaded curves are for discrete signal averaging, Equation (7) for the two resolutions in the case of EP imaging. Wedge shaped hatched regions correspond to regimes applicable to all three methods but set minimum imaging time limits for PR and 2DFT imaging.

resonance frequency; 4.0, 6.0 and 8.0 MHz. Practical values for the constant K are obtained from detailed analysis given elsewhere (1).

The straight solid lines of Figure 2 show R vs T at 4.0 MHz for the 3 mm and 6 mm resolution. These resolutions correspond respectively to a 128 x 128 and a 64 x 64 pixel array in a practical whole body imaging system with an object field of 38.4 x 38.4 cm^2. In all cases the slice thickness taken is 10 mm. Each solid line starts at $T = T_o$ = 30 msec and corresponds to what I consider the shortest practical imaging time in, say, a single shot EP experiment.

4. DISCRETE SIGNAL AVERAGING

If the data accumulation time could be continuously increased, then R follows the straight line in Figure 3. However, in all three planar imaging methods (except PR using SSFP), a delay T_d between shots is mandatory. This is illustrated in Figure 4 where it is assumed that data are taken in during period T_o in the most efficient manner possible, i.e. continuously, thereby following Equation (1) and the straight lines in Figures 2, 4 and 5. For the purposes of illustration only, I have taken the shortest practical delay to be T_d = 100 msec. The data acquisition period is taken to be T_o = 30 msec for all the planar imaging methods considered. (In some experiments T_o may well be shorter, but times much greater than 30 msec become progressively more difficult to achieve through T_2 limitations. Magnet inhomogeneity may restrict this still further). In this case, for a two or more shot EP image, we hop over from the 30 msec imaging time (T_o) which lies on the continuous curve, Figure 2 and Equations (1) and (2), to the discrete imaging time curve (shaded) given by

$$T_i = mT_o + (m - 1)T_d \qquad (5)$$

where the integer m = 1,2,3.... denotes the number of shots or experiments. The corresponding discrete signal/noise ratio R_i is related to the initial value R_o by the expression

$$R_i = \sqrt{m}\, R_o \qquad (6)$$

Equations (5) and (6) may be combined to yield

$$T_i = (R_i/R_o)^2 (T_o + T_d) - T_d \qquad (7)$$

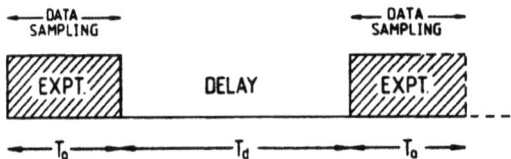

Figure 3. Generalized repeated data acquisition experiment in which data recorded in the sampling window T_o are discretely averaged in successive coadditions interspersed with wait periods or time delays T_d.

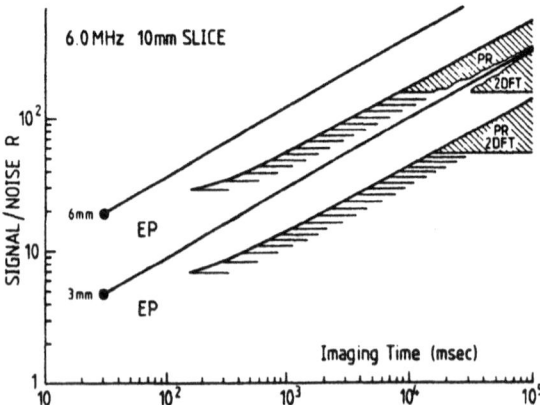

Figure 4. As for Figure 2 but calculated at 6.0 MHz. See text for more detail.

The horizontal shading in Figure 2 is intended to emphasize that T_d is an arbitrary parameter in Equation (7) so that for a given signal/noise improvement T_i may be longer depending on T_d.

An important distinction between EP and other planar imaging methods is clearly evident in Figures 2, 4 and 5, namely that there is a minimum imaging time for both PR and 2DFT corresponding to a minimum value of m in Equation (5).

For a 128^2 matrix $T_{i min}$ = 16.54 sec while for a 64^2 matrix $T_{i min}$ = 8.22 sec where T_d = 100 msec in both cases. (The wedge-shaped hatched regions on Figure 2 are intended to emphasize that for given R_i/R_o, T_i may be arbitrarily long, depending on T_d). At these times Figure 2 indicates the corresponding signal/noise ratios as approximately 26.5 and 75.0 respectively, whereas the single shot 30 msec EP experiment gives R = 2.33 and R = 9.32 for 3 and 6 mm resolution respectively. To obtain a 128^2 image with R = 10 would take at the very least 3.0 sec from Figure 2.

Figures 4 and 5 indicate considerable signal/noise ratio improvements for higher Larmor frequencies. At 6.0 MHz, for example, the corresponding signal/noise ratios for a 30 msec imaging time are R = 4.7 and R = 19.0 for 3 and 6 mm resolutions respectively, while at 8.0 MHz, we obtain R = 8.0 and R = 30.0 for the same two resolutions.

Equation (7) and the above discussion regarding multishot EP imaging and PR and 2DFT imaging applies equally well to Figures 4 and 5. A glance at the imaging times in these curves leads one inevitably to ask the question already hinted at previously, namely, what use is very large R if the object is moving?

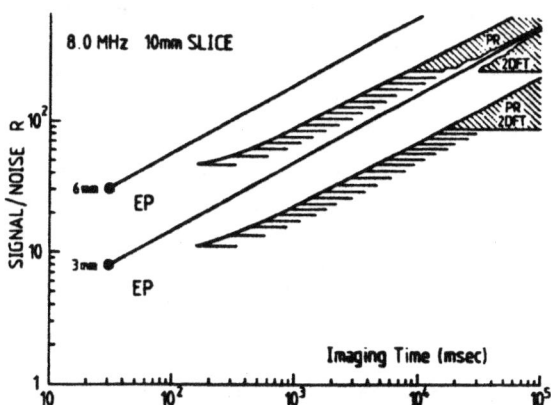

Figure 5. As for Figure 2 but calculated at 8.0 MHz. See text for more detail.

Remember also, that in practical PR and 2DFT imaging, T_d is often closer to 500 msec making the imaging times in all figures longer by almost a factor of five.

The clear message contained in Figures 2, 4 and 5 is that time-wise it does not pay to signal average because there is no imaging method yet devised which allows continuous collection of signal data at full equilibrium signal amplitude. To achieve something close to full signal height it is necessary to repeat experiments with delay times which are invariably much longer than the actual data accumulation time. This process is extremely inefficient and costly of time.

5. OBJECT MOTION

Our discussion of picture quality so far has assumed a static object. Naturally, for whole body work in vivo, involuntary motions occur in the subject being imaged and the question, totally ignored by most practitioners of NMR imaging is: what happens to an image when such motions are present? More fundamentally, we may enquire whether the word 'resolution' as usually defined has any relevance.

It is helpful to invoke a photographic analogy, though we emphasize that this has only limited applicability. Suppose we wish to photograph a swinging pendulum. Being regular oscillatory motion, the pendulum bob will spend on average more time at the displacement extrema and very little time in the vertical position where it is travelling fastest. An exposure which takes several pendulum periods will therefore yield an image of not one bob but two at each displacement extreme with blurring between. To catch the pendulum anywhere in the cycle requires an exposure much shorter than the intrinsic swing period.

Of course, when motion of an object is aperiodic, the image is completely blurred. The basic resolution of the camera in terms of the lens aperture, photographic grain size, etc. has remained the same in all pictures, but the spatial resolution of the picture has clearly degraded.

Theoretical analysis shows that our photographic analogy corresponds to the slow motion case, i.e. when there is relatively little motion during the data acquisition period. When there is significant motion during the data sampling process, this leads to a broadening of the pixel point spread function, producing image blurring.

In whole body imaging, all motional regimes exist to varying degree within the body, especially the trunk region. The presence of both static regions and irregularly fast moving regions can clearly lead to a deceptively good image quality and overrated claims for resolution. The reality is that resolution as measured with a phantom, is only obtainable if object displacements are less than one pixel during the imaging process.

Typical adult abdominal wall motion due to breathing alone is of the order of 10 mm. Breathing will also introduce corresponding displacements of all vital organs. For these reasons, despite the apparent quality of NMR whole body images and the claimed resolution, what we see, by and large, is high quality blurred images. These images may, nevertheless, be valuable medically, but it is clearly nonsensical to look for soft tissue detail in organs like the stomach, intestines, liver and kidneys. Bone is another matter and so is the head. But even the head, or at least the contents, are moving and this leads us to question the claims for high resolution head pictures.

6. CONCLUSIONS

Three methods of planar imaging have been examined. All have ostensibly the same imaging efficiency but two methods, PR and 3DFT have minimum imaging times, which under the most favourable conditions are around 10 and 20 secs for 64^2 and 128^2 arrays respectively. In practice these times are more like a factor 5 higher putting the 64^2 array image time at 50 sec and that of the 128^2 array at about 1.5 min. The pixel size in the latter case is 3 mm. Our main conclusion is that an imaging time of 1.5 min is, in general, inconsistent with 3 mm resolution whole body imaging. It may be that parts of the image which correspond to static regions of the subject have 3 mm resolution. However, there seems little basis for going much beyond 64 x 64 arrays in PR and 2DFT especially when considering soft tissues in vital organs.

In contrast, EP imaging may be performed with high efficiency over any time scale from single shot 30 msec imaging to an arbitrarily long time. For short times, especially single shot, therefore, genuine resolution is obtainable although at some sacrifice of signal/noise ratio. However, the single shot S/N expectation at 6.0 MHz, for example, is ~ 5 for 3 mm and ~ 19 for 6 mm resolution (15,16).

All three planar imaging methods are able, with suitable modifications, to measure T_1, T_2 and continuous flow. However, only one method, EP imaging, is able to image movement in an ungated real time manner.

Acknowledgement

The author wishes to thank the Editors of the Bowman Gray International Symposium on NMR Imaging (Ref. 17) for permission to reproduce the figures and some text used in this paper.

References

1. Mansfield, P., Morris,P.G. NMR imaging in biomedicine. In; Waugh, J.S., ed. Adv. Magn. Reson. Suppl. 2. Academic Press N.Y. 1982.
2. Hinshaw, W.S. Spin mapping: applications of moving gradients to NMR. Phys. Lett. (1974), 48;87-88.
3. Damadian, R., Minkoff, L., Goldsmith, M., Stanford, M., Koutche J. Tumour imaging in a live animal by field focusing NMR (FONAR). Physiol. Chem. Phys. (1976), 8:61.
4. Gordon, R.E., Hanley, P.E., Shaw, D., et al. Localization of metabolites in animals using P-31 topical magnetic-resonance. Nature (1980), 287:736-738.
5. Hinshaw, W.S. Image formation by the nuclear magnetic resonance sensitive point method. J. App. Phys. (1976), 47:3709-3721.
6. Mansfield, P., Maudsley, A.A., Baines, T. Fast scan proton density imaging by NMR. J. Phys. (E)(1976), 9:271-278.
7. Lauterbur, P.C. Image formation by induced local interaction; examples employing nuclear magnetic resonance. Nature (1973) 242:190-191.
8. Kumar, A., Welti, D., Ernst, R.R. NMR Fourier zeugmatography J. Magn. Reson. (1975), 18:69-83.
9. Mansfield, P. Multi-planar image formation using NMR spin echoes. J. Phys. C (1977), 19:L55-58.
10. Garroway, A.N., Grannell, P.K. and Mansfield, P. Image formation in NMR by a selective irradiative process. J. Phys. C (1974), 7:L457-62.
11. Edelstein, W.A., Hutchison, J.M.S., Johnson, G., Redpath, T. Spin warp NMR imaging and applications to human whole-body imaging. Phys. Med. Biol. (1980), 25:751-756.
12. Doyle, F.H., Pennock, J.M., Orr, J.S. et al. Imaging of the brain by nuclear magnetic resonance. Lancet (1981), ii:53-57
13. Taylor, D. (1981)(private communication).
14. Maudsley, A.A. Multiple line scanning spin density imaging. J. Magn. Reson. (1980), 41:112-126.
15. Rzedzian, R., Mansfield, P., et al. Real-time nuclear magnetic resonance clinical imaging in paediatrics. Lancet (1983), ii:1281-1282.
16. Rzedzian, R., Doyle, M., Mansfield, P. et al. Echo planar imaging in paediatrics: Real-time nuclear magnetic resonance. Ann. Radiol. (1984), 27:2-3, 182-186.
17. Proceedings of an International Symposium on NMR imaging (1981 (Eds. R.L. Witcofski, N. Karstaedt and C.L. Partain). Pub: Bowman Gray School of Medicine of Wake Forest University, Winston-Salem, North Carolina, U.S.A.

CLINICAL NUCLEAR MAGNETIC RESONANCE IMAGING

C.L. Partain, M.D., Ph.D, M.V. Kulkarni, M.D., M.R. Mitchell, M.D.
J.A. Patton, Ph.D, M.P. Sandler, M.D., A.E.James, Jr, J.D., M.D.
Department of Radiology and Radiological Sciences, Vanderbilt University Medical Center, Nashville, Tennessee, U.S.A.

INTRODUCTION

The emphasis in this presentation will involve a discussion of tissue characteristics as potentially observed and recorded by nuclear magnetic resonance imaging. Several different pulse sequences are available to the NMR imaging physician and scientist. This results in a multitude of different NMR scan parameters each yielding significant tissue contrast differentiation, and it is essential to attempt to understand these differences on a theoretical and physical basis, as well as to extend this understanding to the biochemical and pathophysiological significance of the resulting changes in tissue contrast appearance. Assuming this is possible, a data base will be generated allowing the intelligent choice of pulse sequences and pulse sequence parameters which will yield maximum diagnostic information in minimal time and with minimal cost. This approach may lend itself to computer based diagnostic planning as a function of clinical presentation and be one valuable component of a logical diagnostic workup that is increasingly necessary as a result of the expansion of high technology medical applications in response to increasing regulatory control in many countries.

TECHNIQUE

The two most commonly utilized pulse sequences at our institution are spin echo and inversion recovery. These sequences are discussed and illustrated from the viewpoint of the physical and mathematical basis, instrumentation, image production and resulting clinical applications, requiring the identification and interpretation of soft tissue contrast variations. Parametric variables that are defined for the spin echo sequence include the pulse echo time (TE) and the pulse repetition time (TR). Inversion recovery pulse sequence parameters include inversion time (TI) and the previously described TE and TR parameters. A photograph and schematic representative of the 0.5 Tesla superconducting MRI system at Vanderbilt University Medical Center is shown in Figure 1.

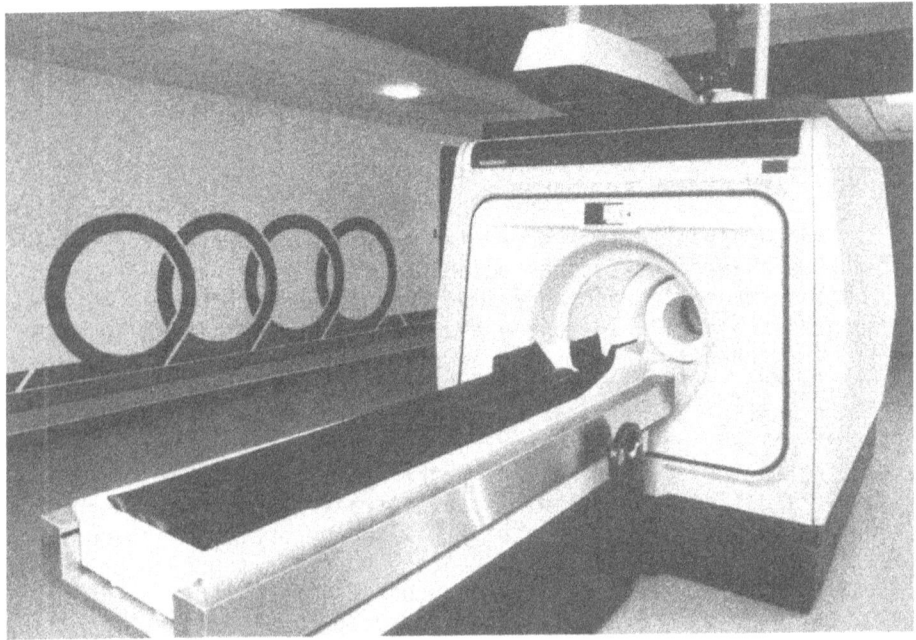

Figure 1. MRI system. A. Photograph of 0.5 Tesla superconducting total body scanner, Technicare, Solon, Ohio, USA.

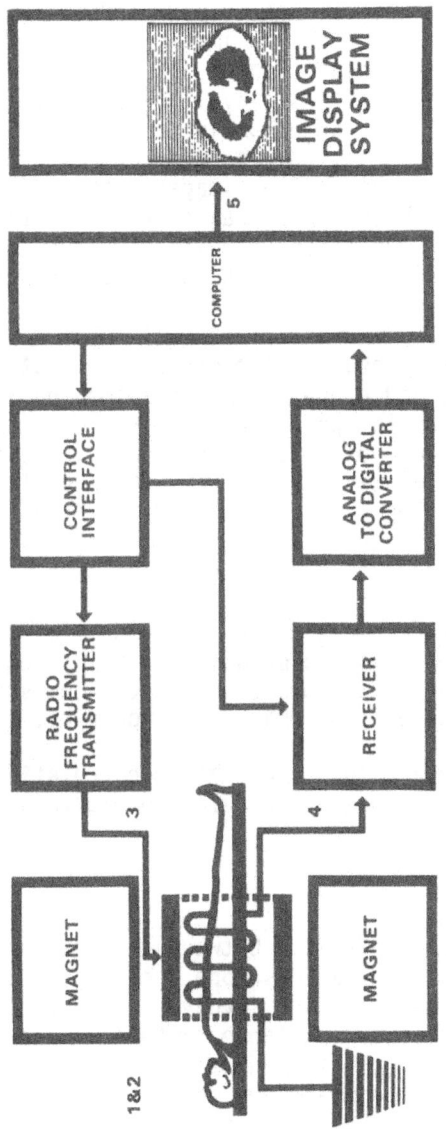

Fig. 1B. Schematic diagram

CORRELATIVE IMAGING

The clinical correlation of multiple imaging modalities is increasingly important because of the accelerating complexity of instrumentation and because of the growing pressures of government control which demand optimal use of high technology based medical diagnostic equipment. Today's imaging instrumentation allows the generation and presentation of diagnostic images based upon information not previously available by alternative techniques and with less risk to the patient. These images tend to be quantitative, tomographic, thin section and, sometimes, dynamic, high-resolution magnification images without ionizing radiation or any known adverse biological effect. In addition, there is an unprecedented explosion of multiformatted digital images which must be displayed, reviewed, and appropriately archived and retrieved.

Many pressures come to bear in the proper application of computer based, complex, and expensive medical imaging instrumentation. There is the need to appropriately distribute this equipment in ways that are medically, economically, socially, and politically feasible. Beyond that, there is the need for continuing research and development in spite of significant limitations of funding bases for these investigations. It is also abundantly clear that cooperative teams of physicists, engineers, computer scientists, physiologists, biochemists, and physicians are and will be required to realize the full potential of the newer metabolic functional imaging modalities including, in particular, magnetic resonance imaging, single photon emission computed tomography, and positron emission tomography.

Following are example cases illustrating correlative principles of magnetic resonance imaging in relationship to other imaging modalities.

Nuclear Medicine

An intriguing comparison exists between conventional radioisotope imaging and the newer radioisotope techniques of SPECT and PET and that of MRI because each involves quantitative functional imaging using isotopes: unstable isotopes in the first case and stable isotopes in the second case. In particular, there is a special opportunity to compare and correlate the pathophysiological significance and metabolic/biochemical basis for imaging in magnetic resonance imaging and positron emission tomography. These two modalities are described by some as the only true physiologically based imaging modalities and are already generating significant new data providing fresh insights into disease processes and response to therapeutic modalities (1, 2).

One disease process in which conventional nuclear medicine and magnetic resonance imaging have teamed together in a study of relative sensitivity and specificity is the orthopaedic problem of avascular necrosis of the femoral head. Multiple centers are evaluating the relative role of these modalities in this entity. There is continuing debate about whether MRI or nuclear medicine is more sensitive for the diagnosis of AVN. Most investigators claim that MRI is more sensitive. In our experience, nuclear medicine has been more sensitive in two cases out of ten. Figure 2 illustrates an abnormal coronal MRI view through the femoral heads in pediatric and adult patients with avascular necrosis in this region. The bone scan was also abnormal in this region. Another example of the correlation of nuclear medicine and MRI is in the evaluation of the single "cold" palpable nodule and is shown in Figure 3.

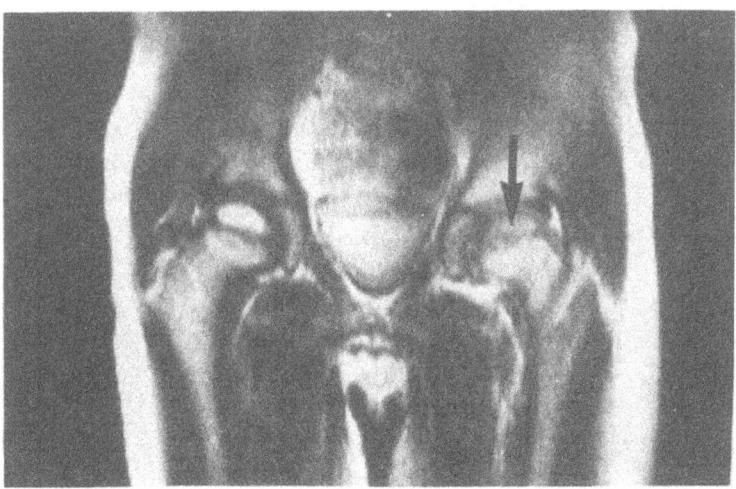

Figure 2. Avascular necrosis left femoral head (arrow), coronal MRI, SE 30/500. A. Pediatric patient.

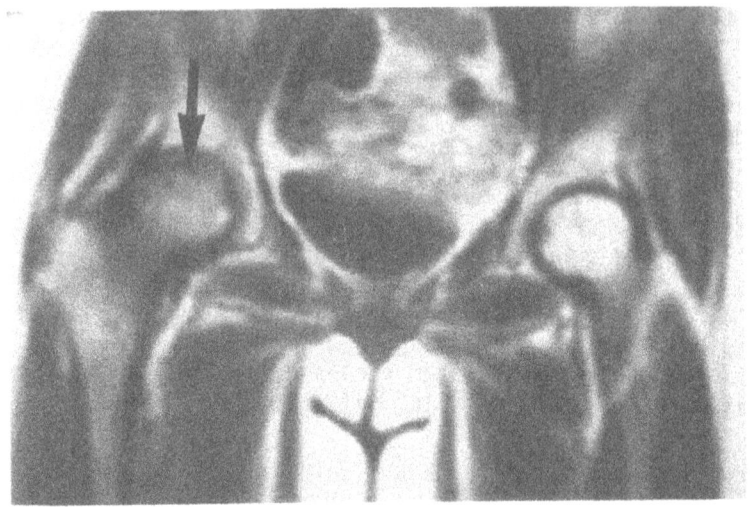

Fig. 2B Adult patient.

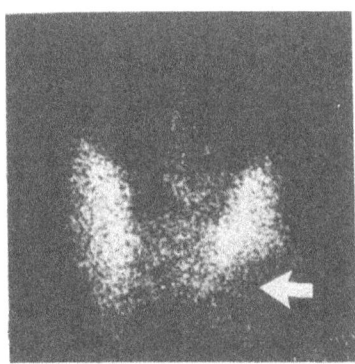

Fig. 3 Single "cold" thyroid nodule, adenoma.
A. Technetium 99m pertechnetate thyroid scan "cold" nodule (arrow).

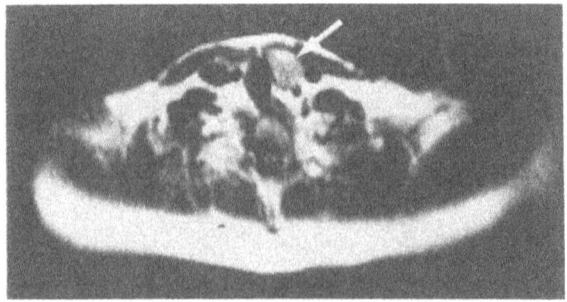

Fig. 3B Transverse MRI, 30/500.

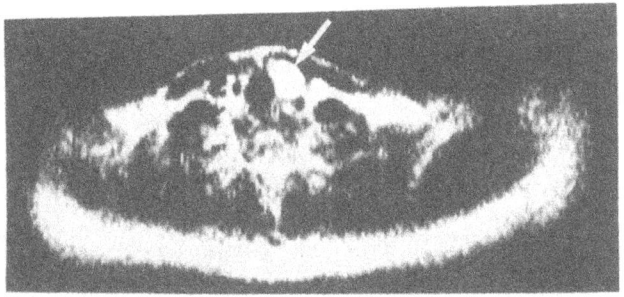

Fig. 3C   Transverse MRI, SE 120/1000.

A patient with renal cell carcinoma is imaged in Figure 4 with comparison of nuclear medicine, x-ray computed tomography, and magnetic resonance imaging. Superior anatomical resolution is provided in the coronal plane by MRI. Additional functional imaging capability may be added in the future with dynamic contrast enhanced renal MRI using a bolus injection of Gd-DTPA which is handled 100% by glomerular filtration.

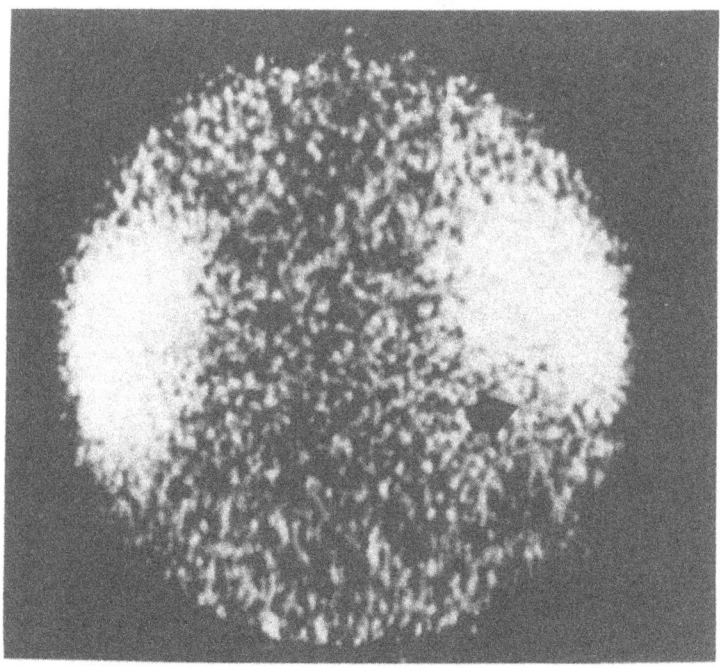

Figure 4.   Renal cell carcinoma, right kidney. A. Nuclear medicine renogram, I-131 hippuran.

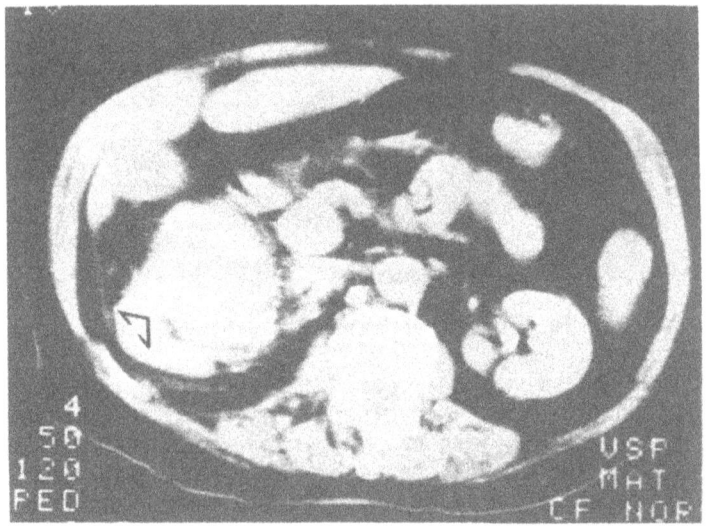

Fig. 4B X-ray computed tomography, contrast enhanced.

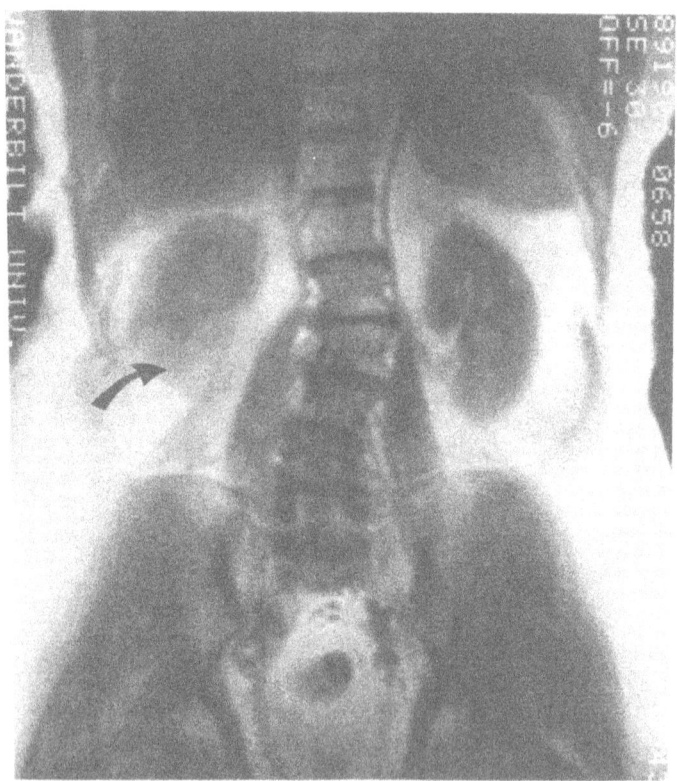

Fig. 4C Coronal MRI, SE 30/500.

Brain tumors may be imaged with exquisite anatomical detail at any viewing angle as is illustrated in Figure 5, where nuclear medicine and MRI are compared. Metastatic breast carcinoma to the L-4 vertebral body was imaged by nuclear medicine bone scan and further characterized by MRI sagittal image, Figure 6.

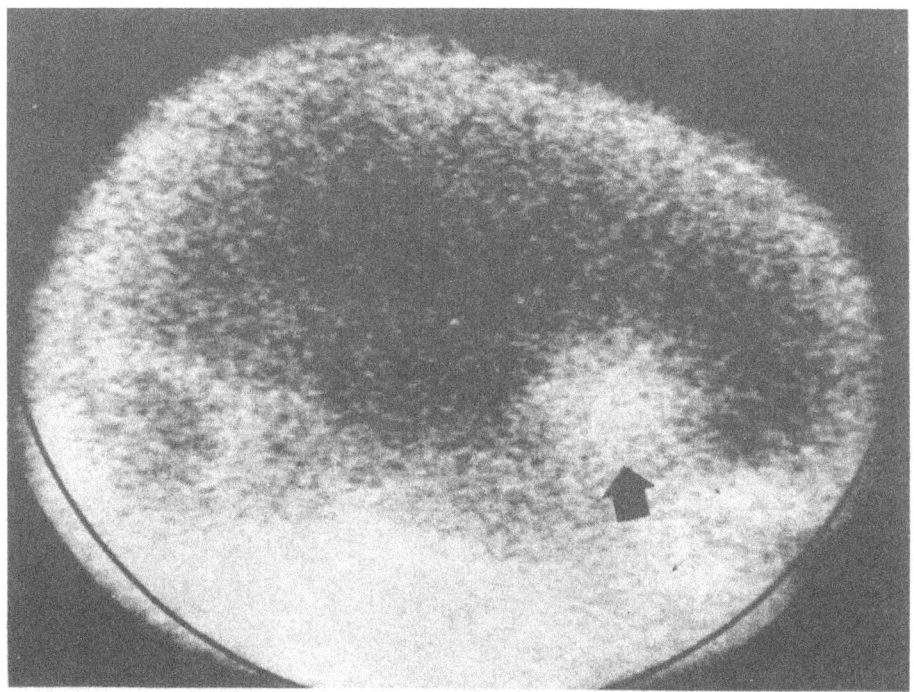

Figure 5. Brain tumor, schwannoma, 5th cranial nerve.
A. Nuclear medicine with Tc-99m gluco-heptonate, tumor (arrow).

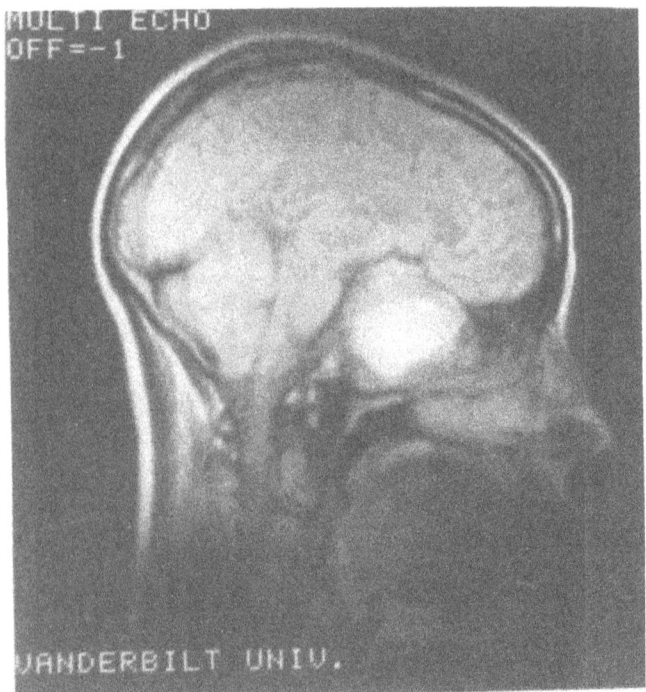

Fig. 5B

Sagittal MRI, SE 60/1000.

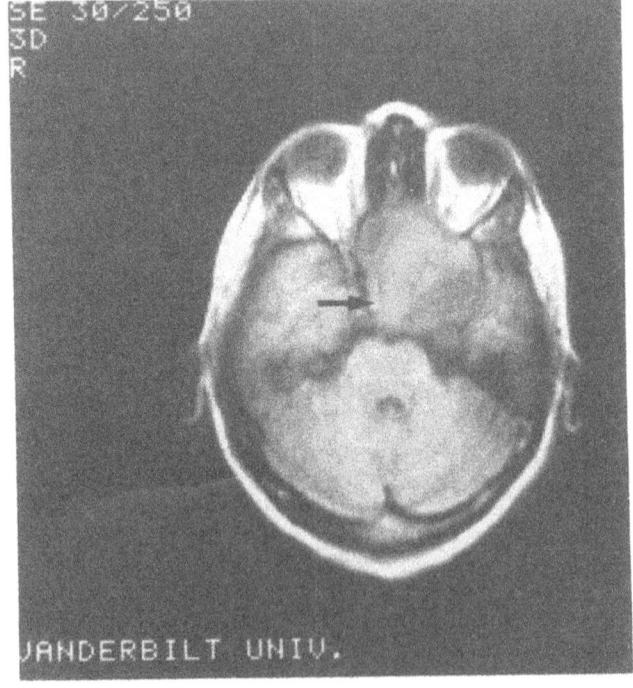

Fig. 5C

Transverse MRI, SE 30/250.

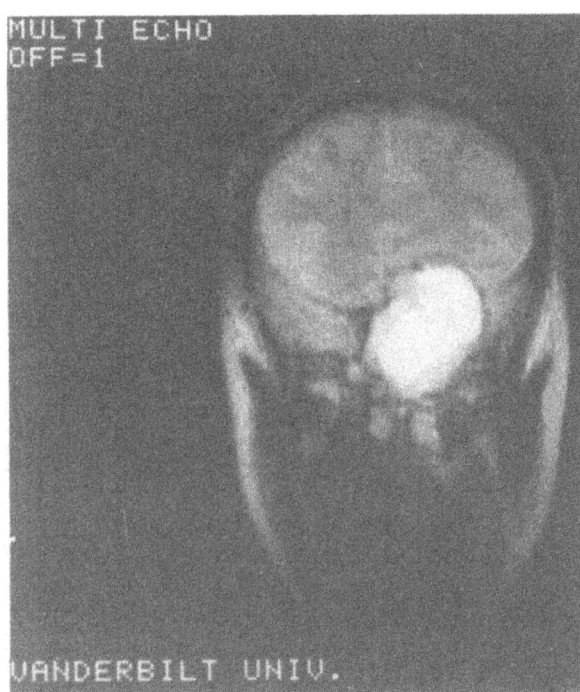

Fig. 5D

Coronal MRI,
SE 120/1000.

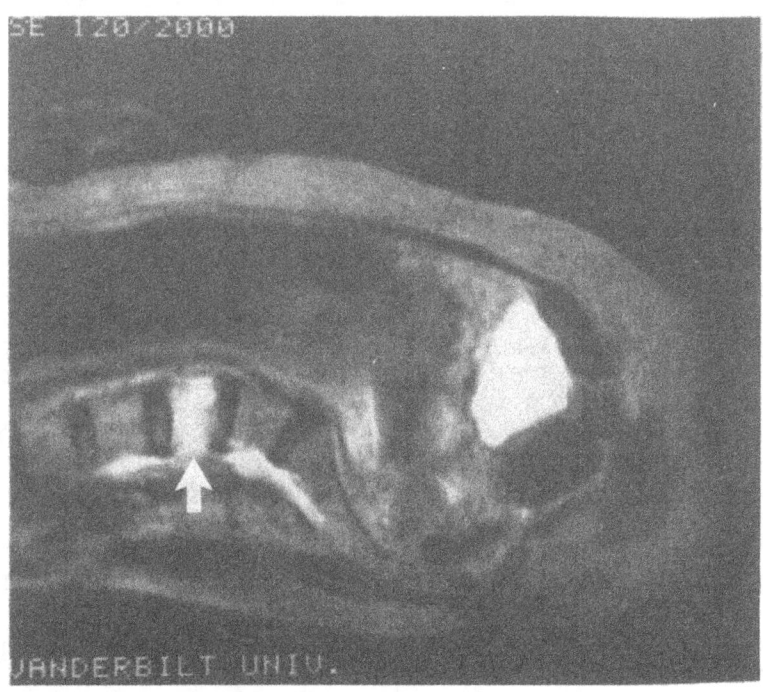

Fig. 6 Metastatic breast carcinoma to L-4. A. Sagittal MRI,
SE 120/2000, L-4 metastatic lesion (arrow).

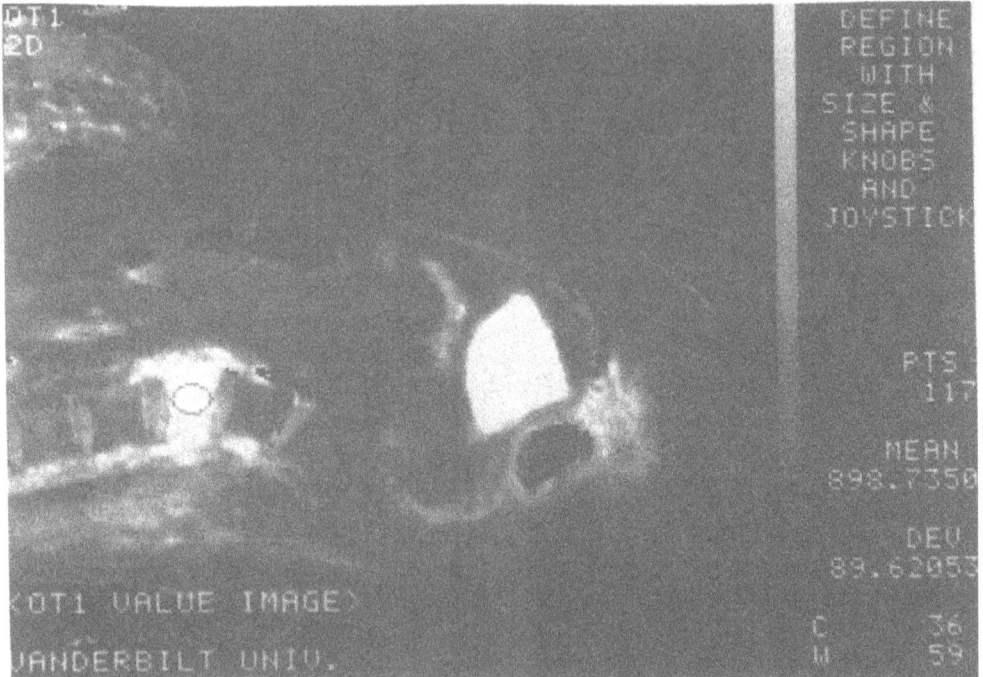

Fig. 6B Calculated T1 MRI sagittal image with average T1 elevated at 899 msec.

Ultrasound

The absence of ionizing radiation and ease of utilization make both ultrasound and magnetic resonance imaging attractive modalities from the viewpoint of patient safety. Clinical areas of potential correlative imaging include the evaluation of cystic structures and the evaluation of intrauterine pregnancy. Ultrasound and MRI comparative studies of breast disease are in progress in multiple centers (3,4). An example case of a normal breast by MRI surface coil imaging is illustrated in Figure 7. One clinical area where MRI appears possibly more sensitive than ultrasound is in the detection of placenta abruptio illustrated in Figure 8. A coronal MRI of third trimester intrauterine pregnancy is shown in Figure 9. Example application areas in MRI studies of the pregnant patient include: a) placental insufficiency; b) placenta abruptio; c) pelvimetry; d) intrauterine fetal anomalies; e) assessment of fetal subcutaneous fat in intrauterine growth retardation; and f) assessment of fetal lung maturity.

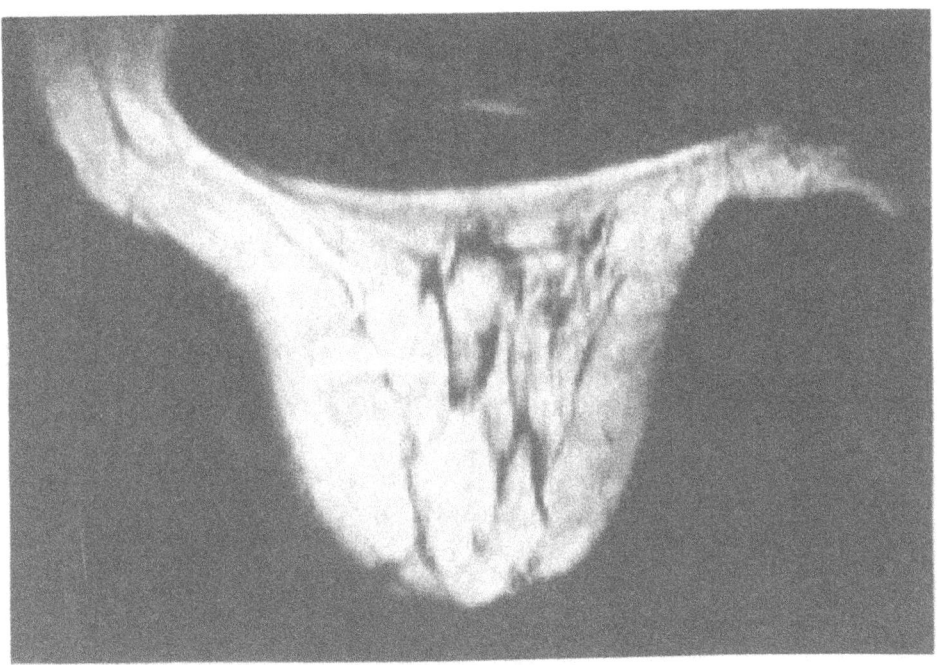

Fig. 7 Normal breast, MRI surface coil image, SE 30/250, 0.5 cm slice thickness.

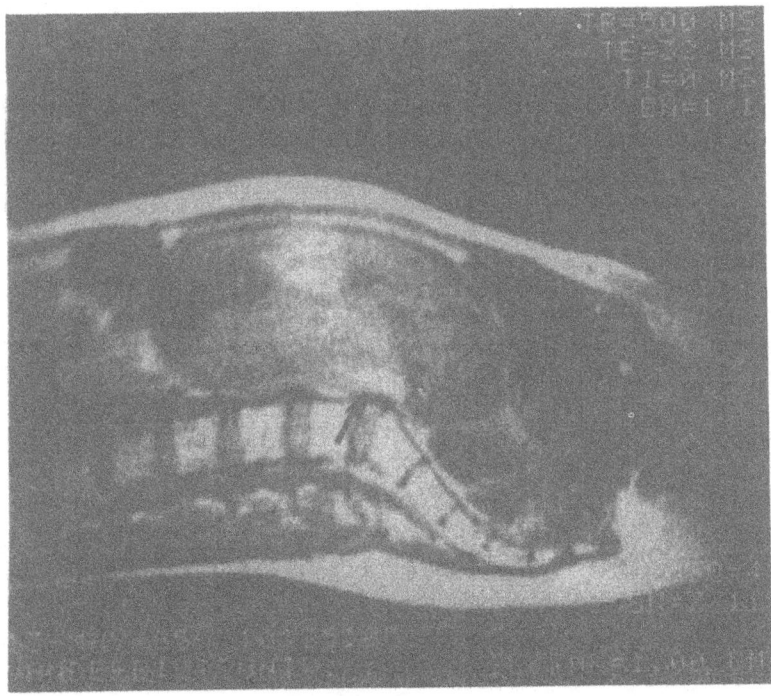

Fig. 8 Placenta abruptio, hematoma (arrow), MRI sagittal, SE 32/500

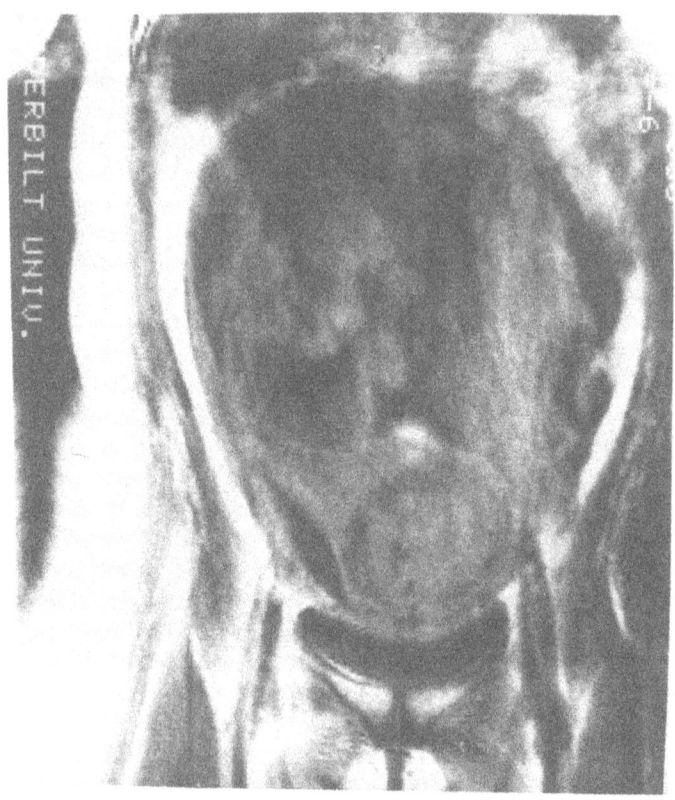

Figure 9. Normal third trimester pregnancy. Single fetus, vertex presentation. Coronal MRI image, SE 30/500.

Mammography

Complementary roles are apparent in the evaluation of breast masses using conventional mammography and MRI (4, 9). A benign adenoma is illustrated in Figure 10, and a carcinoma in Figure 11. MRI demonstrates excellent soft tissue sensitivity in a breast composed primarily of fat, but initial results are disappointing if the breast tissue has significant fibrocystic disease.

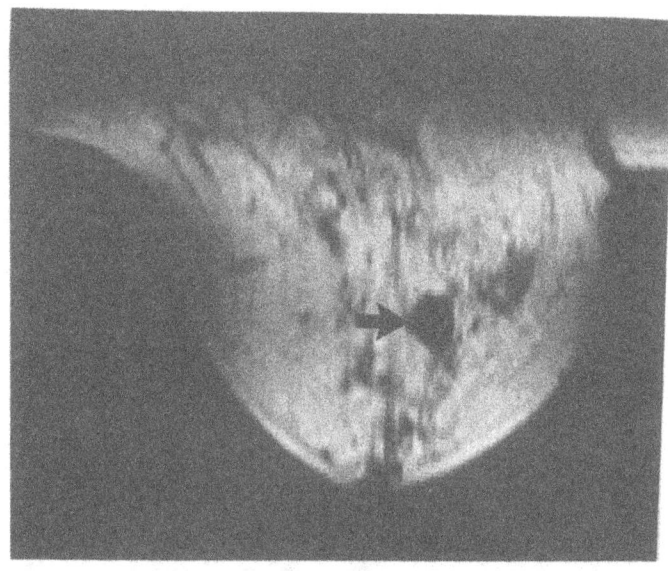

Figure 10 Benign breast adenoma (arrow), MRI transverse, surface coil, SE 30/500.

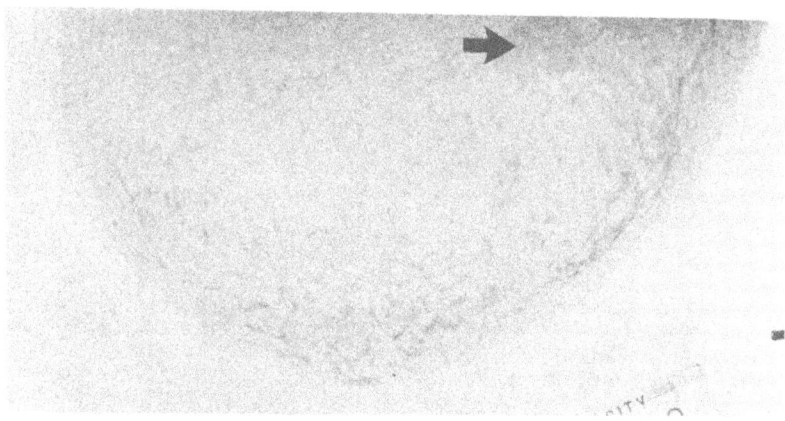

Figure 11 Carcinoma of the breast (arrow). A. Craniocaudad mammogram, mass (arrow).

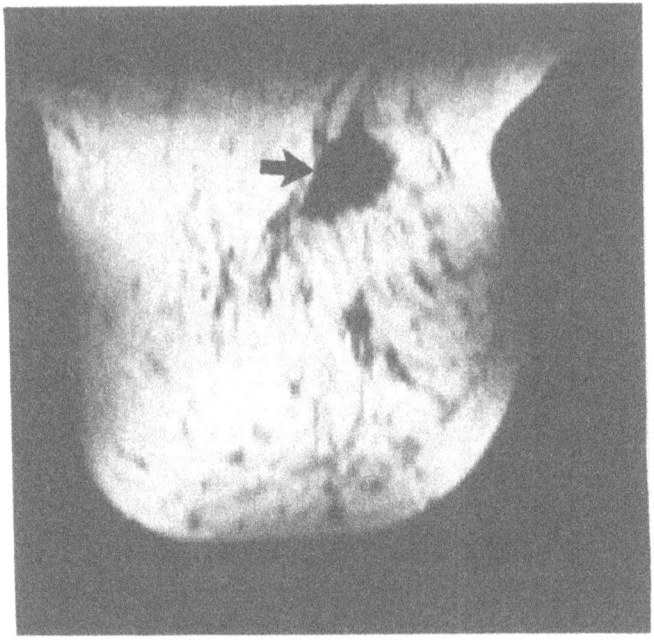

Figure 11B Transverse MRI, surface coil image, tumor (arrow), SE 30/250.

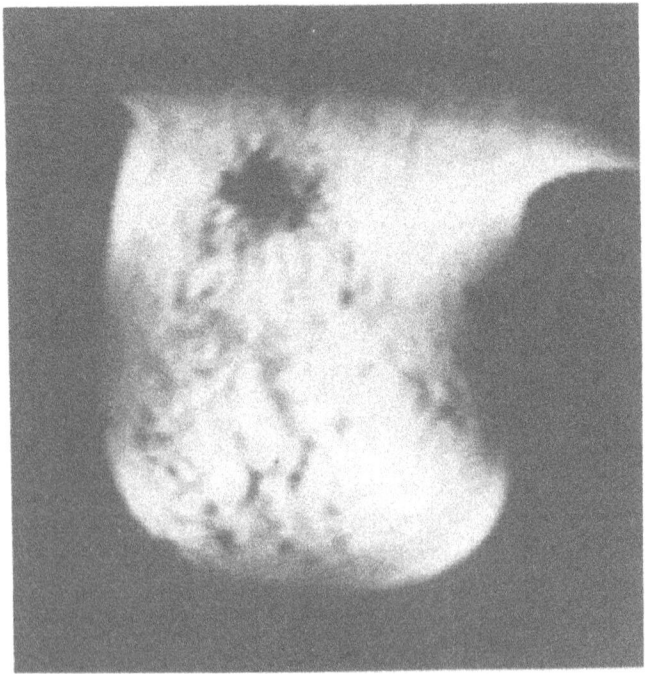

Figure 11C Sagittal MRI, SE 30/250.

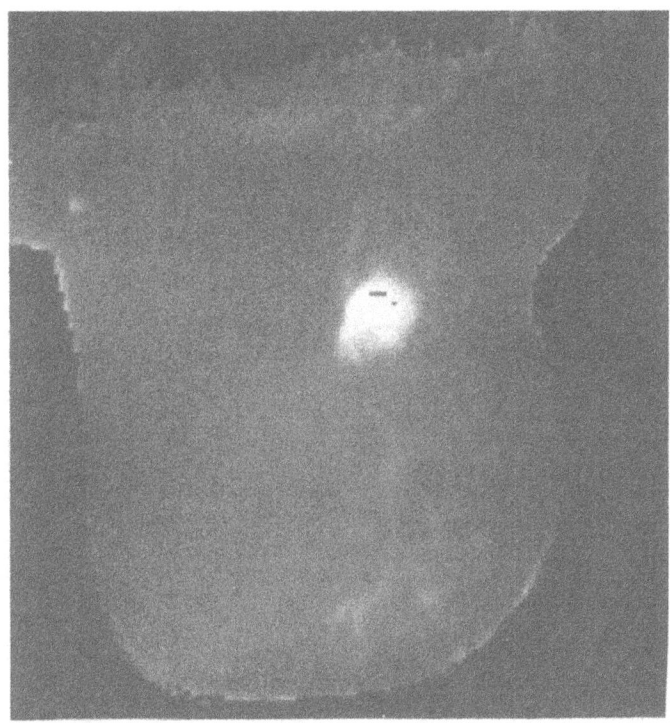

Figure 11D Transverse calculated T1 image. Tumor has elevated T1=670 msec, significantly greater than adjacent fat.

Computed Tomography

The tomographic imaging capability in the transverse plane of computed tomography has been equalled in most parts of the body, except the mesentery and bowel, using magnetic resonance imaging. This position is likely to be solidified with the recent developments in MRI of contiguous thin-slice, multislice, multiecho imaging where slice thickness now approaches 1 mm. This presumes that there are no contraindications for magnetic resonance study where obviously CT would be required. These contraindications include cardiac pacemaker and aneurysm clip.

The continuing evolution of relative roles of CT and MRI is actively under investigation at multiple centers (5,6). It is our view that most moderate sized community hospitals and, certainly, medical centers need x-ray computed tomography as the first tomographic imaging modality with high anatomical resolution. Beyond that, the second tomographic unit probably should be magnetic resonance imaging because of the metabolic and biochemical basis for imaging which is possible with this technique.

A comparison of MRI and CT in primary brain tumor is shown in Figure 12. The coronal image was not available by CT. Normal spine in coronal view is shown in Figure 13. Midline sagittal imaging in a child with meningomyelocele and a multicompartmental syringomyelia is shown in Figure 14. A myelogram and CT were not needed in this case.

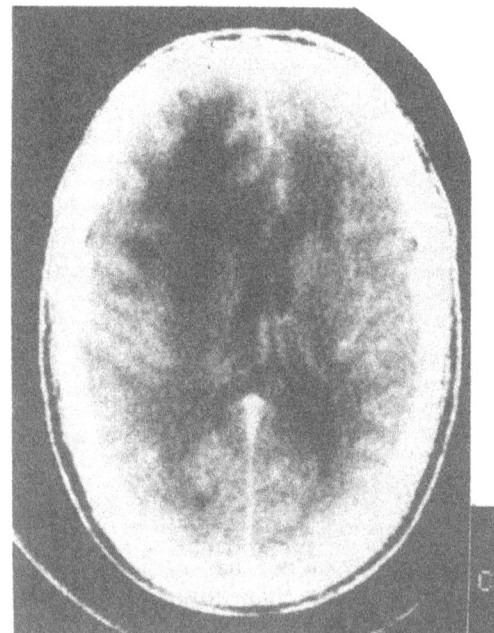

Fig. 12 Glioma. A. CT non-enhancing mass.

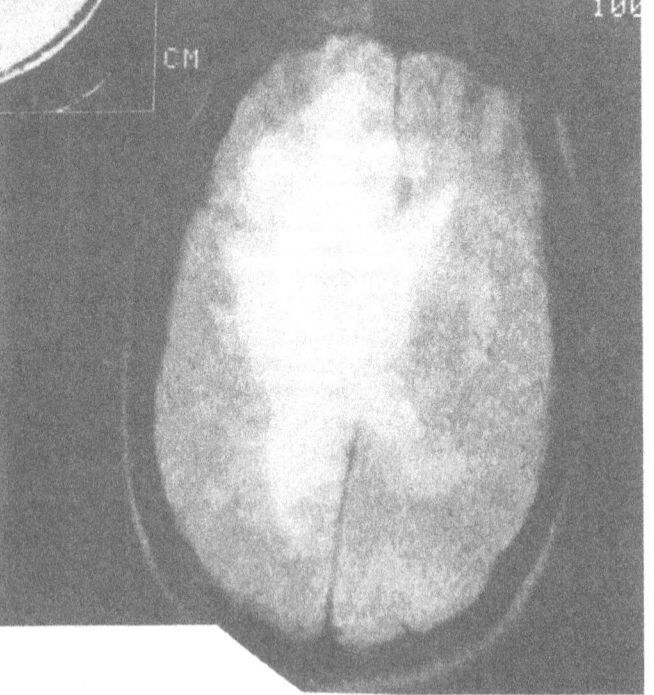

Fig. 12B MRI transverse, SE 120/2000.

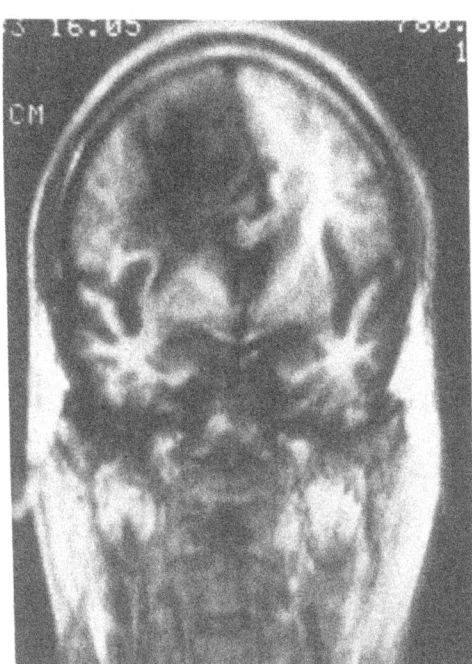

Fig. 12C MRI coronal, inversion recovery, 30/450/1500.

Fig. 13 Normal spinal cord visualized to the conus medullaris.

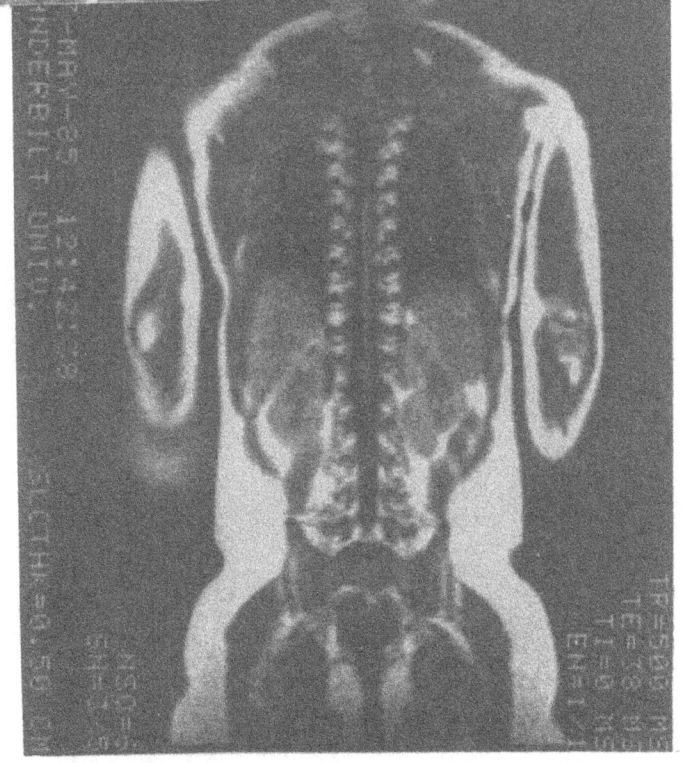

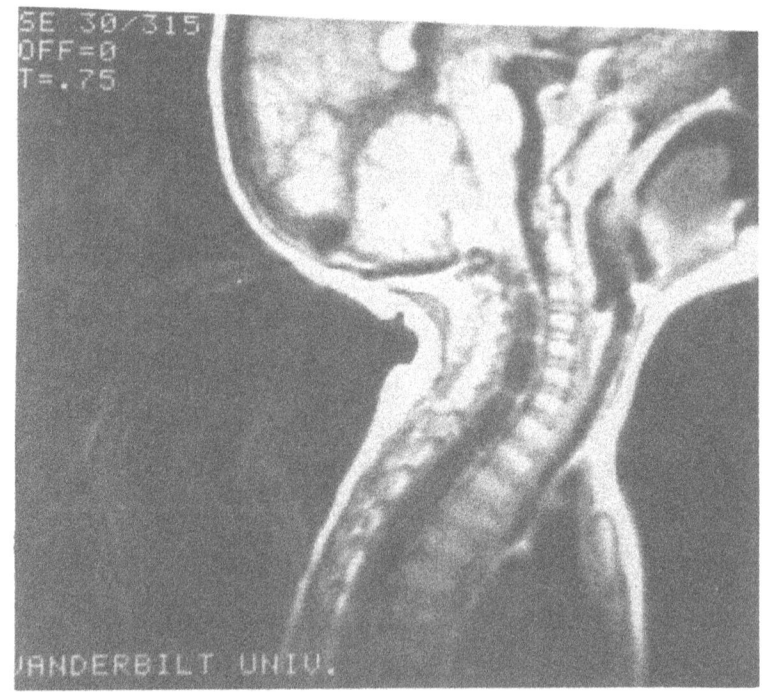

Fig. 14 Meningomyelocele with tethered cord (arrow) and syrinx.
A. Sagittal MRI, cervical spine, SE 30/315.

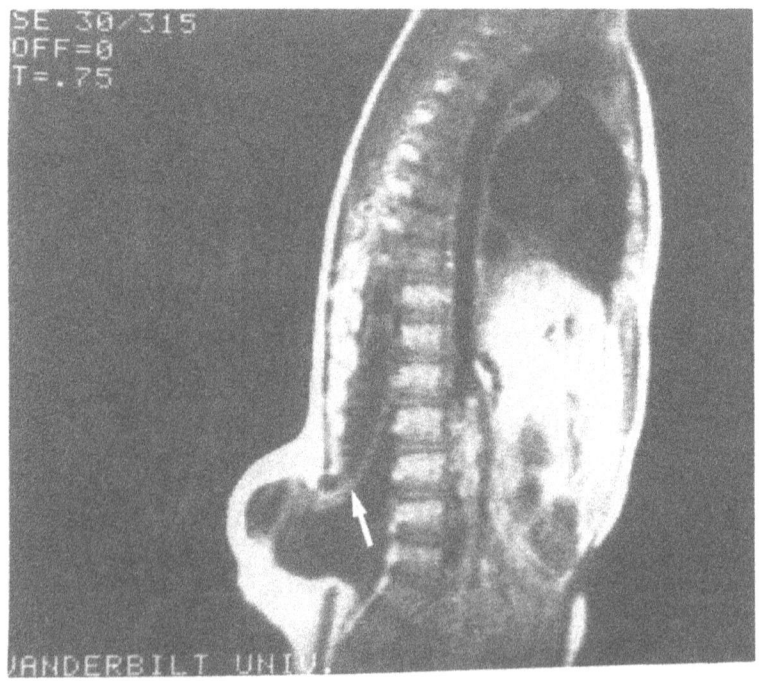

Fig. 14B Sagittal MRI, lumbar spine, SE 30/315.

Fig. 14C   Sagittal MRI, lumbar spine, SE 90/2000.

The dramatic soft tissue contrast for the abnormal plaque of multiple sclerosis in a patient with a negative CT is illustrated in Fig. 15. Other recent results in patients with neurological disease include a cystic astrocytoma, Fig. 16; recurrent craniopharyngioma, Fig. 17; acoustic neuroma, Fig. 18; and Arnold Chiari malformation, Fig. 19.

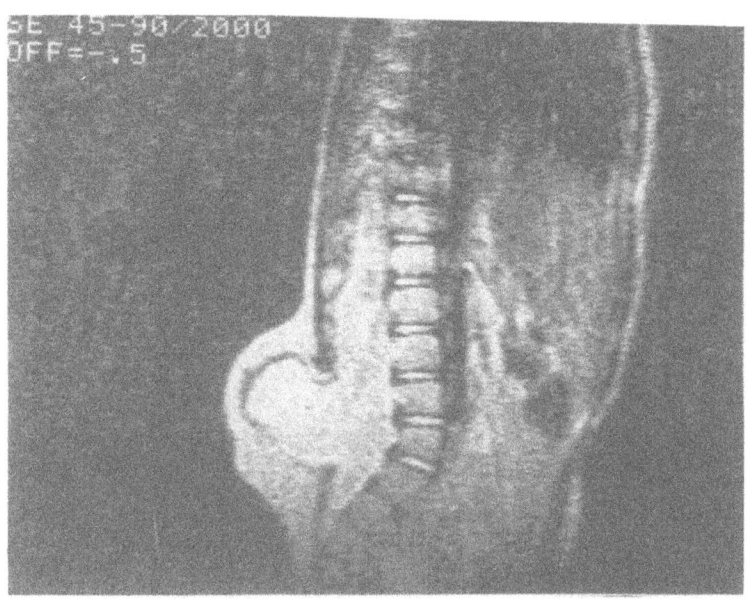

Fig. 15 Multiple sclerosis. Abnormal plaques have increased intensity (see arrows for typical abnormalities). Transverse MRI, SE 120/1000.

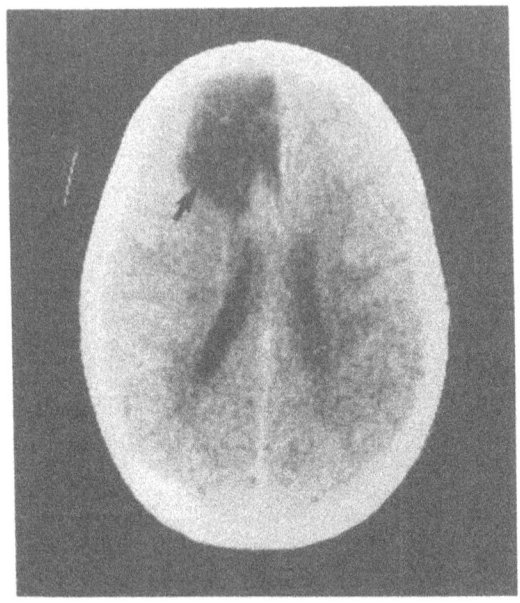

Figure 16. Cystic astrocytoma, right frontal lobe.
A. Contrast enhanced CT.

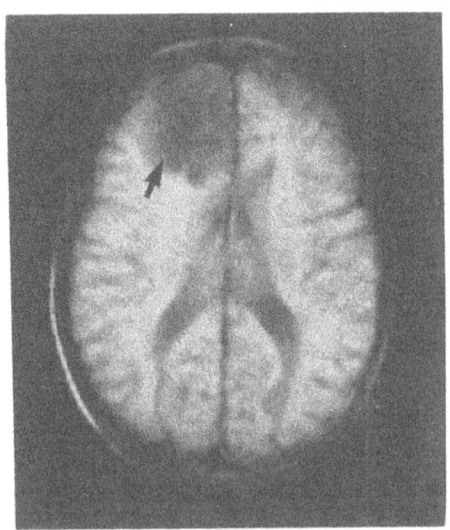

Fig. 16B   Transverse MRI, SE 30/500.

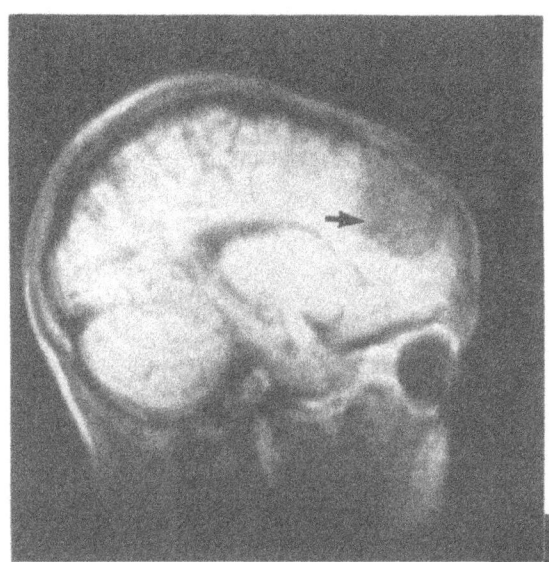

Fig. 16C Sagittal MRI, SE 30/500.

Fig. 16D Transverse MRI, SE 120/1000.

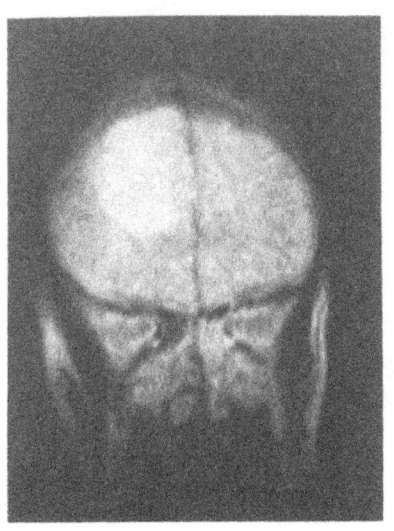

Fig. 16E Coronal MRI, SE 120/1000.

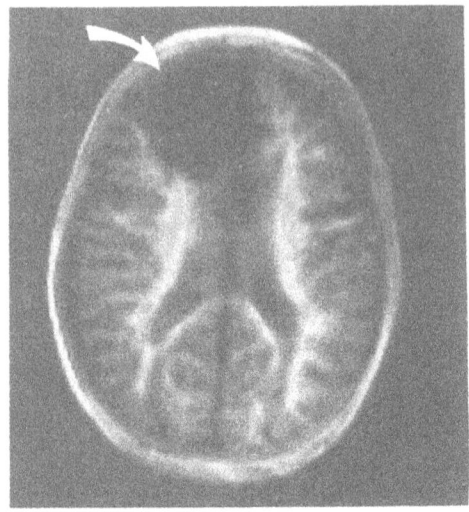

Fig. 16F   Transverse MRI, IR 30/450/1500.

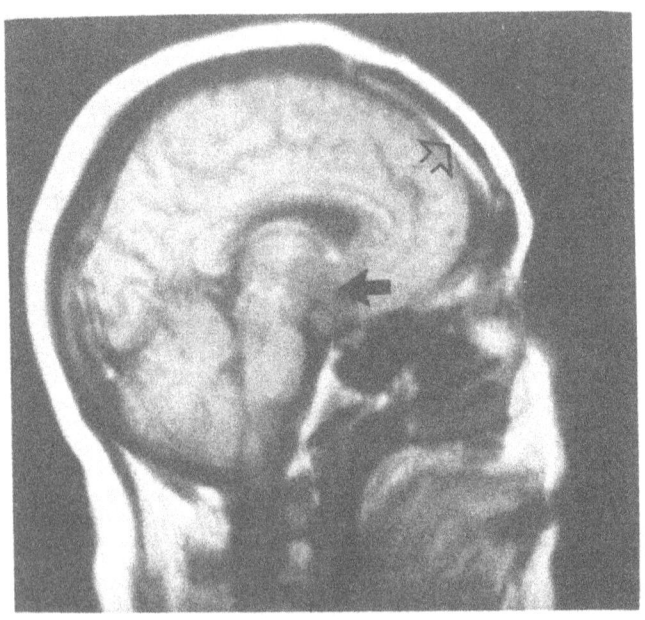

Figure 17. Recurrent craniopharyngioma. A. Sagittal MRI, SE 30/500, tumor (closed arrow), subdural hematoma (open arrow).

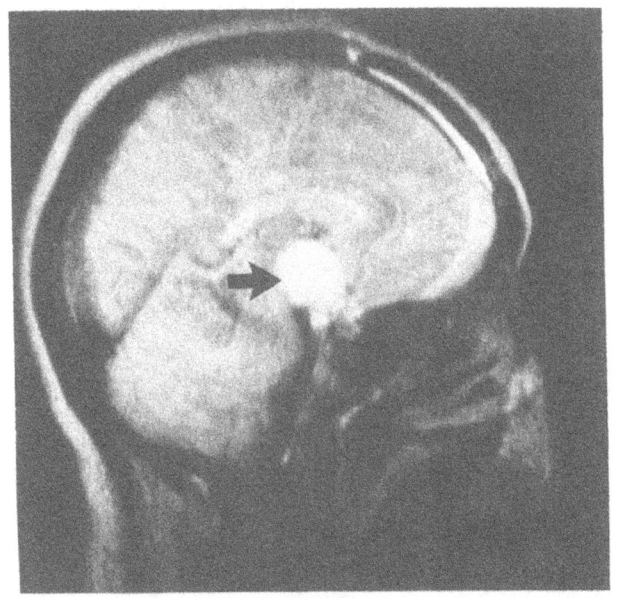

Fig. 17B   Sagittal MRI, SE 120/1000.

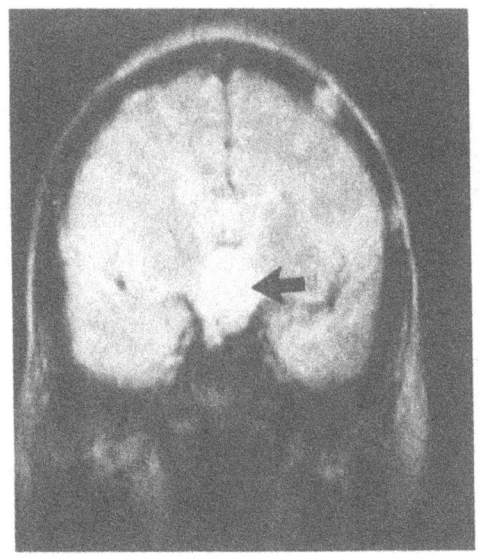

Fig. 17C   Coronal MRI, SE 120/1000.

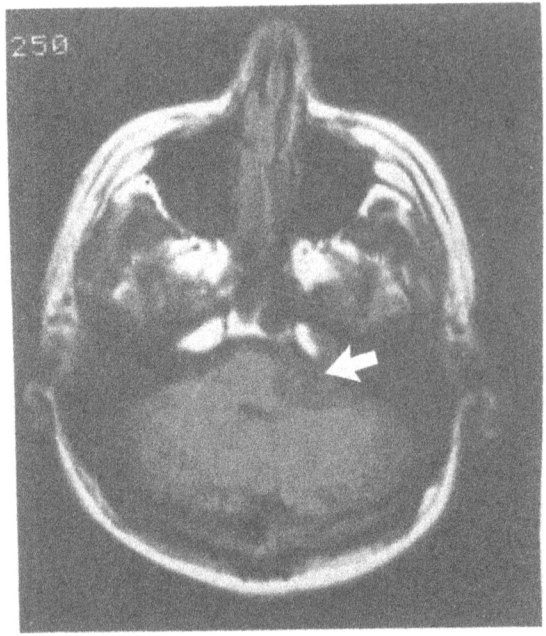

Figure 18. Acoustic neuroma. A. Transverse MRI, SE 30/250, tumor (arrow).

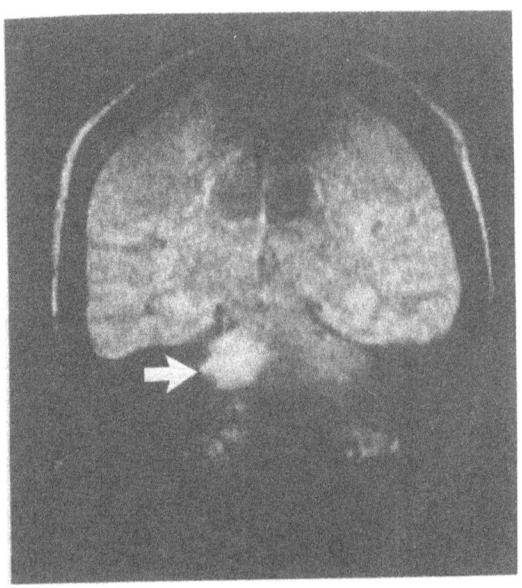

Figure 18B Coronal MRI, SE 120/1000, tumor (arrow).

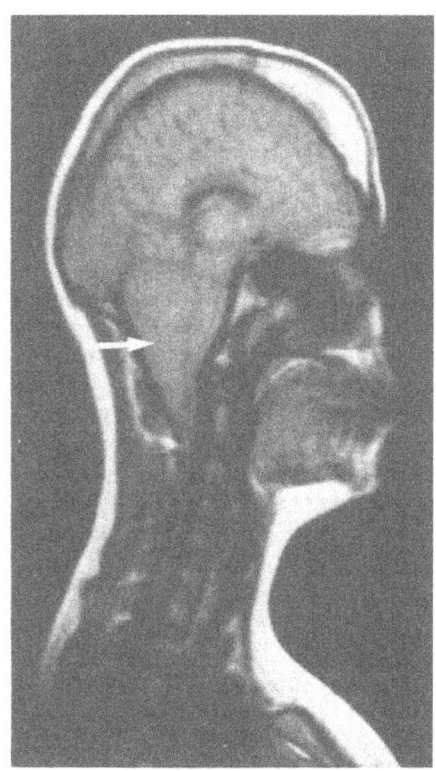

Fig. 19 Arnold Chiari malformation.

A. Sagittal MRI, SE 30/500.

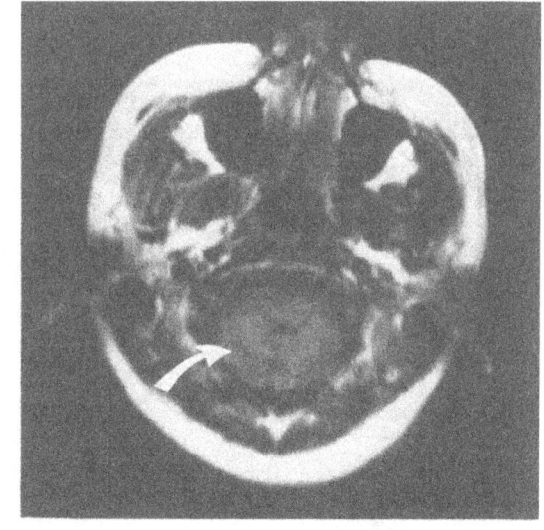

Fig. 19B Transverse MRI, SE 30/500.

Cardiac gated MRI results from patients with diseases of the thorax include lymphoma with mediastinal mass (Figure 20), coarctation of the aorta (Figure 21), pericardial cyst (Figure 22), repaired tetralogy of Fallot with right sided aortic arch (Figure 23), and single cardiac ventricle (Figure 24). It is apparent that thoracic MR imaging with cardiac gating is superior to CT in evaluating mediastinal masses, major vessels, and cardiac anatomy. Functional imaging of the myocardium will be considerably enhanced by the further development of thin section, oblique, and cine-mode imaging with the supplementary data from in vivo NMR spectroscopy at high field strengths using C-13, Na-23, and P-31 as complementary information to hydrogen (proton) MR imaging.

MRI clinical results in the abdomen include patients with Wilm's tumor, right kidney (Figure 25), and polycystic kidneys (Figure 26). Limited utility has been demonstrated in imaging of the bowel and mesentery due to peristaltic motion. However, the remainder of the abdomen and pelvis may be imaged quite well using MRI techniques.

Surface coil techniques are a powerful new development and provide high resolution magnified images as is illustrated by the orbital image using a 16 cm circular surface coil (Figure 27). Surface coil imaging is already a powerful tool in the evaluation of the entire spine because of the availability of thin section (1 mm) magnified imaging coupled with the full range of pulse sequence selection and resulting soft tissue contrast. Great potential exists for additional application of surface coils to joints, arteries, the orbit, the fetus, the breast, the scrotum, gated cardiac studies, and in vivo NMR spectroscopy.

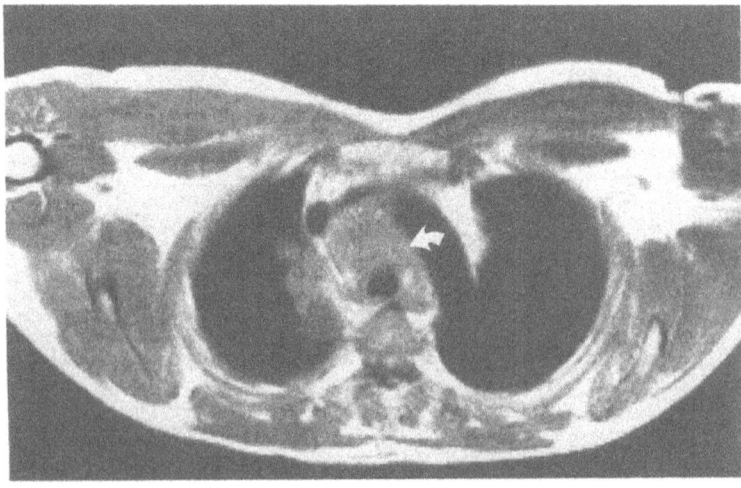

Figure 20. Lymphoma with mediastinal mass (arrow). Transverse MRI, SE 30/500.

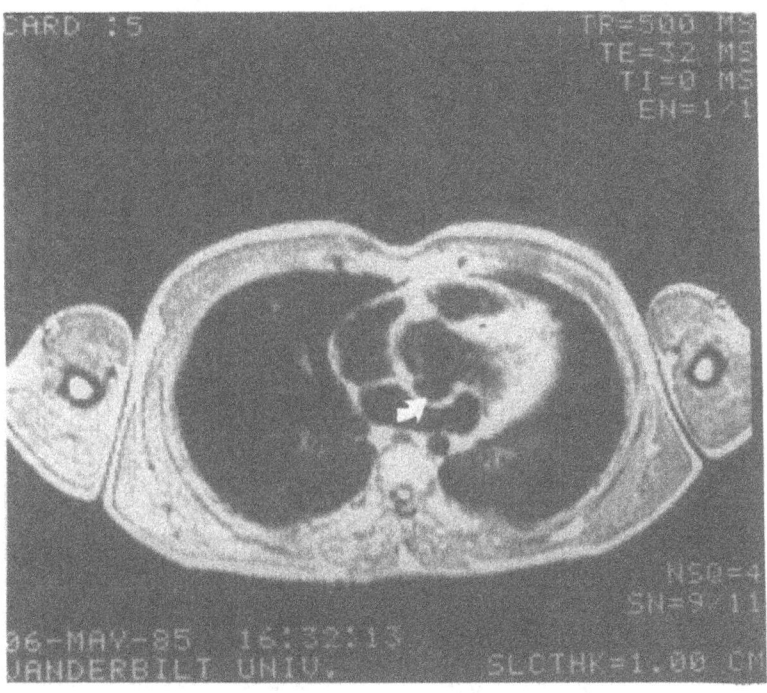

Fig. 21 Coarctation of the aorta. A. Cardiac gated transverse MRI, SE 30/500.

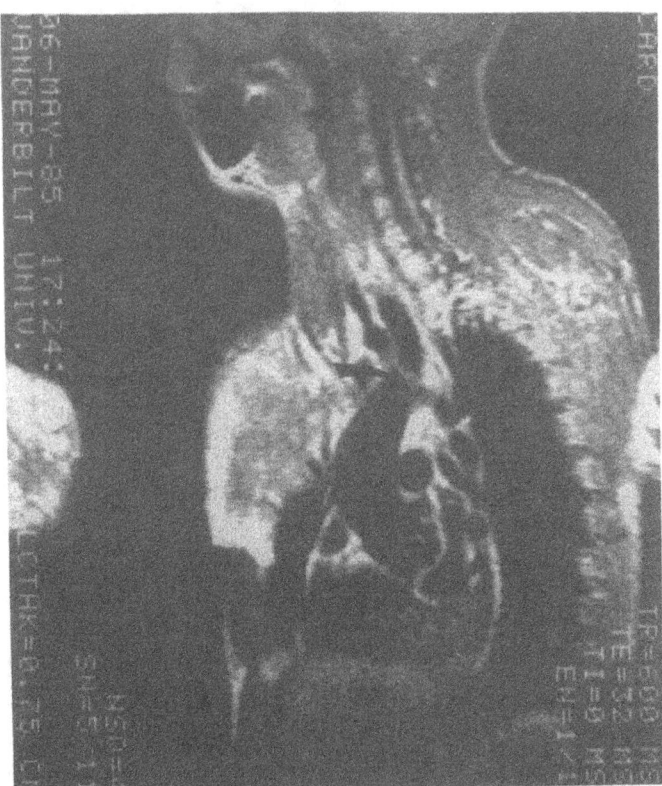

Fig. 21B

Cardiac gated oblique MRI, SE 32/500, arrow at coarct.

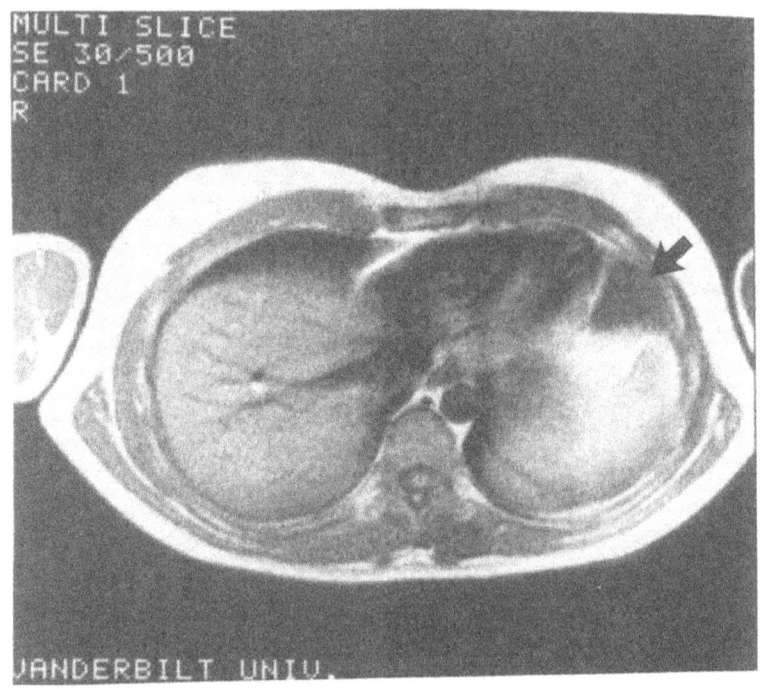

Fig. 22 Pericardial cyst (arrow), cardiac gated transverse MRI, SE 30/500.

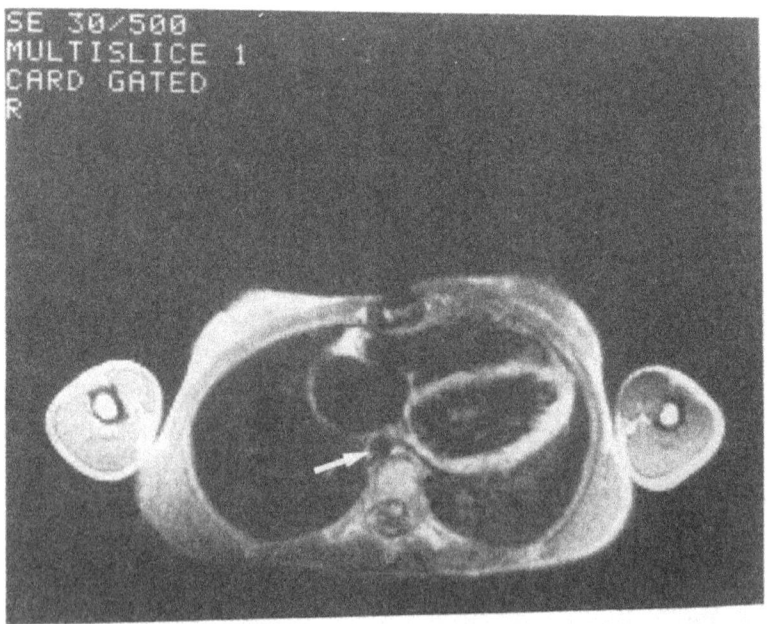

Fig. 23 Surgically repaired tetralogy of Fallot with right sided aortic arch (arrow). Gated transverse MRI, SE 30/500.

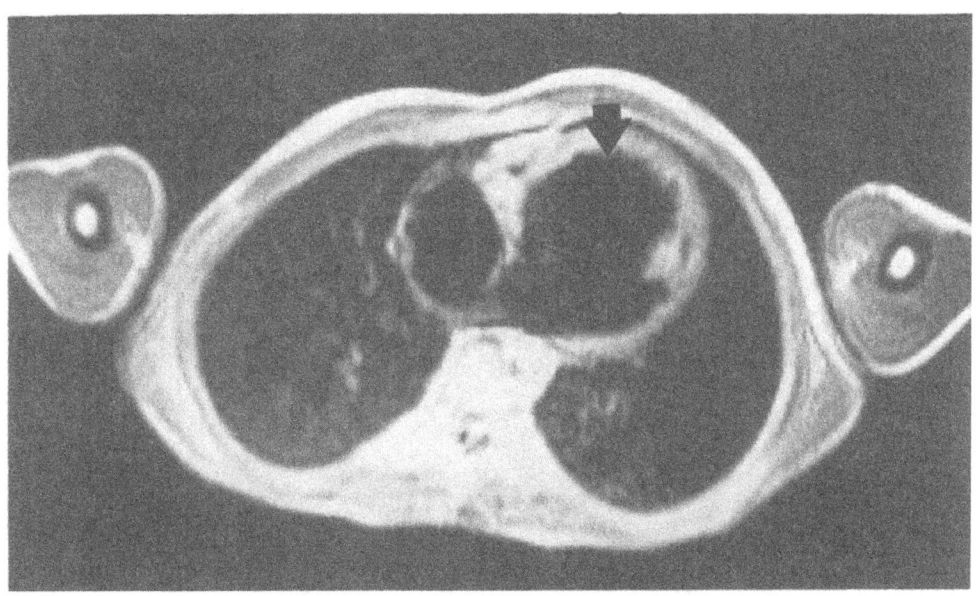

Figure 24. Single cardiac ventricle, gated transverse MRI, SE 30/500.

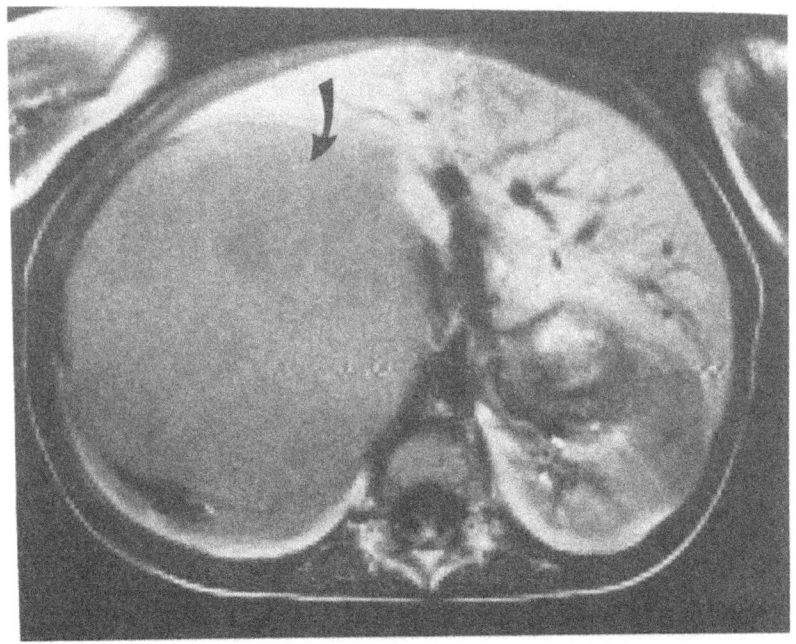

Figure 25. Wilm's tumor in child. A. Transverse MRI, SE 30/500, tumor (arrow).

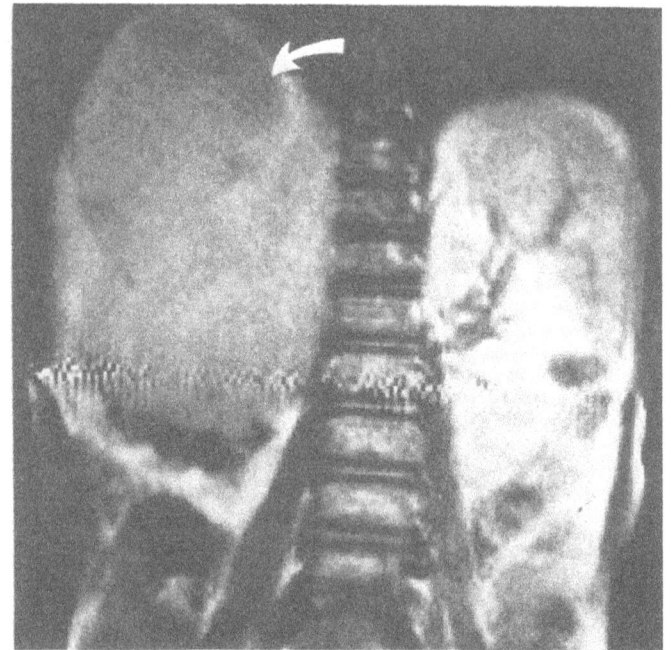

Fig. 25B Coronal MRI, SE 30/500, tumor (arrow).

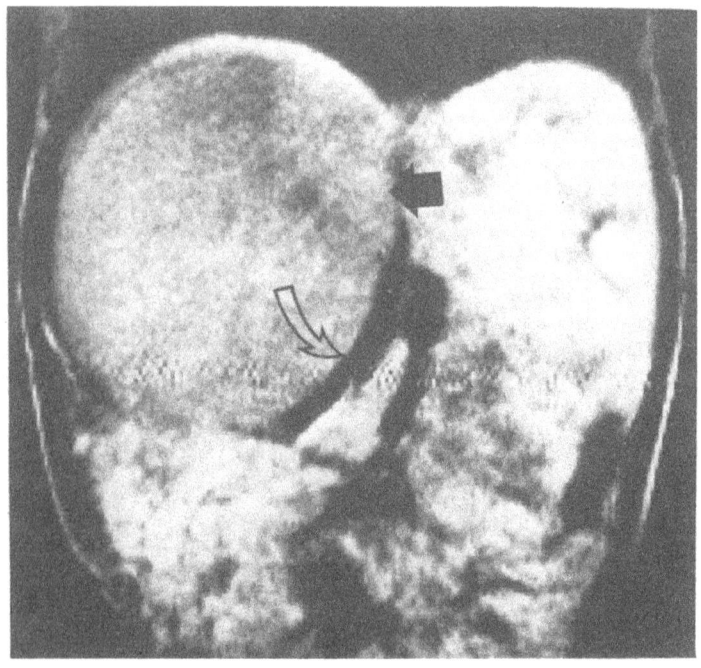

Fig. 25C Coronal MRI, SE 120/1000, tumor (closed arrow), deviation inferior vena cava (open arrow).

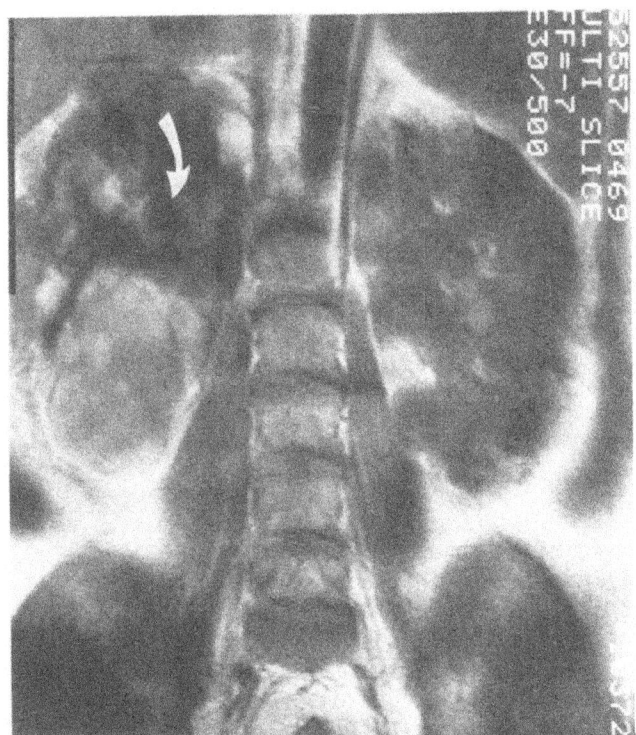

Figure 26.
Polycystic kidneys.
A. Coronal MRI,
SE 30/500, cyst
(arrow).

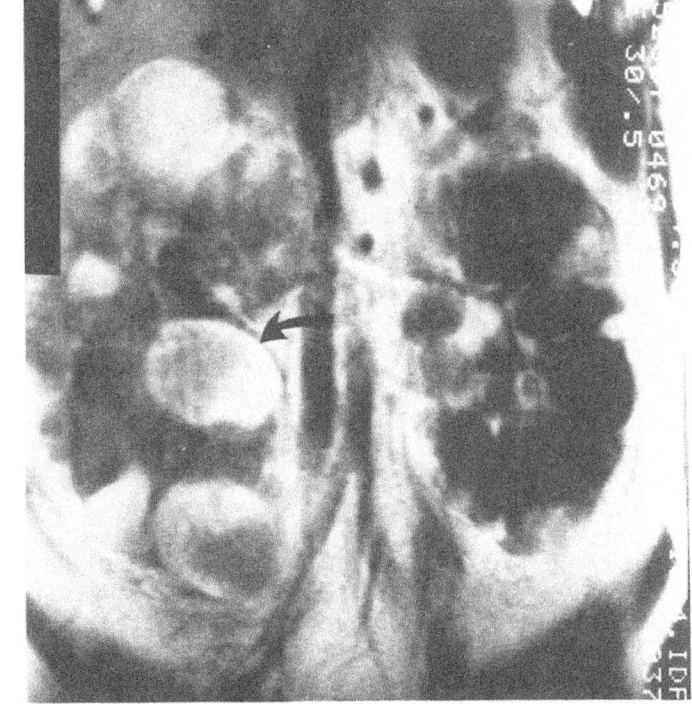

Fig. 26B

Coronal MRI,
SE 30/500,
hemorrhagic
cyst (arrow).

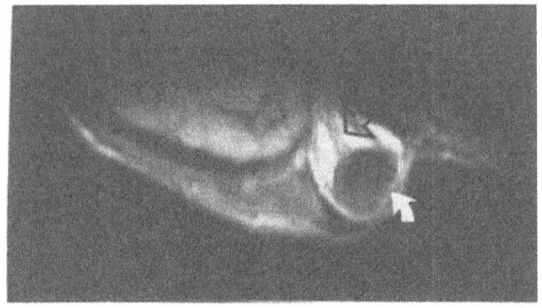

Figure 27. Normal orbit, surface coil, thin section 0.5 cm, SE 30/250, lens (closed arrow), optic nerve (open arrow).

CONCLUSION

Tomographic, thin-section, quantitative, dynamic medical imaging is revolutionizing once again the diagnostic tools of the physician. Magnetic resonance imaging is evolving as a powerful modality which is the first line of defense in several entities in patients who can tolerate an imaging procedure taking several minutes in the evaluation of such diseases as intracranial mass and spinal cord abnormality (7,8). Tomographic viewing at multiple angles allowed by MRI lends itself very well to correlative imaging with other modalities including functional nuclear medicine and anatomic images from CT and ultrasound (10-1

Acknowledgments

Acknowledgment is made of the editorial assistance of Margaret Moore, the photographic assistance of John Bobbitt, and the technical assistance of Jill Craig and Oscar Wolfe.

REFERENCES

1. Brownell GL, Budinger TF, Lauterbur PC, McGeer PL. Positron tomography and nuclear magnetic resonance. Science 215, 4533: 612-626 (1982).

2. Kulkarni MV, Sandler MP, Shaff MI, Jones JP, Patton JA, Partain CL, James AE. Clinical magnetic resonance imaging with nuclear medicine correlation. J Nucl Med 26(8) (1985).

3. Cole-Benglet C, Soriano R, Pasto M et al: Solid breast mass lesions: Can ultrasound differentiate benign & malignant? In Jellins J and Kobayashi T (eds): Ultrasonic Examination of the Breast. New York, John Wiley & Sons (1984).

4. Partain CL, Kulkarni MV, Cook LT et al: Nuclear magnetic resonance imaging of the breast: Functional T1 and three dimensional imaging. In Adams D (ed): Nuclear Magnetic Resonance Imaging: A Special Issue, Cardiovascular and Interventional Radiology, Vol. 8 (1985).

5. Stark DD, Moss AA, Goldberg HI, et al: Magnetic resonance and CT of the normal and diseased pancreas: A comparative study. Radiology 150 (1):153-162 (1984).

6. Dooms GC, Hricak H, Crooks LE et al: Magnetic resonance imaging of the lymph nodes: Comparison with CT. Radiology 153 (3):719-728 (1984).

7. Margulis AR, Higgins CB, Kaufman L and Crooks LE: Clinical Magnetic Resonance Imaging. San Francisco, Radiology Research & Education Foundation, UCSF (1984).

8. Partain CL, James AE, Rollo FD and Price RR: Nuclear Magnetic Resonance (NMR) Imaging. Philadelphia, W.B. Saunders Co. (1983).

9. El Yousef SJ, Duchesneau RH, Alfidi RJ et al: Magnetic resonance imaging of the breast. Radiology 150:761 (1984).

10. Sandler MP, Patton JA, Partain CL: Clinical Thyroid Imaging. Norwalk, CT, Appleton-Century-Crofts (1985).

11. Sandler MP, Patton JA, Kulkarni MV, Shaff MI, Partain CL: Nuclear Medicine, Magnetic Resonance, and Correlative Imaging Modalities. Baltimore, William & Wilkins Co. (1986).

12. Partain CL, Price RR, Patton JA, Kulkarni MV and James AE Jr: Nuclear Magnetic Resonance (NMR) Imaging, 2nd Edition, Vol I & II. Philadelphia, W.B. Saunders Co. (1986).

SESSION ON PRINCIPLES AND APPLICATIONS OF NUCLEAR MAGNETIC RESONANCE IMAGING

DISCUSSION

M. Waller:

How many snapshot images were used to produce your computed T_1 maps?

P. Mansfield:

In our T_1 procedure we usually take 32 images in a given plane. Half of these are taken with a repetition period of 200 ms, the remaining half with a longer period of 1.4 s. The total procedure takes about 30 s per slice.

S. Petersen:

Do you think that it will also be possible to obtain T_2 information in echo-planar imaging, realizing that gradient switching has a different impact on the phase of stationary, diffusing, perfusing and flowing spins?

P. Mansfield:

In regions where there is bulk flow, the measurement of T_2 by EPI is likely to be rather difficult. However, in static regions we believe that T_2 will be measureable. Of course, the EPI gradients will complicate matters and 'T_2' will possibly include some diffusion component. However, my feeling is that diffusion effects are relatively small..

S. Petersen:

Could you use the chemical shift imaging method to compensate for the inherent inhomogeneities in the magnetic field?

What was the maximum gradient strength and dB/dT used?

Have you tried calculating the ejection fraction in the cardiac studies?

P. Mansfield:

The EPSM technique can be used to compensate for magnet inhomogeneities.

The maximum gradient strength used was 0.5 G cm^{-1} and dG/dT = 200 T $m^{-1}s^{-1}$.

We have not tried calculating the cardiac ejection fraction but it is planned.

R. Guzzardi:

The comparison of the heart cross-sectional images should be with X-ray, CT fast tomography and not with digital readiology which is a 2D technique.

P. Mansfield:

Yes, I believe this would be a better comparison since digital radiology produces projection images whereas we are, of course, producing three dimensional images.

A. Todd-Pokropek:

What are the FDA regulations about NMR/MRI in obstetrics?

P. Mansfield:

I do not know what the FDA regulations are. However, I can say something about the NRPB guidelines. These have been prepared for NMR imaging in Britain. In foetal scanning the general rule is that it is alright to scan within the first trimester provided that the foetus is subsequently aborted. In late pregnancies there seems to be no problem. In addition to satisfying the NRPB guidelines it is also clearly necessary in Britain to obtain permission from the local Ethical Committee.

PART IX APPLICATIVE PROBLEMS AND FUTURE DIRECTIONS OF NMR FOR IN VIVO STUDIES

Chairman: Peter Mansfield (U.K.)

STATE OF THE ART MAGNETIC RESONANCE IMAGING

Joseph D. Weissman, M.D., Ph.D.

Technicare Magnetic Resonance Clinical Research Program

Solon, Ohio

In less than a decade Magnetic Resonance Imaging (MRI) has evolved from a laboratory demonstration to a safe and effective technique for clinical diagnosis. This evolutionary process continues. At this time 2-D and 3-D imaging of the head and body is firmly established in clinical use. Surface coil imaging, two-component chemical shift imaging, in-vivo spectroscopy and flow imaging are currently in various stages of development.

The present state of the art of MRI is a function of an array of technologies: magnet, Rf coil, Rf pulse amplifier, gradient coil and driver, pulse programmer, A/D converter, computer system architecture, array processors and mass storage (both magnetic and optical). The overall product design is the result of a complex process which balances the advantages and disadvantages of each component for optimal system performance and flexibility. The design of a MRI system is a great technical challenge, since there are many interactions between the components. The overall result must be tested by use in the clinical setting.

I will discuss the organization of a state-of-the-art MRI system. Several examples of the kinds of system interactions affecting design choices will be given. At the conclusion some of the exciting imaging methods now in advanced development will be mentioned.

One fact is and will remain constant: all MRI devices must have strong magnets large enough to admit the area of the body to be imaged and be of sufficient homogeneity for imaging applications. For H-1 imaging this translates into several tens of parts per million (ppm) across the useful portion of the magnet bore. For spectroscopic applications the requirements are much more stringent: the homogeneity over one voxel must be 1/2 or so of the desired chemical shift resolution - in absolute terms 0.1 ppm (H-1 chemical shift spectroscopy/imaging).

There are three types of magnets in current use: permanent, resistive and superconductive. Permanent magnets (PM) have been used in MRI and magnetic resonance spectroscopy (MRS) applications for many years. Their chief advantage is low cost of operation as they require neither cryogens nor large amounts of electricity. PM's are limited in field strength and are subject to small fluctuations in magnetic field which can be difficult to correct. They are also impossible to shut off, which may pose certain safety problems. The weight and cost of the 100 tons of magnetic material for a whole body MRI is the greatest drawback for PM's. The potential of PMs for specialized limited field of view MRI scanners is intriguing.

Resistive magnets (RM) have been used in MRI and MRS applications for over 30 years and currently operate at maximum field strengths of 0.15T to 0.25T for whole body systems. Their field strength and operating cost are determined by energy dissipation (heating) in the magnet coils. A temperature-stable coil cooling system is essential for optimum operation. Magnetic field homogenity suitable for MRI (or MRS in analytical scale instruments) is achieved. Resistive MRI scanners are currently the most cost-effective and easiest to site MRI units. Some available resistive units are 1/2 the cost of superconducting units.

Superconducting magnets for MRI applications are air- core solenoids and can attain the highest field strengths. These magnets are very uniform and stable since they are wound with fine superconducting wire, run at constant temperature and require no power supply. The maximum available field strengths for these magnets (currently available 1 m bore magnets have fields in excess of 2.0 T) probably exceed that which is optimal for whole body proton imaging. The question of optimal magnetic field strength is complex and the most contentious one in MRI.

The optimal magnetic field strength for H-1 MRI depends on the area to be imaged, required resolution, motion effects and siting considerations. A multiplicity of assumptions about the significance of signal, noise, contrast, interpreter perception, chemical shift, pathological changes, imaging time, operational characteristics, and energy deposition are also involved.

The simplest approach to the optimal field question examines signal and noise without any of the considerations of imaging, i.e., on the same terms as for "analytical" MRS of small, homogeneous liquid samples. In the case of MRS of such samples it has been found that performance improves with field strength to the 1.0 to 1.5 power. In MRI various considerations, as discussed below, limit the improvement of performance to the 1.0 or less power of field strength.

The additional interactions required for MRI and the need to study "samples" as large, inhomogeneous and "nonideal" as the human body make higher magnetic fields relatively less attractive than they would be in MRS. These additional imaging-related interactions represent design challenges in some cases and absolute physical limits in others.

The gradient pulses used for spatial encoding in spin-warp imaging induce eddy currents in surrounding conductive loops. Eddy currents interfere with the imaging process by altering the effect of the gradient pulses and distorting the signal phase within the imaged volume. These loops may be within any structure of the magnet assembly: gradient coils, shim coils, Rf coils, magnet housings, magnet windings or the patient transport system. This represents a considerable design challenge. Eddy currents can be alleviated with the use of passive shimming and other similar measures. Although eddy current interactions are present during operation at all field strengths, at high field strengths their interactions are more of a problem because stronger gradients are needed to suppress chemical shift artifacts.

The excitation phase of the MR process involves exposure of tissue to radiofrequency magnetic fields and the deposition (conversion to heat) of a fraction of this radiation via inductive and capacitive (dielectric) interactions. This energy deposition increases with the square of the operating frequency or magnetic field. This amount of energy is much greater than that absorbed due to magnetic resonance. Measurements made at 1.5T confirm that Rf energy deposition in multi-slice multi-echo operations can exceed the current US FDA Rf energy deposition guidelines. If operation of a system at 1.5T, for example, is restricted such that current guidelines are not exceeded, then the relative performance of the "high" field system is reduced compared to that of a low-field system.

A further complication of operation at high fields is the phenomenon of "chemical shift artifact", the formation of separate fat and water images along the frequency encoded axis. The water and fat components are nearly superimposed on each other at low fields. The separation of the water and fat images increases proportionately with field strength, provided that all other operational parameters are maintained constant. This chemical shift artifact is an unwelcome form of information in the image. At 1.5 T the water and fat separation is several image pixels wide and could affect image interpretation. The chemical shift artifact can be overcome by increasing gradient strength. This increases the system bandwidth but signal power remains constant. The S/N decreases proportionately as a result. If the chemical shift artifact is maintained constant over field strength with increased gradient strength, then the S/N advantage of higher fields is largely lost. A better approach is to either accept chemical shift artifacts or to select the water or fat component (as described below) and display the image without artifacts.

While Rf energy deposition is a potential safety problem, particularly in undervascularized, sensitive tissues such as the lens of the eye, another safety factor related to field strength is a more immediate concern. To my knowledge no individual has been injured by a ferromagnetic object drawn into the magnetic field of a MR imager in a clinical setting. Nonetheless, there have been a number of serious industrial accidents involving personnel working on large magnets (the majority of which are permanent or electromagnets used for metal separation). Thus the potential exists for "ballistic" interactions with any MR imager. The energy of these interactions increases with the square of the magnetic field strength until the ferromagnetic object is fully saturated. After this point the ballistic kinetic energy increases proportional to the field strength.

In our clinical experience with a number of MRI systems operating at 0.15, 0.3, 0.6 and 1.5T it appears that the 1.5T images, in areas such as the head (and possibly other areas of detailed anatomy which are not subject to physiological motion) seem "prettier" than their low field counterparts when the images are made under comparable conditions. Controlled clinical evaluations suggest that this difference in appearance does not reveal itself in the increased detection of lesions, assuming comparable efforts are made to optimize operation at each field strength.

Magnetic Shielding

The installation of a MRI system requires that magnetic field intensity be at or below a certain level in nearby areas where public access cannot be controlled or sensitive devices are installed. In such situations magnetic shielding is required.

There is no magic to magnetic shielding, contrary to general expectations. It is basically the precisely engineered placing of ferromagnetic material around the magnet to shorten the flux return path. The amount of ferromagnetic shielding material required is roughly a linear function of the magnet field strength and largely independent of the shield shape or distance from the magnet. A flexible approach to shielding is best, using only the minimum shielding necessary to accomplish the task. Thus one wall adjacent to a restricted area may be shielded with a single plate of ferromagnetic material. For uniform contraction of the field profile a three or four sided mirror shield is an effective design, combining ease of magnet servicing and low cost of construction.

Gradient System

The gradient system of a MRI system applies spatially linear magnetic field gradients to the imaged volume during MR signal evolution. This causes the phase of spins at different coordinates to differ from each other in a predictable way, hence the terms "phase encoding" and "spatial encoding". As we shall see, more than space can be encoded for in MRI. The maximum span of phase encoding over the observed area must be less than 180 degrees, since further spin encoding would cause degeneracy and image rollover.

Phase encoding does not increase the amount of MR

signal available from the sample or patient, it only fractionates the existing signal according to space, velocity, acceleration, etc.. If the resolution of a system is doubled along one axis by doubling the number of phase encoded steps, the signal from each voxel (and the SNR) is halved. To recover this loss in S/N, assuming the rest of the MR system is maintained constant, requires a quadrupling of imaging time.

Phase encoding may be used for more than spatial discrimination. Basically, a gradient pulse with a nth time moment can encode for the nth time derivative of distance. This is consistent since the zeroth time derivative of distance is distance itself. The number of resolved points along the phase encoded axis is determined by the number of gradient steps. Each step of the gradient differs from the previous step by a constant amount. In any case the static and dynamic magnet irregularities must be less than the step between the successive gradient pulses.

The magnetic field gradients applied during signal readout cause the observed resonance frequencies of spins at different locations to differ during readout, hence the term "frequency encoding". Usually the signal is phase detected with a reference signal at the resonance frequency of the system with all gradients turned off. The resolution along the frequency encoded axis is determined by the number of A/D conversions during each acquisition. The maximum frequency encoding of any spin must be less than 1/2 the A/D conversion rate, since further frequency encoding would cause aliasing and image rollover (but along the frequency-encoded axis.)

For both frequency and phase encoding the accuracy of gradients is important. The resolution of the system is not derived from the absolute magnitude of the system gradients but from the ratio of the amplitudes to intrinsic (bulk susceptibility, chemical shift) and extrinsic (magnetic field) inhomogenities. The magnitude of gradients during readout determines signal bandwidth and hence the SNR. Thus optimal resolution is best obtained by using the most homogeneous magnet possible before increasing gradient strengths.

Rf

The Rf coils and associated receivers and transmitters are the "front end" of the MRI system and present some unique technical challenges. With these the signal is created and read out. For transmit functions the most important consideration is spatial uniformity of tip angles within the area to be imaged. Efficiency and quality factor are not as important. On the other hand, sensitivity to the emitted signal is the most important criterion for reception. Spatial uniformity is less important.

These issues are demonstrated in the high quality surface coil images which are characterized by their lack of uniformity and their high sensitivity. Typically in surface coil operation a modified body coil is used to transmit and a simple surface coil design function as a receiver. Saddle, half-saddle, solenoid and single turn surface coils have been used in various clinical applications. These coils appear to provide improved performance when a directed study of a region of detailed anatomy is needed. With surface coils gradient zoom operation becomes feasible, as the system bandwidth is limited by the localized sensitivity of the surface coil. The decrease in SNR associated with surface coil operation is more than compensated for by the improved sensitivity of the surface coils.

For whole-head and whole-body imaging applications, coil with greater spatial uniformity are used. These may be transmission line, saddle or slotted tube designs. It is important that these have a large useful area to permit multi-slice operation.

Computer Architecture

A modern MRI system must perform many tasks simultaneously: image acquisition, data archiving, hardcopy generation, image post-processing, reconstruction and patient data entry. Typically these are very stereotyped and a multicomputer design with multiple data links between the components is more effective than a single large mainframe computer. Some operations, such as archiving data on magnetic tape are limited by the existing 8-bit serial interfaces. In the future industry-standard optical disk systems will offer the best opportunity for efficient data storage. It is prudent to wait for industry standard hardware and interfaces for these systems to ensure availability and reliability. In the meantime magnetic tape represents a system that we know works.

At any stage of MRI system design there is always

the temptation to restrict flexibility at a given stage, such as in the selection of pulse sequence timing parameters. This has the advantage of simplifying quality assurance, but the disadvantage is that the system operation is restricted before the value of different modes of operation can be fully evaluated. A more effective approach is to offer a standard set of operational parameters in a "foreground" mode but to allow the experienced and investigational operator flexibility in "background" mode.

New Imaging Modes

More so than any other imaging modality, MR offers the possibility of physiologically relevant data collection. Currently flow imaging, chemical shift imaging and paramagnetic contrast agents are being evaluated in research and clinical settings.

Flow Imaging

The interaction of flowing spins and magnetic field gradients has been reasonably well understood for more than 20 years and provides the basis for flow imaging and for flow artifacts with conventional MRI. A number of approaches are possible. We have implemented an approach where a three dimensional data matrix is collected. Two dimensions are spatial - a single slice of tissue is studied using conventional selective excitation methods. The data matrix is expanded in a third direction according to the velocity of the spins normal to the selected plane. The spin velocities are separated into n velocity ranges by n velocity phase encoding steps. Flow phase encoding pulses are biphasic and contribute signal phase proportional to velocity.

A flow imaging system developed at this institution was used with cardiac gating to measure the flow of blood in the carotid and jugular vessels of a normal volunteer. Phantom measurements were also made. A transverse section through the image matrix yields a spatial image of a given velocity range of spins. The zero-velocity plane image corresponds to a conventional MRI image with total "flow- void" effect. A selected coronal plane through the image data matrix is actually a flow profile across a given line across the carotid and jugular vessels. The flow pattern through the neck vessels was well demonstrated and the laminar flow within the phantom was confirmed.

Two - Component Chemical Shift Imaging

The differences in resonant frequency between fat and water can be exploited to yield separate fat and water images. The conventional spin-echo image with short TE represents a sum of fat and water components. By uncentering the 180 degree pulse and maintaining TE constant an "out of phase" image can be generated with a signal intensity equal to the difference of the fat and water components. The addition and subtraction of image data obtained from these images results in the formation of "water" and "fat" images. In our particular implementation of this technique a hybrid pulse sequence with alternating in and out of phase images is acquired and processed to maintain object registration. The clinical utility of this method is yet to be established, however preliminary results indicate that useful information about involvement of the marrow space with tumor, inflammation and other processes may be obtained.

Contrast Agents for MRI

Paramagnetic contrast agents or "magnetopharmaceuticals" (MPs) offer the possibility of increased specificity of MRI diagnostic information. At present several classes of MPs are being evaluated. Soluble chelates of paramagnetic transition element metal ions reduce the relaxation time of adjacent water protons and thus alter image contrast. Substances like gadolinium DTPA reside predominantly within the intravascular space and appear to delineate areas of edema and blood-brain barrier leakage.

Conjugates of paramagnetic transition element chelates with antibody molecules offer the chance to target the relaxing effect of these complexes to cell surface ligands on tumors, bacteria and other sites in normal and pathological states. This represents a marriage of monoclonal antibody production techniques and protein chemical modification methods. At present there have been several intriguing demonstrations of antibody directed MRI contrast enhancement. There remains much to be demonstrated and researched in this area, particularly in the methods for increasing the numbers of paramagnetic sites per antibody molecule. Further developments include specialized software for the quantification and isolation of these contrast effects.

The Future of MR

Despite the flurry of research and development activity in MR, there are limits to this method which cannot be surmounted with technology. Chief among these is the limit on sensitivity imposed by physical laws. There is no question that in-vivo spectroscopy (IVS) will be a major area of research interest and an effective tool for many research centers. Most likely the information obtained from IVS will help improve medical therapy in a general sense. The application of this technology to clinical diagnosis on a patient-by-patient basis is problematic.

The history of magnetic resonance has been one of continual development and increasing scope. Almost certainly this will continue in the future where MR seems certain to provide direct and indirect benefits to medical care.

PANEL ON APPLICATIVE PROBLEMS AND FUTURE DIRECTION OF NMR FOR IN VIVO STUDIES

DISCUSSION

P. Mansfield:

In chemical saturation procedures one cannot use arbitrarily long pre-saturation pulses because the line you are trying to saturate will recover due to competitive T_1 effects. Does this mechanism present difficulties with current experiments? Does the RF power level present a power deposition problem in a patient at the frequencies used? Does the T_1 recovery during the imaging procedure present a problem, perhaps by introducing unwanted signal artefacts in the final image? In other words, in a water image, how much of the signal is coming from fat?

D. Shaw:

The question raises several points; firstly, the question of RF energy dissipated into the patient. The power used in a chemically selected pulse is very low since its objective is simply to apply a 90° pulse to the single line of water as opposed to excite a large bandwidth. The width of the selective pulse is determined by the line width which is to be saturated, i.e. the water line, and is therefore typically a few msec in duration thus being 10 times larger and one tenth the power of a normal 90° pulse. A chemically selective pulse typically therefore increases the power used by a few percent.

Finally, the question of T_1 recovery; it is only the magnitude of M_2 at the time of the 90° excitation pulse that influences signal intensity in the image. Since the chemically selective pulse immediately proceeds the 90° pulse relaxation during the few msec delay between these two pulses is negligible.

A. Todd-Pokropek:

With respect to fitting FIDs in spectroscopy using a set of Lorentzian lines, we have been troubled both in the frequency and time domain by errors in the first few points and the FID, the hump in the frequency domain. Could you suggest ways to avoid this?

D. Shaw:

Removal of 'hump' and phase artefacts from high resolution spectra is standard on commercial software. Hump or base line roll effects are removed by convolution, usually with a sinc function and/or base line fitting with polynomials. Specific functions have been proposed for special cases, e.g. the effect of phospholipids on in vivo ^{31}P brain spectra or when using some localising techniques. The topic is well reviewed for example in J.C. Lindon and A.C. Ferridge, Prog. NMR Spectroscopy, 14 (1980) 27.

S. Derenzo:

Can you say anything regarding the health effects of the RF fields required to saturate a particular chemical species or to decouple protons?

D. Shaw:

The power needed for saturation of a particular chemical species is very small. The maximum allowable power of 0.4 W/kG in the U.S.A. and the maximum allowable temperature rise is $1°$ in the U.K. Proton decoupling requires significant power levels and is not suitable for routine diagnostic measurements. The research applications are significant, however, as humans undergoing proton decoupling do not report discomfort.

P. Mansfield:

Some of the expressions you develop for moments C_e in terms of the $a_m b_n$ products look very much like cumulants which have been used to describe NMR decay functions. However, more usually the FID can be expressed rigorously as a moment expression in time, i.e.

$$f(t) = 1 - \tfrac{1}{2} M_2 t^2 + M_4 t^4/4! + \ldots$$

This is an infinite series in which M_2, M_4 ... are the even moments of the absorption line shape $g(\nu)$. That is to say

$$M_n = \int \nu^n g(\nu) d\nu.$$

Because of time reversal symmetry, the odd terms vanish in the series expansion. For special cases, for example when $g(\nu)$ is a Gaussian function, there is a derivable relationship between M_2 and M_4, i.e. $M_4 = 3M_2^2$. More usually, however, especially in liquid like systems, $g(\nu)$ is not Gaussian but approximates to a Lorentzian shape. In the time domain this approximates to an exponential function for long times. How do you see your analysis fitting in to the framework of NMR or NMR imaging? Do you see it as an alternative method of describing the FID process itself or as a way of describing the physiological object of imaging?

A. Rescigno:

The moments have the physiological meaning described in section 2 of my paper "Image Analysis and the Method of Moments" (these proceedings). Section 7 shows how to analyze them to get information pixel by pixel. Because physiological processes are strictly irreversible, odd moments do not vanish in this case; the only simple relationship among successive moments is the one shown in section 5 for a simple compartment. Of course, the multidimensional moments described in section 15 incorporate other physical properties of the signal and can be treated as terms of an integral transform.

M. Waller:

Could anyone comment on whether there is yet any evidence for MRI (NMR) being able to offer earlier diagnosis of disease states?

J. Weissman:

I am a physician who works for a manufacturer of MRI devices, Technicare. Thus I cannot speak from the viewpoint of a practising clinician. Still, I will address certain aspects of this issue.

No manufacturer can yet claim that cancer can be detected with MR before CT, etc. as there is yet no study which would support this in a strict sense. At Technicare we have, as part of our successful FDA premarket approval submission, accumulated a significant body of clinical information which shows that MRI is as or more sensitive than CT, nuclear studies, conventional radiography, etc. in many applications. These include imaging of the head, (especially posterior fossa), spinal cord, pelvis and mediastinum.

Controls have been included in the design of these studies to minimise the effect of prior knowledge of diagnostic information from other modalities.

In general, patients were selected for these studies in some light of clinical history or diagnostic findings. The studies also include a significant proportion of normal controls. As a result of a certain amount of prior knowledge bias in patient selection these initial study results are inherently biased against MRI, since some patients were selected with prior knowledge of corroborative or correlative data.

A. Ozman:

What order of magnitude of accuracy is achieved in the homogeneous (static) magnetic field?

How does the introduction of human body effect the field?

P. Mansfield:

It rather depends on the size and type of magnet. For 0.5 T supercons with 1 m bore we can expect better than 10 ppm homogeneity over a 3 T cm special volume.

S. Petersen:

Has anybody commented on the possibility of measuring perfusion as distinguished from flow and diffusion?

P. Mansfield:

I am not sure whether perfusion would manifest itself in NMR imaging in a manner different to slow flow. Certainly there are many techniques to measure flow and a British group at the University of Guildford have very recently produced pure diffusion images.

M. Waller:

Is there an adequate model for the dielectric behaviour of the body to allow satisfactory answers to questions of safety in RF power deposition and field switching?

P. Mansfield:

The electrical characteristics of human tissue have been measured over a very wide range of frequencies and the dielectric behaviour is well documented. A group in Utah, under C. Durney, have made calculations of RF absorption in the far field case. Their computer modelling includes studies of non-homogeneous discretely distributed systems to simulate organs within the body. This approach will go a long way to answering questions regarding safety, etc. but needs to be modified for the near field case.

S. Derenzo:

There is some concern about 'hot spots' caused by high local RF absorption, and a difficulty in understanding the detailed dielectric properties of the human body. Would it be possible to design an imaging procedure that is sensitive to RF absorption similar to the grid-dip NMR method used to measure magnetic fields?

P. Mansfield:

Durney is extending his simulation studies to finer grids using finite-element analysis. This work should lead to an understanding of the problem of 'hot spots'.

In a sense, we already have such image procedures since static image phase artefacts contain RF penetration information.

Power deposition was also discussed and a figure of 0.4 W kg^{-1} was mentioned as the FDA upper limit. Some concern was expressed regarding power deposition in saturation type experiments designed to highlight particular components of chemical shift in proton images.

The question of free radicals was raised and Mansfield gave a brief introduction to the topic of free radical pairs and the effects of static magnetic fields. It was pointed out that static fields and local fields or gradients could convert radical pairs from a non-magnetic singlet state to a magnetic triplet state. However, this would require fairly high static fields. The consequences of this could be a slowing of chemical reaction rates. In biological systems this might affect enzyme reactions. Although theoretically possible there seems to be no evidence so far for static biomagnetic effects of this sort.

The question of achievable resolution in spectroscopic imaging was raised and it was pointed out that at very high fields bulk susceptibility of the patient, around 1 ppm, would influence line shapes. Techniques for curve fitting (and deconvolution) of overlapping lines were mentioned.

The panel was asked if NMR imaging could be used to measure blood perfusion (see specific questions). It was thought that this might be possible by observing washout of suitable contrast agents.

Of the commercial imaging equipment itself, important factors were identified which would affect customers' choice, including cost and mean time between failures. However, the panel was unspecific in its comment.

PART X   NUCLEAR MEDICINE AGENTS AND INSTRUMENTATION

Chairman: Richard C. Reba (U.S.A.)

RADIOPHARMACEUTICALS FOR IN VIVO DIAGNOSIS - CURRENT TOPICS AND
FUTURE PROSPECTS

PETER H. COX

Rotterdam Radio-Therapeutic Institute
Dept. of Nuclear Medicine
Rotterdam, The Netherlands

1. INTRODUCTION

The realisation that nuclear medical techniques could be used to
study pathophysiological processes in vivo gave rise to a demand
for high purity target organ specific radiopharmaceuticals with a
reproducible biodistribution. This in turn has led to the emergence
of radiopharmacy as a recognisable subdiscipline of nuclear medicine
and during the last few years programmed research has largely
replaced serendipity as the source of new in vivo reagents.
    The basic requirements for a successful radiopharmaceutical
are that it should show a high specificity for the organ or tissue
to be investigated, have biodistribution characteristics which
relate to the physiology of that organ, that it should give a low
radiation dose to the patient and be of low toxicity. Chemical
toxicity is seldom a problem because the carrier molecules are
usually used at nanomol concentrations. The most common adverse
reaction is an allergic one which may be severe but which nevertheless is quite rare. Radiation effects are also seldom a problem
but with some labels in common use, Thallium-201 and Indium-111 for
instance, this is a potential problem due to the fact that they
emit Auger electrons which give a high local radiation dose. In
cases where the labelled compounds penetrate the cell membrane
nuclear damage may result with possible mutagenic effects. For this
reason alone it is necessary, when using a radionuclide which emits
Auger electrons, to carry out biodistribution studies at the cellular level to determine the risk of nuclear damage (1).
    In general, however, radiopharmaceuticals can be considered as
non toxic whereby the restrictions applied to drugs are largely
irrelevant.
    It is self evident that the most suitable reagent to evaluate
organ function is a natural metabolite which has been labelled in

such a way that its biodistribution remains unaffected. The most
effective manner to realise this is to utilise positron emitting
nuclides, such as C^{11}, N^{13} and O^{15}, which can be incorporated into
organic molecules without affecting the chemical structure.

Unfortunately the installation and operation of an clinically
useful positron production and scanning unit is so costly that they
are restricted to a few specialised centres. The current economic
situation also precludes their introduction on a wider scale in the
near future. It would therefore appear that single photon emitters
will remain the primary source of radiopharmaceuticals for some
time to come.

2. GENERAL CONSIDERATIONS

Before we consider the relative merits of single photon emitters in
the light of recent developments there are a number of general
considerations which apply to all radiopharmaceuticals. The majority
of gamma emitting radionuclides available to nuclear medicine are
not represented in the elements occurring in biological systems.
Hence the labelling of suitable carrier molecules is either accomplished by tagging or by substitution labelling. In tagging a radioactive element is added to the molecule either alone or protected
by organic groups to prevent enzymatic or chemical degradation in
vivo. With substitution labelling a radioactive analogue of a
naturally occuring element in the molecule, such as Selenium-75 for
sulphur, is incorporated into the carrier.

Both labelling methods can significantly alter the biodistribution characteristics of the carrier molecule. Methionine, for
instance, is an essential amino acid for the synthesis of biologically active peptides. It can be labelled by substituting Selenium-75 for sulphur and the resultant seleno-methionine is readily taken
up by cells which are synthesising peptides. In some way it is
recognised by the cell as being different from natural methionine
and is not utilised for protein synthesis. A similar effect is
observed in the case of iodinated cholesterol in the suprarenals.

With tagging additional problems may be encountered. The degree
of iodination of fibrinogen affects the rate of blood clearance
(2), the greater the degree of iodination the more rapid it is.
Different nuclides bound to the same carrier endow the carrier with
entirely different biodistribution characteristics. Human serum
albumin labelled with Cr-51 has a half life of ± 6 hours for its
transport via the lymphatics from a subcutaneous injection site.
Iodine-131 labelled HSA using albumin from the same source has a
half life of ± 120 hours under the same conditions (3). Electrophoresis of the two compounds shows that different molecular weight
fractions are labelled.

In view of these factors it is not surprising that the bulk of
radiopharmaceuticals in use today are based on non physiological
carrier molecules which have been identified as having suitable
biodistribution characteristics to provide clinically useful
information on organ function or to identify focal lesions. Let us

now have a look at some recent developments

3. POSITRON EMITTERS

The use of C^{11}, O^{15} and N^{13} has made it possible to label compounds without affecting their biological behaviour. This in turn has led to a considerable advance in our knowledge of organ function and in particular of the brain (4-6).

The positron emitting halogens are also emerging as a potential source of a wide range of new radiopharmaceuticals (7-10). F^{18} for example is of interest not only because of its chemical reactivity but because its relatively long half life makes it possible to produce radiopharmaceuticals in a central location for distribution to hospitals in the region.

The major drawback of positron emitters is cost. The economics of installing and operating a cyclotron and positron scanner is such that they are unlikely to become cost effective enough to be considered for routine hospital use and as such will remain the perquisite of a few research centres. The future development of positron cameras suited for both positron and single photon emission will open the way for the exploitation of halogen labelled compounds and generator produced nuclides such as Gallium. Until this is realised the bulk of nuclear medicine will be based, as now, on single photon emitters.

4. ULTRA SHORT LIFE GENERATORS

There has been a great deal of interest in recent years in the use of ultra short life nuclides to measure physiological activities in vivo. Such compounds have the advantage of high photon flux coupled with low radiation dose to the patient. A further advantage is that repeat studies can be carried out at short intervals. Two generators have become available on a regular basis which produce nuclides falling into this category; the mercury/gold and the fluid rubidium/krypton generators.

$Gold^{195}$ produces a high photon flux suitable for multiple first pass cardiological studies which can be repeated at three minute intervals. The three minute interval is a limitation imposed by the regeneration time of the generator. The disadvantages are that the energy $Gold^{195}$ is only fully exploitable if a multicrystal camera is available, there is a relatively high radiation dose to the personnel, the number of repeat studies per patient is limited to about ten because of the mercury breakthrough. The generator is nevertheless useable for three days.

The fluid Kr^{81m} generator on the other hand is only useable on the day of manufacture. Kr^{81m} is eluted in 5% glucose solution and can be eluted continuously for long periods. It is idealy suited for organ perfusion and has been used with great success for direct intracoronary perfusion to study changes in the intracoronary blood pool during pacing or following the administration of drugs. We have also used this generator for liver perfusion studies to monitor cytostatic drug distribution to intrahepatic tumours.

5. TECHNETIUM-99m

Technetium still remains the work horse of nuclear medicine and there has been much interest in developing new compounds during the last few years. This has primarily centered around the development of synthesised compounds rather than stannous chelates with the advantage of a clearly defined chemical entity. Examples are the cationic complexes developed by Deutsch (11) for myocardial scintigraphy or the anionic DADS complexes developed by Davison (12) for renal studies (fig. 1). A problem with this approach is the lack of knowledge of structure activity relationships and the problem of biodistribution variation between man and other animal species. To date no synthesised Technetium compound is in routine clinical use and all of the compounds under investigation were discovered by serendipity and so called blind screening.

The possibility of developing lipophylic complexes has become a real one which offers high hopes for the development of a reagent which passed the blood brain barrier (13). It is not unreasonable to hope that the knowledge which is being garnered at present will lead to the development of Technetium complexes which have been designed for a particular function.

Traditional methods of Technetium labelling have not yet lost their utility and during the last year we have seen the introduction of nanocolloids for bone marrow scintigraphy, Aprotinin for function-

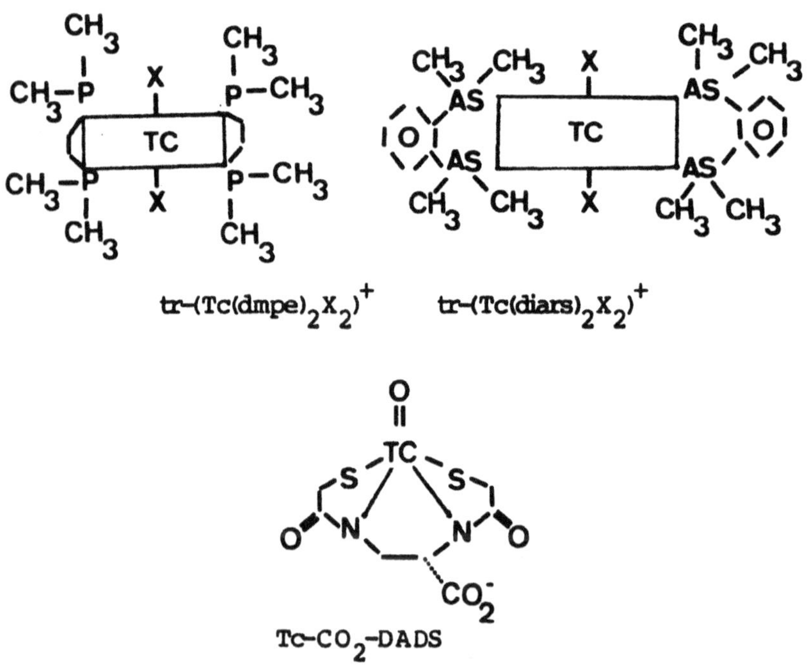

$tr-(Tc(dmpe)_2X_2)^+$ $tr-(Tc(diars)_2X_2)^+$

$Tc-CO_2-DADS$

Fig. 1. Synthesised Technetium complexes.

al renal scintigraphy using static images, Thiodiglycollic acid as a hippuran substitute and an antimelanoma monoclonal antibody fraction for tumour imaging.

The use of solid phase labelling to label sensitive compounds has produced plasminogen activator for thrombosis detection (14) and glutamate for tumour localisation (15).

6. IODINE-123

Despite the relative high cost Iodine-123 has continued to flourish and a number of new compounds have been introduced on a commercial basis during the last year: Iodoamphetamine and HIPDM for brain, Methyliodobenzylguanidine for phaeochromocytoma, Plasminogen for thrombosis and of course improved w-fatty acids for the myocardium.

These are all, however, costly products and not surprisingly a number of in house labelling kits have appeared which will enable an optimal use of Iodine. At the present time kits are available to prepare hippuran, antipyrine and iodoamphetamine which are based on iodine exchange reactions. In the case of hippuran and amphetamine this leads also to the formation of an Iodo-Copper complex which raises the background activity.

A further development which we have in clinical trial at the present time is a solid phase labelling kit to label bleomycin at room temperature without the need for heating. This should become available in the new year.

Finally it is interesting to note that other chemically active nuclides are beginning to arouse interest for instance a Thallium complex with diethyldithiocarbamate has been reported as a potential reagent for brain scintigraphy recently.

REFERENCES

1. Cox, PH. Radiopharmaceuticals Toxicity and Safety. In: Radiopharmacy and Radiopharmacology Yearbook, vol. II, Cox, PH and King CM, (eds), London, New York, Gordon and Breach, (1984) (in print).

2. Rhodes, BA, Croft BA, In: Basics of Radiopharmacy, St. Louis, USA, CV Mosby Comp. (1978) 69-70.

3. Cox, PH, The kinetics of macromolecule transport in lymph and colloid accumulation in lymphnodes. In: Progress in Radiopharmacology, vol. II, Cox, PH (ed), Amsterdam, Elsevier/North-Holland Biomedical Press, (1981), 267-292.

4. Kearfott, KJ et al,C-11-Dimethyloxazolidinedione Biodistribution J. Nucl. Med. (1983) 24:805-811.

5. Raichle, ME et al, Brain blood flow measured with H2 15O. J. Nucl. Med. (1983) 24:790-798.

6. Herscovitch, P et al, Brain blood flow measured with intravenous H2 15O. J. Nucl. Med. (1983) 24:782-789.

7. Garnet, ES et al, L-Dopa distribution in man. Nature (1983) 305:137-138.

8. Friedland, RP et al, Labeled choline and phosphorylcholine: body distribution and brain autoradiography. J. Nucl. Med. (1983) 24:812-815.

9. Scholl, H et al, Bromine 75 labelled 1:4-Benzodiazepines. J. Nucl. Med. (1983) 24:417-422.

10. Crawley, JWC et al, Dopamine receptors displayed in the living human brain with 77-Br-Bromospiperone. Lancet ii (1983) p 975.

11. Deutsch, E. Recent developments in Technetium chemistry as applied to the generation of new radiopharmaceuticals. In: Radiopharmacy and Radiopharmacology Yearbook, vol. I, Cox, PH (ed), London, New York, Gordon and Breach,(1984).

12. Davison, A et al, A new class of oxotechnetium (5+) chelate complexes containing a Tcon2s2 core. Inorg. Chem. (1981) 20: 1629-1632.

13. Kung, HF et al, Synthesis and biodistribution of neutral lipid soluble Tc99m complexes that cross the blood brain barrier. J. Nucl. Med. (1984) 25:326-332.

14. Cox, PH et al, Tc-plasminogen activator, a reagent for thrombosis detection in vivo. Eur. J. Nucl. Med. (submitted for publication) (1984).

15. Campos de Cremer, E et al, Tc-glutamate, a comparative study of stannous and solid phase labelling. 4th Congr. Brazilian Soc. of Biol. and Nucl. Med., Porto Alegre, (abstr.) (1984).

SINGLE PHOTON IMAGING: STATE OF THE ART, LIMITATIONS AND FUTURE NEEDS

A Todd-Pokropek

Dept. of Medical Physics
University College London, U.K.

ABSTRACT

Single photon imaging may currently be divided into two main classes, those of planar imaging and tomography. Two key issues are: which sampling strategy to use, and how efficient is the system that results. Thus the imaging problem can be generalised as trying to estimate activity values within a volume, trying to optimise both the statistical **reliability** of any given estimate and its **robustness** (e.g. parameter estimation). Gains in reliability have been achieved by improved efficiency, for example of collimator and detector. Gains in robustness can be achieved by improving the sampling scheme, both the spatial and energy resolution, and in the elimination of various distortions. Scatter rejection is of particular importance.

Major, current issues in Single Photon Emission Computerized Tomography (SPECT) are the correction of degradations caused by scatter, non-uniform sampling, and attenuation with the aim of enabling quantitative estimates of activity distributions. Monte Carlo methods provide powerful tools for performing such corrections, which must be independent of the object distribution. SPECT is very photon limited, and a variety of single and multiple slice machines are being developed to improve sensitivity. Multiple angle coded aperture imaging also appears very promising. The current 'state of the art' for each of these approaches is presented.

1. INTRODUCTION

Single photon imaging covers the area of all systems based on the detection of gamma photons obtained by emission from a radioactive tracer administered to a patient, with the exclusion of imaging systems based on the detection of pairs of coincident photons obtained by emission from positrons. The two main subdivisions are normally considered to be planar imaging, e.g. obtaining a projection image as in conventional radiography from a given angle, and tomography, conventionally called Single Photon Emission Computerised Tomography (SPECT).

The fundamental problem is (as usual) how to obtain the best estimate of the activity distribution in 3-D within the patient. However, there may be considerable divergence in the interpretation that is placed on the term 'best estimate'. Muehllehner [1] has shown that, for a given object distribution, it may be possible to obtain images of high quality by aiming for the images with the most (reasonable) resolution, at the expense of sensitivity. He has stated that, for an image composed of hot spots at various spacings, an image at 4mm resolution and 100K events might be of equal image quality to one at 8mm and 3.2M events, but estimates of image quality are very object dependent. In general any detection system needs to be optimised in terms of sensitivity and resolution. However, this tends to ignore the question of how the data should best be sampled.

Two related concepts may be considered: **reliability** or the statistical accuracy of a measurement, and **robustness**. These terms must be defined. Let us consider a point in space. At that point, within the patient, there exists a certain (true) activity concentration t expressed in terms of activity per unit volume. Let an estimate e of the activity concentration be made. Then we would like e to be (at least) proportional to t. By the statistical accuracy of e we mean the error associated with e (assuming no bias) given by repeated measurements under similar conditions, that is, essentially the error related only to the statistical nature of the process. By robustness, we mean the error given by e associated with changes in the measurement conditions, in particular, when other values of activity concentration within the patient change.

When considering planar imaging, the statistical accuracy of a particular measurement is given by the Poisson nature of the number of counts collected from that region, while the robustness is affected amongst other things by the activity lying along the 'line' of measurement, but at other positions than the point in question. In tomography, it is sometimes found that the robustness of the technique is greater since the influence of surrounding activity is reduced, but that the statistical accuracy is worse, since the signal to noise ratio in tomography,

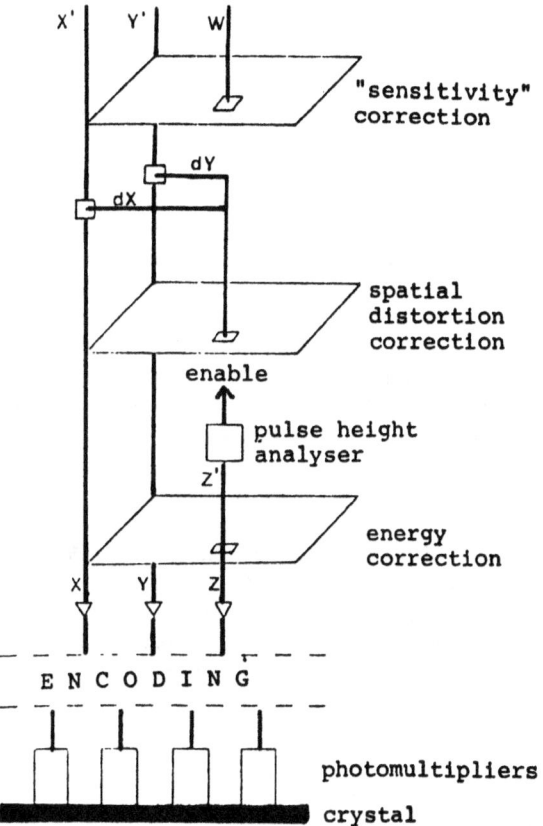

Fig. 1

The flow chart corresponding to a modern gamma camera with digital correction for energy, spatial distortion and "sensitivity"

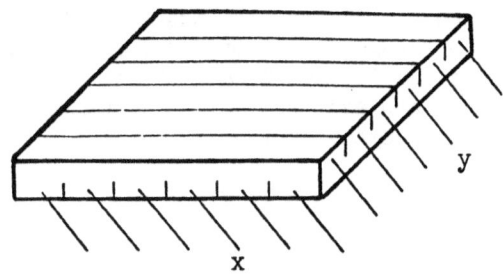

Fig. 2

The encoding scheme for a solid state camera showing orthogonal strips such that one set can be used for determining the x coordinate, and the other, the y coordinate

for a given number of detected counts, is considerably degraded. The sampling strategy used clearly alters both parameters, not necessarily in a simple manner. What we would like to find is a strategy which minimises the overall error.

In particular, it is possible to define a generalized system response function (SRF) as follows. Let an activity distribution be defined as **A** being the activity at every point m in image space. Then also define **R** as the response observed at every point n in detector space. These spaces could be simply some Cartesian space in x,y or they could be more complex including energy, angle of incidence etc. Care needs to be taken when defining the norm of such spaces. The system response function is then defined using the relationship

$$R = SRF\ A$$

where SRF(m,n) is the probability that an event emitted from point m is detected at point n. If SRF is independent of the position m, then the definition tends towards the conventional definition of a Point Spread Function as normally used. Note that the integral of the set of values SRF is equal to the system sensitivity.

2. CONVENTIONAL DETECTORS

The most commonly employed system used for detection of 'single photons' in vivo is the gamma camera [2]. A considerable improvement of such detectors has occurred, primarily as a result of the availability of analogue and, more commonly nowadays, digital correction circuitry. These are illustrated diagrammatically in Fig 1. A photon is incident at estimated coordinates x,y. At each level of the correction system, a correction factor is stored, dependent on the current value of x and y. Thus, for example, to correct for spatial distortion, a table of correction factors DX and DY are stored for values of x and y such that a new estimate of the current origin of the photon x',y' is generated from

$$x'=x+DX(x), \qquad y'=y+DY(y).$$

In practice, the number of stored coefficients may vary, and measurements must be taken to avoid digitization errors in the calculation [3]. Similarly, the apparent energy E of a photon detected at x,y may be tested against a pair of values ELOW(x,y) and EHI(x,y) such that the event is only included in the image forming process if

$$ELOW(x,y) < E < EHI(x,y).$$

Actual methods of implementing this correction may vary [4,5,6]. The availability of such techniques permits systems to be designed to optimise sensitivity and resolution, normally by maximising the number of light photons detected for each gamma photon, and ignoring any problems of the uniformity of response. Thus photomultipliers may be placed directly in contact with scintillators, which may themselves be thinner to improve resolution, but at the expense of sensitivity and uniformity.

However, such correction systems do not eliminate all sources of error, for example, changes in the responses (gains) of individual photomultipliers (PMTs). For this reason several different 'autotune' methods have been proposed [7,8]. If the response of individual photomultipliers may be determined to a known input, the change with respect to 'calibration' may be found, and the system 'recalibrated'. The known impulse might be the light from a single LED coupled to the scintillator, from a set of LEDs each coupled to each PMT, or from a radiation source. In general, we have a set of observations O from the set of detectors (for each gamma camera PMT). We wish to know C, the set of changes that need to be applied to this set of detectors. Thus assuming that it is possible to establish a matrix equation of the general form

$$O = A C$$

where A is a matrix of system constants, then, by determining A^{-1}, the desired corrections C may be evaluated. This leads to the so-called parallel tuning algorithm [9], as distinct from the serial tuning algorithm which is essentially an iterative solution to the above equation. All such correction techniques require that the 'known' input is considerably more stable than the variations which might be expected from the detectors which are to be corrected.

This approach may be generalized, as suggested by the definition of the system response function SRF in section 1, by extension to a multi-dimensional space which includes energy, scatter etc. Thus, from an observation of a set of values O, a maximum likelihood estimate can be made of detection position and photon energy.

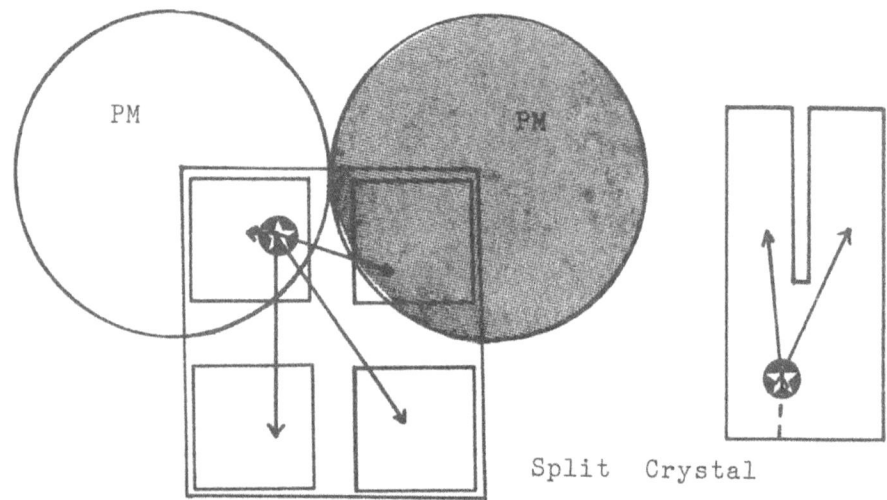

Fig 3 A split crystal design, coding the region of the crystal in which an event was detected by the relative amounts of light detected by several PMs.

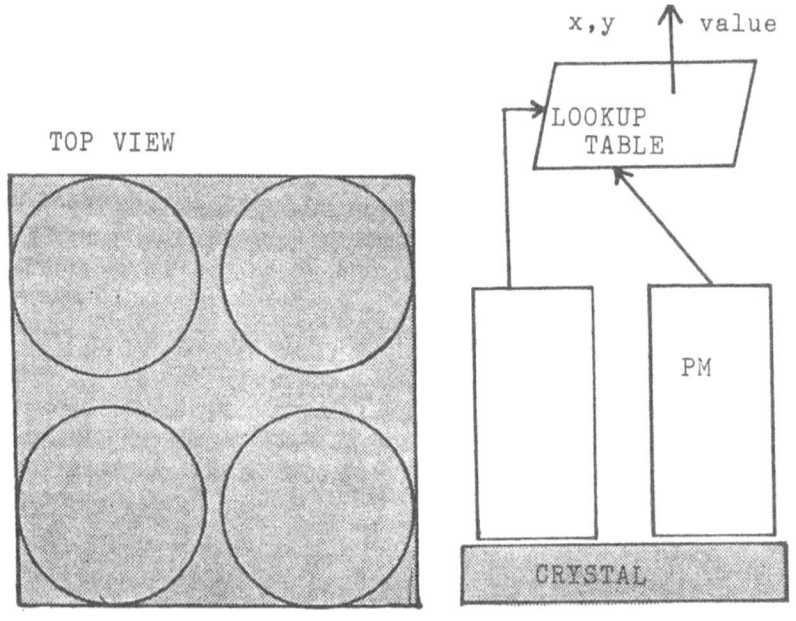

Fig 4. A modular gamma camera design, where the output from several PMs is used to select an address in a lookup table containing x,y.

3. OTHER PLANAR DETECTORS

The gamma camera is based on the use of a large scintillating crystal. Many other types of gamma photon detectors have been proposed, but are (to say the least) not in widespread use. A number of groups have worked on cameras using intrinsic Germanium semiconductor detectors, with suitable coding schemes to extract positional information [10], as shown in Fig 2. While prototypes have produced encouraging results, no large field of view devices appear to have been constructed.

An alternative, which is now being tested in the form of full scale prototypes [11,12] is the Multi-Wire Proportional Chamber (MWPC). The chamber, filled with a suitable gas, records on pairs of electrodes the passage of a gamma photon, or often an electron emitted from a suitable converter attached to the chamber. Such devices have, in principle, very good intrinsic resolution, but rather poor efficiency, e.g. sensitivity. Likewise, although the chamber itself may be quite cheap to produce, suitable encoding electronics are required for each electrode (as for the Ge camera). Other more esoteric devices have been proposed, for example the use of superconducting granules [13], gamma photon sensitive image intensifiers etc.

However, several more practical designs have been made for extended detectors using discrete scintillating crystals. One such design, the so-called Baird-Atomic camera, uses individual crystals and PMs in an array [14]. This has been improved by sectioning the crystal as shown in Fig 3, such that the 'part' of the crystal in which the photon was detected can be determined by evaluating the relative amount of light seen by several PMs [15]. A further generalisation of this idea is that of the modular gamma camera as described by Barrett et al [16] and illustrated in Fig 4. Here each crystal is observed by a (small) number of PMs, and the position of the event within the crystal located. Conventional electronics would not perform this task adequately since considerable distortions and edge effects exist. However, by a combination of suitable analogue preprocessing and a large digital lookup table, as indicated in the previous section, such effects can be largely eliminated. Thus an array of such detectors may be used in various geometrical configurations. Such a system can be considered in a very abstract manner. For example, let the signals from the four photomultiplier for each camera module be called a,b,c and d. It is required to find a best estimate for the spatial coordinates x and y (and possibly the energy). This can be treated as a parameter estimation problem, and the probability distributions for a-d for a known x,y can be determined, such that a maximum likelihood (or other) estimate of x,y can be determined for an observed a-d. This is an example of a true digital camera where encoding is performed at the level of individual photomultipliers, rather than after

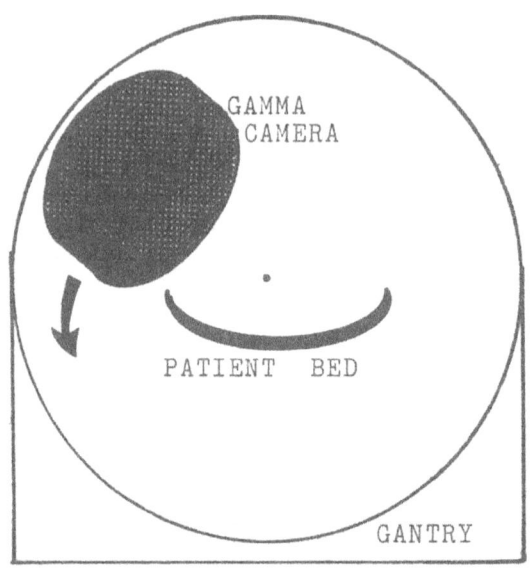

Fig 5. The conventional rotating gamma camera SPECT system.

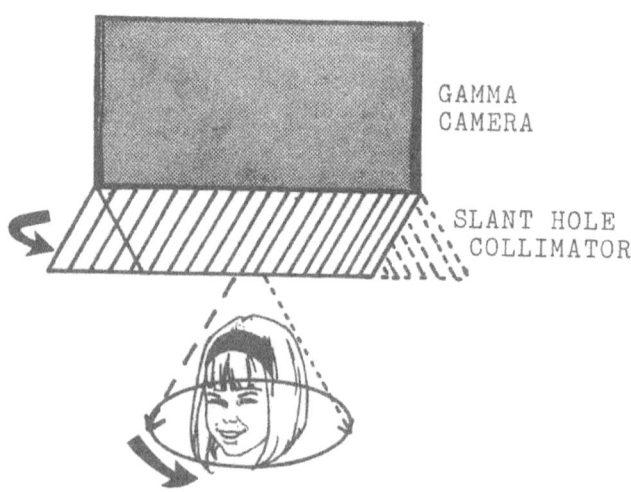

Fig 6. Tomography performed using a rotating slant hole collimator.

some analogue encoding stage.

4. TOMOGRAPHY- ROTATING GAMMA CAMERAS

The sampling strategy for conventional planar detectors is to observe the activity distribution only for a few orthogonal views such as anterior, posterior, left and right laterals. An alternative approach is to perform complete angular sampling, and view the image from a complete set of angles uniformly spaced around the object (patient). It may be readily shown [17,18] that N_{theta} the number of angles required to obtain adequate angular sampling is of the order of

$$N_{theta} = \pi D/d$$

where D is the diameter of the field of view and d is the resolution of the system. Hence for D=36cm and d=1.2cm, N_{theta} should be about 90. In fact most systems work with far fewer samples, typically 32 in 180°, i.e. 64 in 360°. In any analysis, it is reasonable to assume that the total amount of time spent collecting data is constant, and that therefore, as the number of angles increases, the length of time spent at any given angle decreases, and that therefore the statistical accuracy of the image at any given angle is worse. However, the overall signal to noise after reconstruction is largely independent of the number of angles, although resolution tends to be worse, and streak artefacts tend to be seen, when fewer angles are used.

By far the most common system for performing this type of tomography is the rotating gamma camera as illustrated in Fig 5. Such SPECT systems are very photon limited. It is suggested [19] that when a total number of counts N_{tot} are detected for a given slice, and then reconstructed into N_{pixel} pixels containing data, the signal to noise ratio S/N at a point is

$$S/N = K \cdot N_{tot}^{1/2} / N_{pixel}^{3/4}$$

$$= K' / FSD$$

where K and K' are constants and FSD is the coefficient of variation (the fractional standard deviation) of the reconstructed image at a (central) point. For example, for N_{tot} equal to 400K and N_{pixel} equal to 800, reasonably typical values, the value of S/N is about 4, and FSD is about 25%. These are rather poor values. See also the review papers [20,21].

For this reason many methods have been used to try to improve sensitivity. The simplest device has been to use two opposed heads, as shown. This improves sensitivity by a factor

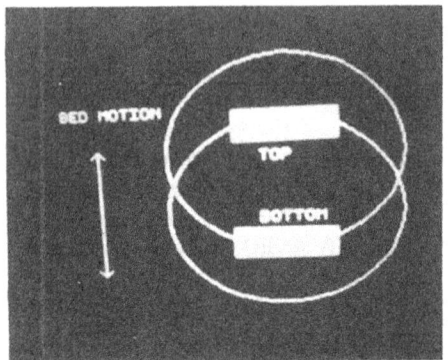 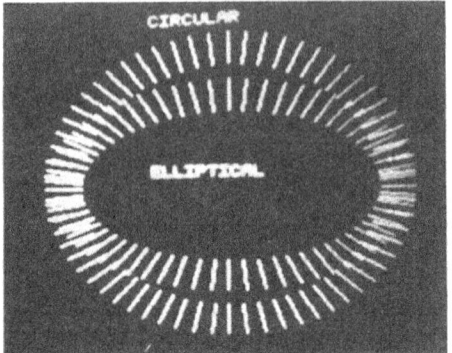

Fig 7. Non circular orbits may be achieved by various methods, for example by moving the bed up and down to give, as shown on the right, an elliptical orbit relative to the patient.

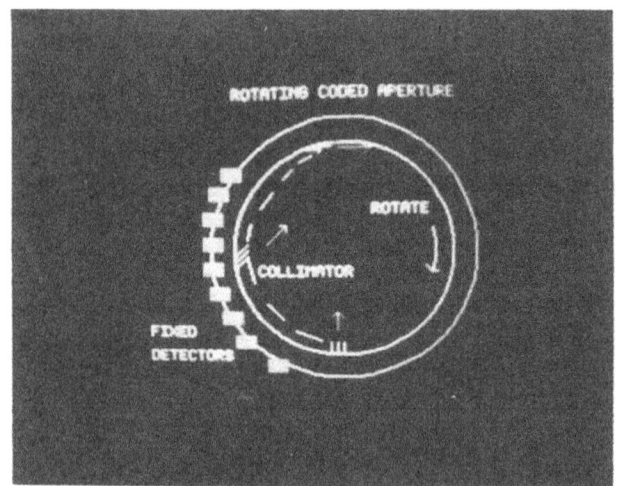

Fig 8. Various designs of rotating ring systems have been designed where some code, here a slant hole with a tilt varying with angle, is rotated in front of a fixed detector array.

of two, has no other advantages, but requires much more care is setting-up. An experimental system using three heads in the form of a triangle has also been described [22]. Converging collimators increase the solid angle and therefore can improve both sensitivity and resolution, at the expense of the field of view. The use of a slant hole collimator, as illustrated in Fig 6, permits the rotating cameras to approach a patient's head more closely than a conventional parallel hole collimator with circular orbit [23]. The uniformity of such collimators (the variations between the angle of slope of the set of holes) is often not very satisfactory. However, such effects can presumably be measured and then corrected.

A number of systems now exist which can perform non-circular orbits: by moving the bed up and down, by moving the detector head up and down, or by moving the detector gantry from side to side, while a normal circular orbit is performed [24]. As shown in Fig 7, such a system results in a non-circular orbit, the form of which can be controlled by the translation motion superimposed. Such system can approach the patient more closely, and thereby improve resolution, and can eliminate some of the effects of non-uniformity artefacts. Some systems attempt to achieve the same results by physically moving the detector head closer to or further away from the patient, while rotating. Considerable efforts must be made to ensure patient safety.

More specialised devices are those using coded aperture, and the many variations on single and multiple slice geometry, as described below.

5. SPECT SINGLE/MULTIPLE SLICE SYSTEMS

As in Positron ECT, many workers in the field have felt the urge to optimise SPECT systems by using a geometry based on optimising performance within one or several slices, rather than within a volume such as defined by the rotating gamma camera. Such systems have in common the feature that the solid angle of detector used, for a given slice, is much greater than that of a gamma camera. They are therefore (for that slice plane) much more sensitive. The cost of such a design aim is the loss of volume sensitivity. It appears to be very difficult to compare the performance of such systems with the more conventional rotating gamma camera systems, since performance within a slice cannot easily be compared to performance within a volume without invoking a rather arbitrary 'equivalent number of slices' for the volume. In addition, sensitivity must be compared for an equivalent resolution, in all three directions. Many (single and multiple) slice systems have rather variable resolution, particularly perpendicular to the slice plane.

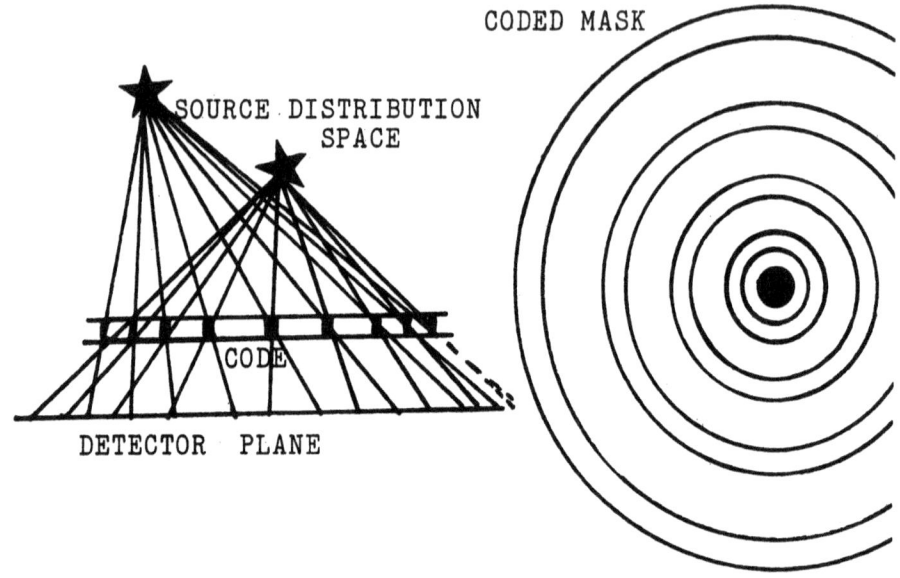

Fig 9. A coded aperture detector system imaging a distribution of point sources using a mask to generate a shadow for each point source.

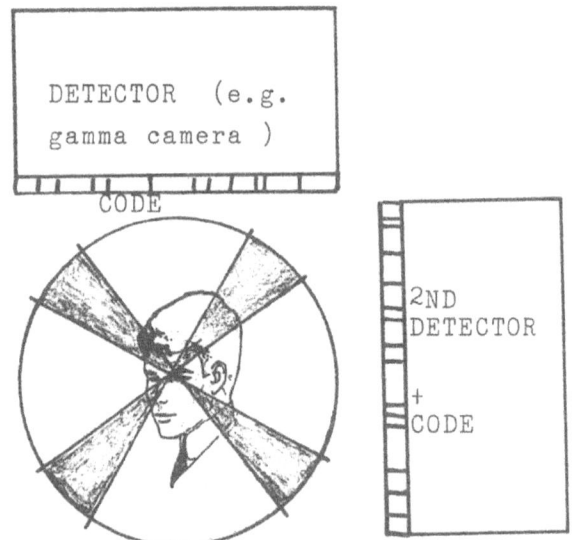

Fig 10. A dual orthogonal coded aperture system design. The grey areas in the circle indicate the angular frequencies which are missing after the data collection.

One of the earliest designs for such a system was that of Kuhl et al [25,26]. Here, a set of detectors collected data by the method, familiar from X-ray CT, of 'translate rotate'. Such a system may be extended by increasing the amount of detector material, so that no translations are necessary. Examples are those described by Moore [27] and Stokely [28] (also discussed by Hill and Rommer in these proceedings).

An alternative design is shown in Fig 8. Here a ring of detectors is used, while a specially designed collimator rotates between the ring and the patient to give the sampling pattern [29]. This is rather similar to some of the coded aperture techniques discussed later.

A further extension to this is to extend the ring of detectors in the perpendicular direction, that is, to produce a cylinder of detector material, as described in the MUMPI system [30]. More or less conventional Anger type electronics have been proposed for this system, although considerable care in the design of the correction circuits will be required. The form of the collimator to use also requires care.

6. CODED APERTURE

Basically all collimators are forms of coded apertures. Single photon systems require apertures to select direction since (unlike conventional x-ray systems) the emission process is intrinsically isotropic. Extreme examples of collimators are pinholes, and parallel hole collimators, both with an approximation to a unique one-to-one mapping between projection and image. In between, there are numerous other schemes where, for the gain of an increase in the number of detected photons, a mapping is used where detected photons could have originated from more than one position, and the image must be 'reconstructed' by eliminating the smearing and superimposition caused by the aperture. Such a process increases noise. The total gain (or loss) of signal to noise ratio/ resolution is both dependent on the efficacy of the algorithm used, and of the form of the object.

Common examples of coded apertures range from the simple annular aperture, via the Fresnel zone plate [31] (on and off axis), to a so called random code. An example is shown in Fig 9. In all cases, the desire is to increase the number of events detected (the 'mark' to 'space' ratio of the code), while maintaining an efficient code. The multiple pinhole [32] is in fact an example of such a a system, having a one-to-one mapping between image and object, but with a considerable gain in sensitivity over the single pinhole as a result of the increase in aperture. However, such systems cannot reconstruct the image independently of depth. The mapping for a multiple pinhole, as for the other coded aperture systems, changes with (is a function of) distance from the aperture. Thus reconstruction must be performed in 3-D rather than in 2-D for a planar projection. This necessarily degrades the signal to noise ratio. In addition, such systems normally have very limited angular sampling. As a result the reconstruction problem is effectively ill-posed, and very unstable. This also means that the reconstructions tend to be very noisy.

One method suggested to improve the performance of such algorithms is to use two orthogonal coded detectors. This is illustrated in Fig 10. If, for a given slice, the Fourier reconstruction plane is considered, then, for a single detector, the space labelled 'A' contains known values. Thus the remaining space needs to be determined by some method (extrapolation!) and as a result, the reconstruction becomes very noisy. Addition of a second orthogonal detector fills the space labelled 'B' which should considerably reduce the instability of the problem. It may be noted that in 3-D, rather than for a single slice, the volume of data for which Fourier coefficients are known remains very small in comparison to the total Fourier space.

Several worker have been actively pursuing research in this area. Bizais et al have investigated the dual orthogonal 7-pinhole system [33]. Barrett et al [34] have pursued the dual orthogonal random coded aperture, and Rodgers et al have investigated the rotating coded aperture ring system SPRINT [35].

7. SCATTER CORRECTION

In all the systems so far discussed, the presence of scattered events degrades the image [36]. The effect of scatter is to reduce contrast. It would therefore be desirable, if possible, to eliminate such effects. The most common method is of course to use an energy window (the nuclear medicine equivalent to the use of a screen in conventional radiology). However, at the relatively low energies normally used, and the energy resolution of the systems involved, it is not possible to eliminate completely all scattered events. Thus dual energy techniques seem to be attractive. The scatter contribution can be measured at a lower energy window, and then eliminated. In fact such scattered events, being correlated with the form of the activity distribution, contain information which could be exploited. The corollary is that a simple 'background subtraction' is inadequate, since the scatter contribution in an image has shape and form. Thus in general, it is desired to find $p'(x,y)$ the corrected photopeak image from $p_i(x,y)$ the observed images at various energies. One method which has been described [37] is to obtain $p'(x,y)$ from

BEFORE

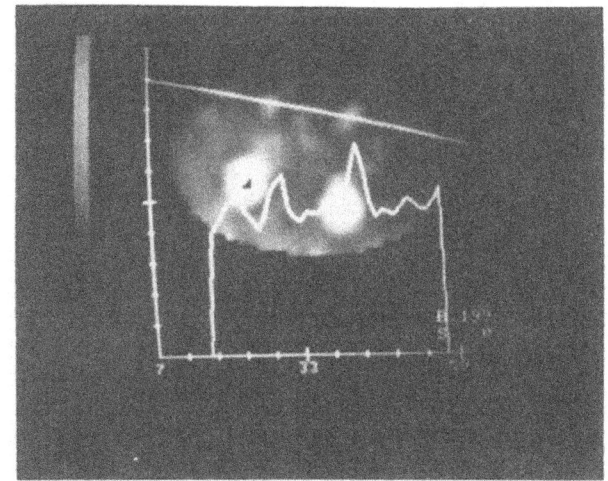

AFTER

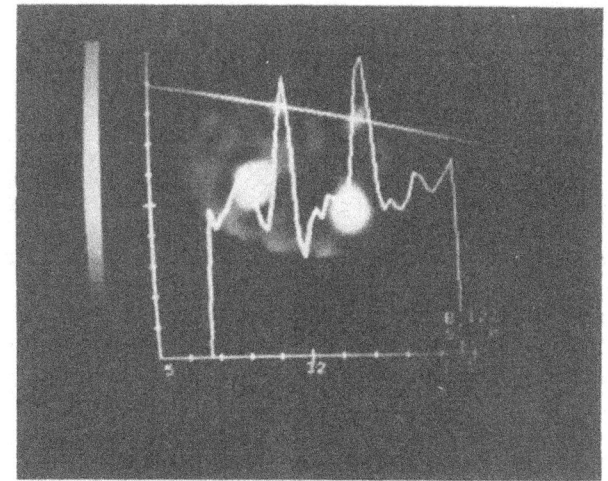

Fig 11. The result of scatter correction on an image with four hot spots in a uniform background. Note the considerable increase in contrast.

$$p'(x,y) = \sum_{i\ x'\ y'} p_i(x-x',y-y') \cdot w(i,x',y')$$

where $w(i,x',y')$ is an appropriate set of weights, assuming the process to be stationary. An alternative operation would be to look up a value of $p'(x,y)$ from a set of values of $p_i(i,x,y)$ in the neighbourhood of x,y. However, the condition of stationarity is still required.

Several authors [38,39] have used Monte Carlo models to investigate these effects. A model is supposed of the activity distribution within some attenuating scattering medium. Events are followed until either they are detected or they fall below some energy threshold. For any energy window, the history of any events (unscattered, single/multiple scatter) is known. Thus the inverse process, reconstruction of the true activity process for various 'contaminated' observations can be studied. One general technique, unfortunately impractical, is to perform an ART-like iteration, making guesses at the true activity distribution, generating by Monte Carlo methods the expected observed event distributions, correcting the activity distribution using error terms etc. However, an analytic form of the inverse process should be a good solution to include the scatter correction operation. One suggested method is to obtain the generalized system response function as discussed previously, by simulating a point source at every position within the object to be reconstructed, and then to solve the inverse problem by Maximum Likelihood methods [39,40].

The approximate methods previously suggested, however, can produce a spectacular improvement in image quality, as shown in Fig 11. Here filtered scatter data, collected using an energy window in the Compton region, has been subtracted from raw tomographic data (from the photopeak window) before reconstruction. The gain in contrast is considerable. In addition, it appears to be much easier to quantitate the resulting data [34].

8. DISCUSSION- LIMITATIONS AND FUTURE TRENDS

In the previous sections, an implicit assumption was that the desired end product of an imaging system was an image, and that the system should be optimised is the sense of image quality. However, if the desired end product was the estimation of, for example, concentration of some label within some possibly large volume, the design constraints become quite different. It may still be necessary to produce an image, such that the volume region of interest may be defined; however, the estimating of concentration may proceed directly from the original observed data rather than from the image(s). Such an approach using 'parameter estimation algorithms' could be very powerful.

At present, although tomographic systems were expected to revolutionise Single Photon Imaging, this is not the case. The images have often been of poor quality, contaminated with considerable artefacts, noisy, and requiring longer acquisition times than for conventional planar images.

In tomography, artefacts have been of considerable annoyance since the tomographic process tends to amplify these effects [41]. Great care is required to ensure the linearity and stationarity of the system. Such effects can be eliminated by the measurement of distortion, for example, of the error in the observed centre of rotation as a function of angle, for example the change in uniformity as a function of angle, of energy, of collimator etc. However, the low signal to noise ratio remains a problem, when images are considered.

It is often stated that the ability to quantite in Emission Tomography is the desired end point. Provided that several other effects, notably those of scatter, partial volume, and sampling of objects close to the system resolution in size are eliminated, then quantitation in SPECT can be achieved, possibly with a reasonable signal to noise ratio for the estimates. However, such estimates cannot be obtained for very small volumes, unless there is very great contrast between those volumes and the surrounds. Thus the uptake of a very specific label into a very small tumour could (theoretically) be quantitated accurately. However, the difference (if small) between, say, the pelvis and the parenchyme of the kidney, does not appear to be accessible to quantitation with presently available spatial resolution. Temporal resolution may assist, but often (for example in tomography) at the cost of spatial resolution. Thus, as in many other imaging techniques, the fundamental limitation in numbers of quanta available bound overall system performance, defined in terms of a combination of spatial, temporal and contrast resolution.

Future trends therefore suggest that Single photon emission imaging can be improved by the following methods. Firstly, gains in contrast can be achieved by improvements in radiopharmaceuticals. Secondly, gains in spatial resolution (in 3-D) can be exploited by greater care in instrument design (elimination of artefacts). Thirdly, gains in sensitivity (or resolution v. sensitivity) need to be made by increasing the sensitive volume of detectors, and improving the sampling strategy. Fourthly, temporal resolution needs to be exploited (if the sensitivity is adequate). Fifthly, considerable gains are possible from improvements in algorithms, both for imaging and for quantitation.

BIBLIOGRAPHY
1. Muehllehner, G., Colsher, J.G. and R.M. Lewitt. A hexagonal bar positron camera: problems and solutions. IEEE Trans. Nucl. Sci. NS-30 (1983) 652-660.
2. Anger, H.O. Scintillation camera. Rev. Sci. Instr. 29 (1958) 27-33.
3. Todd-Pokropek, A. Image processing in nuclear medicine. IEEE Trans. Nucl. Sci. NS-27 (1980) 1080-1094.
4. Muehllehner, G., Colsher, J.G. and E.W. Stoub. Corrections for non-uniformity in scintillation cameras through removal of spatial distortion. J. Nucl. Med. 21 (1980) 771-776.
5. Knoll, G.F. and M.E. Schrader. Computer corrections of camera nonidealities in gamma camera systems. IEEE Trans. Nucl. Sci. NS-29 (1982) 1272-1279.
6. King, S.E., Jih, F., Lim, C.B., Chaney, R. and E. Gray. Spectral-spatial-sensitivity distortion trends and accurate correction methods in scintillation gamma cameras. IEEE Trans. Nucl. Sci. NS-32 (1985) 870-874.
7. General Electric Inc., Technical Literature, GE400A Gamma camera.
8. Elscint, Technical Literature, Digital Gamma camera, and Personal Communication.
9. Digitrac for Scintiview system. Siemens Publication 710-002810, 1985
10. Ewins, J.H., Armantrout, G.A., Camp, D.C., Kaufman, L. et al. A clinical high purity germanium gamma camera. In Medical Radionuclide Imaging, (IAEA, Vienna, 1977) 1 149.
11. Lim, C.B., Chu, D., Kaufman, L., Perez-Mendez, V., Hattner, R. and D.C. Price. Initial characterization of a multi-wire proportional chamber positron camera. IEEE Trans. Nucl. Sci. NS-22 (1975) 388-394.
12. Jeavons, A., Shorr, B., Kull, K., Townsend, D., Frey, P. and A. Donath. A large area stationary positron camera using wire chambers. In Medical Radionuclide Imaging, (IAEA, Vienna, 1981) 1 49-72
13. Hueber, D., Valette, C. and G. Waysand. Superheated superconducting granules as high spatial resolution detectors. In Information Processing in Medical Imaging, ed DiPaola, R., (INSERM, Paris 1979) 88 661-672.
14. Bender, M.A. and M. Blau. Autofluoroscopy: the use of a non-scanning device for tumor localization with radioisotopes. J. Nucl. Med. 1 (1960) 105.
15. Heydat, D.W. and R.H. Jones. Scinticor: TM A new digital gamma camera. J. Nucl. Med. 25 (1984) P22.
16. Milster, T.D., Selberg, L.A., Barrett, H.H., Easton, R.L., Rossi, G.R., Arendt, J. and R.G. Simpson. A modular scintillation camera for use in nuclear medicine. IEEE Trans. Nucl. Sci. NS-31 (1984) 578-580.
17. Gilbert, P.F.C., The reconstruction of a three dimensional object from its projections and its application to electron microscopy II, direct methods. Proc. Royal. Soc (Lond)

Biol. 182 (1972) 89-102.
18. Snyder, D.L. and J.R. Cox, Jr. An overview of reconstructive tomography and limitations imposed by a finite number of projections, in Reconstruction tomography in diagnostic radiology and nuclear medicine, eds Ter-Pogossian, M.M., Phelps, M.E., Brownell, G.L. et al, (University Press, Baltimore, 1977) 3-32.
19. Budinger, T.F., Derenzo, S.E., Greenberg, W.L., Gullberg, G.T. and R.H. Huesman. Quantitative potentials of dynamic emission computed tomography, J. Nucl. Med. 19 (1979) 309-315.
20. Larsson, S.A. Gamma camera emission tomography- development and properties of a multi-sectional emission computed tomography system. Acta Radiologica Supp. 363 (1980).
21. Budinger, T.F., Gullberg, G.T. and R.H. Huesman. Emission computed tomography, in Image reconstruction from projections: Implementation and applications, ed Herman, G.T., (Springer Verlag, New York, 1979) 32 147-246.
22. Lim, C.B., Gottschalk, S., Walker R., et al. Triangular SPECT system for 3-D total organ volume imaging: design concept and preliminary imaging results. IEEE Trans. Nucl. Sci. NS-32 (1985) 741-748.
23. Chang, W., Lin, S.L. and R.E. Henkin. A rotatable quadrant slant hole collimator for tomography (QSH): a stationary scintillation camera based SPECT system. In Single Photon Emission Computed Tomography and Other Selected Computer Topics, ed Sorenson, J.A., (Soc. of Nucl. Med., New York, 1980) 81.
24. Todd-Pokropek, A. Non-circular orbits for the reduction of uniformity artefacts. Phys. Med. Biol. 28 (1983) 309-313.
25. Kuhl, D.E. and R.Q. Edwards. Image separation radioisotope scanning. Radiology 80 (1963) 653-662.
26. Kuhl, D.E., Edwards, R.Q., Ricci, A.R., Yacob, R.J., Mich, T.J. and A. Alavi. The MARK IV system for radionuclide computed tomography of the brain. Radiology 121 (1976) 405-413.
27. Moore, S.C., Brunelle, J.A. and C.M. Kirsch. Quantitative multi-detector emission computerized tomography using iterative compensation. J. Nucl. Med. 23 (1982) 706-714.
28. Stokely, E.M., Sveinsdottir, E., Lassen, N. and P. Rommer. A single photon dynamic computer assisted tomography (DCAT) for imaging brain function in multiple cross sections. J. Comput. Assist. Tomog. 4 (1980) 230-240.
29. Kanno, I., Uemura, K., Miura, Y., Miura, S., Hirose, Y., Koga, K. and H. Hattori. Headtome: a hybrid emission tomograph for brain. In Medical Radionuclide Imaging, (IAEA, Vienna, 1981) 1 153-164.
30. Logan, K.W. and R.A. Holmes. Missouri university multi-plane imager (MUMPI): a high sensitivity rapid dynamic ECT brain imager. J. Nucl. Med. 25 (1984) P105.
31. Barrett, H.H., Wilson D.T. and C.D. De Meester. Fresnel

zone plate imaging in radiology and nuclear medicine. Opt. Eng. 12 (1973) 8-12.
32. Vogel, R.A., Kirsch, D., LaFree, M. and P. Steele. A new method of multiplanar emission tomography using seven pinhole collimator and Anger scintillation camera. J. Nucl. Med. 18 (1978) 648-654.
33. Bizais, Y., Rowe, R.W., Zubal, I.G., Bennett, G.W. and A.B. Brill. Coded aperture tomography revisited. In Information Processing in Medical Imaging, ed Deconinck, F., (Nijhoff, Boston, 1984) 63-93.
34. Barrett, H.H., Barber, H.B., Ervin, P.A., Myers, K.J., Paxman, R.G., Smith, W.E., Wild, W.J. and J.M. Woolfenden. New directions in coded aperture imaging. In Information processing in medical imaging, ed Deconinck F., (Nijhoff, Boston, 1984) 106-129.
35. Rodgers, W.L., Clinthorne, N.H., Stamos, J., et al, SPRINT: a stationary detector single photon ring tomograph for brain imaging. IEEE Trans. Medical Imaging, MI-1 (1982) 63-68.
36. Pang, S.C. and S. Genna. The effect of Compton scattered photons on emission computerized transaxial tomography, IEEE Trans. NS-26, (1980) 2772-2774.
37. Todd-Pokropek A., Clarke G. and R. Marsh. Preprocessing of SPECT data as a precursor for attenuation correction. in Information processing in medical imaging, ed Deconinck F., (Nijhoff, Boston, 1984) 130-150.
38. Beck, J.W., Jaszczak, R.J., Coleman, R.E., Starmer, C.F. and L.W. Nolte. Analysis of SPECT including scatter and attenuation using sophisticated Monte Carlo modeling methods, IEEE Trans NS-29 (1982) 506-511.
39. Floyd, C.E., Jaszczak, R.J. and R.E. Coleman. Inverse Monte Carlo: a unified reconstruction algorithm for SPECT. IEEE Trans NS-32 (1985) 779-785.
40. Shepp, L.A. and Y. Vardi. Maximum likelihood reconstruction for emission tomography. IEEE Trans MI-1 (1982) 113-122.
41. Todd-Pokropek, A.E. Artefact creation and non-uniformity in tomography. Proc. Symp. American College of Physicians, Emission Computer Tomography: The Single Photon Approach, (BRH, Washington, 1981) 302-310.

DIGITAL IMAGING IN NUCLEAR MEDICINE

Dr. J.SALOMON

ELSCINT European Operations
40, Rue Jean Jaurès
93170 Bagnolet, France

SUMMARY

First pioneered by Elscint in the area of nuclear detectors, the concept of digital imaging in Nuclear Medicine has greatly evolved to encompass today nearly all aspects of clinical computing, namely quality assurance, on-line diagnostics, new NM imaging modalities, as well as picture archiving and communication systems, largely due to the systematic "uptake" of microprocessors by the medical computing community.

It is our goal to try and review various aspects of the impetus of this technology, with its possible after-maths in newly evolving (or to-be-created) modalities within and beyond today's N.M. frontiers.

IMPACT OF MICROPROCESSORS TECHNOLOGY

From the manufacturer's point of view, the scope of activity in Nuclear medicine was traditionally split between detectors (gamma cameras) and clinical processors. Competition is particularly fierce in the latter area, especially since the introduction of microprocessors in current end-station computing, from 8-bit micros to the 16-32 bits main frames of today.

A more thorough analysis of trends of "observed vs. expected" results can be found elsewhere (1).

DIGITAL NUCLEAR MEDICINE AXIOMS: THE CONSTRAINTS

What needs to be stressed is the continuous decrease in the main frame hardware prices (cpu, array processor), against the spiralling costs of software development, even in a discipline where many clinical processing breakthroughs have already been achieved and published (2).

Nowadays cost-containing requirements have, therefore, induced the design of N.M. equipment aiming at high imaging performance with a long system "half life".

A THREE-STEP SOLUTION

Pooling the Microprocessors

The starting axiom of digital imaging, as introduced by Elscint with its Apex line 4 years ago, has been the pooling of computing resources around a network of microcomputers, accepting a priori the very high software overhead involved in the design of a truly integrated camera/computer system.

Targeting the product at superior performance led, for example, to the definition of new hardware standards, including 512 X 512 acquisition, 1-2 MBytes addressing, parallel independent multi-displays, standard array processor in configuration, etc...

The actual block diagram of this system can be found on Figure 1, where one can identify a multiple bus structure effectively networking the main frame (Intel 8086) with its ancillary micro processors (Intel 8089 for I/O, Intel 8085 for display, AMD 2901 for acquisition), while the Anger detector itself acts merely as an "ordinary" peripheral to the system.

Digital Software-driven Handling of the Physics of Image Acquisition.

The second axiom lies in the potential of the computing system, especially through its in-board bit slice/array processor.

The dual "genetic diseases" of Anger cameras are well known. Their deleterious effects (3) are materialized by :

- the variable off-peaking of the crystal/PM's response across the detector face (local energy windows).

- and the misalignment of photon events with under-the-PM's
- crowding effects that produce linearity artifacts (4).

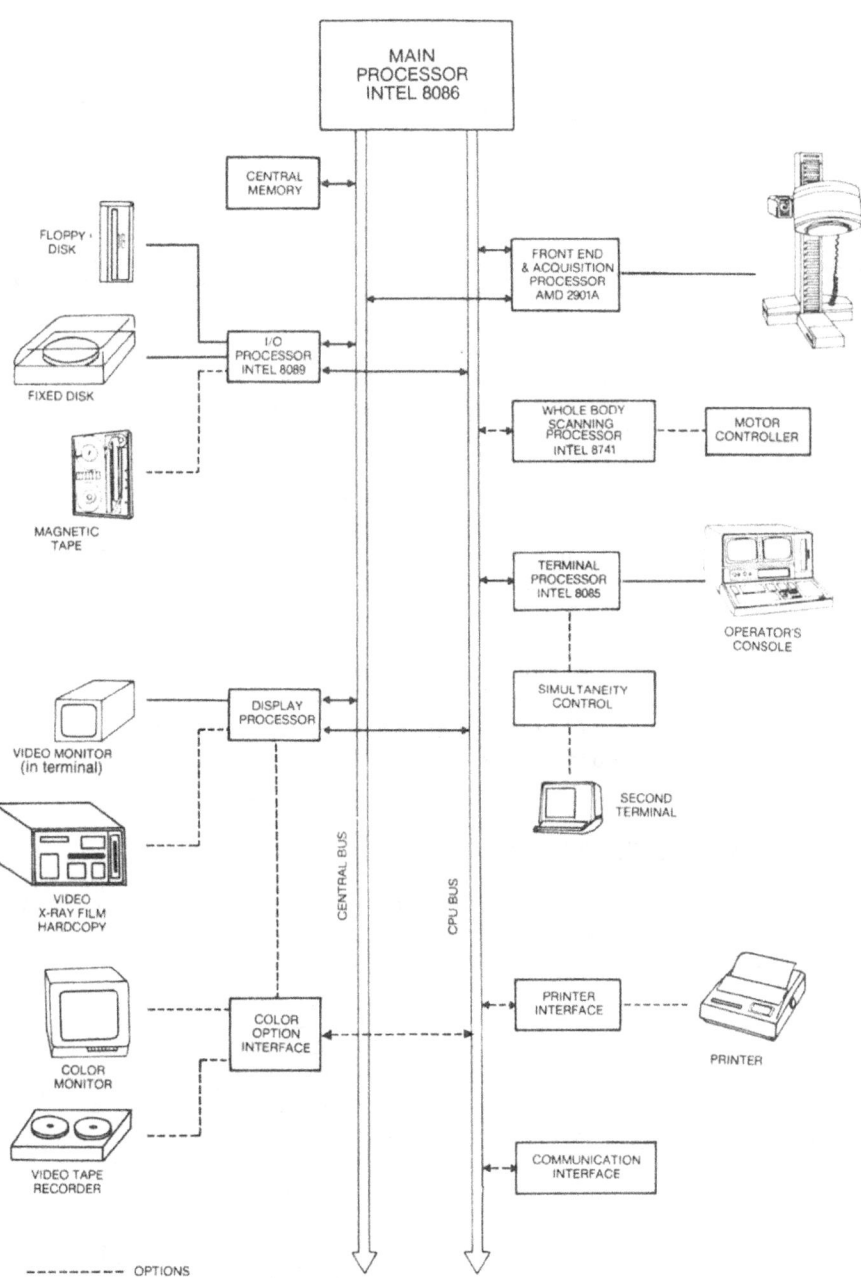

Fig. 1: Apex Digital Gamma Camera Block Diagram

Hardware analog circuitry that can counteract these intrinsic mistakes has long been produced by many NM manufacturers (5).

Till today, however, it is noteworthy that despite a most recent endorsement by major companies, the Elscint design still retains some unique features and benefits from its fully digital (software) approach.

It features the dynamic (software) loading of a fine-tuned correction circuitry prior to each acquisition, merely by loading large software correction tables into the array processor's internal memory. Acquisition then proceeds, and corrections are done on-the-fly. Thus, sharp tuning is possible for all types of scans, since the system disk can hold scores of different correction tables: a set for each isotope, and even for each desired count rate range per radio-element (<u>in particular</u> for demanding fast gold or Tc cardiac first passes).

This software process has obvious advantages over fixed circuitry: it is easy to tune, to change, and to expand to any newly introduced isotope, simply by appending a set of customized tables to the disk (also erected by a simple software program).

Increasing evidence for the need and benefits of this unique feature of optimizing the detector response has originated from today's most demanding N.M. area: SPECT, especially for multi-isotopes (6) and asymmetrical windowing (7), where other approaches led to serious difficulties (8).

Digital Control over the Head

The impact of the third digital processing breakthrough introduced by Elscint in N.M., and by now largely imitated in the market (even if only partially) is perhaps the most important one.

Whatever correction scheme has been adopted, none of it is effective unless it stays valid over months of regular work. Thus, a crucial element in the design of a digital N.M. system should be the monitoring and control over the detector response, including not only PM gains (as in other market brands), but other preamplifiers, X and Y offsets and energy gains, etc..., in order to keep the detector tuned over an extended period of time.

As can be seen in Figure 2, this system is equipped with the so-called "calibration package" which uses a sourceless acquisition simulator (L.E.D.'s) to be run at idle camera times, in order to restore, among others, PM gains to the reference "birth date" values depicted.

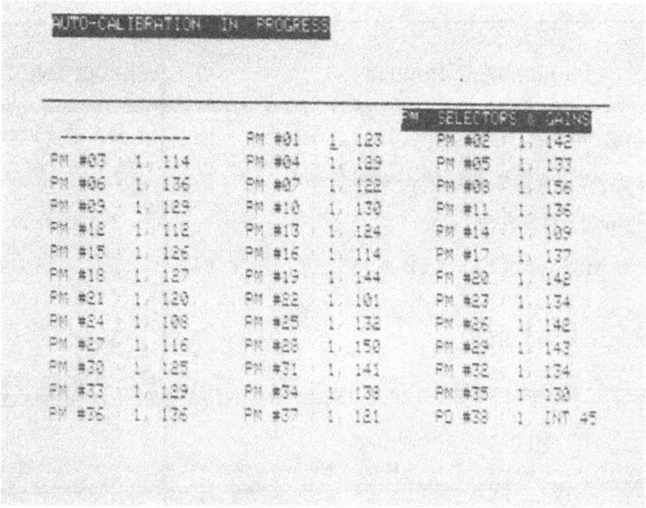

AUTO-CALIBRATION IN PROGRESS

PM SELECTORS & GAINS

--------------	PM #01 1, 123	PM #02 1, 142
PM #03 1, 114	PM #04 1, 129	PM #05 1, 133
PM #06 1, 136	PM #07 1, 122	PM #08 1, 156
PM #09 1, 129	PM #10 1, 130	PM #11 1, 136
PM #12 1, 112	PM #13 1, 124	PM #14 1, 109
PM #15 1, 126	PM #16 1, 114	PM #17 1, 137
PM #18 1, 127	PM #19 1, 144	PM #20 1, 142
PM #21 1, 120	PM #22 1, 101	PM #23 1, 134
PM #24 1, 108	PM #25 1, 132	PM #26 1, 142
PM #27 1, 116	PM #28 1, 150	PM #29 1, 143
PM #30 1, 125	PM #31 1, 141	PM #32 1, 134
PM #33 1, 129	PM #34 1, 138	PM #35 1, 130
PM #36 1, 136	PM #37 1, 121	PD #38 1 INT 45

Fig.2: PM gains as references for automatic calibration; last value is that of LED pin-diode (simulator).

This number-crunching iterative algorithm performs in seconds, thus virtually at each user request, and involves extensive use of the array processor to exercise a tight feed-back loop over the detector via in-board digital-to-analog converters.

SUBSEQUENT ADVANTAGES OF A FULLY DIGITAL GAMMA CAMERA

So far, we have examined the "raison d'être" of the design of a fully digital gamma camera. There are, of course, associated benefits that enable its use to be synergized in order to make it a tool of general interest in Nuclear Medicine.

Choice of the Operating System

It is well recognized today that traditional real-time operating systems -especially those running under 16-18 bits cpu's- are rather unable to cope with current performance requests from the Nuclear Medicine community, either because of lack of memory (e.g. lower matrix sizes and dynamic frame rates limits), or because of limited multitasking facilities (e.g. no possibility to reframe a cardiac gated list mode on-the-fly).

Thus, an early process of "matchmaking" had to take place in order to ensure the most intimate and powerful overlap between the overall hardware design (see Figure 1) and driving software.

PROCESSING MODULE	EXECUTION TIME (SEC.)
Scrolling (H or V)	0 (on-line)
Frame rotation by degree and zoom	< 1
W.B. zipper elimination	2 (automatic)
E.C.T. trans. slices (60 proj. X 64 X 64)	2.4 /slice
1-2-1 spatial or temp. smoothing (64 frames X 64 X64)	3
CLINICAL PROCEDURE	
PVC Post processing for arrhythmia in cardiac list mode	0 (on-the-fly)
Representative cycle for 1st pass	1 / cycle
Fourier coefficients (Phase + Amplitude) any harmonic for 60 frames X 64 X 64	7
Multislice profiles of ECT Tl 201 (Bull's eye) for 16 sl. X 128 X 128	13
MTT and flow functional images for 60 frames X 64 X 64	<35
Fully automated cardiac package (auto-ROIS, REFI, Paradox, Fourier, PER, PFR) for 60 frames X 64 X 64	<150

Table 1.: Typical Apex processing performance .

The choice by Elscint of Intel's IRMX-86 to fully support the hardware stems from the great extent of multitasking resources offered by this operating system, its mail boxes , dynamic task creation and killing facilities, as well as its own powerful development tools (9).

Clinical Processing Performances

The same acquisition tool that enables high spatial and temporal resolution to be maintained even at high count rates can be made available, during idle array processor time, for standard data analysis. Quantitative results, see Table 1, show typical execution speeds for some by-now "classical" N.M. procedures (10).

This gain in performance, hence in work throughput, could be achieved owing to the natural computing reservoir of the architecture, serviced by the proper software (i.e. no system redesign or add-on whatsoever).

Quality Control Improvements (11)

A typical fringe benefit from the "do - it - digital" capacities of those N.M. systems lies in periodical automatic maintenance features -say of a whole body attachment- for which two distinct parameters can be checked: repetitive sampling of the velocity of the bed during scanning (i.e. velocity calibration) to correct post factum bed speed irregularity, as well as the parallelism of the head to the bed motion (i.e. torsion calibration). Figures 3 and 4 show a sequence of both quality control programs. Statistically significant deviations from previously authorized standards are - if accepted- taken into account for real-time image optimization during subsequent whole body scans.

System Friendliness

A non-less typical -and unique- example is the standard interaction with user during the evaluation of ECT reconstruction,as depicted in Figure 5 (12). A 3-D effect is obtained by rotating the raw data while the reconstruction of any slice progresses.

At the same time and on the same display the system is also able to show and separately contrast enhanced multiple views (i.e. coronal, sagittal, and transaxials), as well as to track dynamically (with markers) the level of the cuts.

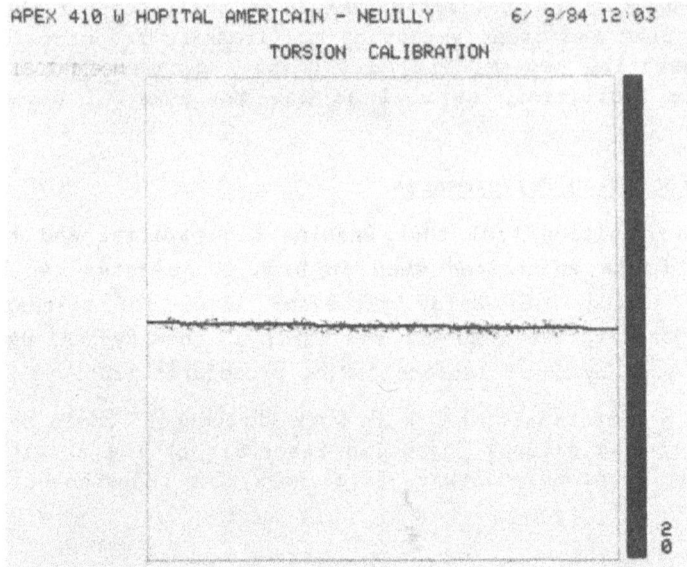

Fig.3: Torsion scan to outline precise motion trajectory of point source on bed.

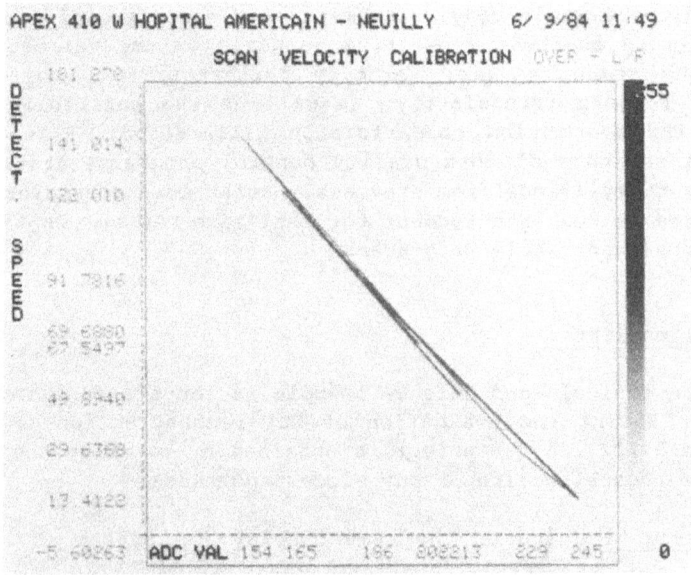

Fig.4: Velocity scan with plot of various bed speeds vs control sensor references.

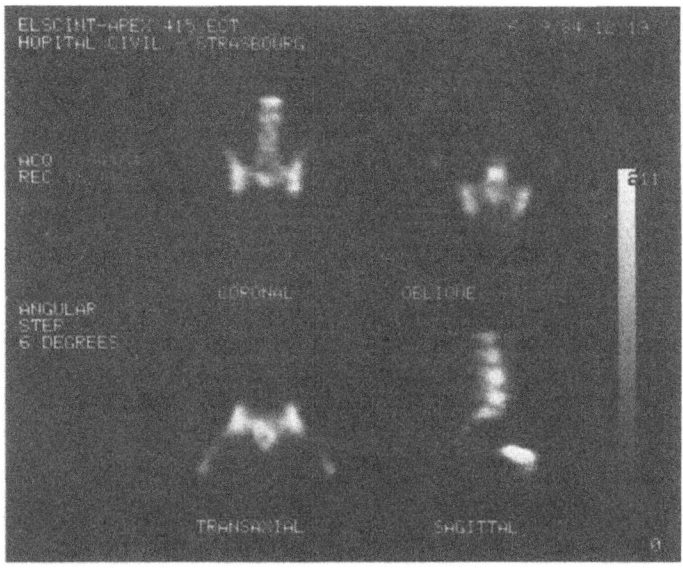

Fig.5: Multiple ECT slices on single display with separate contrasts.

Ease of Program Development

The use of CLIP, a fully Elscint developed BASIC-like interpreter with its own interface to Nuclear Medicine imaging, enables even for the novice user the development of sophisticated clinical protocols with full parameter passing, as well as structured programming statements.

Because of the vast computing power resources, CLIP has some unique features that distinguish it from other manufacturers counterparts. For example, it features fault-tolerant teaching sessions, during which the machine "learns" the clinical protocol to-be-built: extensive and interactive syntax checking prevents errors from being learned during the interactive operations. Hence, no off-line programming with a standard editor is required from the novice user.

It can be seen from Table 1 that, despite the huge software overhead involved (friendliness has its price!), the clinical protocols designed as a collection of CLIP macros still provide very fast execution times.
Such an achievement throughout the various operating system overhead interfaces (especially in I/O) is indeed a breakthrough in itself.

CONCLUSION : A GLANCE TO THE FUTURE

All in all the development of integrated digital Nuclear Medicine systems has largely stimulated other manufacturers efforts toward the improvement of their own product line.
The natural outcome of the digital approach is twofold.

On one hand, the heavy R & D companies investment could (and is!) utilized for instrumentation in neighboring areas: similar microprogrammed cpu's for "simple" echocardiography, functional imaging for MRI spin echo sequences, patient archiving, and regional function quantification in DSA, etc... Vice versa, one-way borrowings are already available, such as isometric and life 3-D displays from the CAD/CAM repertoire. A clear prerequisite for it is a common intermodality company development program.

On the other hand, use can be made of the existing architecture to further extend the concept of networking to other user terminals in separate clinical departments, aiming at a PACS system around the achieved N.M. breakthroughs, via standard serial / parallel interfaces or through local networks (e.g. Ethernet architecture, in Elscint's case)

What is -or should be- the center of gravity of tomorrow's imaging stations is not yet clearly defined.
One thing remains sure: the need for versatile, friendly and easy-to-maintain systems, intrinsically able to accomodate 'foreign" developments (e.g. gate arrays, optical disks), in an ever tightening control over one's operating costs.
There is, today, no substitute for fully digital systems to accomodate all these seemingly conflicting requirements in the Nuclear Medicine environment.

REFERENCES

(1) Pretchner, D.P., European J. of Nucl. Med.,5, 175-184 (1980).

(2) "Digital Imaging: Clinical Advances in Nuclear Medicine", P.D. Esser, Ed., Society of Nuclear Medicine, Inc.,N.Y., 1982.

(3) Hasegawa, B.H., D.L. Kirch, M.T. Le Free, R.A. Fogel, P.P. Steele, and W.R. Hendee, J.Nucl.Med.,22, 1075-1080

(4) Koral, K.F., M.E. Schrader, and G.F. Knoll, J.Nucl.Med.,22, 1069-1074 (1981).

(5) Muehllehner,G., R.H. Wake, and R. Sano, J.Nucl.Med.,22, 72-77 (1981).

(6) Todd Pokropek, A., Nuclear Med.Comm.,5, 421-437 (1984).

(7) Jaszczak R.J, K.L. Greer, C.E. Floyd,Jr.,C. Craig Harris, and R.E. Coleman, J.Nucl.Med.,25, 893-900 (1984).

(8) Jahangir, S.M., A.B. Brill, Y.J.C. Bizais,and R.W. Rowe, J.Nucl.Med,24, 356-359 (1983).

(9) Introduction to the IRMX-(TM)86 Operating System, O.N. 980312403, Intel Corporation, Santa Clara, Ca (1982).

(10) Tallia R., P. Morello, and G. Castellano, J.Nucl.Med.,25, 608-612 (1984), corrected in J.Nucl.Med.,25, 904 (1984).

(11) Raff,U., V.M. Spitzer, and W.R. Vendee, J.Nucl.Med.,25, 679-687 (1984).

(12) "Emission Computed Tomography: Current Trends", P.D. Esser, Ed., Society of Nuclear Medicine Inc., N.Y., 1983.

DISCUSSION SUMMARY

PANEL ON NUCLEAR MEDICINE AGENTS AND INSTRUMENTATION

During the panel several questions were raised. Adelstein was interested in knowing, with respect to the labeling of cancer chemotherapeutic agents other than Bleomycin, which chemotherapeutic agents Cox felt to be most amenable to the labeling, and which purposes they could be used for. The answer was that, according to Cox's knowledge, only Bleomycin and Adriamycin have been labeled. These and Gallium Nitrate have been used for tumor detection. The only other virtue of such labeling is to monitor uptake of cytotoxic drugs in tumors as a way to predict response, and perhaps to monitor tumor response. The potential advantage of I-123 Bleomycin, as a nonspecific tumor localizing agent, is that the optimum scanning time is 1-2 hrs post injection instead of 24 to 48 hrs. Radiotracer concentration by the spleen has been used to predict the efficacy of splenectomy for certain hemolytic conditions and tumor uptake to predict tumor response to treatment with varying results, primarily false positives. Reba asked which was the evidence that labeled antibiotic chemotherapeutic agents would be reliable indicators for the success of chemotherapy. According to Cox, only that documentation of uptake would suggest the potential for therapeutic response while if no significant uptake occurs, treatment with the unlabeled compound will probably not be useful. It had been suggested that Au-195m was a good agent for cardiac imaging in children. Edward asked for a comment, particularly with regard to radiation dose problem. Cox answered that the main problem is not Au-195m but Mercury breakthrough, which cannot be completely prevented. The critical organ for Hg is the kidney and he recommended considerable caution with respect to pediatric use of this generator system. The maximum number of bolus injections in an adult is ten. This will be much less in children, and therefore the main question was if the limited number of boli would give satisfactory diagnostic information. The Osmium/Iridium generator seems to be a better proposition. Then the problems associated with the future development and diffusion of new radiopharmaceuticals for single photon tomography imaging were considered. Guzzardi asked for a comment about the spreading use and the cost of I-123 compounds and the possibility of labeling new molecules with Tl-201. Cox replied that I-123 is indeed relatively expensive but its effective use can be promoted by the use of labeling kits, several of which are already available in Europe. Some examples are hippuran, amphetamine and Bleomycin and expansion of the form of radiopharmaceuticals is expected during the next few years. Further areas for development lie in the field of Thallium and Gallium chemistry plus, of course, Technetium and Indium. Thallous ion is a very reactive species and has not yet been exploited as a radiolabel. A potential problem with Tl-201 and In-111 is the possibility of damage to the cell nucleus due to Anger electrons. With these two nuclides, products should be developed to obtain minimal binding to the cell nucleus. Along with these photon emitters, the possibility of developing Ga-68 generator product together with rubidium and flourine compounds bring positron imaging within the realistic expectation of being available within general hospitals. Russell asked which function was used for the Novak reconstruction. The results are taken from some, as yet unpublished, work at G.E.. The strategy by Novak is a negative exponential weight determined as a function of distance from the collimator face. Allemand asked for a more detailed comment about the optimal weighting functions used to improve the signal to noise ratio. Todd Pokropek would not use such a (relatively) coarse algorithm, but rather try to optimize a more general approach such as Maximum Entropy or a maximum likelihood method | in which the collimator PSF function can be included. Any such optimization is , however, object dependent, which is an argument against the so-called Novak approach. Viergever wished to discuss the slices of images obtained at different resolution and sensitivity values (experiment by Muehllehner). It resulted of prior importance to strive for high resolution and to consider high sensitivity as a secondary objective. Viergever has an opposite experience with time-coded aperture imaging, a form of multiplexed coded aperture imaging. Given limitations provided by pinhole spacing, pinhole viewing angle ($\geq$ maximum angle of incidence of gamma rays) and plate thickness needed for absorption of unwanted photons, it was found that a coarse pinhole, i.e. the largest possible pinhole diameter, gave better results than those achieved with a fine pinhole. (Van Giessen JW, Viergever MA: IEEE Trans. Med. Ins. 3: 1-9, 10984). The question was if it was possible that the difference was due to the difference in imaging modalities since coded aperture techniques have a poor sensitivity. Todd Pokropek stated that this was quite object dependent and is probably reconstruction method dependent as well. Therefore, the problems are not exactly comparable and the mathematics of the evolutions should be carefully examined before giving a precise answer. ART is very non-linear and it may not be easy to compare with these results those for filtered back-projection. It was stated that orthogonal Coded Aperture Imaging (CAI) has great advantages compared to non-orthogonal CAI because a large part of the Fourier space is covered by the projections. In this regard, Viergever wished to know if a reconstruction could be done in the Fourier space or, for example, using a convolution method. Todd Pokropek pointed out that the problem was considerably less ill-posed, which made it easier to perform the reconstruction. Viergever commented that limited angle tomographic systems have a field of view of typically one steradian or less. It has been shown (Tam K-C, Perez-Mendez V, MacDonald B: IEEE Trans. Nucl. Sci. 26: 2797-2805, 1979) that at considerably worse levels at least one-quarter of the entire Fourier space, i.e. (steradians) is needed to perform reconstruction based on the inverse Randon transform. Most orthogonal view systems do not meet this requirement, having a field of view of two steradians or less. Therefore, for this kind of imaging, iterative algorithms are more suitable. ART, which has the best performance for the most problems, is not extremely sensitive to the degree of ill-posedness of the system. Todd Pokropek replied that the above comment referred to 3-D imaging. For a given 2-D slice reconstruction, the game is such that in the Fourier space, almost all frequencies have been sampled, thus the problem is no longer badly ill-posed. The intention was not to suggest that such data should be directly reconstructed in the frequency domain. The 2D-FFT analogy was used to indicate to what extent the problem was ill-posed. Barret T et al (Tucson) suggest very considerable gains, albeit a very different algorithm (Annealing), and the results from Brookhaven (Brill et al) were also encouraging. As for collimators, Wolf added that he had tried depleted uranium collimators but they had not worked. Todd Pokropek replied that there would appear to be some materials supposedly self-shielded which should be worth testing. Then Guzzardi asked some questions to Salomon. Firstly he wished to know if the digital camera would actually digitize X, Y, Z and not each individual P.M. event. Secondly, which was the clinical validity of the 3-D and profile display of the tomographic images of Tl-201 distribution. Lastly how the count-rate corrections were applied when a variable factor following acquisition of the actual count rate was applied. The answer was that Elscint was still concerned with Anger camera. A photon can be digitized but not a scintillation! However, as soon as possible, the event, the energy and the position will be "grabbed" and processed by software,

including any postprocessing through the same computer system and by way of its particular input peripheral - Anger detector. Then with regard to the second question, there are two potential strategies for 3-D representation, i.e. morphology and function. The morphology part is merely an adaptation of CAD/CAM isometric and shadowing techniques. It has iconographic advantages, as long as there is a live display. The functional aspect has some perspective potentials. For example if the stacked slices have intrinsic functional content, e.g. quantity of tissue or regional blood flow, such a display will help in digitizing the global function. None of these techniques, however, are intrinsically able to solve the problem of true distribution because of the error in determining the true attenuation of the radionuclide. The techniques are, however, performing as visual tools. With regard to multi-slice concentric representation (bull's eye), one needs a precise indication of depth, as, for example, in case of massive scar tissue. The advantage of this type of presentation is the possibility to use it as a single functional image to compare in one image, several stress/rest slices or several ED/ES slices, i.e., multi slice regional ejection fraction. In principle, this technique offers the same amount of information as a full set of planar images. We have to wait to gather more clinical data to determine how this method of presentation will be accepted. As for the last question, the correction scheme, in the APEX system it is user-selected. For example, loading the appropriate 'fast' correction tables is requested before each cardiac first-pass study. The optimum detector response is guaranteed, as spatio-temporal resolution is preserved. This has nothing to do with the optional use of a dead-time correction circuitry. Due to the camera performance, it has been found that count losses, if any, are very low, even at 100 kilocounts/second with a window, as determined during a clinical first-pass study. Thus, the dead-time is not usually selected, although it is available. If one wants to study it, it will follow the actual count rate and 'increase' the count numbers recorded. Fusco wished to know Salomon's opinion about the problem of the so-called 'user open software'. In other words, if it is better to allow users to make up general protocols by themselves while the machine simply provides a number of basic commands. Or if it is better to enclose with the software package a sort of library containing the main functions requested for a Nuclear Medicine system. The answer was that one would be able to provide both.
Since general protocols are made by including basic functions and allowing free parameter passing in a top-to-bottom way, it is enough

to provide the capability to edit or upgrade any existing protocol, to have it reviewed or customized by each user. There is a potential danger in using 'closed' protocols if they refer to internal (absolute) references. As an example, a thallium set of 'normals' may depend on risk factors of patients studied which may vary in the different hospitals. Therefore, prior validation at the site is preferable. Subsequently, one can always 'freeze' the protocols and make them available via the menu or the functional key, regardless of their true complexity.

TRANSIENT CHANGES IN RENAL UPTAKE RATE OF 99mTc DMSA AS POSSIBLE INDICATORS OF CHANGES OF RENAL FUNCTION DURING STRESS

S. Ghione*, E. Fommei*, C.R. Bellina**, C. Palombo*, P. Meconi*, L.S. Palla*, C. Rosa*
* C.N.R. Clinical Physiology Institute
** Istituto di Patologia Medica, University of Pisa, Pisa (Italy).

INTRODUCTION

99m Tc dimercaptosuccinic acid (DMSA), a widely used renal imaging agent, represents a good substitute for organic radiomercurials with which it shares the property to accumulate in renal cortical tubular cells (1).. As for radiomercurials (2), their use has also been recommended for quantifying individual renal functions by the measurement of the percentage of the dose accumulated by the kidney after two to four hours (3-5). To our knowledge, however, no studies have been performed on the use of the measurement of accumulation rate of DMSA before attaining plateau as a possible index of renal function. The aim of this brief paper is to report our observation that DMSA accumulation rates may undergo transient modifications during stress tests.

MATERIALS AND METHODS

Six essential hypertensives and one normal subject were studied by means of a large field-of-view gamma camera (Selo KR7) and a dedicated computer (Medusa 12B Sepa). Five to fifteen minutes after dose injection (DMSA, Sorin; 2 mCi), counts over the kidneys' region were acquired with a high sensitivity collimator at a rate of 1 frame every 30 seconds for 45 minutes. The patient remained motionless in the prone position for the whole study which comprised of periods of quiet rest for at least 10 minutes alternated with an isometric exercise and a mental arithmetic test. The isometric exercise consisted of a handgrip at 30% of the individual maximal force for three to four minutes. The mental arithmetic test was represented by difficult subtractions given by voice by one investigator while the patient was urged to answer as quickly as possible and lasted eight to ten minutes. In addition, DMSA uptake was also measured in three cases without any stimulation (care was given to avoid noise or other disturbing factors during the test).

Time/activity curves for each kidney were obtained after selection of suitable regions of interest (ROI) and a careful check in all frames for any inadequacy of the ROI due to possible minor body motions.

RESULTS

In non-stimulated subjects DMSA uptake increased smoothly. On the other hand, in each case studied, both isometric and mental effort induced an abrupt reduction of the uptake rate which resumed its normal course after the end of the test. In each instance

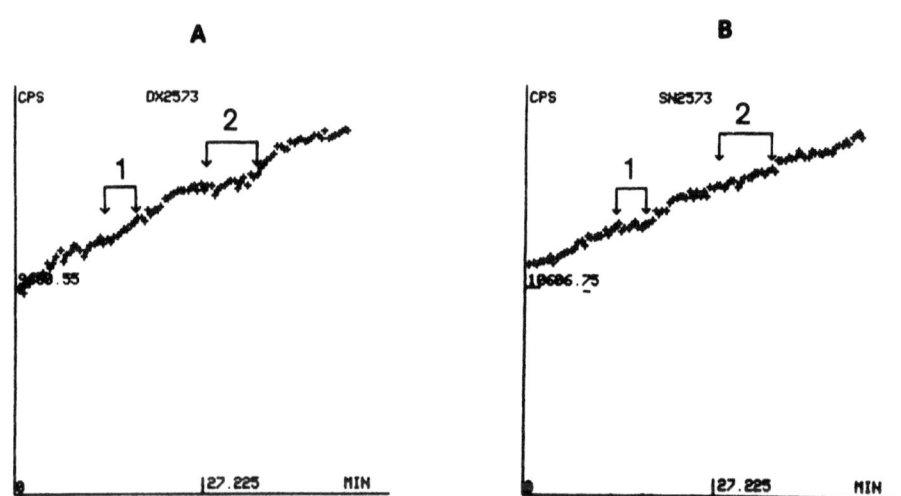

Fig.1: Effect of physical (1) and mental (2) exercise on 99mTc DMSA renal uptake rate.
A = Right Kidney
B = Left Kidney

onset and discontinuation of the test closely corresponded to points of inflection of the time/activity curves (Fig.1). The average decrease of the time/activity slope was 55% (range 36-73%) for the handgrip and 52% (range 32-64%) for the mental arithmetic test. Interestingly, the response of the two kidneys was not always equal.

DISCUSSION

The observation of clear reductions in DMSA renal accumulation rate during stress tests cannot be easily explained since factors determining renal DMSA uptake rate may be multiple and their relation to renal function complex and only partially understood (6-7). Possible conditions which can induce a transient reduction of the accumulation rate of DMSA are a reduced delivery to the kidney and a reduced fractional uptake by the tubular cells. In the first case a reduced renal blood flow would have to be assumed, in the second a change in tubular handling of 99m Tc DMSA. In addition, since a minor fraction of DMSA passes through the kidneys and is excreted in the urine, a further possibility of explaining our observations is in terms of an increase of renal excretion of DMSA. Finally, renal accumulation rate might also change because of geometric reasons, such as a displacement of the kidney during the tests either to a more distant position from gamma camera or out of the ROI. However, the first explanation appears to us highly unlikely and, as regards the adequacy of the ROI to include all the renal parenchima, extreme care was adopted to avoid the possibility of the renal image in any frame, being out of the borders of the ROI.

At present we have no direct evidence as to whether the reduction in DMSA accumulation rate observed during stress is due to a reduction in renal blood flow, to a reduced uptake by the tubular cells, to an increased urinary excretion or to some combination of these factors. The most likely explanation appears to us to be that of a reduced renal blood flow. This would fit with the observation reported in a recent paper by Hollenberg (8) which confirmed earlier observations by other Authors (9-10) of a marked renal vasoconstriction during emotional response, especially in hypertensive patients. Further studies are however necessary to confirm this hypothesis, which, if validated, could offer an easy and non-invasive method for the evaluation of transient changes in renal blood flow.

REFERENCES

1. Lin, T.H., A. Khentigan, H.S. Winchell. A 99m Tc-chelate substitute for organo-radiomercurial renal agents. J.Nucl.Med., 15: 34, 1974.
2. Raynaud, C., A. Desgrez, C. Kellershohn et al. Measurement of renal mercury uptake by external counting: separate functional testing of each kidney. J. Urol., 99: 248, 1968.
3. Daly, M.J., W. Jones, T.G. Rudo, J. Tremann. Differential renal function using technetium 99m dimercapto-succinic acid (DMSA): in vitro correlation. J.Nucl.Med. 20: 63, 1979.
4. Beekhuis, H., W.H.J. Van Luyk, D.A. Piers. Differential renal function using technetium 99m dimercapto-succinic acid (DMSA); in-vivo correlation. J.Nucl.Med. 20: 898, 1979.
5. Kawamura, J., S. Hosokava, O. Yoshida. Renal function studies using Tc99m dimercapto-succinic acid. Clin. Nucl. Med. 4: 39, 1979.
6. Yee, C.A., H.B. Lee, M.D. Blaufox. Tc-99m DMSA renal uptake: influence of biochemical and physiologic factors. J.Nucl.Med. 22: 1054, 1981.
7. Vanlic-Razumenic, N.M., D.A. Gorcik. Studies on chemical and biological properties of 99m Tc DMS (dimercaptosuccinic acid) - renal imaging agent. Eur.J.Nucl.Med. 1: 235, 1976.
8. Hollenberg, N.K., G.H. Williams, D.F. Adams. Essential hypertension: abnormal renal vascular and endocrine responses to a mild psychological stimulus. Hypertension 3: 11, 1981.
9. Wolf, S., J.B. Pfeiffer, H.S. Ripley, O.S. Winter, H.G. Wolff. Hypertension as a reaction pattern to stress: variations in blood pressure and renal blood flow. Ann.Int.Med. 29, 1056, 1948.
10. Smith, H.W. The physiology of the renal circulation. Harvey Lect. 35: 166 [60], 1940.

Poster Session

OPTIMIZATION OF RIGHT VENTRICULAR EJECTION FRACTION MEASUREMENTS
FROM FIRST PASS AND GATED BLOOD POOL SCINTIGRAPHY

D.Neglia, C.Marcassa, O.Parodi, C.R.Bellina, P.Marzullo, C.Michelassi, S. Berti, C. Contini and A. L'Abbate
CNR Institute of Clinical Physiology and Istituto di Patologia Medica I, University of Pisa, Pisa, Italy

INTRODUCTION

The scintigraphic evaluation of the left ventricular (LV) function is well established (1); on the contrary the complex geometric shape of the right ventricle (RV) and its superimposition with other vascular structures have delayed the quantitative functional evaluation of this chamber. Two main scintigraphic approaches have been used for the calculation of the RV ejection fraction (EF): the first pass technique (2,3) and the equilibrium radionuclide angiography (RNA) (4,5,6). The first pass is theoretically the most valuable method, avoiding some problems which still remain for RNA: the definition of the RV contours, separating the chamber from the right atrium and the pulmonary artery, the choice of the correct background regions (BK). The main problem in the validation of these measures is however the lack of a reliable reference method. In order to optimize the RVEF measurements from both scintigraphic techniques in this study we compare the values computed by three different methods applied to first pass and RNA data. Moreover we studied the role of different BK subtraction on RVEF values determination. Finally, we tested the accuracy of each method in separating patients with RV dysfunction from normal subject and from patients with LV dysfunction.

MATERIALS AND METHODS

Patients. We studied 15 patients: 5 were normal , 7 had dilated cardiomiopathy and 3 had previous myocardial infarction. All the patients were studied by 2D-echocardiography, showing normal biventricular function, (5pts) (Group 1) evident LV dysfunction, (5pts) (Group 2) or evident RV dysfunction (5pts) (Group 3).

Radionuclide technique. The first pass study was performed in basal condition by a bolus injection of 20 mCi of 99mTc, 20 min. after the injection of 0.2 mg/Kg of pyrophosphates through an intravenuos catheter positioned in the superior vena cava. Data were acquired in list mode (anterior-posterior projection) with ECG syncronism by a large field Gamma-camera (SELO KR-7) equipped with a low energy high resolution collimator. After the completion of the FP, a RNA was performed in LAO " bestseptal " projection, using frame mode acquisition for about 6 min.

Data analysis. Two methods were applied to the analysis of FP data and one to RNA data. Method 1: RVEF was computed from the slope of the RV washout curve (Newman method) (7). Three different curves were obtained from different RV ROIs outlining: a) the whole RV; b) the apical region; c) the efflux region. Method 2: a gated reconstruction of FP data was performed and RVEF was computed by a count-based method, taking particular care in drawing the RV ROI with the use of phase image as a guide; systolic and diastolic BK subtraction was performed from three different BK regions: BK1) close to the right atrium, BK2) close to the right atrium and RV, BK3) near the left border of LV. Method 3: RVEF was computed from RNA using a modified Maddahi method, outlining carefully the RV and separating it from the right atrium and the pulmonary artery (we used isolevel contours, cine-mode display and phase image). Three different BK regions were chosen, similar to those used for Method 2. Statistical analysis was performed using the variance test for multiple comparison with Newman-Keuls procedures (8).

RESULTS

In the people examined the RVEF values inside each method were not significantly different. However, in Method 1 the RVEF values derived from the ROI, encompassing the whole RV, were always intermediate between those from the efflux (higher values) and the apical region (lower values). These values were chosen for comparison with the other methods. For Method 2 RVEF values were superimposable and we took the mean as the representative value. These results demonstrated that RVEF calculated from gated FP is independent from BK selection. Moreover, RVEF from method 2, together with LVEF from RNA and the analysis of biventricular wall motion from FP and RNA clearly divided the population studied into 3 groups according to the echocardiographic data. In Group 1 with normal wall motion, normal biventricular EF were demonstrated (RVEF=57.4+8, LVEF=56.4+9.4); Group 2 with echocardiographic LV dysfunction demonstrated lower LVEF (p. 0.05) than normal subjects and normal RVEF (RVEF=58.8+9.6, LVEF=26.6+13.3) (Fig. 1); Group 3 with echocardiographic and scintigraphic evidences of RV wall motion abnormalities showed RVEF values significantly lower than Group 1 and 2 (p. 0.01) (RVEF=24.2+9.3, LVEF=56.8+6. According to these results, we chose the mean RVEF from Method 2 as reference, to correlate with the other two methods. Method 1 provided values significantly lower than the reference values and it was not possible to differentiate the 3 groups of patients. Within Method 3 only values from BK1 and BK3 subtraction were well correlated with the reference values (r=0.81 and r=0.82 respectively, n=15), being RVEF values from RNA always lower than FP values. Moreover, RVEF calculated with BK1 substraction separated more accurately patients with RV impairment from the other (p 0.01) than RVEF's calculated with BK3 substraction (p 0.05).

DISCUSSION

Because of the complex geometric shape of RV, no other available technique (contrast angiography, echocardiography) (9, 10) can be taken as reference. Therefore, we decided to compare the 3 scintigraphic methods and to test the reliability of the RVEF values obtained from each of them by assessing their efficacy in separating patients with prevalent RV or LV dysfunction from normal ones. Moreover, we studied the importance of ROI selection and different BK subtraction in affecting RVEF measurements. Our results indicate that the RVEF values, derived from Method 2, are completely independent from BK subtraction and can correctly separate the 3 groups of patients together with LVEF values from RNA. This method looks to be theoretically

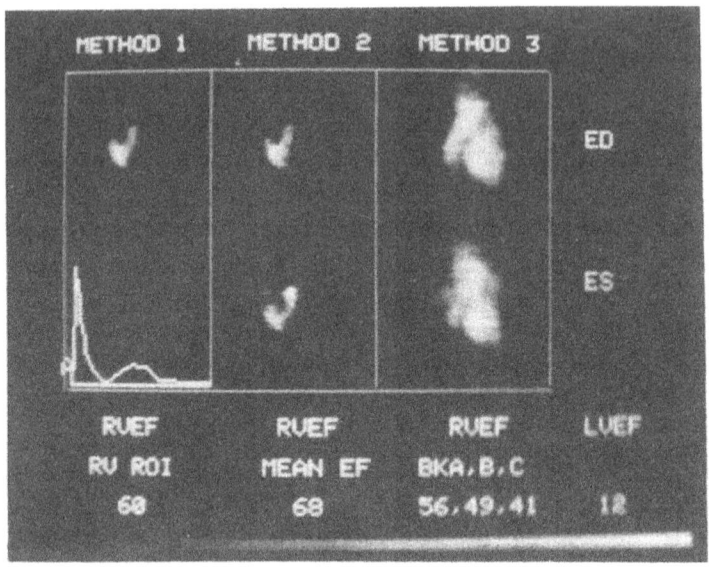

Fig. 1) The three methods RVEF calculation are represented for a patient with prevalent LV dysfunction (Group 2). In Method 1 the RVEF is computed from the RV washout curve; the RV ROI outlining the whole RV has been chosen. For Methods 2 and 3 the end-diastolic and end-systolic frames respectively obtained from the FP and RNA reconstructed cycles are represented. They show normal RV wall motion and a diffuse impairment of LV. LVEF value from RNA is very low while the RVEF value is normal with the three methods. It is important to observe the good correlation between RVEF values from FP data and the value obtained from RNA using BKA substraction.

and practically the best in evaluating the RV function and therefore it was chosen as reference. The results derived from the analysis of RV washout curves during the FP demonstrated, according to data previously published by Maseri, that the RV is not a chamber of homogeneous mixing (single compartment) and that the apical region has slower washout rates while the efflux region has a faster one. This is probably the reason why values from RV ROI do not correlate with the reference and cannot separate the groups of patients. As we have demonstrated Method 2 offers the best evaluation of RVEF. For clinical purposes however, it could be more useful to use the LAO equilibrium RNA for the simultaneous measurements of LV and RV function. Although Maddahi proposed a valuable method for RVEF estimation from RNA, some problems still remain as far as the correct definition of RV ROI and BK selection is concerned.

In order to optimize these measurements, we employed the Maddahi method, modified by the use of isolevel contours, cine-mode display and phase image, to carefully define the RV ROI.

Furthermore we tested the influence of different BK selection on RVEF values. Our results suggest that with proper BK selection, RVEF values from RNA show a good correlation with FP values and can properly separate together with LVEF values obtained from the same acquisition, patients with functional impairment of single or both ventricles from the others. We conclude that:

1) RVEF from the gated reconstruction of the FP data provides the best evaluation of the RV function in different clinical settings;

2) RNA in LAO projection can be used for the simultaneous assessment of the RV and LV function.

REFERENCES

1) Schelbert HR, Verba JW, Johnson AD, Brock GW, Alazraki NP, Ross FJ, Ashburn WL: Non Traumatic Determination of LVEF by Radionuclide Angiography. Circulation 51 (1975): 902.
2) Donato L, Lewis ML, Giuntini C, Harvey RM, Courand A: Quantitative Radiocardiography. III. Results and Validation of Theory and Method. Circulation 26 (1962): 189
3) Johnson LL, MacCarthy DM, Sciaca RR, Carmon PJ: RVEF during Exercise in Patients with Coronary Artery Disease. Circulation 60 51979): 1284.
4) Maddahi J, Berman DS, Matsuoka DT, Waxman Ad, Stankus Ke, Forrester J, Swan Hj: A new Technique for Assessing· RVEF Using rapid Multiple Gated Equilibrium Cardiac Blood Pool Scintigraphy. Circulation 60 (1979): 581
5) Slutsky R, Hooper W, Gerber K, Blatter A, Froelicher V, Ashburn W, Karliner J: Assessment of Right Ventricular Function at Rest and during Exercise in Patients with CAD: A new Approach Using Equilibrium RNA. Am. J. Cardiol. 45 (1980): 63
6) Legrand V, Chevigne M, Foulou J, Rigo P; Evaluation of Right Ventricular Function by Gated Blood Pool Scintigraphy. J. Nucl. Med. 24 (1983): 886
7) Strauss B, Pitt J: Cardiovascular Nuclear Medicine. V ed. Mosby ed. 1979
8) Snedecor GW: Statistical Methods. Iowa State Un. Press, V ed. 1956
9) Jugdutt BI: Right Ventricular Infarction by Echocardiographic evaluation. Am. Heart J. 107 (1984): 505
10) Ferlings J: Measurements of Right Ventricular Volume in Man from Single Plane Cineangiograms. A Comparison to the Biplane Approach. Am. Heart J. 94 (1977): 87

PART XI STATE-OF-THE-ART AND FUTURE TRENDS IN SINGLE PHOTON TOMOGRAPHY

Chairman: S.James Adelstein (U.S.A.)

EMISSION TOMOGRAPHY USING ROTATING CAMERAS

G. van Oortmarssen

Siemens Gammasonics B.V., Uithoorn, The Netherlands

In the last decade, numerous investigations have been conducted in the nuclear medicine field, in the use of tomography as a means to-
a) improved diagnostic imaging, and
b) assessment of quantitative information

Rotating gamma cameras connected to computers as a method of performing tomography seem to be the system of choice in most institutions.

The performance of such systems is far more critical in clinical imaging than in conventional planar imaging. The diagnostic advantage using ECT can be lost quite easily, and become a disadvantage over planar imaging, due to technical problems which are not immediately obvious. Many technical considerations must be made and solved before a system can be used successfully in a routine setup.

Continued quality control must be performed to assure correct functioning. For an ECT system in a routine setup, these functions have to be automated, making use of appropriate hard and software. An ECT system must therefore be designed as an integrated computer-detector-gantry system.

Apart from extremely linear detectors, a stable mechanical setup and state-of-the-art software with a relatively powerful computer using an array processor is required to handle a vast amount of data in an acceptable time. If these criteria are met, an ECT system based on a rotating gamma camera detector will be a powerful diagnostic tool which replaces planar imaging totally in a number of cases.

It has taken a decade of engineering and clinical research from the
early experimental stage to the widespread acceptance of Single
Photon Emission Computed Tomography (SPECT) in Nuclear Medicine.
With today's gamma camera performance and computer technology, SPECT
is now rapidly moving from clinical evaluation into routine application.

Planar images provide a two-dimensional map of the three-dimensional
distribution of a radionuclide within an organ. Planar images provid
limited information about the true distribution of the radionuclide,
and moreover suffer from low image contrast due to source activity
surrounded by background activity. SPECT yields tomographic images
in which background activity is virtually removed, resulting in high
image contrast, and which reflect the true three-dimensional distribution activity (see Figure 1).

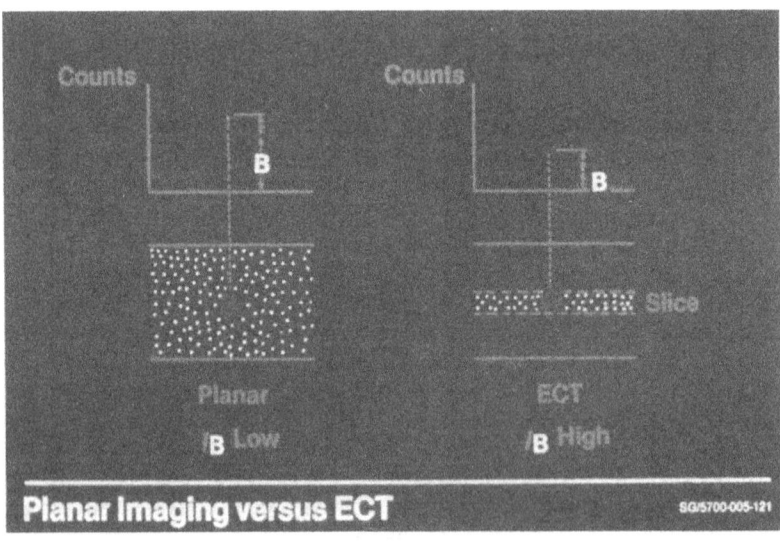

Figure 1

Many different techniques for emission tomography have been suggested and evaluated. Some of those techniques, such as rotating slant hole collimators, pinhole collimator tomography or PhoCon whole body tomography, produce tomographic slice images by blurring overlaying and underlaying activity rather than removing it.

Other methods, e.g. seven pinhole, quadrant slant hole collimator or coded aperture tomography provide computed tomograms but suffer from limited angular sampling like the former methods. Any of these techniques could be used in special applications but are limited with respect to the full spectrum of nuclear medicine applications.

The technologies which have moved SPECT into clinical nuclear medicine are rotational detector systems and the availability of computers with appropriate software. While the camera rotates around the patient in a circle or a half-circle, it acquires a sequence of projection images, e.g. one image every three degrees (see Figure 2). From the projection data, tomographic images are reconstructed using filtered back-projection algorithms. The reconstructed images are initially transverse slices having the same orientation as transmission CT. Since the camera scans a volume rather than a single slice during its rotation, a set of slices can be reconstructed from one orbit. The image data represented by this set of slices can be re-organized into any orientation yielding coronal, sagittal (see Figure 3) or oblique slices.

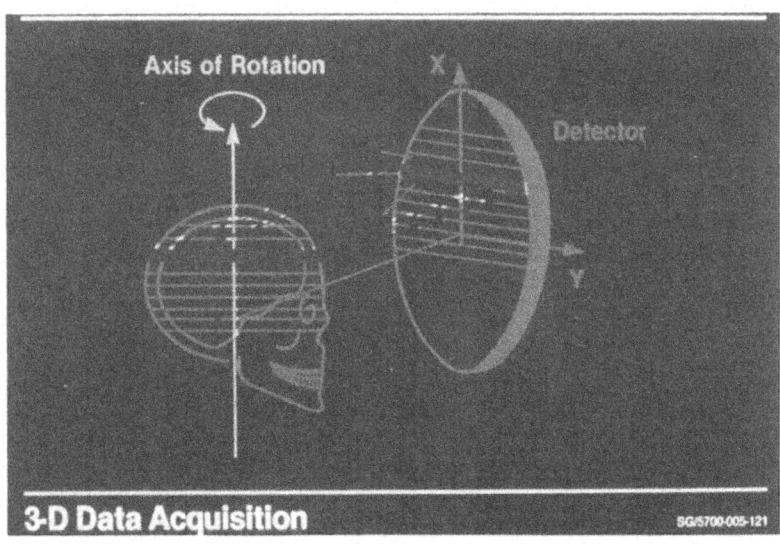

Figure 2

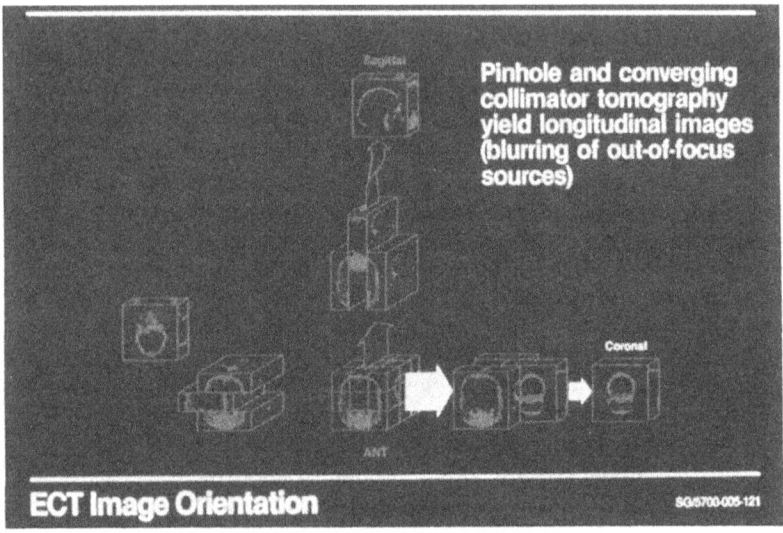

Figure 3

The following will present an overview of the hardware and software requirements for rotational SPECT systems. The principles of SPECT image reconstruction and impact of various correction procedures on SPECT image quality will be reviewed in detail.

Requirements for Rotational SPECT Systems

A rotational SPECT system consists of a rotating, single or dual detector gamma camera (see Figures 4 and 5), a computer with appropriate reconstruction software, and a camera/computer interface to control the detector rotation. The first single and dual detector SPECT systems being developed and evaluated in the late 1970's identified specific performance requirements for emission tomography affecting the camera as well as the computer and associated software

SPECT is much more sensitive to non-uniformities and non-linearities than conventional planar images. Detectors with good intrinsic uniformity and linearity characteristics are a prerequisite for high quality SPECT (see Figures 6 and 7). The introduction of ZLC detectors was a breakthrough in providing this performance.

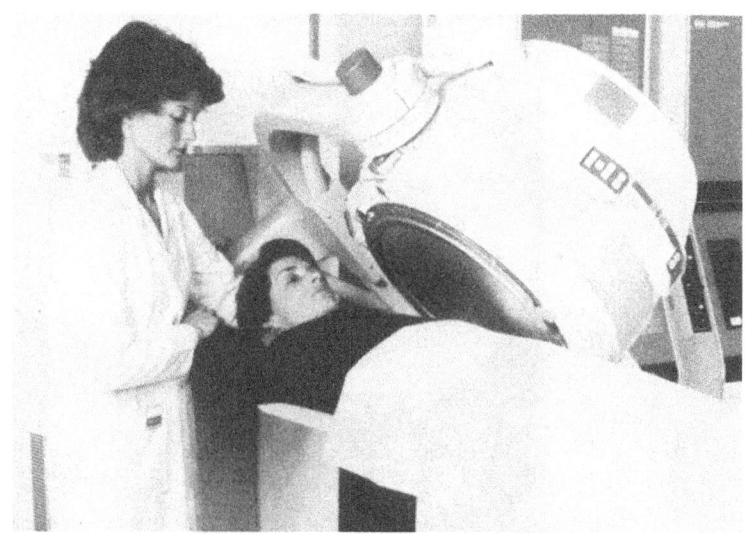

Figure 4

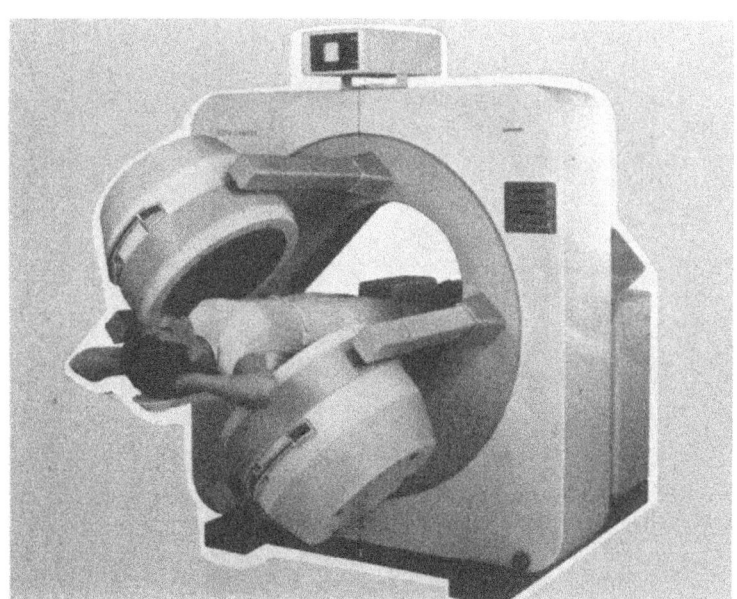

Figure 5

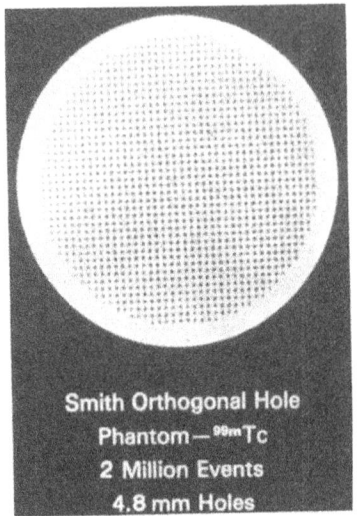

Figure 6

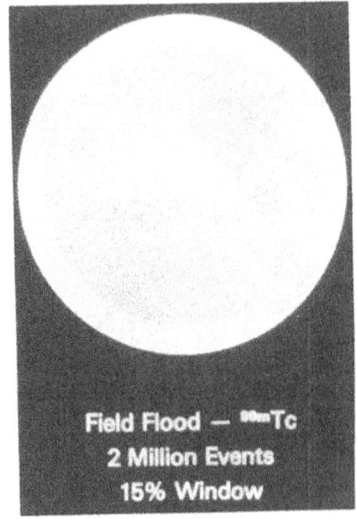

Figure 7

However, as regional sensitivity variations are caused by both detector and collimator, additional uniformity correction must be applied to the raw image data.

Mechanically, the gantry supporting the detector must provide a stable center of rotation and accurate tracking during rotation in order to preserve resolution in the SPECT image. The alignment of the mechanical and electrical center of rotation, or offset correction, is another indispensable quality assurance procedure to be implemented in SPECT software.

Finally, events from the center of the body are attenuated before reaching the detector. Attenuation correction must be applied during or after reconstruction in order to obtain images with an accurate map of the radionuclide distribution - essential for future image quantitation.

Principles of SPECT

The major SPECT data processing characteristics, which will be discussed and illustrated in this chapter, include the method of filtered back-projection and filter section, the role of linear and angular sampling, the corrections for uniformity and center-of-rotation offset, as well as attenuation correction.

The effect of these characteristics on resolution, lesion detectability and uniformity in SPECT images is best demonstrated in phantom studies. Phantom studies provide an advantage over clinical studies because they are not limited in the number of counts acquired, are free of motion blurring, and offer a priori knowledge of the true activity distribution (see Figure 8).

A high resolution SPECT phantom (Data Spectrum Corporation, Chapel Hill, N.C., U.S.A.) was employed in testing SPECT system performance. The phantom consists of a uniform activity compartment, six sectors of cold or hot rods with diameters between 12.7 mm. and 4.8 mm. with a center-to-center spacing of twice the diameter, and six cold spheres, 31.8 mm. to 9.5 mm. in diameter. The phantom was imaged using a ZLC 7500S camera with a parallel ultra-high resolution and a high resolution collimator. The phantom was filled with 35 mCi Tc-99m. Unless otherwise specified, 180 projection images over 360 degrees were acquired at a radius of rotation of 13 cm. Matrix sizes of 64 x 64, 128 x 128 and 256 x 256 were utilized for both acquisition and reconstruction. 5.000.000 counts per view were collected, resulting in a total of 90 million counts per study.

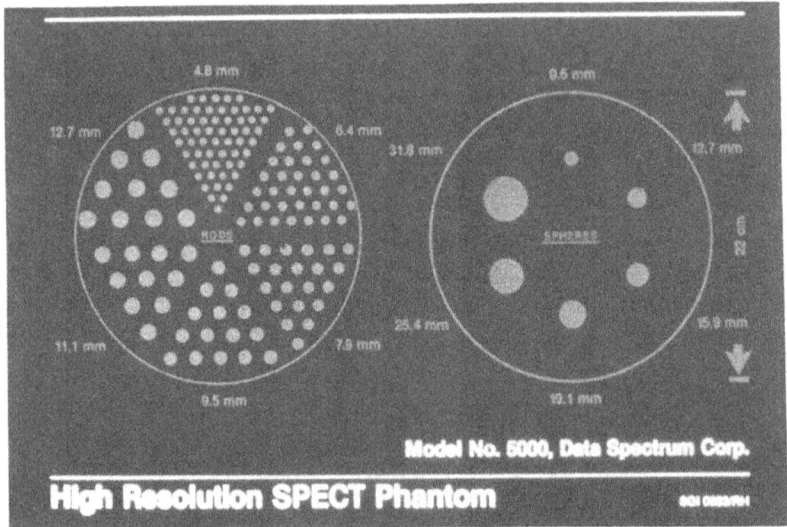

Figure 8

With such a high number of counts, statistical noise in the reconstructed image is reduced to the point where the full range of resolution becomes visible.

The ECT Processor utilizes, as most presently available SPECT software, back-projection algorithms for image reconstruction.
Figure 9 illustrates the principle of simple, i.e. unfiltered back-projection. Planar projection images of the object are acquired from several angles around the object. These data are then back-projected slice by slice into an image matrix which represents a reconstructed slice image. Since the projection data does not contain any information regarding the depth of the source, the number of counts measured in each projection is equally distributed over the depth. The result is a reconstructed image of the source, but is intolerably blurred unless appropriate filtering is applied.

In order to obtain unblurred, sharp images, "filtered back-projection" algorithms are applied. Rather than back-projecting the unprocessed image data, the projections are first filtered, or convolved. Each point in the filter is calculated from all the values in the original projection weighted by a function which is called the "convolution kernel" or "filter function" (see Figure 10).

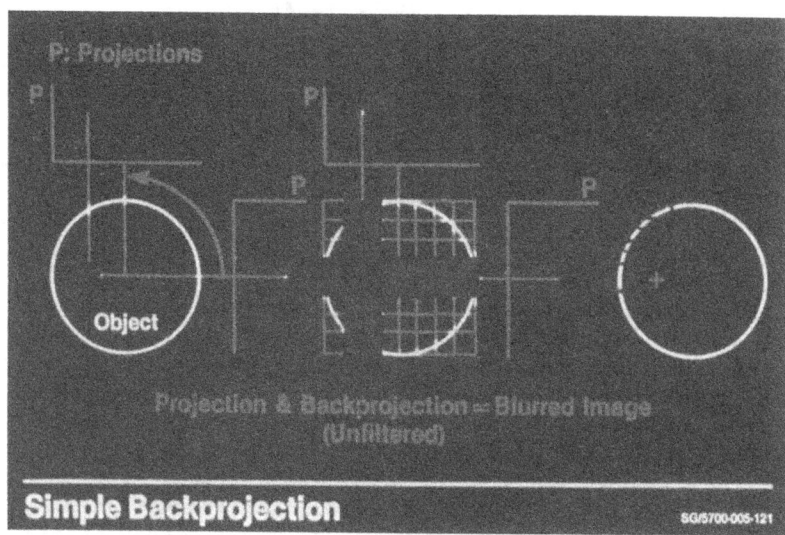

Figure 9

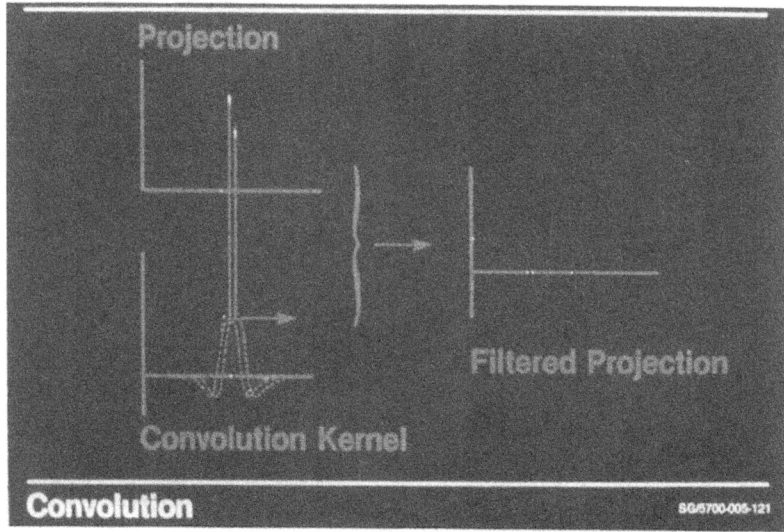

Figure 10

In SPECT applications, the operator selects an appropriate filter function dependent upon the number of counts expected in the study. Figure 11 demonstrates four examples of filter functions represented in the spatial frequency domain. The cut-off frequencies are 1.0 and 0.5 times the Nyquist frequency, respectively. The Nyquist frequency is half the inverse pixel width and reflects the pixel resolution in the image matrix. The Ramp filter is the sharpest and gives the best spatial resolution, but emphasizes noise and is therefore used only in count abundant studies as e.g. the phantom studies presented here. The Shepp-Logan-Hanning filters are the smoothest and are recommended for most clinical studies. Figure 12 demonstrates how spatial resolution in SPECT images is affected by the choice of convolution filter. The loss in resolution in the cold rod phantom images with increasing filter degree can easily be appreciated. The Ramp and Shepp-Logan filters are definitely the filters of choice for high count phantom studies. Using the same filters for the reconstruction of the cold sphere section of the phantom, Figure 13 shows that five of the six spheres can be detected independent of the choice of the filter. The sphere section is used to study lesion detectability in SPECT images (five), which is a trade-off between spatial resolution and signal-to-noise ratio. Although resolution is sacrificed by utilizing a smooth filter, thes images indicate that lesion detectability may not be negatively affected. This result explains and justifies the Shepp-Logan-Hanning filters as being appropriate for most clinical applications.

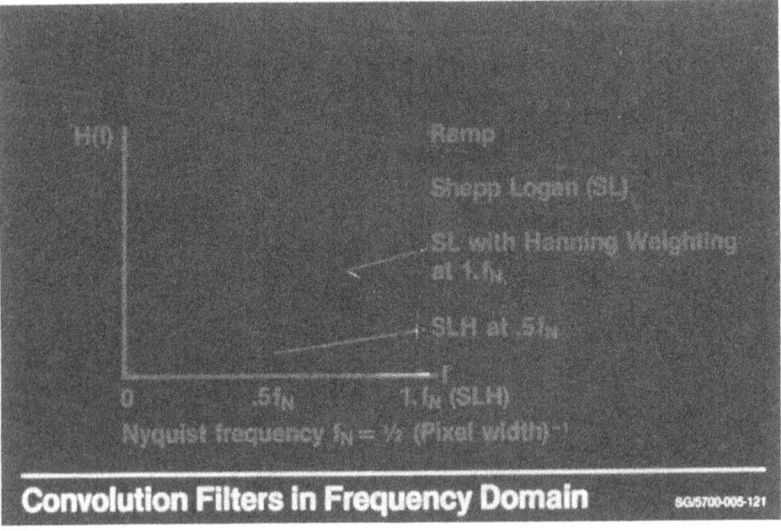

Figure 11

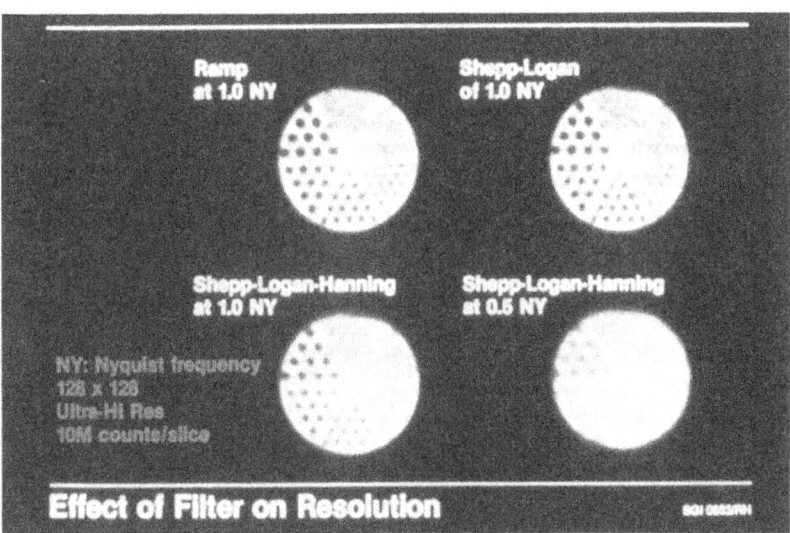

Figure 12

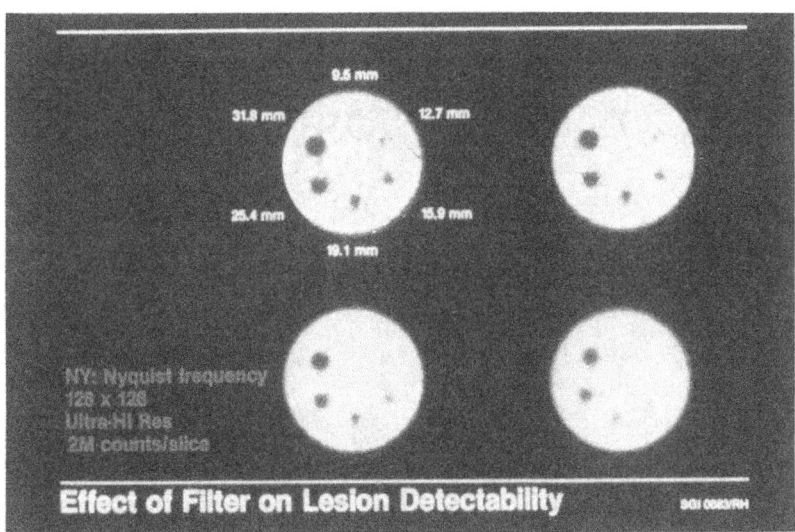

Figure 13

Linear and Angular Sampling

Other than statistical noise, linear sampling or matrix size is another severe limitation of SPECT resolution. The sampling theorem requests that in digital imaging, the pixel resolution is at least twice as good as the best system resolution. Figure 14 compares the pixel widths of 64 x 64, 128 x 128 and 256 x 256 matrixes to the FWHM system resolution at the radius of rotation and the collimator selected. Sampling with a 64 x 64 matrix obviously does not match system resolution, whereas both the 128 x 128 and 256 x 256 matrix do.

The cold rod phantom images in Figure 15 confirm that sampling with a 64 x 64 matrix does not take advantage of the system resolution of the camera. The use of 256 x 256 appears to be most appropriate and demonstrates that the ZLC 7500S camera is capable of resolving even the smallest, 4.8 mm. rods. A 256 x 256 matrix, however, requires excessive image memory and computation time. The best compromise appears to be a 128 x 128 matrix.

With this choice, system resolution is fully matched by pixel resolution, and, with the array processor of the ECT Processor, computation time is still very short.

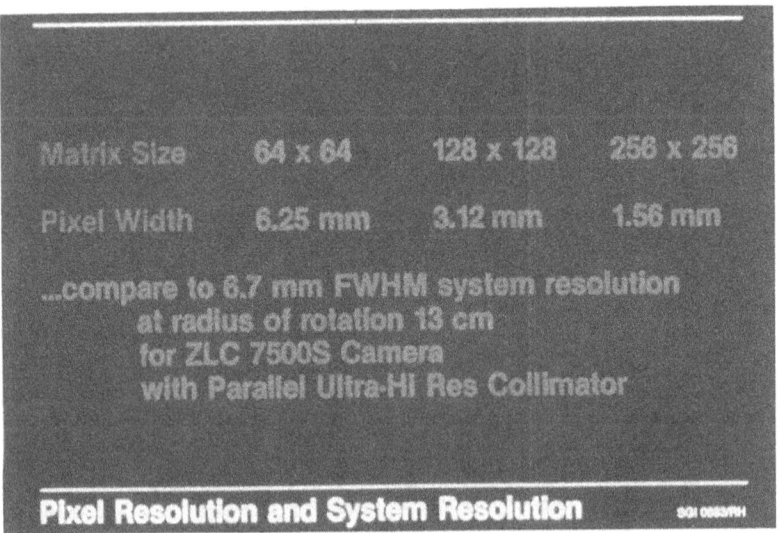

Figure 14

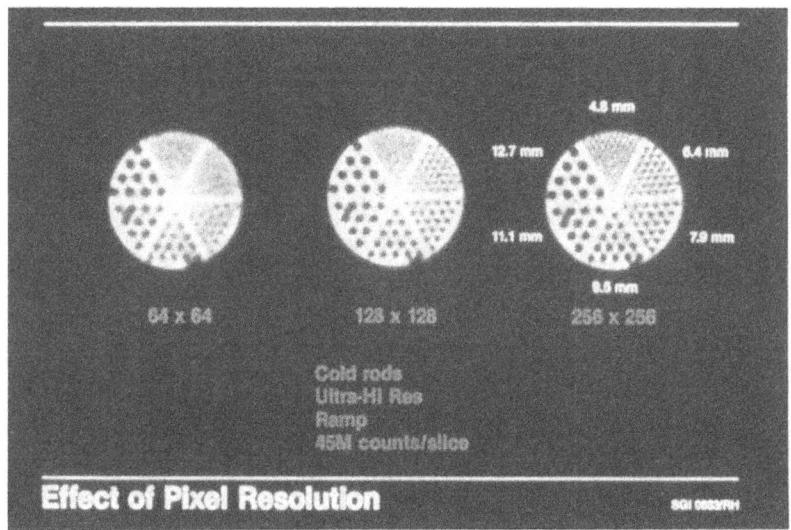

Figure 15

Uniformity and Offset Correction

Good detector uniformity and linearity, provided by ZLC detectors, are fundamental for high quality SPECT imaging. However, SPECT is extremely sensitive to residual regional variations in detector and collimator sensitivity, which must be corrected to avoid image artifacts.

Figure 16 illustrates the effect of regional sensitivity variations. A camera with an element of increased sensitivity would create a distorted projection image of a centered source. As this element scans different areas of the source during rotation, these distortions may result in a typical ring artifact in the reconstructed image.

Uniformity correction of the projection images prior to filtered back-projection reduces the effect of regional sensitivity variations. Flood images with 30 to 100 million counts are typically acquired to calculate a flood correction matrix.

The effect of center-of-rotation misalignment is illustrated in Figure 17. The center of the reconstructed image represents the mechanical system's center of rotation.

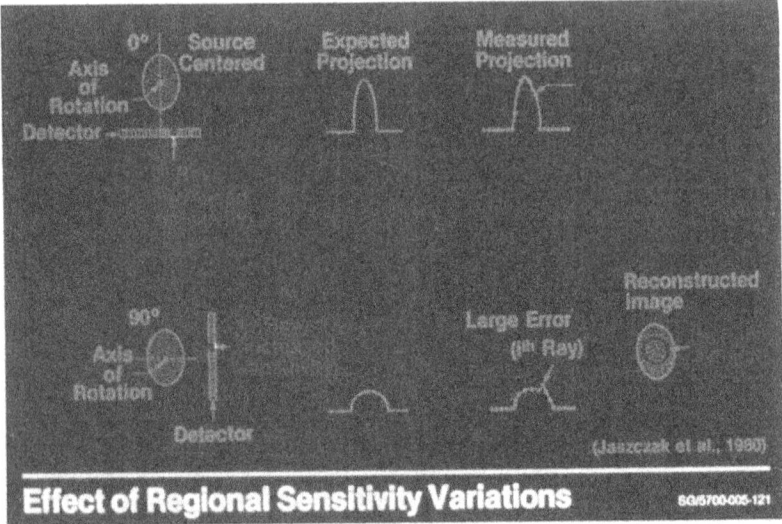

Figure 16

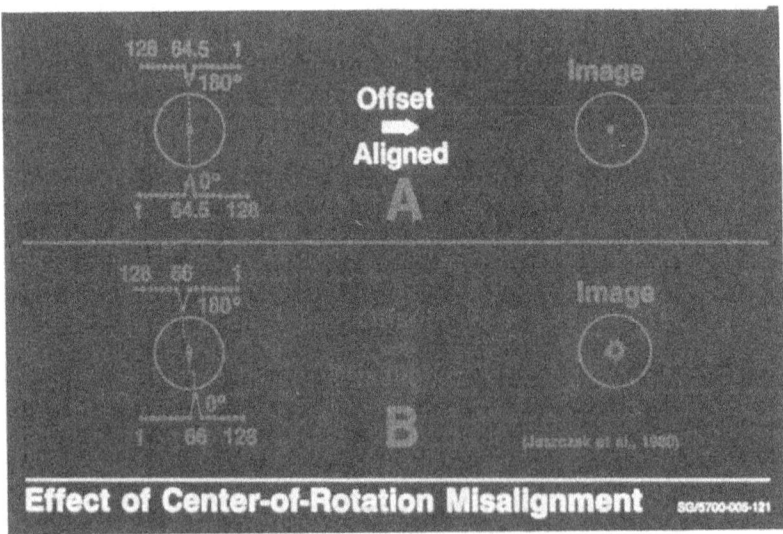

Figure 17

If mechanical and electrical center of rotation are well adjusted, the SPECT image accurately represents a point source without any distortions. If there is an offset between mechanical and electrical center of rotation, the SPECT image of the point source will demonstrate a ring artifact rather than a point image, and resolution is significantly reduced.

Offset correction realigns the mechanical and electrical center of rotation. Point of line source images are acquired to calculate the offset, and to correct the projection images before reconstruction.

Attenuation Correction

Photons emerging from the center of an object are attenuated more than photons near the edges. As a consequence, the projection profile of an object with uniform distribution of activity is flattened compared to the profile expected without attenuation (see Figure 18). Photon attenuation follows the well-known exponential law with μ being the attenuation coefficient. As a result of attenuation, the profile of the SPECT image shows higher peripheral and decreased central activity (see Figure 19). The goal of attenuation correction is to restore uniformity in the SPECT image.

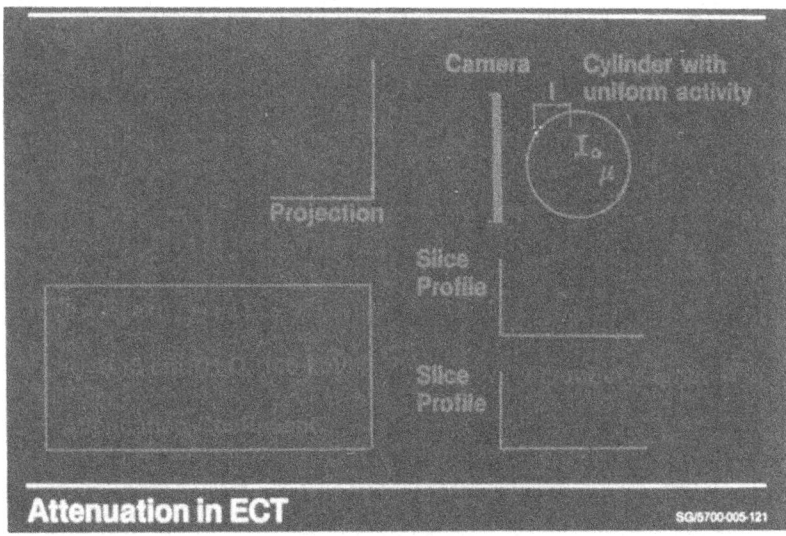

Figure 18

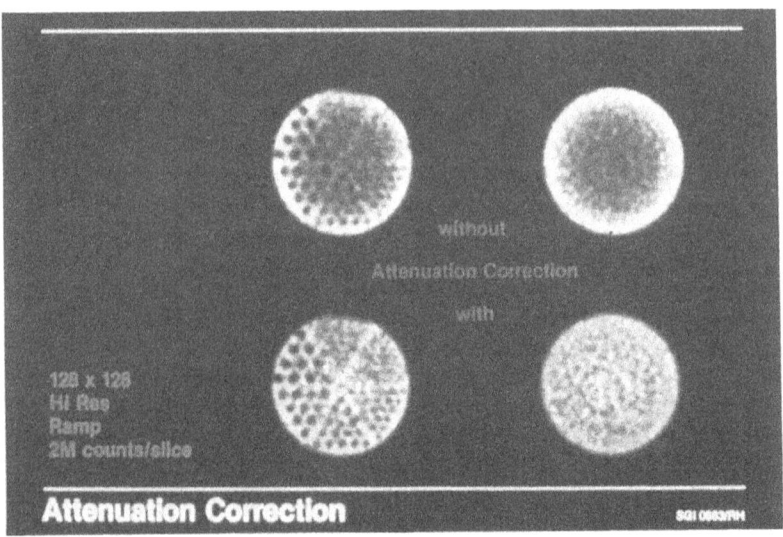

Figure 19

A proven method for attenuation correction is the multiplication of each reconstructed slice by a suitable correction matrix. The calculation of attenuation correction matrixes assumes constant attenuation throughout the body and knowledge of the body's contours (see Figure 20). Body contours can be calculated automatically if Compton scatter images are acquired simultaneously with the peak images (see Figure 21). Conventional nuclear images are created with unscattered photons detected within a small window around a photopeak. Photons scattered within the body are normally rejected using pulse height analysis. In SPECT imaging, Compton scatter image can be acquired simultaneously with peak images using a second analyzer. The body boundaries for each projection and slice are calculated from the scatter images with automatic boundary detection These contours are then employed in the calculation of the attenuation matrixes.

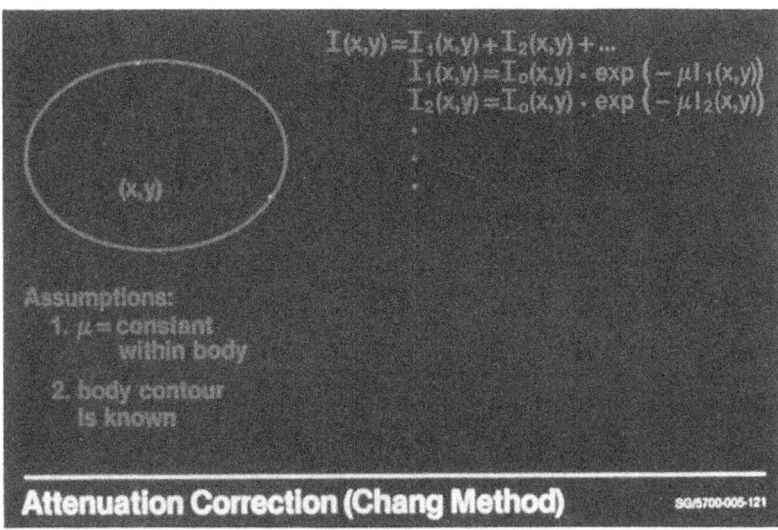

Figure 20

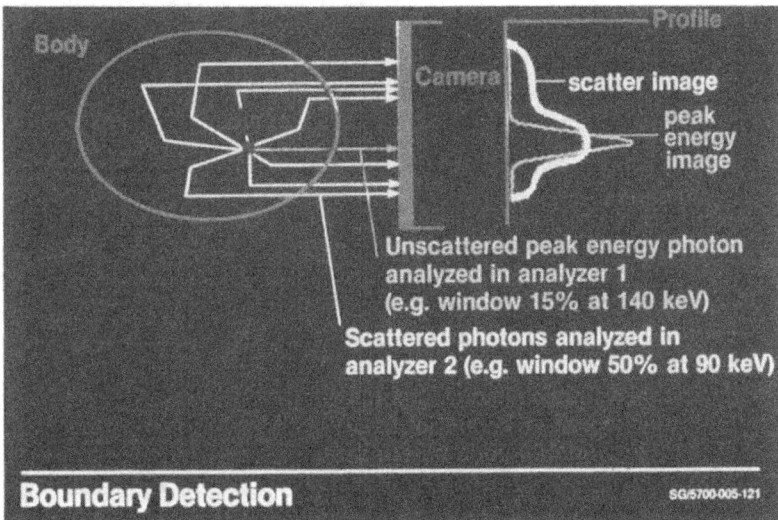

Figure 21

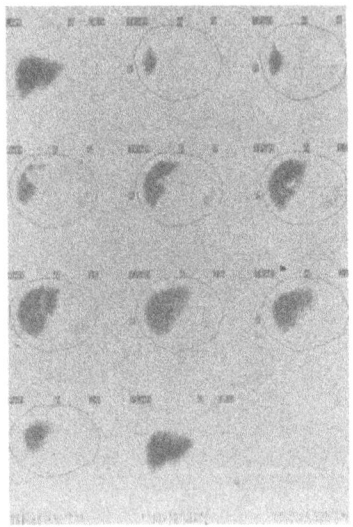

Figure 22

Figure 22 shows a sequence of transverse slices of a liver study with an overlay of the contours. The images were attenuation corrected with the correction matrix method described above. An attenuation coefficient of $\mu = 0.13$ cm^{-1} was selected in these images, which resulted in good uniformity throughout the organ.

Figures 23, 24, 25 and 26 with SPECT brain, liver and heart (Thalliur images demonstrate the quality obtainable with a good SPECT system.

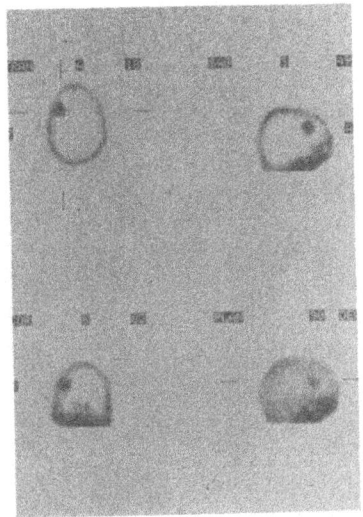

Figure 23

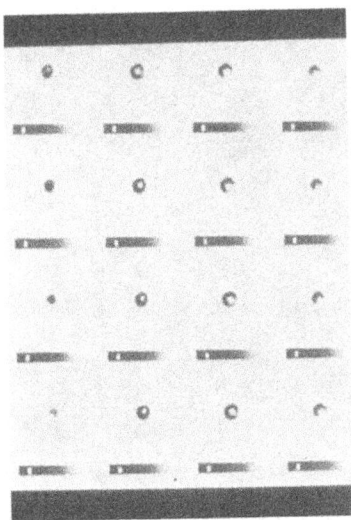

Figure 24

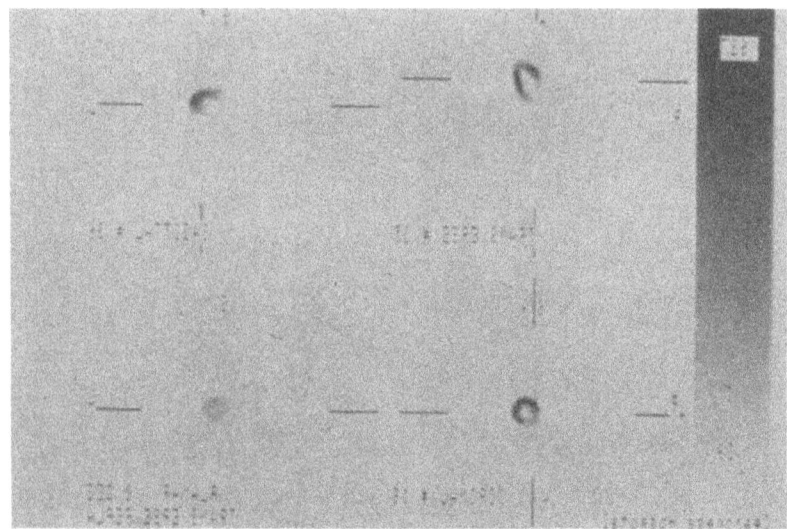

Figure 25

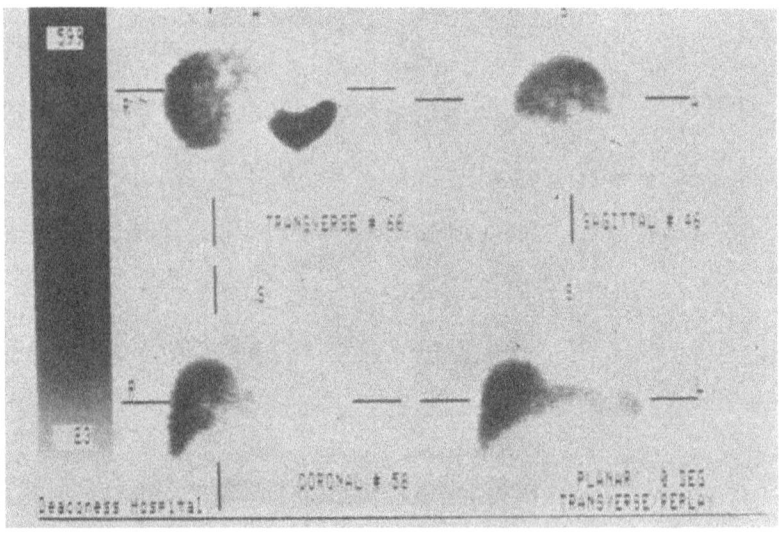

Figure 26

Limitations and Outlook

Rotational SPECT has become attractive because it does not require special, dedicated equipment. State-of-the-art, all-purpose gamma cameras can be upgraded for SPECT. There are, however, limitations which should be briefly discussed.

With reasonable acquisition times up to 30 minutes per scan, SPECT suffers from a limited number of counts, making SPECT images sensitive to noise. Smoothing techniques such as the user-selectable reconstruction filters described previously are needed to suppress noise contributions, at the expense of spatial resolution. The call for dual detector cameras to increase the overall system sensitivity originates because of the need for more counts.

The scan time required to acquire a sufficient number of counts limits rotational SPECT to static imaging and presently does not allow the performance of dynamic SPECT studies. Gated blood pool imaging with SPECT is being investigated and may become the exception.

The time requirements for the reconstruction of SPECT images has been another limitation which is presently being overcome by employing array processors, reducing the processing time to only seconds per slice.

Data management, or the interactive selection of transverse, sagittal, corinal and oblique slices from a three-dimensional data set for display, hard copy and filing, has become more convenient with today's SPECT software.

While state-of-the-art SPECT systems fulfill the basic requirements of high quality and clinically reliable SPECT imaging, there is ample room for future improvements and developments. The design of special collimators will address the need for higher system sensitivity. The availability of faster processors will make SPECT even more time-efficient and will allow the implementation of more sophisticated reconstruction and post-processing software. Non-circular tracking will permit moving the camera closer to the patient's body surface and may result in improved resolution and uniformity. Dynamic SPECT imaging of the heart may become feasible with gated data acquisition.

Beside continuing technical improvements, SPECT is expected to initiate the development of new clinical protocols for image quantitation and to promote the development and evaluation of new pharmaceuticals.

References :

1. Budinger,F.; Gullberg, G.T. : 3-Dimensional Reconstruction in Nuclear Medicine Emission Imaging. IEEE Trans. Nucl. Sci., NS-21 (1974), 2.
2. Keyes,jr., J.W.: Orlandea, N.; Heetsderks, W.; Leonard, P.F.; Rogers, W.L. : The Humangotron - A Scintillation Camera Transaxial Tomograph. J. Nucl. Med. 18 (1977), 381.
3. Burdine, J.A.; Murphy, P.H.; DePucy, E.G. : Radionuclide Computed Tomography of the Body using Routine Radiopharmaceuticals. II. Clinical Applications. J. Nucl. Med. 20 (1979), 108.
4. Jaszczak, R.J.; Chang, L.T.; Stein, N.A.; Moore, F.E. : Whole-Body Single-Photon Emission Computed Tomography using Dual, Large Field-of-View Scintillation Cameras. Phys. Med. Biol. 24 (1979), 1123.
5. Soussaline, F.P.; Todd-Pokropek, A.; Zurowski, S.; Huffer, E.; Ranaud, C.E.; Kellershohn, C. : A Rotating Conventional Gamma Camera Single-Photon Tomographic System : Physical Characterization. J. Comput. Assist. Tomog. 5 (1981), 551.
6. Buell, U.; Kirsch, C.M.; Roedler, H.D. : Die Single-Photon Emissions-Computertomographie (SPECT) : Prinzipien, Ergebnisse, Ausblick. Fortschr. Roentgenstr. 138 (1983), 391.
7. Jaszczak, R.J.; Whitehead, F.R.; Lim, C.B.; Coleman, R.E. : Lesion Detection with Single-Photon Emission Computed Tomography (SPECT) Compared with Conventional Imaging. J. Nucl. Med. 23 (1982), 97.
8. Keyes, jr., J.W. : Perspectives on Tomography. J. Nucl. Med. 23 (1982), 633.
9. For a review see : Single Photon Emission Computed Tomography and Other Selected Computer Topics. Ed. J.A. Sorenson. The Society of Nuclear Medicine, New York (1980).
10. Barrett, H.H.; Swindell, W. : Multiplex tomography, in : The Theory of Image Dormation, Detection, and Processing, Vol. 2. Academic Press, London (1981).
11. Muehllehner, G.; Colsher, J.G.; Stoub, E.W. : Correction of Field Nonuniformity in Scintillation Cameras through Removal of Spatial Distortion. J. Nucl. Med. 21 (1980), 771.
12. Rogers, W.L.; Clinthorne, N.H.; Harkness, B.A.; Koral, K.F.; Keyes, jr. J.W. : Field-Flood-Requirements for Emission Computed Tomography with an Anger Camera. J. Nucl. Med. 23 (1982),162.
13. Greer, K.L.; Coleman, R.E.; Jaszczak, R.J. : SPECT - A Practical Guide for Users. J. Nucl. Med. Tech. 11 (1983),61.
14. Jaszczak, R.J.; Greer, K.L.; Coleman, R.E. : SPECT System Misalignment : Comparison of Phantom and Patient Images, in : Emission Computed Tomography : Current Trends. Ed. P.E. Esser. The Society of Nuclear Medicine, New York (1983), 57.
15. Greer, K.L., Jaszczak, R.J.; Coleman, R.E. : An Overview of a Camera-Based SPECT System, Med. Phys. 9 (1982),455.

16. Jaszczak, R.J.; Coleman, R.E.; Whitehead, F.R. : Physical Factors affecting Quantitative Measurements using Camera-Based Single Photon Emission Computed Tomography (SPECT). IEEE Trans. Nucl. Sci. NS-28 (1981),69.
17. Hawman, E.G. : Impact of Body Contour Data on Quantitative SPECT Imaging. Proceedings 3rd World Congress of Nuclear Medicine and Biology, Vol. 1, Paris (1982), 1038.
18. Haerten, R.L.; Bieszk, J.A.; Hawman, E.G.; Malmin, R.E. : Evaluation of SPECT Phantom. Proceedings of the 30th Annual Meeting of the Society of Nuclear Medicine. J. Nucl. Med. 24 (1983), 58.
19. Hounsfield, G.N. : Computerized Transverse Axial Scanning (Tomography) : Part 1 : Description of the System. Br. J. Radiol. 46 (1973), 1016.
20. Budinger, T.F.; Gullberg, G.T. : Transverse Section Reconstruction of Gamma-Ray Emitting Radionuclides in Patients, in : Reconstruction Tomography in Diagnostic Radiology and Nuclear Medicine. Ed. M.M. Ter-Pogossian, University Park Press, Baltimore (1977), 315.
21. Todd-Pokropek, A. : The Mathematics and Physics of Emission Computerized Tomography : Current Trends. Ed. P.E. Esser. The Society of Nuclear Medicine, New York (1983), 3.
22. Schardt, M.A. : Standardization of Performance Measurements of Scintillation Cameras. Electromedica 3/81 (1981), 169.
23. Jaszczak, R.J.; Coleman, R.E. : Selected Processing Techniques for Scintillation Camera Based SPECT Systems, in : Single Photon Emission Computed Tomography and Other Selected Computer Topics. Ed. J.A. Sorenson, The Society of Nuclear Medicine, New York (1980), 45.
24. Chang, L.T. : Attenuation Correction and Incomplete Projection in Single Photon Emission Computed Tomography. IEEE Trans. Nucl. Sci. NS-26 (1979), 2780.
25. Coleman, R.E.; Greer, K.L.; Drayer, B.P.; Albricht, R.E.; Petry, N.A.; Jaszczak. R.J. : Collimation for I-123 Imaging with SPECT, in : Emission Computed Tomography, Current Trends. Ed. P.D. Esser. The Society of Nuclear Medicine, New York (1983), 135.
26. Prigent, F.; Friedman, J.; Maddahi, J.; Bietendorf, J.; Garcia, E.; Areeda, J.; Van Train, K.; Waxman, A.; Berman, D. : Comparison of Rotational Tomography with Planar Imaging for Thallium-201 Stress Myocardial Scintigraphy. Proceedings of the 30th Annual Meeting of the Society of Nuclear Medicine, J. Nucl. Med. 24 (1983), 18.
27. Tamaki, N.; Mukai, T.; Ishii, Y.; Yonekura, Y.; Yamamoto, K.; Kadota, K.; Kambara, H.; Kawai, C.; Torizuka, K. : Multiaxial Tomography of Heart Chambers by Gated Bloodpool Emission Computed Tomography using a Rotating Gamma Camera. Radiology 147 (1983), 547.
28. Gottschalk, S.; Salem, D. : Effect of an Elliptical Orbit on SPECT Resolution and Image Uniformity. Proc. 3rd World Congress of Nuclear Medicine and Biology, Paris (1982), 1026.
29. Todd-Pokropek, A. : Non-Circular Orbits for the Reduction of Uniformity Artefacts in SPECT. Phys. Med. Biol. 28 (1983) 309.

HIGH EFFICIENCY MULTISLICE APPROACH FOR SINGLE PHOTON TOMOGRAPHY OF THE BRAIN

Per Rommer, John Ryding Olsson, and Niels A. Lassen[*]

Medimatic A/S, DK-2900 Hellerup, and [*]Department of Clinical Physiology, Bispebjerg Hospital, DK-2400 Copenhagen NV, Denmark

1. ABSTRACT

Dynamic functional brain studies with a single photon computerized tomography (SPECT) can only provide detailed and reliable information when the studies are performed with a single photon tomograph designed exclusively for the brain investigations.

This paper describes TOMOMATIC 564, a camera constructed especially for brain studies. This dynamic SPECT instrument is used for cerebral blood flow (CBF) measurements after Xenon-133 inhalation as well as after intravenous injection of IOD-123 Amphetamine.

Illustrative examples of investigations performed with both the above-mentioned isotopes show that it is only possible to image CBF if one has a sensitive dynamic SPECT instrument as the TOMOMATIC 564 at one's disposal, which in 5 slices can collect more than 3 million counts in a short acquisition time of 4 minutes.

It is furthermore emphasized that IOD 123 Amphetamine, usually after the initial phase (10 min. after iv), does not have the same isotope distribution as in the later phase (especially in infarcted areas). Therefore, a short aquisition time of a maximum of 5 minutes taken just after intravenous injection is a necessity.

2. INTRODUCTION

During the last decade Medimatic has been developing single photon camera systems for dynamic functional measurement of the cerebral and the peripheral vascular circuit. Medimatic has always worked with the Xenon isotope, especially for brain imaging, because it is suited to rCBF imaging, with the gamma camera technique, the single detector technique and the tomography emission technique.

In 1973 traumatic single hemisphere rCBF measurements were carried out with the DYNAMATIC 254 system (1), and the CT technique became more and more common and consequently reduced the amount of angiographic examinations. The CBF technique was finally made atraumatic (2) in 1974 by means of the single detector system INHAMATIC 33, which carried out CBF measurements with inhalation of Xe-133 instead of injection of Xe-133 in the punctured carotid, which is also often carried out in connection with angiography.

In 1978 the idea of an industrially available single photon tomograph was realized by the release of Medimatic's dynamic Xenon tomograph TOMOMATIC 64 (3,14) which was based on Kuhl's ideas.

Later on, in 1982/83, Medimatic released the TOMOMATIC 32 system. Compared to the TOMOMATIC 64 system, this one was a smaller single photon emission tomograph, also based on Xenon inhalation (5). Unlike TOMOMATIC 64, TOMOMATIC 32 has a better energy resolution, Therefore, it could be to the advantage of a closer discrimination of the primary energy. This system costs only half as much as Tomomatic 64 and it is at the same price level as the computerized rotating gamma camera.

The characteristic feature of all Medimatic's emission tomographs is their ability to measure the dynamic sequential functions due to their exceptional high sensitivity. This high sensitivity allows the camera to collect a great number of counts in a very short acquisition time. This can be used either for brain flow studies, such as in cases of Xenon-133 CBF (9), or to reveal the existing non-steady state of the isotope distribution of IOD-123 (10). Only the very short initial phase (maximum 5 minutes) gives true information about CBF, particularly in infarcted areas when using IOD-123 Amphetamine.

3. FIVE-SLICE DYNAMIC SPECT: TOMOMATIC 564

A continuation of the work carried out in connection with the development of the 3-slices single photon tomograph TOMOMATIC 64, which was finally developed in 1980 (3), has resulted in the development of a dynamic single photon emission tomograph, the TOMOMATIC 564 (T564) (Fig. 1).

T564 by no means renders T64 superfluous. In some aspects it is an improved version configurated as a considerably larger and more user-oriented instrument. Apart from the camera itself, the T564 consists of a processor, in which the vital part is a DEC MicroVAX 1-computer unit with direct access to the imaging system. Additionally, the T564 has a specially designed isotope gas distribution unit, originally developed for measurement of the regional cerebral blood flow (rCBF).

3.1 Camera System Design Considerations

T64 has typically been an instrument used directly by the target group: neurophysiologists, neurosurgeons, and neurologists. The aim, with the T564, is to interest experts in the field of Nuclear Medicine. The instrument is selectively designed for measurement of dynamic regional brain function in 5 slices, and will introduce a new era due to its high sensitivity, even when used with other isotopes than Xe-133.

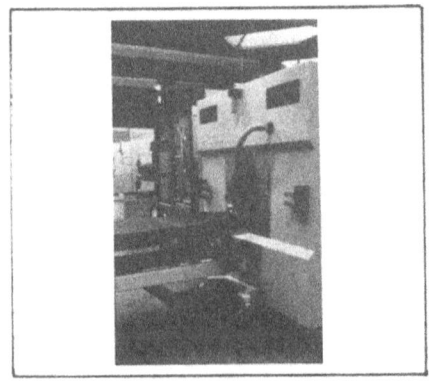

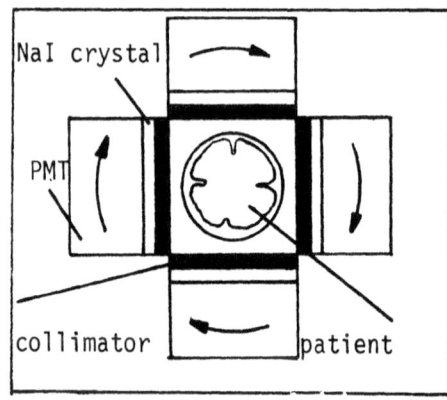

Fig.1
TOMOMATIC 564. Developed from the experience of TOMOMATIC 64 (1)

Fig.2 Detector system in T564. 4 rotating cameras, each consisting of 16NaI crystals, PMTs and exchangeable collimator.

Among the new features are the detectors and the collimators, which are placed in a square around the head and are designed to record activity distribution images with low energy isotopes, up to 200 KeV. In addition to 4 camera units, each consisting of 16 half - inch rectangular NaI crystals completely covered by PMTs, the camera is provided with interchangeable collimators, which can be used with different isotopes and for different examination purposes (fig. 2).

Fig. 3 shows the sensitivities and resolutions of the camera depending on the type of collimator used (10).

The main feature of the camera is its sensitivity. T564 is probably the only single-photon camera in the world which has a sensitivity of approximately 200,000 cnts/sec./µCi/ml for I-123. The electronics of the camera are basically the same as those of T64 (3), but due to a considerably improved energy resolution of the single detector (approximately 18% at 81 keV), it is possible to use the sequential event processor (static system) with more narrow individual window discrimination.

Fig. 4 shows the FWHM for the axial line spread function for the standard collimator measured at 81 KeV.

Fig. 5 shows the line spread function in air, and as can be seen from the figure, the FWHM increases with the distance to the collimator.

TOMOMATIC 564 COLLIMATOR SYSTEM. FIG. 3. (10)				
TYPE	Spat. resolut. FWHM. mm	Max no. of slice.	Slice width mm	Max total sensitivity. Kcnts/s/uCi/ml.
UHS	21	5	20	250
MHS	16	3/5	20	190
MHR	11	3	15	30
UHR	8	3	20	15
With Xenon-133 is the sensitivity 1/3.				

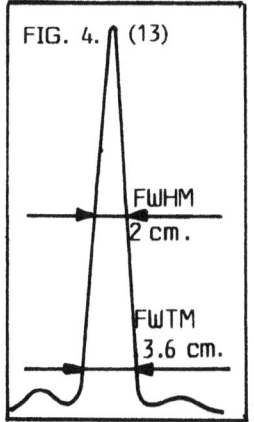

FIG. 4. (13)

FWHM 2 cm.

FWTM 3.6 cm.

Fig. 3. The T 564 collimator system with different sensitivity and resolution. FIG. 4. Measured line spread function with Xenon-133 and the MHS collimator measured in the center (r = 0). (13).

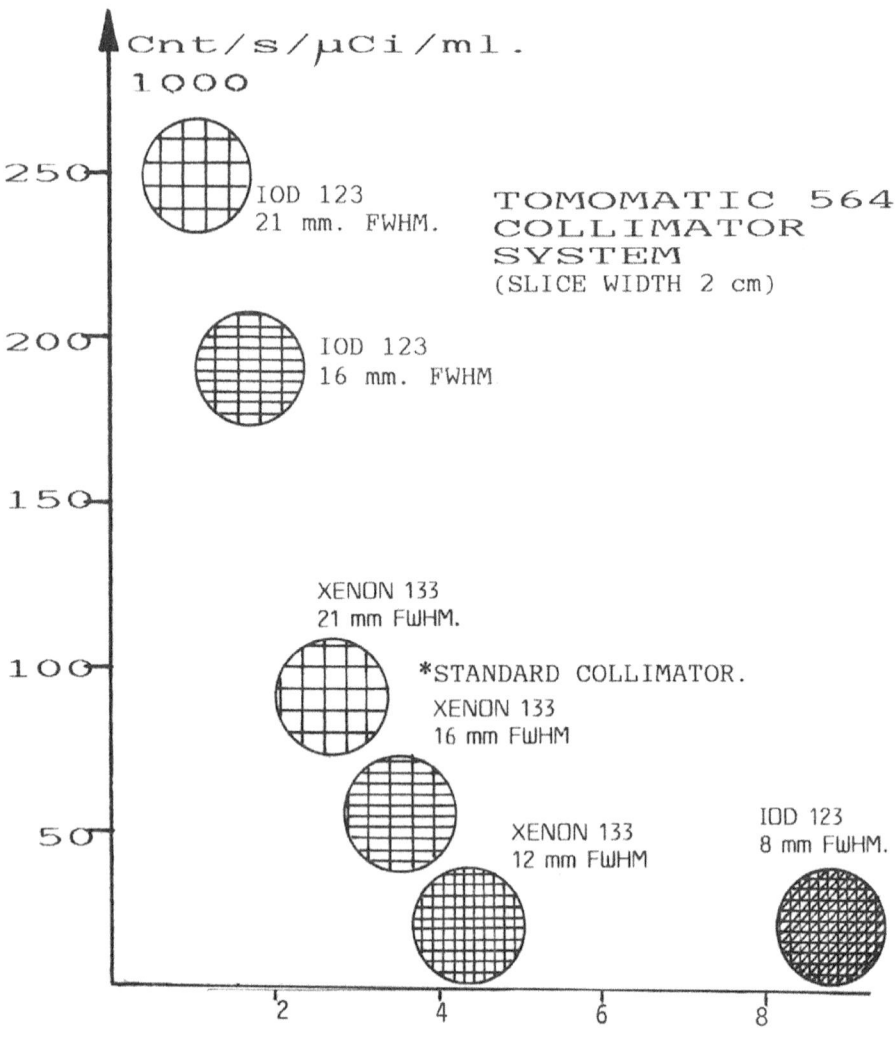

Fig. 3A   ACQUISITION TIME (MIN)

Fig. 3A shows how great a sensitivity is lost for an improved spatial resolution down to 8 mm FWHM in the T 564 collimator system. Reasonably functional studies, giving spatial resolution from 16 - 12 mm in the very uniform T 564 reconstructed image matrix, have been described.

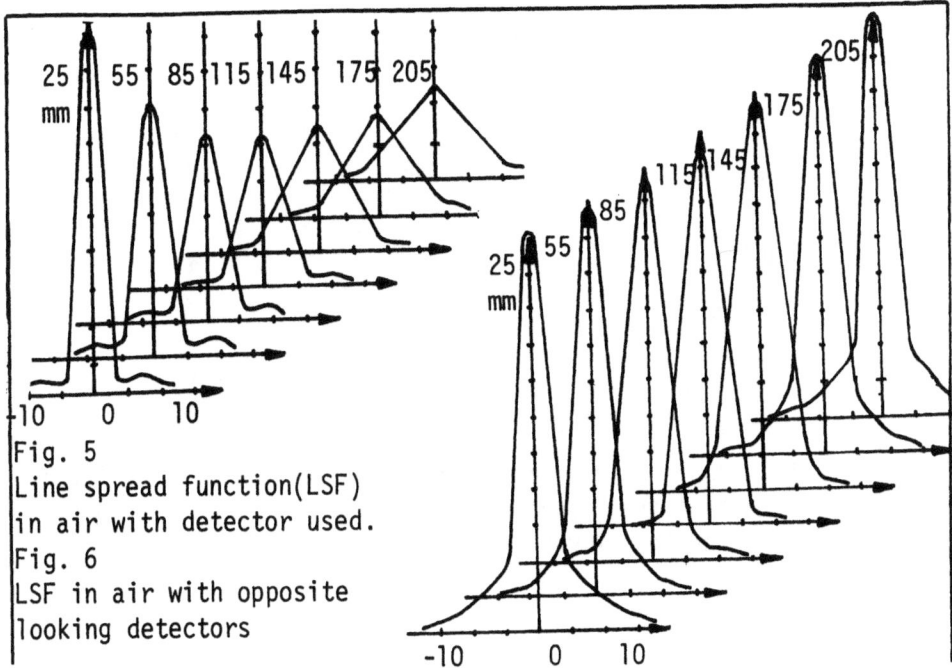

Fig. 5
Line spread function(LSF) in air with detector used.

Fig. 6
LSF in air with opposite looking detectors

If the source is simultaneously seen and recorded by the opposite detector, the result will be a line spread function where the FWHM is relatively constant throughout the distance from one detector to the opposite one.(Fig 6)This is due to the focusing of the <u>standard collimator</u> which results in a uniform reconstructed spatial <u>resolution</u>, when using two opposite detectors.

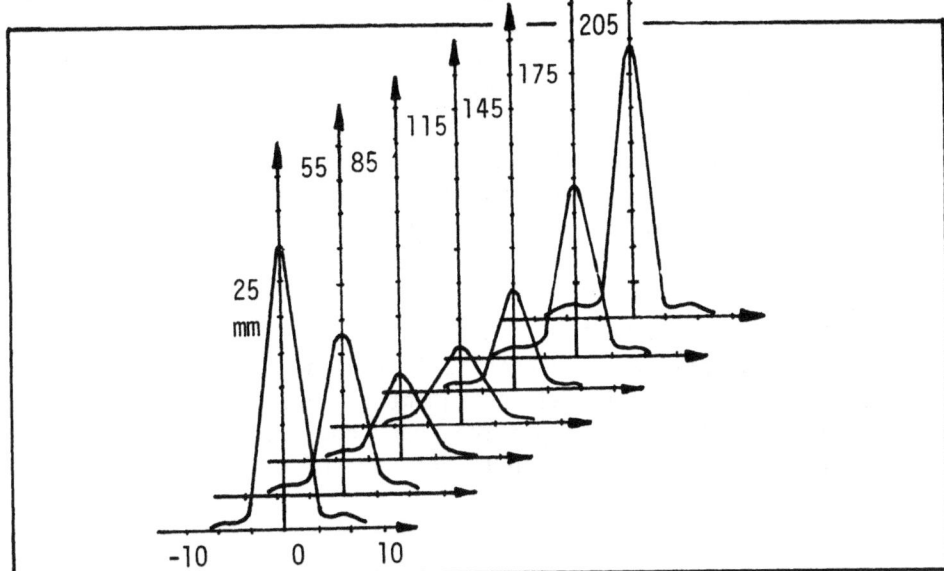

Fig. 7. LSF in water with opposite looking detectors. The T 564 standard collimator and Xenon 133 are used.

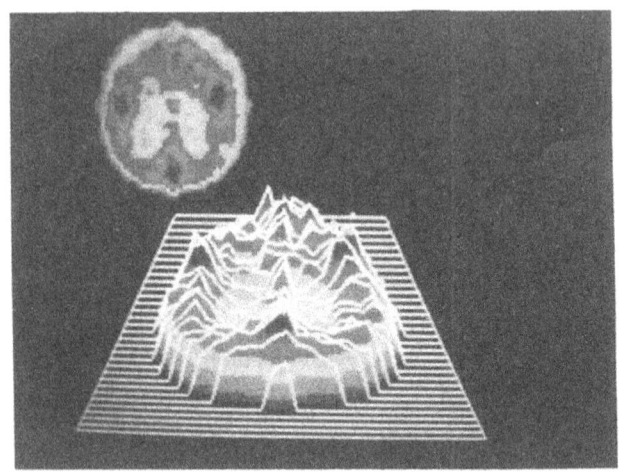

Fig. 8. The colours in the image show the rCBF values in ml/100gm/min. The "tops" of the "mountain" show the differences in density in the CT-scan and the flow values.

3.2 Computer and Imaging System

The T564 is equipped with a DEC computer system, a 32 bit MicroVax type 610qc-xz. This unit is configured with a memory of 1 Mb, 28 Mb discs and 2 x 400 Kb floppy disc. A further option is a 10 Mb hard disc in connection with a so-called image processor computer. There is also access from the computer systems to the image system. Another feature is a 16 colour display system, which can show alphanumeric data as well as patterns with a number of rasters corresponding to a 256x256 raster with extension possibilities up to a 512x512 raster each in 16 colours and 16 grey tone levels. With the optional software package it is possible to show three-dimensional brain flow maps for revealing differences between a CT-scan and a Xenon rCBF tomogram. (Fig. 8)

In Fig. 9 the standard softward package for Tomomatic T564 is specified. The specification shows that the instrument is especially designed and adapted to be a practical, routine research instrument as well as a routine clinical instrument for daily use. Peripheral units such as the graphical printer, hard copy camera and colour monitor which can display the results are part of the standard package.

Fig. 9. The T 564 software package for noninvasive rCBF investigation includes:

a) Operating system
b) Collection of basis functions
c) Calibration programme
d) Data collection programme
e) Sorting and sensitivity correction
f) Reconstruction algorithm with correction for tissue attenuation and noise reduction routines
g) Flow calculation programmes
h) Image display programme library for visual presentation of results as colour coded images, test edition etc.
i) Statistical image processing functions
j) Patient data base (storage of approx. 1000 patient data)
k) Maintenance and system check programme

3.3   The Xenon Administration System

The TOMOMATIC was, from the very first phase of development, conceived as a routine clinical instrument, and it has been of great importance to base the instrument on a standard method, which contrary to the positron instruments (PET) can make low cost examinations. When using the PET cameras each single patient examination costs approximately $5,000-10,000, but with the Tomomatic T564 an examination resulting in the imaging of 5 slices of the rCBF costs less than $100. This is due to the fact that Xenon-133 gas is a standard isotope, and the instrument is much cheaper to purchase than the PET instrument and the complete installation, particularly the instrument, based on single photon techniques, can be operated by a tenth of the personnel required to perform a PET study.

Xenon-133 is an isotope with a half-life of 5-1/2 days and can be delivered on a "call and you get it" basis; that is, Monday to Friday and around the clock. It is very cheap and extremely clean as a radioisotope with a low gamma energy of 81 keV, which only necessitates thin lead shields for effective protection and collimation.

The most important feature of this inert gas is that it is immediately diluted in atmospheric air; a feature which assures that it almost totally disappears from the body through the lungs after the first circulation.

Fig. 10
The Xenon Administration System consists of two parts:
a rebreathing part and a refill (storage) part.
The rebreathing part consists of a closed loop system to which a patient may be connected by means of 3-way valves. These valves are controlled by electronics.
The rebreathing bag has a capacity of 4 liters and the total capacity of the rebreathing system is 5 1/4 liters. The storage part consists of a 2 liter pressure tank connected to a vial gun system.

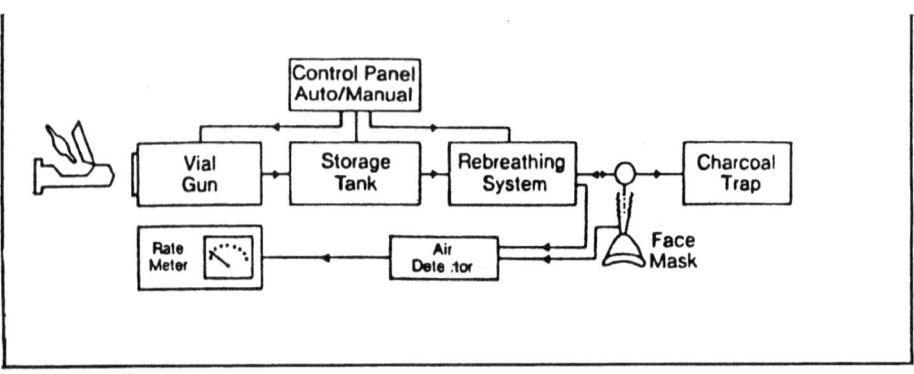

When the Xenon system is used (Fig. 10), a study is carried out with a concentration of 20 mCi Xenon-133 per l/air in the closed respiration system, which has a total volume of 4 l. A patient breathing from this closed system will have a concentration of 10 mCi/l in the lungs after having breathed for 1.5 minutes. This involves an absorb radiation dose per study of 6 mGy in the lungs and 0.6 mGy in the gonads (6). Compared to other imaging techniques the radiation dose of the T564 is very low. Xenon-133 was deliberately chosen to be so low in order to allow repeated studies on normal healthy adults without risk. The window discrimination, according to the primary energy of the isotope, is easily changed by pressing a button. The control panel is shown in Fig. 11. The same control panel informs one of which collimator is in use.

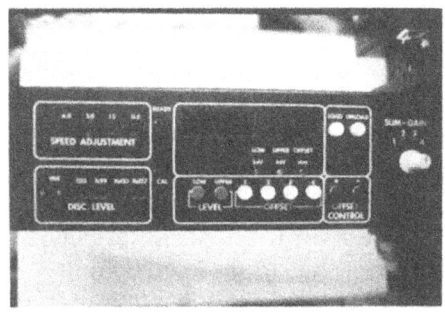 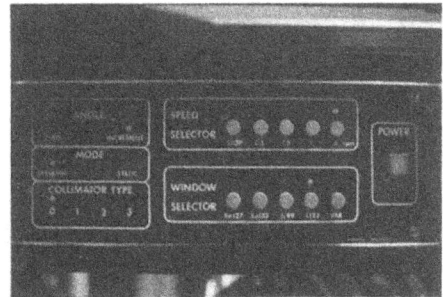

Fig. 11
Front panel of the T 564 camera unit. Discrimination levels can be changed on this pannel. It has preset buttons for Xe 133, Xe 127, I 123 and Tc99.

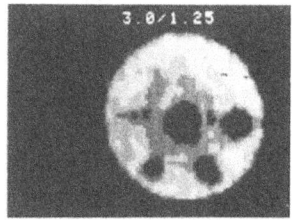

Fig. 12
Phantom studies with a Phelps phantom. The T 564 standard collimator has been used.

3.4 Instrument Performance

First of all, the T564 has a high sensitivity of 200,000 cts/sec./ μCi/ml for I 123. This permits either very fast recordings of dynamic Xenon flow studies or high collimation of, for examnle, I-123 or Tc99m studies which can results in reconstructed images with a high spatial resolution down to 8 mm (3). T564 has been improved with regard to energy resolution, in comparison to T64, so that it is possible to effectively carry out electronic discrimination.

3.4.1 Phantom Study. Fig. 12 shows the results of a phantom study, performed on a Phelps phantom (8). We measured the cold lesion detectability of the T564 detector system. The phantom consists of a 20 cm diameter cylinder, 6 cm thick, containing Lucite rods parallel to the axis of 25mm, 20mm, 15mm, 10mm, 7.5mm and 5mm. The center rod is 30mm in diameter. The standard acquisition conditions for T564 and Tc99 are used and the total number of counts is 3,068,890. In this case the standard T564 collimator with a spatial resolution of 16mm FWHM has been used. The image shows that the 15mm cold spot is distinct and that the 10mm cold spot can be recognized. With the T564 it is possible to obtain the spatial resolution of 8mm FWHM.

3.4.2 Blood Volume with Tc99 m-labeled RBC. Fig. 13 shows blood volume recorded with Tc99m labeled RBC with the high resolution collimator (UHRS). In the PA territory a vessel with its branches can be seen; the diameter of this vessel is less than 10mm. The total number of collected counts is 2,640,000. The spatial resolution is 8 mm FWHM.

3.4.3 Tumor with Tc99m. Another example recorded with the T564 HRS collimator is Fig. 14. This image shows a small tumor in the left hemisphere. The image is the second slice out of 5 slices, and each of the 4 collimators is displaced 1/4 of a detector width. The spatial resolution is 8 mm FWHM. The skull can be seen as a result of the use of Tc99m.

3.4.4 Stroke with Xenon 133 rCBF. The T564 has been especially designed and developed to comply with the high sensitivity requirements for imaging dynamic Xenon studies. Fig. 15 shows a stroke case recorded with Xenon-133 with a recording time of 4 min. The image is the third of 5 slices simultaneously recorded. A total of 2,500,000 counts have been sampled in the period of acquisition. The slice thickness is 20mm and the T564 standard collimator

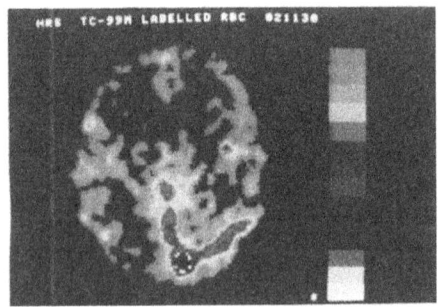 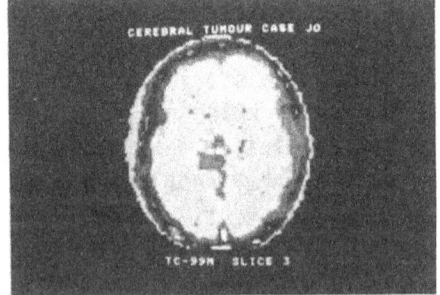

Fig. 13
T 564 study of blood volume with Tc99 m-labeled RBC (FWHM=0.8 cm)

Fig. 14
T 564 study of a tumor case with Tc99m(FWHM=0.8 cm)

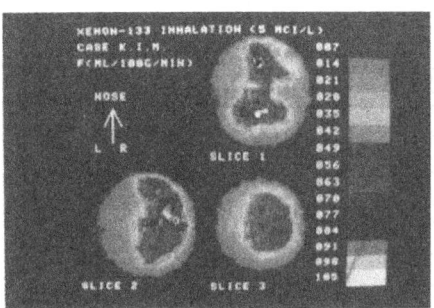 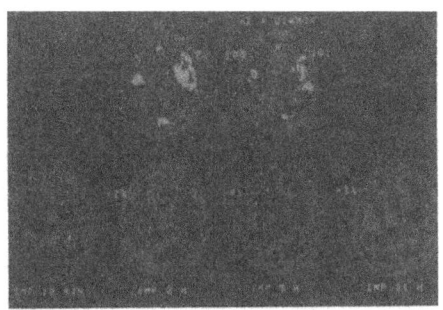

Fig. 15 T 564 study of a stroke using Xenon-133 in CBF. Standard collimator was used.

Fig. 16.The IMP distribution over 21 hours after I.V. injection(C. Raynaud et al,Paris)

has been used with a displacement of the collimator by half a detector width every second.

3.4.5. Neurofibroma with I-123 Amphetamine. Neurofibroma with multiple neuromas. On CT scan, lateral ventricles appear dilated predominantly on the left occipital horn. The IMP distribution may be considered as normal, except on the left occipital area. The IMP distribution demonstrates the non-steady state conditions over 21 hours in intervals of 10min, 2, 5 and 21 hours after I.V. injection. The IMP concentration is initially seen in the grey matter(PCA and MCA areas) and later in the ACA area.

4. BASIC THEORY OF CBF TOMOGRAPHY

The individual brain segment, recorded by our detector can be described as in Fig. 17 where the input goes through the arteries to the grey and white cerebral matter. It then returns to the heart through the veins. Such a circulation system can be described with its input, its system-response function and with its output.The output will always be a function of the input and the response function. In the measuring situation the input is Xenon saturated blood with a known concentration of Xenon. The output from the individual brain segment is the blood quantity as a function of the time. The blood quantity can be measured directly by our detector system as the blood is saturated with Xenon. Output from individual brain segments can be measured by Xenon radiation, which is the function of the time. Therefore,the process can be described by the following mathematical model:

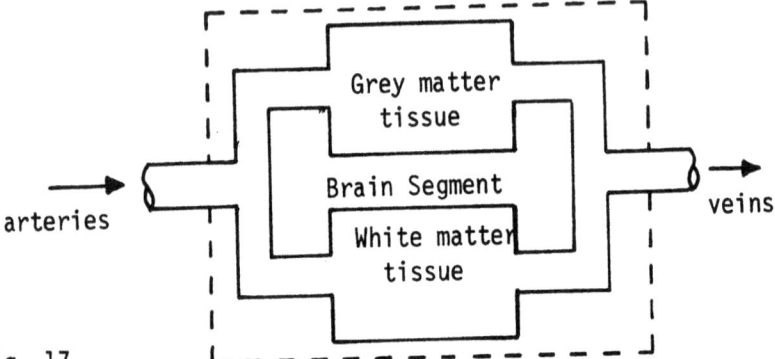

Fig. 17
Model of a brain segment with arterial flow, grey and white matter tissue and outflow through the veins.

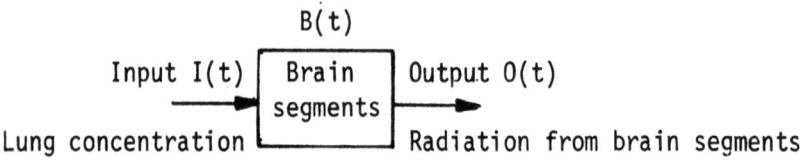

Fig. 18
Brain model with indication of method to measure input and output (Xenon is used as a tracer).

Input can be measured as the lung concentration of Xenon-133, output can be measured as the concentration of Xenon-133 in the individual brain segments. The principle is expressed as a mathematical calculation in the following way:

$$I(t) * B(t) = O(t) \qquad (1)$$

where the convolution of I (t) and B (t) is equal to O (t).

The blood flow in the individual segment B (t) can be found as a deconvolution of formula (1)

$$B(t) = \text{deconv} \frac{O(t)}{I(t)} \qquad (2)$$

4.1 Injection Studies

In the case of injection of Xenon, the input function will be a so-called bolus or mathematically expressed dirac. Such a unit impulse has the ability of I (t)=1, after integration from 0 to infinity. Therefore, the term in formula (2) will be:

$$B(t) = 0(t) \implies B(t) = 0(t) \qquad (3)$$

This means that in the case of injection the measured radiation is a function of the time, equal to the blood flow. On the basis of such measurements it has turned out that the unit response function is an exponential function which can be described as:

$$B(t) = K_{grey} e^{-(f_g/\lambda_g)t} + K_{white} e^{-(f_w/\lambda_w)t} \qquad (4)$$

where the first exponential part is a contribution from the grey matter flow, and the second part is the contribution from the white matter flow. λ is the local tissue/blood partition ratio, with the unit $[gr/ml]$. K is a product of the counting rate measured over the lung, and a scaling factor (9). f/λ is known as k_i (9) and this is the value to be calculated in order to find the blood flow. The total model for injection can be shown in Fig. 23.

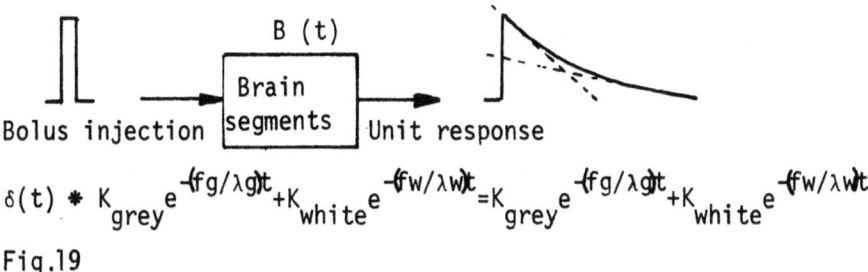

Fig.19

4.2 Inhalation Studies

In the case of inhalation studies the picture cannot be determined simply by calculating the slope of the curve, due to the fact that the inhalation should be considered as an integrated series of clearance curves, displaced in time (Fig.20)

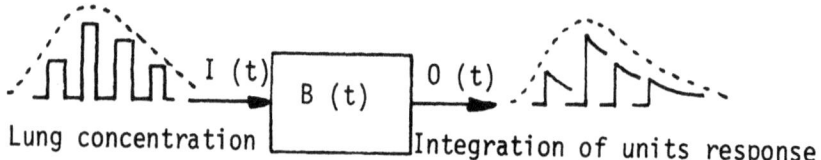

Lung concentration — Integration of units response

When I (t) is a δ (t) it follows that the integral from 0 to infinity is 1. If we assume that the input is a series of δ (t) the output will be a series of regular time intervals. T is the time intervals. Then every output will be T(I(nT)xf(t-nT)). The sum of all outputs will be $\sum T(I(nT) \times f(t-nT))$. If T→0 and we integrate from time 0 to t, we have the convolution integral

$$\int_0^t I(\tau) \times f(t-\tau) d\tau$$

Fig.20

The sum of all these curves corresponds to what is called the convolution integral, when integrated from the time 0 to T. Thus, when using the inhalation method, it is not possible to calculate the transfer function in a simple way, from the output response. The transfer function can only be found by deconvoluting the input function with the output function.

4.3. The Actual Calculation Method for rCBF

Calculation of blood flow in Tomomatic T 564 is based on the method developed by N.A. Lassen and Kanno (10,11). Once a lung curve has been recorded, it is possible to calculate the theoretical outputs if the flow is for example 30, 40, 50, 60 etc., enabling the computer to produce a table of the theoretical outputs at different flow values (Fig. 21). For example if the flow is 30 ml/100gr/min, A1 would have the theoretical value of 38%, A3 the theoretical value of 80% and A4 the theoretical value of 59%. Then the actual output is normized and the number of counts is equal to 100% in the period of 60-120 seconds A2. The percentage of A1, A3 and A4 is calculated in each specific case. The table shows that A1 corresponds to a value of 29ml/100gm/min., A3 to a value of 35ml/100gr/min., and A4 to a value of 25 ml/100gr/min. All calculations are carried out by the computer for every single pixel in the image.

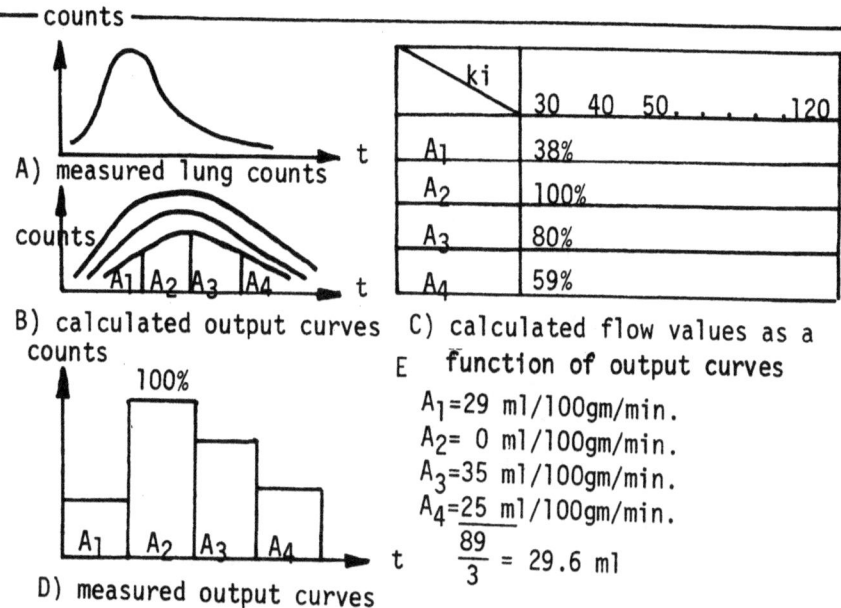

Fig. 21. rCBF calculation in T564. A)Lung curve is measured. B)From the lung curve some theoretical outputs are calculated. C)From the theoretical output in B, a table of flow values corresponding to different curves are developed (curves are normalized with $A_2=100\%$). D)After finding the different flow values from A_1, A_2 and A_3 we take the average, in this case 29.6ml/100gm/min.

With the use of IMP-123 the model for blood flow calculation is very simple. The promising agent n-isopropyl-p-Iodoamphetamine has a brain uptake of 1.3% of the injected dose at 2 minutes; 1.9% at 60 min. and 1.5% at 180 min. These components meet both the demand for optimal imaging and for high initial uptake with retention of the tracer within the brain parenchyma (7). The initial distribution of IMP-123 is correlated with CBF (Kuhl, 1981, 7). 5 min. after injection, there is a good correlation to CBF but IMP-123 concentration makes an underestimation of the true flow with a factor of correlation of 0.86 (7).

5. SENSITIVITY AND RESOLUTION

5.1. Lack of Sensitivity Causes Reduced Spatial Resolution

In dynamic Xenon studies, the sequence in a flow calculation is based on 1 minute Xenon distribution images. Tomomatic 564 has a sensitivity for Xenon 133 of 70,000 cts/sec/μCi/ml and for Iod-123 of 200,000 cts/sec/μCi/ml. These are the absolute minimum sensitivities necessary for making dynamic functional studies with reasonable spatial resolution. Increased spatial resolution requires increased collimation, and increased collimation with single photon camera systems causes reduced camera sensitivity. If, for instance, one wants to make functional flow CBF measurements with a resolution in the area of 1.5-1.8 cm, this can only be done with a sampling time of 3-5 minutes, both for Xenon and Iod-123. This is sufficient presuming that the patient lies completely still and that one wants to reveal areas which, in the initial phase, have a different isotope distribution from the subsequent phases, particularly in an infarcted area. When one wants to make use of Xenon and when it is a question of clearance measurement, a sufficient number of counts is required within each data sample. This is necessary in order to make a reconstruction of statistically good activity distribution pictures. If these pictures are not well dimensioned, when statistically viewed, calculations made on the basis of sequences of such pictures will be completely wrong. When looking at a patient study (Fig. 22) made by Dr. Claude Raynaud in Orsay, Paris (12), the following can be observed:

A 50-year old man with symptoms of a left MCA-infarct has an improved hypofixation 13 days after the infarct. This hypofixation can be observed in the IMP image, 3 to 8 minutes after iv. injection. After only 2 hours this infarcted area is already remarkably reduced but is, however, still visible. After 5 hours the infarct can only be traced in the deeper parts. When the corresponding CBF-Xenon study is watched in the upper part of the picture, one can observe that

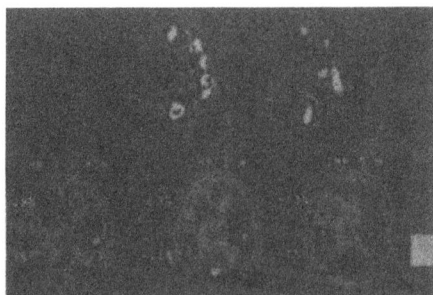

Fig. 22.
IMP-123 CBF measurement compared with Xe-133 CBF. IMP-123 CBF has no steady state value, therefore a fast acquisition is necessary (12).

the entire left hemisphere in the resting state is infarcted and after a dose of a dilating substance, such as Diamox, the area of the infarct is considerably increased indicating that the arteries in the left side and the collateral circulation in the left side cannot dilate in spite of Diamox.

As can be concluded from observation of this picture, which is by no means a unique case, it is extremely important to be able to measure with a very short sampling time, if one wants to reveal an infarct or reduced regional functions at a very early stage with I-123 amphetamine. With a sampling time, which with a conventional gamma camera would have been 20-40 minutes, the infarct, as observed in the first picture from 3-8 minutes, would have been reduced in size and intensity by 8%, from 19% to 11%. If, however, the measurement is carried out using Xenon, one gets a very distinct impression - maybe a somewhat exaggerated impression - of the size of the infarct. When using Xenon it is also important to get a sufficient number of counts per measuring period, in this case one minute. These measurements were made by a T 564 standard collimator, with the above-mentioned camera sensitivity. It is of course a fact that if one wants images with higher resolution, this can be achieved by means of T 564 by replacing the collimator with a high resolution collimator, which gives resolutions as low as 8mm FWHM in the reconstructed picture, but with considerably increased data sampling times. This is thus a compromise between the wish for measurements of reduced or increased regional function with short data sampling times or with long data sampling times to measure the very small dimensions of regions in the brain, often with anatomic changes.(See Fig 3 A)

5.2 Proposal for an Alternative Geometrical Configurated Single-Photon Camera or Single Photon Camera Based on Alternative Scintillators to Sodium Iodide

It is relatively simple to estimate, for instance, for a brain scanner, the maximum count rate with a specific isotope, dosed in a said amount, by placing the head in a Well counter. In this way an uncollimated Well counter will be able to detect how many counts can be collected per second without collimation. A simple calculation shows that in this case a camera sensitivity of more than 4,000,000 cnt/sec/μCi/ml would be needed. It could, of course, be tried, if something other than NaI-crystals proved more effective as stopping power of a specific strength; but at present the sodium iodide

being the sodium iodide scintillator is a reasonably efficient using low energy isotopes. A factor of at least 20 is lost by collimation It is thus mainly a question of collimation and distance to measuring object, which determines the sensitivity of a given camera.

In T 564 a configuration has been chosen, whereby a collection of detectors have been placed in a square around the object that is to be reconstructed. It has, of course, been considered how each detector tray could be designed, the detector tray being a group of crystals, referred to here as a camera. Individual crystals have the advantage of being able to collect a greater number of counts per second without significant loss of counts, compared to a single large crystal, which is able to cover the object more efficiently. In this way no area is wasted by lack of covering crystal. It is our intention to continue working with the geometrical form, with which we have worked until now, as we still find many possibilities of increasing the camera sensitivity by improving the collimation and reducing the distance to the object being measured.

6. DATA PROCESSING

6.1 Data Sampling

The data collection from T 564 is performed in sequences corresponding to 1.5°, 3° or 4.5° while the tomograph rotates. As the two cameras are displaced one-half detector width in proportion to each other, only a one-half rotation is necessary to achieve a complete set of data. Each data sampling carried out per 4.5° consists of 80 projections per revolution and consequently 40 projections per half revolution corresponds to a complete set of data. Consequently, each time the camera rotates a full turn, 2 sets of data have been sampled. In this way during the first minute of the data processing, for example, 12 sets of data will be sampled.
For normal Xenon flow studies a total processing time of 4 to 4-1/2 minutes is used. This means that during the first 1 to 1-1/2 minutes 18 data sets are sampled and during the following 3 minutes 12 data sets per minute. From this data sampling, 4 reconstructed matrices of the activity distribution are created per slice. After 1 to 1-1/2 minutes we have, thus, the raw data which create the background for a reconstruction of the activity distribution of the first 1 to 1-1/2 minutes, and the following minutes similarly.
In order to have acceptable imaging in sequences of 4, upon which

the flow can be calculated, it is necessary to have a count rate of
approximately 2.5-3 mill counts per 4 to 4-1/2 minutes. If one does
not operate with a count rate of this size, a statistically good
quality is not achieved and if bad images are used for the calculation of flow, the flow-calculation is spoilt by too many errors and
too much noise.

6.2 Sorting

After the data sampling is completed the data are sorted and made
ready for the reconstruction. Thus a reconstruction of the past
4 and 1/2 minutes means a total of 20 activity distribution slices
plus 5 calculated CBF slices.

6.3 Mathematical Treatment

The images are usually reconstructed according to the Filter Back
Projection Principle (FBP), but there are also algorithms for arithmetic reconstruction technique (ART). The latter, which in the on-
line version takes longer time, is more suitable for subsequent attenuation correction, according to the iterative attenuation techniques. After reconstruction, well-know filter techniques are used
for refinement of the images before the flow calculation can start.

7. DATA CORRECTION TECHNIQUES

The philosophy behind the Tomomatic family is to give the best primary information by means of a very sensitive detector system. In
this way, measurements with a very high counting rate can be performed and thus good statistics of the images can be achieved. The
above is fundamental for high quality imaging. However, not all the
problems are solved with this, as there are some physical relations, such as attenuation in the brain, uniformity in the
various photomultiplier tubes (PMT) amplifications and non-uniform
speed, which can influence the final quality of the images. Therefore the signals must be processed in the camera controller and DEC
computer system.

7.1 Attenuation

A reduction in attenuation has already been attempted by arranging
two detectors one in front of the other viewing the same brain region

(Fig. 7). Line spread functions for Xenon standard collimators show that in spite of these arrangements, the maximum values decrease by 68% from the circumference to the center. We talk about a very big attenuation of signals from these regions of the brain which are the farthest points from the detector. Therefore, mathematical compensation for this attenuation is carried out by T564 reconstruction software. After this compensation there are only a few percentage points of influence in the attenuation. The effect of the attenuation compensation is shown in Fig.23. A recording of a homogen phantom study is shown where the calculated number of counts results as a function of the distance from the circumference to the center. The difference between the maximum number of counts and the center is 8%, which mean that the actual deviation in the particular points is below 4% from the theoretical result. This is a result of the applied method causing an overestimation in the circumference and an underestimation in the center. Fig. 24 shows a 20 cm cylindrical phantom where half of the phantom is filled with Tc99m in water. It shows the sharp border line between the filled and unfilled part of the phantom.

7.2 Uniformity of the Reconstructed Distribution Matrix

Besides the attenuation problem, some other physical problems are problematic, for example: amplification variations in PMT, factors due to the non-uniformity in rotation. Many methods of preventing this problem have been tried. First of all, the detector arrangement is designed in such a way that amplification variations have a minimal influence. Each of the 4 rotating cameras consists of 16 separate NaI detectors. Because of this, there are no problems with the

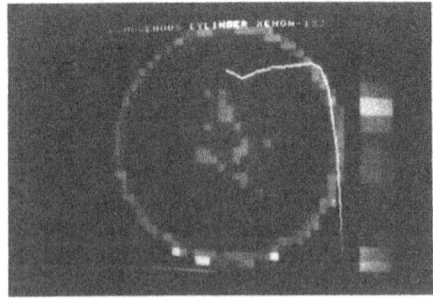

Fig. 23
Phantom study with a uniform phantom. The white curve shows the attenuation effect (13).

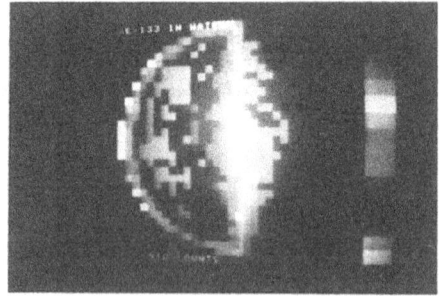

Fig. 24

Phantom study with half of the field filled with tracer (13).

geometrical determination of scintillations in the single slices. The slice separation is performed on each of these 16 NaI detectors as in an Anger camera. In T 564, the 5 slices are separated with a heavy collimator so that the crosstalk is limited within a relatively large amplification variation. In addition, the software package is supplied with programs which make it possible to move the spectrum for the separate channel, in such a way that variations arising during the day can be eliminated. The above, combined with a very simple calibration procedure, gives a uniformity that varies by only a few percentage points from the theoretical values, a uniformity which counts less than 0.2 cm over the whole reconstructed image. Finally, the Tomomatic software is supplied with a program for elimination of systematic errors, which normally cause ring artifacts. Combined with the modular construction of each single camera, this means that the error occurring in one of the NaI crystals of the PMT does not disrupt the measurement. This secures a very reliable instrument, which can be kept running even with minor errors, thus avoiding the possibility of a total halt in operation.

7.3 Noise Filter

A Xenon-133 rCBF measurement with T 564 is recorded during 4 minutes, thus the dynamic image is produced on the basis of 4 static images, 0-60 sec., 60-120 sec., 120-180 sec. and 180-240 sec. In the second period from 60-120 sec., usually 1,200,000 counts are recorded for the whole camera. This is normally necessary in order to obtain good quality pictures. Fig. 29 shows the noise level as a function of different counts. As can be seen, it is possible to

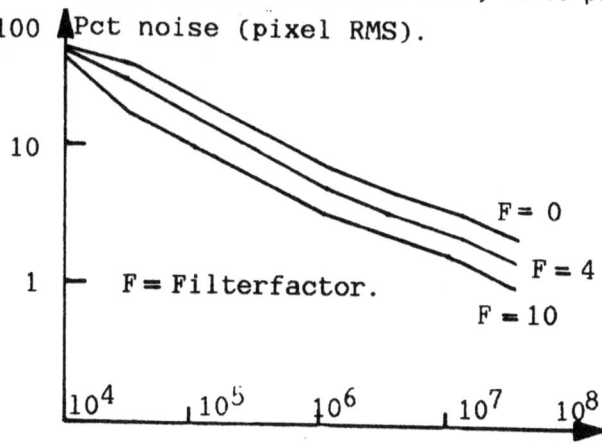

Fig. 25
Noise as a function of collected counts (13).

improve an image, despite the presence of noise, by use of the T 564 noise suppressing filtration program. For example, an image recorded with 1,000,000 counts can be improved from 8% noise without a filter to below 5% by using filter factor 10. In a similar way, an image which is recorded with 500,000 counts and a filter factor 10 can have the same quality (taking noise into consideration) as an image with 1,000,000 counts and filter factor 4. However, there are of course certain drawbacks to filtrating the images, since heavy filtration causes part of the information to be lost. However, with appropriate compromises, there is a possibility that the quality of images can be improved significantly.

8. AN ILLUSTRATIVE MEDICAL EXAMPLE

Even for a high sensitivity and consequently a rough collimator such as the collimator used in the Tomomatic 32 (spatial resolution: 2.1 cm FWHM), a very useful result can be obtained. The progress of two patients, suffering from left MCA infarct (middle cerebral artery), was followed closely throughout a long period of illness. This was made possible by the relatively inexpensive investigation method that was used, and the investigations proved particularly useful as they allowed CBF measurements to be made, which could be repeatedly reproduced. It can be concluded from this example that it is possible to foresee the prognosis on a quantitative basis which can be constantly revised and updated, each time a CBF measurement has been performed either with Xenon-133 or with Iod-123 amphetamine. Contrary to other techniques, imaging the "tissue", the single photon technique has the ability to show the effect, rather than just the physical presence of an infarct. An occlusion, for instance, can be of the same size and yet still have a very varied effect in the different patients, depending on whether the collateral circuit is able to take over the blood supply. In other cases the effect of an occlusion after spontaneous recanalization on account of luxury perfusion can be observed, in spite of the fact that the occlusion no longer exists. The example in Fig. 26 (5) shows that the quantitative nature of the single photon emission technique makes a clinical and objective patient follow-up possible so that an evaluation of the prognostic value of a given treatment is possible.

8.1 Normal Rest Flow Picture

Picture A shows a normal flow in an adult at rest (5). Pictures B and C show the blood flow in a patient measured with an interval of

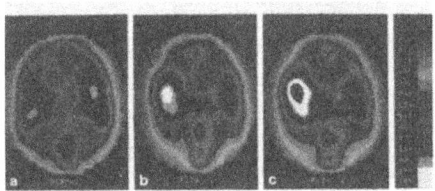
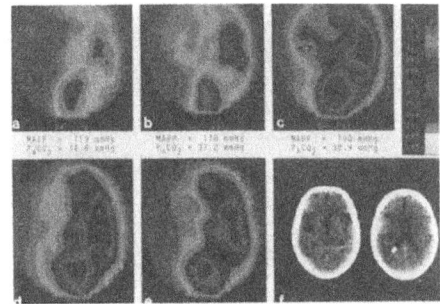

Fig. 26
rCBF in a normal patient compared to rCBF in a patient taken with a 50 min. Interval. (5)

Fig. 27
rCBF in a patient with complete occlusion in left MCA. Patient 1 (5)

50 minutes. The scale to the right indicates the blood flow in ml for 100g cerebral tissue per minute. It is important to notice that it is possible to reproduce any deviation from the norm. Figs. 25, 26 and 27 show a case with 2 patients suffering from occlusion of MCA; the cases, however, have developed differently (5). Here it is not enough to diagnose an occlusion by CT-scan, but it is important in a quantitative way to be able to follow the courses of the disease of the two patients.

8.2 Complete Occlusion of Left MCA-Patient 1

This patient (5) suffers from a complete occlusion of the left MCA, causing a reduced flow in his left side. In pictures B and C the blood flow is improved in the affected area because of improved collaterals, developed during the occlusion in the left MCA. This improvement, however, is transitory, as pictures D and E show. The blood flow eventually decreased. This region will not recover because the blood flow increase came too late.

8.3 Complete Occlusion of Left MCA-Patient 2

This patient (5) has an occlusion of the left MCA, just as in patient 1, but in this case one can find a strong luxury perfusion in the spontaneous recanalization in the left side. The luxury perfusion disappears eventually and the blood flow in the left side decreases to below normal. As the spontaneous recanalization came too late, recovery of this area was therefore not possible.

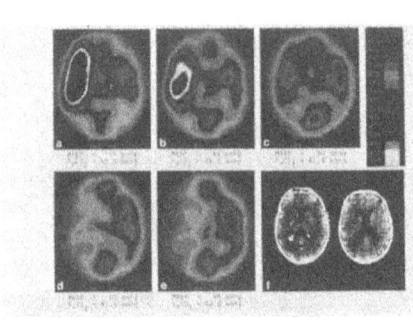
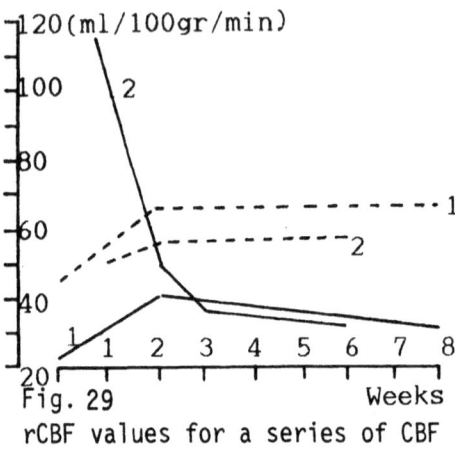

Fig. 28
rCBF in a patient with complete occlusion in left MCA. Patient 2 (5)

Fig. 29
rCBF values for a series of CBF tomograms. Patients 1 and 2 (5)

8.4 Conclusion-Patients 1 and 2 (5)

In patient 1 the flow slowly increases and in patient 2 (in the beginning) there is a heavy luxury perfusion. In both cases, however, the flow ends in the ipsilateral hemisphere of about 30 ml/100gr/ml and in the contralateral hemisphere of about 70 ml/100gr/ml. Repeated CBF measurements by D-SPECT can demonstrate non-invasively and at a low cost the time-dependent alterations of DBF dynamics after onset of cerebral infarction. The states of "misery-perfusion" and of relative or absolute "luxury-perfusion" can be recognized as transient phenomena observed sequentially in the early time course of cerebral infarction before the brain recovers its "matched-perfusion" state in chronic stage. Serials of CBF tomograms allow us to reveal these important aspects of the hemodynamics of larger infarcts, aspects that may be very decisive for the success of active therapeutic cures of medical or surgical nature (5).

9. FUTURE BRAIN SPECT

During the last decade research in the field of Nuclear Medicine and in the fields related to it, has proved that patient examinations with cost in the range of USD 10.000, are bound to be rather limited in the future. Up to now, few centers are able to carry out such examinations routinely, because of their high cost. The important development in radiopharmaceuticals is expected to give effective results, especially in the field of single photon tracers. Therefore, single photon emission tomography will replace the positron emission tomography in the future, when it is a question of both clinical research and clinical routine examination. Already today an examination costs less than USD 150 per patient and before the end of 1985, the examination cost will be reduced to half this price.

The single photon tomographs of the future will, however, be those instruments which can comply with the demand of high sensitivity and a high counting rate. High sensitivity allows, as is well known, collimation - a collimation in terms of multiple slices and collimation leading to high spatial resolution. Medimatic has gone far with its new instrument, Tomomatic 564. No single photon tomograph of the future will be epoch-making unless it has a sensitivity of approximately 150.000-200.000 cts/sec/μCi/ml, as is the case with Tomomatic 564. With 200.000 cts/sec/μCi/ml for the isotope Iod-123, it is possible, as has already been described, to record simultaneous multiple slices with spatial resolutions of less than 10 mm at a sampling time of less than 10 min., which is short enough time for revealing the newly discovered and so very important initial isotope distribution which is already completely changed 1 hour after dosing or injection (12). In a few years, single photon tomographs will have a sensitivity of more than 1/2 million cts/sec/μCi/ml and should thus be able to record 5 slice images with spatial resolution below 1 cm in a sampling time of less than 5 minutes. The industry must now undertake the task of continuing to develop instruments with dynamic SPECT (D-SPECT), so that new SPECT-tomographs will be developed selectively for brain and heart examinations, without wasting time in trying to develop an instrument that is perfect in revealing any defects in all organs simultaneously.

REFERENCES

1. Sveinsdottir, E., Larsen, B., Rommer, P. and N.A. Lassen. A Multidetector Scintillation Camera with 254 Channels. Journal of Nuclear Medicine 18 (1977) 168-174.

2. Risberg, J., Maximillian, A.V. and I. Prohovnik. Change of Cortical Activity Pattern... Neuropsychologia 15, 793-798.

3. Stokely, E.M., Sveinsdottir, E., Lassen, N.A. and P. Rommer. A Single Photon Dynamic Computer Assisted Tomograph... Journal of Comp. Ass. Tomography 4 (1980) 230-240.

4. Kanno, I. and N.A. Lassen. Two Methods for Calculating Cerebral Blood Flow from Emission... Journal of Comp. Ass. Tomography 3 (1979) 71-76.

5. Sugiyama, H., Christensen, J., Olsen T.S. and N.A. Lassen. Cerebral Blood Flow Tomography Measured Repeatedly in Patients with Infarction of Middle Cerebral Artery Territory. (in preparation)

6. Atkins, H., Robertson, J.S., Croft, B.Y., Isui, B., Suskind, H., Ellis, K.V., Loken, M.K. and S. Treves. Estimation of Radiation Absorbed Doses from Radio-Xenon in Lung Imaging. Journal of Nuclear Medicine 21 (1980) 454-465.

7. Hill, Thomas C., Holman, B. Leonard and Philippe L. Magistretti. Emission Computed Tomography of the Brain with Radiolabelled Amines. Computed Emission Tomography. Edited by P.J. Ell and B.L. Holman, pp.419-437 (Oxford, 1982).

8. Phelps, M.E., Hoffman, E.J., Huang, J.C. and D.E. Kuhl. ECAT:A New Computerized Tomographic Imaging System for Positron-Emitting Radiopharmaceuticals. Journal of Nuclear Medicine 19 (1978) 635-647.

9. Lassen, N.A., Stokely, E.M., Sveinsdottir, E., Henriksen, L., Rommer, P. and Goldmann, T. Dynamic Emission CT of Xenon 133 inhalation for Study of Cerebral Blood Flow.Emission Computed Tomography:The Single Photon Approach. BRH (1981) 237-244.

10. Per Rommer et al. Evaluation of a 5 Slice Dynamic Single Photon Emission Computerized Tomograph (D-SPECT) Designed Selectively

for Functional Brain Examination. (in preparation)

11. Celsis, P., Goldman, T., Henriksen, L and N.A. Lassen. A Method for Calculating Regional Cerebral Blood Flow from Emission Computed Tomography of Inert Gas Concentrations:Practical Approach. Journal of Comp. Ass. Tomography 5 (1981) 641-645.

12. Raynaud, C., Rancurel, G., Samson, Y., Kieffer, E., Baron, J.C., Cabanis, E., Lassen, N.A., Comar, D., Rapin, J., Moretti, J.L., Ashienazy, S., Richard, S. and M. Bourdoisseau. Measurement of Oxygen Metabolism, 123-I-IMP Distribution and rCBF-Xe in patients with Ischemic Vascular Disease. Proc. of 31st Annual Meeting of the Society of Nuclear Medicine, June, 1984, Los Angeles.

13. Holm, S., Department of Neuro Medicine, Rogshospitalet, DK-2400 Copenhagen NV. TOMOMATIC 64. Meeting in the Hospitalier Frederic Joliot, Orsay, Paris, March 5, 1984.

14. Lassen, N.A., Sveinsdottir, E., Kanno, I., Stokely, E.M. and P. Rommer. A Fast Single Photon Emission Tomograph for Regional Cerebral Blood Flow Studies in Man. Journal of Comp. Ass. Tomography 2 (1978) 660-661.

DESIGN AND PERFORMANCE OF THE CLEON TWO-DIMENSIONAL,
FOCUSED-RAY GEOMETRY SCANNER FOR SINGLE PHOTON TOMOGRAPHY

Hugh F. Stoddart, Consultant

Groton Design Associates
P.O.Box 200, Groton, MA 01450, U.S.A

1. BACKGROUND

Nuclear medical tomography preceded computer aided x-ray tomography (CAT) by several years. Kuhl[1], in 1963, described a nuclear scanner that consisted of a pair of opposed, collimated detectors which defined a pencil-shaped region of sensitivity between them. The detectors were coupled together and driven in a translate-and-rotate scan pattern that took data from a single "slice" transverse to the axis of the body just like the first x-ray CAT scanners that were to follow.

Initially, Kuhl produced images by simply "backprojecting" his data. Later he developed more sophisticated methods of processing the data to reduce the unwanted buildup of background in the images. But the first use of analytically accurate reconstructions, the mathematical basis of which dates back to Radon[2] in 1917, was in x-ray tomography[3,4]. It was made practical by the availability of sufficiently powerful digital computers at reasonable cost. By analytically accurate reconstructions we mean a mapping of the slice in which the calculated value of a parameter (e.g., radioactivity concentration or x-ray absorption) is the same as the actual value within the body at the corresponding location.

Because radionuclide scanners have the ability to image exceedingly minute concentrations of all sorts of biologically active molecules that can be *tagged* with radioisotopes, positron-emitting radionuclide tomography (PET) and "single-photon" emitter radionuclide computed tomography (SPECT) are unique in mapping *physiological* activity. Other imaging methods including CAT, nuclear magnetic resonance (NMR) and ultrasound, mostly measure *anatomy,* that is, the distribution of major constituents.

In 1974, the Cleon Corporation started a project to design an optimum single-photon radionuclide tomographic scanner for the brain. While the technology of PET was advancing rapidly it was felt that the cost of the equipment and the need for a nearby cyclotron and radiopharmacy would severely restrict its clinical use. Radionuclide tomography using radiopharmaceuticals tagged with the commonly available single-photon emitters seemed to hold more potential for widespread clinical use even though the availability of such radiopharmaceuticals were lagging far behind those available to PET.

The use of PET was viewed as the medical research tool for developing new physiological imaging procedures with SPECT following along with the development of analogous radiopharmaceuticals when clinically efficacious procedures become defined. For example, the earlier PET work on brain function using fluorodeoxyglucose is now being duplicated by SPECT using iodoamphetamin and other new single-photon radiopharmaceuticals.

2. REQUIREMENTS FOR 'SPECT' SYSTEMS

The fundamental requirement for a SPECT system is sensitivity. Poor sensitivity can only produce noisy, low-resolution images. This is especially true since tomographic reconstruction dramatically amplifies the stochastic noise inherent in radioactive decay. The problem is compounded by the need for short data collection times for any one slice. Any patient motion that occurs during data collection invalidates the reconstruction and may create intolerable artifacts in the slice image. *It is therefore absolutely imperative to have the maximum detector area possible around the head and to have it devoted to a minimum number of slices at a time.*

One design possibility considered at Cleon for an optimum SPECT scanner was an extention of Kuhl's concept. (In order to increase sensitivity he had already placed multiple detectors along the transverse scan direction[5].) However, since the thickness of the slice sets the maximum dimension of the detector perpendicular to the slice, the total area of detectors that could view any one slice was geometrically limited to a thin, polygon-shaped ring. While this configuration may be sensitive enough for xenon flow studies in the brain for which a relatively large amount of radioactivity is available for a short time (see Lassen[6]), it becomes marginal at low radionuclide concentrations. Also, like the rotating gamma camera, this design is subject to rotational artifacts.

Another possibility considered was to invoke that ingenuous work-horse of nuclear medicine for the last quarter of a century, the Anger[7] gamma camera, either by rotating the patient in front of the camera or rotating the camera about the patient axis. A little consideration will reveal that this is really identical to the multiple detector versions of the Kuhl geometry but with even less detector area per slice. The only way the Kuhl system detector area can be approached is by using *three or four* gamma cameras completely surrounding the patient.

Now as those of you who have used gamma cameras know, they can be fussy machines. The location of a scintillation caused by an incident gamma ray is deduced by the relative sizes of the light pulses received by nearby photomultiplier tubes. If the gains of the photomultipliers drift, the deduced location will be in error and cause various artifacts in the reconstruction. In the usual "planar" gamma camera applications this location error manifests itself as a field uniformity problem and has been dealt with by computers and "field flattening algorithms" that depend on data taken by exposing the gamma camera to a uniform test source for a long time. However, position accuracy requirements are much more stringent for tomographic applications and the problem is still being struggled with along with the associated rotational artifacts[8].

Between rotating gamma cameras and Kuhl-type systems for dedicated brain scanning the clear choice is the latter; mostly because somewhat more detector area can be brought to bear on a slice due to quite a bit more flexibility in collimator design and detector layout, and also because the instrumentation can be made more robust. (A commercial instrument that adopted and expanded this concept is described in these proceedings[9].)

But remember that the detection geometry of gamma cameras and Kuhl-type systems are basically similar. We will refer to it as the *one-dimensional, parallel (or "fan") ray geometry* since the data collected for each projection is one dimensional. The amount of detector that can be utilized in the axial direction to collect data in any one slice is limited by the slice thickness required. As a consequence, gamma rays originating in the slice that have paths out of the plane of the slice (and this is the vast majority) are thrown away.

Is there a way to increase the detector area to include at least some off-slice gamma rays and, if so, can this data be collected in such a way as to permit an analytically accurate tomographic reconstruction?

3. THE CLEON BRAIN SCANNER

In early 1975, a drastically different radionuclide brain scanner geometry was proposed[10]. The fundamental concept was to abandon the "in slice" detector limitation and to use highly focusing collimators to bring as much detector area to bear on a single slice as possible. In a typical geometry the detectors used to collect data from a single slice had axial dimensions *fourteen times* the slice thickness. The total detector area involved in taking data from a *single slice* was greater than 3000cm^2.

Development of this concept was carried out by the Cleon Corporation research group during 1975 and 1976 and a number of machines were subsequently built by Union Carbide Imaging Systems[11]. These machines are still being used at Harvard Medical School Hospitals and the Middlesex Hospital in London and continue to produce excellent images even though Union Carbide abandoned the nuclear medicine business in 1979 and the design of the systems has never been optimized. Rights to the system were acquired by Photon Diagnostics of Medfield, MA, in 1984 and an updated version using a new computer has been designed.

The detector geometry of all "Cleon-type" brain-scanning machines is basically the same. Twelve, 12.7x20.3cm NaI detectors are equally spaced about the head with centers located in a plane transverse to the patient axis. Unlike the one-dimensional systems, the short dimension of the detectors lies in the tangential direction while the long dimension is parallel to the patient axis. The focusing collimators are 15cm thick and the focus is 10cm from their front face. Thus, each detector subtends an angle of 28° in the plane of the slice and 44° perpendicular to the slice.

Detector motion is in *two dimensions* and confined to the plane of the slice. Each detector makes a set of twelve, linear scans tangent to the slice but at different distances from the center of the slice. The scans are 20cm long and are spaced about 1cm apart in the radial direction. The radial locations of the detectors are such that the *focus* of each detector performs a rectilinear scan of slightly more than the half of the slice closest to it. Since the detectors are uniformly spaced in angle, twelve such scans are produced 30° apart and covering the whole slice. Note that all points in the slice come under the focus of at least six detectors (but not at the same time). We will refer to this unique system as *two-dimensional focused-ray geometry* since the data collected form two-dimensional arrays within a single slice. The data from each of the tangential scan lines is put into 128 "bins" corresponding to 128 elongated "pixels" 1.6x10mm in object space. Thus an array of 1536 data points is accumulated in the slice by each detector during its twelve traverses.

An important consequence is that if all the 18,432 elongated pixels from one slice are simply interpolated and summed onto a 128x128 grid *without reconstruction*, a surprisingly good image of even complicated objects is obtained. The requirements for reconstruction are thus minimized and reconstruction noise amplification is less than for the previously discussed geometries.

One way to look at this is as a *three dimensional* Radon reconstruction of a plane from partial (360° in azimuth but +/- 22° in altitude) angular data, the integration over angle being performed by the detectors with their focusing collimators. In practice, what is done now is to filter each of the twelve scan lines from each detector before backsummation. The filtering kernel was determined experimentally by iterating a best fit to the known radioactivity concentrations in several phantoms that closely approximated the distributions found in brain scans.

There appears to be little doubt that the reconstruction algorithm can be substantially improved and work to that end is underway at Photon Diagnostics, Donner Laboratory, Harvard, and Middlesex Hospital. Researchers at Photon Diagnositics and others at Donner Laboratories under Dr. Budinger are looking at three dimensional reconstructions to produce a first image that can then be quickly iterated to a corrected image. Moore at Harvard has been continuing the work started at Carbide on iterative reconstructions and Jarritt and Dr. Ell at Middlesex have been making extensive use of a maximum entropy reconstruction. Iterative reconstructions appear especially attractive for this geometry since the unfiltered backsummed image is so good that convergence should be quick and uncomplicated.

4. ADVANTAGES OF TWO-DIMENSIONAL, FOCUSED-RAY GEOMETRY

The use of highly focused collimators in the manner of the Cleon brain scanner leads to several important advantages:

A. A high spatial resolution and a tight, point-spread function *that are constant* throughout the slice and determined only by the characteristics of the collimator set being used.

B. The slice thickness is constant throughout the slice for the same reason. No 'lens-shaped' slices.

C. All detector area is invested in one slice at a time providing short, single-slice scan times. Motion artifacts are much less likely compared to rotating gamma cameras that require much longer times to collect the data in a slice. Repeated rapid scans of the same slice permit dynamic studies or they may be added to enhance the image.

D. Two-dimensional scanning by itself produces an image thereby reducing the reconstruction task, attendant noise amplification, and artifacts due to patient motion during slice. Noise reduction may be traded for increased sensitivity.

E. *ROBUST;* no critical adjustments. Relatively very insensitive to detector gain drifts and other instrumental variations.

F. Easier attenuation correction since sampling depth is known. Linear relationship of reconstructed image to radioisotope concentration.

5. PERFORMANCE

Resolution, slice thickness, and sensitivity are determined by the collimators and the reconstruction filter roll-off spatial frequency. The collimators that were shipped with the machines from Union Carbide Imaging Systems gave a resolution of about 9mm and a slice thickness of 15mm. An early high resolution collimator set had a resolution of about 7mm but was poorly constructed giving too low a sensitivity. New collimators in two versions are being developed at Photon Diagnostics. The first will have a millimeter or so better resolution than the present ones but should also have better sensitivity due to improved fabrication techniques. The second will be a high sensitivity collimator with several times the sensitivity of the old ones and a resolution of better than 12mm.

The machine has multiple slice capability by computer controlled indexing of the bed. This is feasible since it only takes several minutes to scan each slice. Moore and the Harvard Group have modified one of their machines to do a single scan in less than a minute in order to do dynamic studies with some new radiopharmaceuticals.

Drs. Hill, Holman, and Clouse, in another paper at this meeting[12], describe the performance of the machine and present interesting clinical results and comparisons with rotating gamma cameras. Dr. Ell has done similar studies at Middelsex.

While caution should be exercised in making parametric comparisons between systems so different in their workings as this two-dimensional focusing geometry and the various one-dimensional geometries, judgments by experienced diagnosticians of the relative *clinical* value of images obtained in a routine medical environment must be considered significant.

6. ACKNOWLEDGEMENTS

Many people have made important contributions to the development and design of this new SPECT brain scanner, first at Cleon Corporation, then at Union Carbide Imaging Systems, and now at Photon Diagnostics. Drs. Hill, Holman, and others at Harvard and Dr. Ell at Middlesex have made extensive medical use of the machines, while S. Moore and P. Jarritt have continued to support and enhance the machines at Harvard and Middlesex, respectively, after Union Carbide left the nuclear medical business. Important early contributions to the reconstructions and the design of computer simulations that lead to a clearer understanding of the method were made by H.A. Stoddart (Brown Univ.) who continues to provide valuable insights. Dr. Budinger has contributed important ideas and raised a number of thoughtful questions about the machine[13].

1. Kuhl, D.E. and R.Q. Edwards. Image separation radioisotope scanning. Radiology 30 (1963) 653-661.
2. Radon, J. Über die Bestimmung von Functionen durch ihre Integralwerte längs gewisser Mannigfaltigkeiten; Berichte Sächsische Akademie der Wissenschaften. Leipzig, Math.-Phys.Kl.,69 (1917) 262-277.
3. Cormac, A.M. Representation of a function by its line integrals, with some radiological applications. J.Appl.Phys. 34 (1963) 2722-2727.
4. Hounsfield, G.N. A method of and apparatus for examination of a body by radiation such as x- or gamma-radiation. British patent #1,283,915 (1972).
5. Kuhl, D.E. and R.Q. Edwards. Transverse section radionuclide scanning system. United States patent #3,970,853.
6. Lassen, N.A. and L.Henriksen, O.Paulson. Regional cerebral blood flow in stroke by ^{133}Xe inhalation and emission tomography. Stroke 12 (1981) 284-288.
7. Anger, H.O. Radiation image device. United States patent #3,011,057 (1961).
8. van Oortmarssen, G. Emission tomography using rotating gamma cameras. *These proceedings*.
9. Rommer, P. High efficiency multi-slice approach for single photon tomography of the brain. *These proceedings*.
10. Stoddart, H.F. Nuclear transverse sectional brain function imager. United States patent #4,209,700 (1980).
11. Stoddart H.F. and H.A. Stoddart. A new development in single gamma transaxial tomography: Union Carbide focused collimator scanner. IEEE Trans.Nuc.Sci. NS-26 (1979) 2710-2712.
12. Hill, T.C. and B.L. Holman, M.E. Clouse. Clinical Comparison between detector ring and rotating gamma camera for single photon tomography. *These proceedings*.
13. Budinger T. Revival of clinical nuclear medicine brain imaging. J.Nuc.Med. 22 (1981) 1094-1097.

CLINICAL COMPARISON BETWEEN MULTI-RING DETECTOR AND
ROTATING GAMMA CAMERA FOR SINGLE PHOTON TOMOGRAPHY

T.C. Hill, B.L. Holman, S. Moore, P. Kasulis,
M.E. Clouse
Department of Radiology, Harvard Medical School,
New England Deaconess Hospital and Brigham & Women's
Hospital, Boston, MA, U.S.A.

Our clinical comparison of the multi-ring detector system
and rotating gamma camera for single-photon tomography of the
brain is based on over 200 studies performed on the Harvard
multidetector system and over 30 studies performed on a single-
headed rotating gamma camera system (GE-400T and Siemens 3700).
The advantages of the multidetector system are: 1) improved
sensitivity and resolution; 2) uniform resolution and sensitivity
across the field of view; 3) absence of ring or rotation artifacts;
4) ease of setup for examination; and 5) short scan time.

MULTIDETECTOR SYSTEM

The Harvard multidetector brain scanning system, previously
called the Cleon-710 and currently designated as the Novo SPECT
system, is an instrument introduced by Stoddard and Stoddard using
short-focused, wide-angled collimators together with a fast
scanning pattern within a slice. Its design offers improved
sensitivity and more uniform resolution through the transaxial
slice than that offered by the rotating gamma camera. The head
scanning system consists of a gantry assembly with 12 scanning
detectors. Each detector has a focus collimator, a 20 x 12.5
x 2.5 cm sodium iodide (thallium) crystal, a photomultiplier
tube, (8.7-cm. in diameter) preamplifiers, and a dual pulse-
height analyzer mounted at $30°$ intervals around the 28-cm
opening.

The detectors move in 6 pairs: when one pair of detectors
is scanning tangentially in increments moving toward the center
of the patient opening, the adjacent pairs are scanning tangent-

ially in increments moving away from the center. The focal point of each detector encompasses half of the field of view. Each of the six opposing detector pairs performs a rectilinear scan in the plane of the brain slice from a different angle. Each detector performs 12 tangential line scans spaced at 1-cm intervals, with each line 20 cm long and divided into 128 resolution elements. The spacing of slices can be selected in multiples of 3 mm and controlled by the patient couch movement. The gantry can be tilted up to $\pm 20°$ the vertical, allowing image sections at various convenient angles. The high collection efficiency of the detectors makes rapid scanning (2-5 min) of an entire slice possible.

During data collection the counts are recorded in a matrix as if they had come from the focal point of the collimator. The collimator is recording a blurred image because it also detects counts of the focal point. This blurring function is similar, if not identical, to the blurring function described by Radon (1) in his classic paper on reconstruction of an object when its line integrals or projections are known.

If all the counts from all the detectors were added to produce an image, the result would be the radionuclide distribution convolved with the collimator function. Reconstruction, at least in theory, could be performed by deconvolving the collimator function from the blurred image. In practice, however, for a variety of reasons, it is more practical to adapt the method of Shepp and Logan (2) to this geometry. Each line of back projected data is filtered by what is approximately a ramp in frequency space. The exact coefficients of the filter are chosen empirically, so that a uniform radionuclide distribution reconstructs uniformly after a uniform attenuation correction is performed. In other words, it is assumed that the effect of out-of-plane activity can be ignored and that the reconstruction can be done in a manner similar to that of conventional x-ray CT scanners.

The quantitative ability of this scanner is encouraging because the response to increases in activity is linear. Present algorithms do not fully account for the effects of attenuation. This problem is largely the same for all single photon systems. The current simple attenuation correction is performed on the raw data (data gathered directly from each collimator and before reconstruction) by multiplying each pixel with an exponetial factor based on the distance from the pixel to the edge of the field of view in a direction perpendicular to the scan lines (3). This simple scheme is adequate for most imaging tasks, but quantitation is sensitive to source position. More general solutions to the attenuation problem may be able to improve the quantitative capabilities of the system (4). Relative quantitation is possible for fixed geometry situations, in which the patient serves as his own control (5).

The sensitivity and resolution of the multidetector system compare favorably to other single photon emission tomography instruments (3). Table 1 shows the sensitivity and resolution for SPECT systems. This table shows that there is great promise for a device with a large crystal area.

When I-123 is imaged with this system, additional factors must be considered. Because the I-123 we use for the radiolabel is produced by the Te-134 (p, 2n) ^{23meV} I-123 reaction, 2.1 to 4.6% contamination with I-124 is present at the time of injection. The effects of scatter and so-called lead punch-through by high energy photons from the I-124 contamination are minimized in the images by an approximate background subtraction applied to the raw data by using a scatter mask. This mask was obtained by scanning three cylindrical phantoms representing the head, lung, and liver activity (6). One of the cylinders is filled with 0.04 mCi of pure I-124 and placed in the gantry. The other two are filled with 0.08 mCi I-124 and placed on the patient couch in positions roughly approximating the lung field and lower torso. The mask and subsequent patient studies are all scanned in the dual channel mode with the low energy pulse-height window set at 135-185 keV (surrounding the I-123 peak) and the high-energy window set at 310-360 keV. The two-dimensional projection of intensity distributions recorded in the low-energy window is a close approximation of the intensity distribution from the I-124 background when scanning a patient with I-123. This technique is not an exact compensation for punch-through and does not replace the requirement for pure I-123.

For patient studies, at least one tomographic image is obtained at 2 cm above the orbitomeatal line. Additional images are obtained at 2-cm increments from the initial slice. The injected dose is 5 mCi, and imaging is performed between 20 and 60 min after the injection. To improve the statistical quality of the images, 2 to 6 slices from the same level must be summed for image analysis.

ROTATING GAMMA CAMERA

The alternative method for transaxial reconstruction of externally administered radiotracers uses the rotating gamma camera. From a practical point of view, this approach is the favorite because so many rotating gamma cameras are already available in nuclear medicine laboratories, and most commercial vendors are currently selling versions of them. The realities of imaging I-123 with an Anger camera tend to offset the advantage of availability. The general principles of rotating gamma camera tomo-

TABLE 1

Comparison of Some Single Photon Emission Tomographic Scanners

SYSTEM	USEFUL CRYSTAL AREA (cm^2)	SENSITIVITY cts sec^{-1} uci^{-1} cc	SPATIAL RESOLUTION (mm)
MARK IV (7)	610	15,400	17
CLEON 710	3070	14,000 (130-170 KEV) 22,000 (105-173 KEV)	10
SEARLE Dual Camera	2200	1,100 (126-154 KEV) (ESTIMATED)	16
Anger Camera	500	630 (ESTIMATED)	11

graphy have been reviewed extensively (7), and we discuss here only those features that affect I-123 imaging.

The major constraint on rotating gamma camera tomography is sensitivity. Because of cost and considerations of patient dose, the injected dose of I-123 amines is likely to be in the range of 2-3 mCi. The low sensitivity of the rotating gamma camera is compensated somewhat because it collects volumetric information as opposed to the single slice information obtained with the multidetector system.

Adequate spatial resolution is the second critical element necessary for effective tomographic imaging with the rotating gamma camera and iodine-123. This is a particular problem because most of the iodine-123 presently available in the United States contains I-124 as an impurity. The resulting scatter significantly affects resolution and contrast. Alternatively, iodine-123 can be produced by an indirect method, iodine-127 (p, 5n) xenon-123, iodine-123. This method requires a proton energy of 55-70 meV (compared to 24-28 meV for the direct method) and results in a small amount of iodine-125 impurity (usually less than 0.4%). This method of production is available on a limited basis in the United States and somewhat more widely in Europe.

Meanwhile, can the rotating gamma camera tomography be performed with I-123 derived from the p-2n reaction. In evaluating one such system, the GE-400T Polack showed that the lower energy high-resolution collimator was clearly superior to the medium energy collimator. However, in evaluation of the Siemens 3700, the low-energy collimator was clearly inferior due to the high amount of septal penetration from the I-124 contamination. This most likely is due to the difference in manufacturing these two collimators: the GE-400T Leap collimator is a cast collimator, and the Siemens low-energy collimator is a ribbon collimator. The imaging obtained on the GE-400T was obtained with $360°$ rotation, 64 images and a total imaging time of 40 min. The images obtained on the Siemens 3700 system were obtained with the medium energy collimator, $360°$ rotation with $2°$ angular sampling and continuous rotation for 20 min.

Current rotating gamma camera systems are not optimized for head imaging. Most detectors are too large to permit an axis of rotation close to the head. These detectors must clear the patient's shoulder and are therefore at some distance from the head during imaging. This results in a loss of spatial resolution. Long bore collimators would allow imaging closer to the head but would sacrifice too much sensitivity. Specially designed, smaller diameter detectors will be necessary to improve the quality of brain tomography with I-123. Multiple detectors also may be necessary to improve sensitivity.

CLINICAL RESULTS

Images obtained on the multidetector system in a normal individual clearly show the greatest activity in the strips of cortex along the convexities of the frontal, temporal, parietal, and occipital lobes that correspond anatomically to cortical gray matter. Activity is also high in the region corresponding to the basal ganglia. The region between the basal ganglia and the convexities, corresponding to cortical white matter, has less activity. Activity in the cortical gray matter is uniform in the temporal, parietal, and occipital regions but appears patchy in the frontal regions. The contours of activity are undulating and reflect the gyral architecture observed on transmission CT examinations. Impressions of the interhemispheric and sylvian fissures are also present.

A normal study on a rotating gamma camera fails to delineate the degree of cortical architecture present on the multidetector system. However, large perfusion abnormalities such as those that occur in stroke or the asymmetries seen in varying degrees of cerebral vascular disease can be appreciated on tomographic images from the rotating gamma camera. However, small areas of minimal activity may be undetectable with a rotating head SPECT system as demonstrated in Figure 1A & 1B.

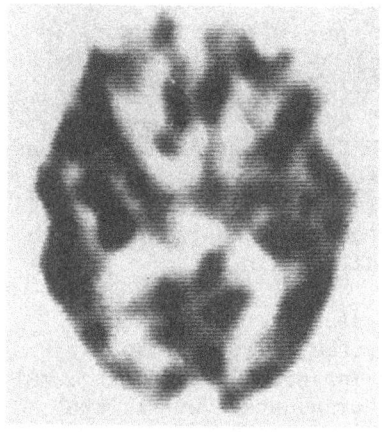
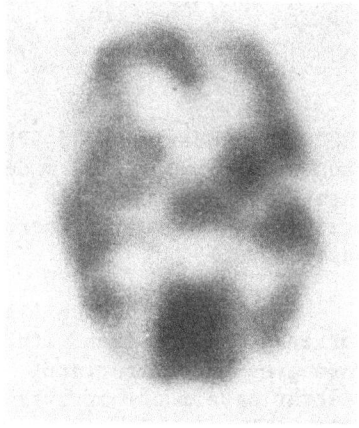

FIGURE 1A Multidetector transverse slice of patient with temporal lobe epilepsy showing an area of increased activity in the right temporal lobe.

FIGURE 1B Rotating head SPECT transverse slice of same patient fails to demonstrate this same area of increased activity.

With perfusion imaging, the anatomic detail and quantitative ability may not be as important for its clinical application as in studies with pharmaceuticals that reflect regional receptor concentration. The ability to discern smaller structures and to accurately quantitate the regional activity will be needed to detect small changes in receptor activity expected in disease states. Fig. 2A shows a study with radiolabeled I-123 QMB reflecting regional receptors in a normal patient. In a study in a patient with Alzheimer's disease, persistent activity at 24 hr is related to the receptor concentration affinity and blood flow in this patient. The rotating gamma camera images of such patients fail to accurately define the regional distribution of these muscularenic receptors (Fig 2B).

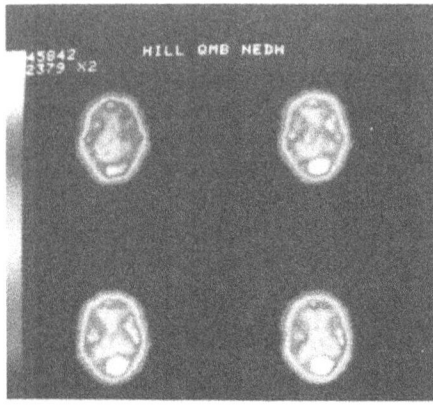 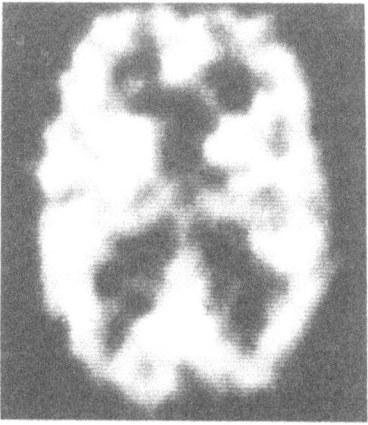

FIGURE 2A Rotating head SPECT transverse slice fails to delineate the same anatomic detail that the multidetector image shows.

FIGURE 2B Multidetector transverse slice demonstrates an increased concentration of the compound in the receptor rich basal ganglia.

With new technetium lipophilic radiotracers that have a shorter resonance time with the brain, faster scan times may prove even more important. Fig. 3 is an animal study with a multidetector system of bat cyclohexane showing uptake within the brain without cortical gray and white matter differentiation. In a study performed with the same compound on a rotating gamma camera, however, the limited sensitivity hampers the image quality to an even greater extent.

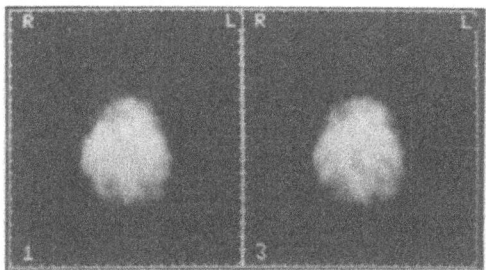

FIGURE 3 Monkey study obtained with a Tc^{99m} labeled BAT cyclohexane. Longer retention is seen with this analog but how much redistribution between grey and white matter is unknown. Slice on left is data collected from approximately 13 min-32 min; slice on right is data collected from approximately 43-60 min.

CONCLUSION

Although the rotating gamma camera appears to be able to do tomography of brain studies, its strenghts will be its wide availability and its multipurpose design that will allow general nuclear medicine departments to get acquainted with SPECT imaging. Its lower sensitivity and poor resolution may limit its usefulness to nonquantitative assessment. A dedicated multidetector system for brain study is clearly needed to exploit the newer radiopharmaceuticals that can show regional receptor concentration and its faster scan time may be needed for the newer technetium lipophilic brain agents. In view of the rapid growth of neuronuclear medicine, dedicated brain systems could be justified at the present time by many larger nuclear medicine departments.

REFERENCES

1. Radon, J. "On the determination of function from their integrals along certain manifolds." Ben Saechs, Akod WSS Leyszeg, Mat. Phys., K.I. 69 (1917), 262-277.

2. Shepp, L., and Logan, B.F. "Fourier reconstruction of a head section." IEEE Trans. Nucl. Sci. NS-21 (1974), 21-43.
3. Zimmerman, R.E., Kirsh, C.M., Lovett R., and Hill, T.C. "Single photon emission computed tomography with short focal length detectors." In: <u>Single Photon Emission Computed Tomography and Other Selected Computer Topics</u>. Society of Nuclear Medicine (1980), 148-157.
4. Gullberg, G.T. "The attenuated radon transform: Theory and application in medicine and biology." Doctoral dissertation, University of California, Berkeley, (1979).
5. Hill, T.C., Lovett, R.D., Zimmerman, R.E. "Quantification of Tc-99m glucoheptonate uptake in brain lesions with emission-computed tomography." In: <u>Single Photon Emission Computed Tomography and Other Selected Computer Topics</u>. Society of Nuclear Medicine, (1980), 169-176.
6. Hill, T.C., Holman, B.L., Lovett, R, et al. "Initial experience with SPECT (Single-Photon Computerized Tomography) of the brain using N-isopropyl I-123 p-iodoamphetamine." Concise communication. J Nucl Med, 23 (1982), 191-195.
7. Keyes, J.W., Jr. "Instrumentation." In: <u>Computed Emission Tomography</u>, edited by P.J. Eli and B.L. Holman, Oxford University Press, Oxford. (1982), 243-262.

DISCUSSION SUMMARY

PANEL ON
STATE-OF-THE-ART AND FUTURE TRENDS IN SINGLE PHOTON TOMOGRAPHY

Several comments were made by the participants in the session. Derenzo considered that in PET of the chest, the attenuation is carefully measured and incorporated into the tomographic reconstruction of the activity distribution. Consequently, if SPECT of the chest is to develop into a quantitative technique, it should be necessary to be able to measure the attenuation and use this information in the reconstruction. In the method of laminar compton scatter imaging described by R. Guzzardi, as the beam is attenuated along its length, the 90° scattering depends on electron density at a well-defined point, and the scattered photons must escape the patient before they can be detected. Then he asked if it was necessary to perform a non-trivial computer fit to all the data to simultaneously determine the spatial distribution of attenuation coefficients. Having great difficulties in trying to estimate the value of µ for constant attenuation problems such as the attenuation of Tc99m photons in water, Todd Pokropek noticed that the basic physical model was poorly represented in such systems.

Van Oortmarssen considered that the Chang attenuation correction technique does not require a constant µ. One possible solution is, as has been used in positrons, to fit a model, using information such as obtained by transmission, or by the method suggested by Guzzardi, to estimate µ from knowledge of the system, for example after a Monte Carlo model, and to use such noiseless values of µ in the attenuation correction. Another method is to estimate µ as part of the reconstruction technique.

Guzzardi clarified that the accuracy in estimate of attenuation coefficients, using both transmission and scattering methods, was 10% and that photons scattered at 90° from frontal section of the chest were used.

Van Oortmarssen noticed that, before back projection, one has to convolve the acquired data in order to avoid blurring of the reconstructed images. He showed four convolution kernels. Fusco asked why he chose just four filters. The answer was that although he mentioned only four filters in his talk, a fifth one was recently added, namely a Shepp-Logan with a cut-off at 0.75 of the Nyquist frequence, and these five filters would adequately cover all the clinical requirements. The artifacts generated by such measures have been evaluated, and in particular how the reconstructed slices were affected by using, as kernel, a special set of numbers, representing the real values that the ideal convolution takes at given points. In addition, Van Oortmarssen evaluated how his reconstructed slices were affected by back projecting the modified projected data, which can assume negative values and thus give a negative result. Then Fusco asked how the reconstructed data had been handled, in order to save regional relative density distributions and to avoid overflow or underflow errors. Finally, it was considered how much the Siemens system would have been improved by using 32 bits, instead of 16 bits. The effects that are possibly created by these filters have been evaluated and it was concluded that in all clinical requirements an appropriate filter can be chosen to minimize these artifacts and to produce very acceptable images. Any negative values that occur during the reconstruction are considered in the calculation. However, when the final value is a negative, the number is set to zero. Overflow and underflow problems have been overcome by using a sufficiently deep memory of 16 bits in addition to careful up/down scaling whenever required or useful. If a 32 bit processor would have been used rather than a 16 bit system, the overall operating system may have been more flexible and faster. However, as the reconstruction and filtering is done in a separate array processor, the advantage would have been minimal. Todd Pokropek stated that it is really unfair to compare the Cleon system with a rotating gamma camera using a medium energy collimator. It may well be that there has been the necessity of using a medium energy collimator since there might have been high energy contaminants in I-123. However, the use of the medium energy collimator has been disregarded, since it <u>destroyed</u> image quality in the tests performed. A general problem with such comparison is that one is not entitled to compare 'state of the art' of one system with the 'garbage' on another system. In general, if the same quality of image is obtained with a medium energy collimator and a low energy hi-resolution collimator, the imaging system should be suspected. T. Hill replied that although many of the images taken with IMP were performed on the Siemen's 3700 the system needed a medium energy collimator because of the high energy contaminants in I-123, and the images shown from the General Electric 400T system were performed with their LEAP collimator. In addition, the images of the distribution of I-123 labeled QNB were made with P5N I-123 and a LEAP collimator on the Siemens' system. In those images the activity within the basal nuclei, particularly the caudate nucleus, was not evident on the rotating gamma camera and was well identified with the dedicated multi-detector system. Since the deep structures are important to identify the muscarinic acetylcholine receptors, it was concluded that these dedicated systems would be necessary to fully exploit these radio pharmaceuticals.The image quality from studies performed with medium energy and LEAP collimators are different as they are performed with a dedicated neuro-SPECT system. However, with filtering and volumetric smoothing, images obtained at coarse resolution can be made to appear aesthetically pleasing.From the panel presentations and subsequent discussion the following points have been presented:

1) SPECT is still an emerging technology that has made significant progress in the past two years but has some remaining problems before confidence in its ability to provide accurate quantitative
measures of regional radioactivity or artifact-free images will be realized. In particular, we need to pay still more attention to the matter of attenuation.
2) Better performance specifications need to be developed for intersystem comparison. These specifications need to take into account the form of the reciprocal relation between resolution and sensitivity as well as other measures such as signal-to-noise, etc. In addition, standardized phantoms should be adopted and some representation of distribution in vivo developed.
3) Advances in radiochemistry and radiopharmaceutical chemistry need to be made concomitant with those in physics and engineering. For example, it is inappropriate to compare systems using iodine-123 contaminated by varying and relatively large quantities of iodine-124. The most promising approaches would seem to be through receptor-avid agents: hormones, drugs, immunoglobulins as well as metabolites and their analogues. The development of labeled substances with the same or similar specificities and affinities as the parent molecules is the real challenge.

POSTER SESSION

EVALUATION OF THE COMPUTER ARTIFACTS
GENERATED IN SPECT RECONSTRUCTION

U. BIADER CEIPIDOR, F. FUSCO and E. MUCIACCIA
Medical Systems Division - EURO-BIT   Rome,Italy

M. A. MACRI'
Department of Neurological Science - University of Rome, Italy

ABSTRACT

Reconstructed images in single-photon emission computer tomography (SPECT) always differ in some way from the original unavailable objects.
Many different factors affect such integrity (i.e. collimation, sampling, filtering, scattering, attenuation, etc.).
In this work a new approach to selecting the artifacts generated by a computer program is presented. Simulated SPECT projection data were made up in order to detect only the degradations in reconstructed slices due to specific computer implementation of filtered backprojection algorithms in the IDRA system.
Some calculations on picture characteristics are described, showing in a qualitative manner the difference, that is the error, between the original model and the computed model.
The results can provide a valid guide for better programming. In addition, a new image correction method is proposed.

1. INTRODUCTION

In the last few years SPECT has been receiving increased interest with regard to the clinical practice of nuclear medicine, particularly for cerebral blood flow and perfusion studies (1) due to improved computer capabilities.
Extensive research on different physical aspects of SPECT has been conducted (2)(3). However, studies on the causes of loss of spatial resolution are presently carried out using synthetic phantoms (4).
Among the factors which affect reconstructed images the computer contribution has seldom been taken into proper account.

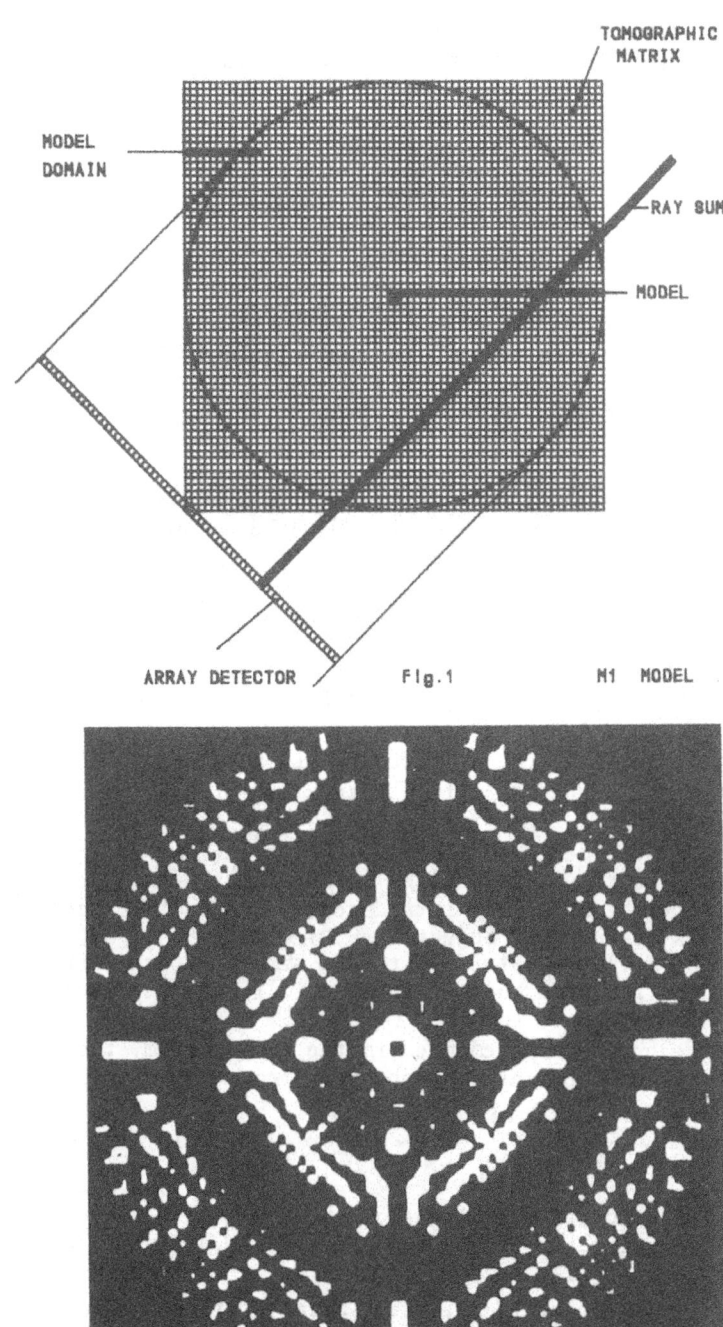

Fig. 2   M1 model reconstruction

In this work we show how one can select and evaluate such errors. In addition a method to correct reconstructed slices is proposed.

2. TOOLS AND METHODS

For our purpose we used a computer simulation of acquired phantom projections.
Some definitions are given below.
A "mathematical model", or simply a model, is a matrix $M=(m(i,j))$ for $i,j=1,64$ with non zero elements only for i,j such that set $y=S-i$ and $x=j-S$, where $S=33$ for $1 \leq i,j \leq 32$ or $S=32$ otherwise, is:

$$x^2 + y^2 = 32^2 + 2 = 1026 \qquad (1)$$

An example of a model is
$M1=(m1(i,j))$ with $m1(i,j)=10000$ for $32 \leq i,j \leq 33$ (fig.1)
A "projection procedure" is an operator $P\sim$ that, given M, generates a projection matrix $P=(p(k,m))$ with

$$p(k,m) = \sum_{ij} c(k,m,i,j) * m(i,j) \qquad (2)$$

where $c(k,m,i,j)$ is the weighting factor for pixel i,j in the k-th pixel of the m-th projection.
A "simple reconstruction procedure" is an operator $R\sim$ that, given P, generates a reconstruction matrix $R=(r(i,j))$ for $i,j=1,64$.
A "reconstruction procedure of order n (n>0)" is the application n times of the ordered sequence $(P\sim,R\sim)$ to matrix M.
The final matrix is called the n-th reconstruction of M.
Applying the terminology introduced by Herman (5), the matrix M defines a discrete 3D object $V=(S,D)$ with $d(i,j,1)=m(i,j)$ and then a phantom F. The P matrix is thus a simulated acquisition of the phantom F, ignoring most of the physical factors which affect reconstruction.
Using the program implemented in the IDRA system, the first and the second reconstructions were obtained from each P matrix.

3. RESULTS

The reconstructed image of the model M1 is shown in fig.2. The differences are due to the artifacts of the reconstruction program.
We note the star artifact, the ringing artifact, a radial asymmetry in background noise and a hole in the center.
Using the FWHM (3) we found that the spatial resolution loss ranges from 1.31 to 2.22.
Fortunately for "real" models, such non correlated artifacts are summed and the final result is acceptable (fig.3).

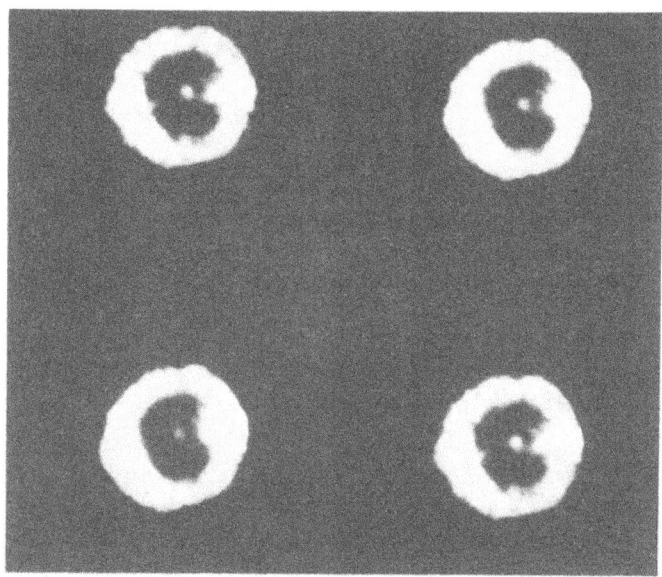

Fig. 3. Human head transverse section. Top: the section (left) and its first reconstruction. Bottom: the second reconstruction (left) and the section with different display parameters.

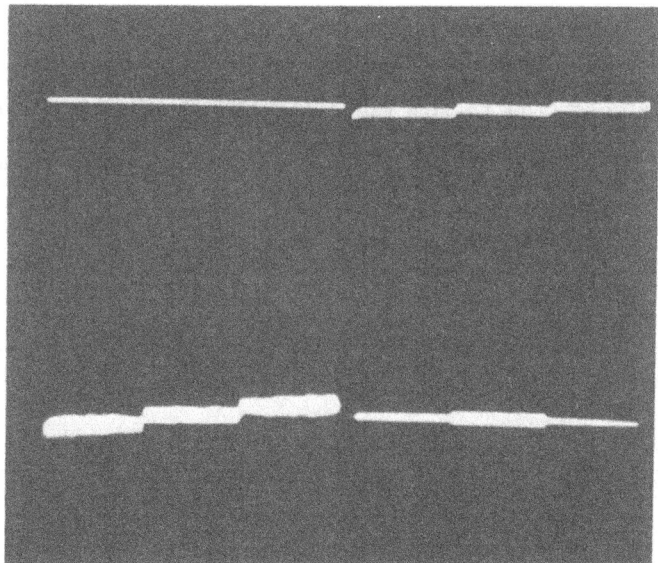

Fig. 4. A correction method example. Top: the model (left) and its first reconstruction. Bottom: the second reconstruction (left) and the corrected reconstructed model.

4. CORRECTION METHOD

We assume that the reconstruction program acts as an operator $T^\sim$ such that: $R = T^\sim (M)$.
We search for an operator $T^\sim$, expressed by a square matrix T, where

$$R = M * T \qquad (3)$$

Applying recursively the 3), with Ro=M, we can write

$$R_{n+1} = R_n * T_n \qquad (4)$$

If Ro is an unavailable object, the succession (Tn), defined by 4), has an unknown To. But if we set To=Tl, then it simply follows from the 4), denoting with R' the inverse of R, that:

$$\char`\^Ro = R_1 * R'_2 * R_1 \qquad (5)$$

By using the Ngan (6) "nmse" value as a measure of the distance between two pictures, we can define that: "^Ro is a corrected version of Rl if nmse(Ro,^Ro) ⟨nmse(Ro,Rl)". Unfortunately the application of 5) to different models does not always give a corrected matrix, so that the To=Tl hypothesis is not general.

5. CONCLUSION

The computer simulation approach described in this work represents a good tool for a reconstruction program test. In fact, removing most of the error sources allows program artifacts to be selected so that design flaws can be isolated. In our case we improved the weighting factor table and the overflow handling. Besides this, we presented a new method for reconstructed image correction. While this method is faster than iterative techniques, it does not always perform well. The determination of the optimal choice for succession (Tn) is under investigation.

REFERENCES

1. P. Gerundini, G. Lenzi, V. Di Piero, A. Savi, F. Triulzi, F. Fazio
   "Studio sulla perfus...", Elettromedicali, spec., pp. 46-50, 1984
2. S. A. Larsson
   "Gamma camera emission...", Acta Radiologica s.363, pp. 5-75, 1980
3. R. A. Brooks and G. Dichiro
   "Principles of computed...", Phy. Med. Biol. 21, pp. 689-732, 1976
4. M. Goiten
   "Three-dimensional density...", Nucl. Inst. Meth., pp. 509-518, 1972
5. G. T. Herman
   "Three dimensional...", Dig. Imag. Proc. in Med., pp. 93-118, 1981
6. K. N. Ngan
   "Image Display...", IEEE Tran. Acoust. Signal Proc., pp. 173-177, 1984

POSTER SESSION

LIMITED ANGLE SAMPLING IN SPECT

Knešaurek K.

Clinic of Nuclear Medicine and Oncology, "Dr. M. Stojanović" Clinical Hospital, Vinogradska 29, Zagreb, SR Croatia, Yugoslavia

The advantages of limited angle sampling in SPECT are a much shorter acquisition time and in some cases a better detectability of lesions. Limited angle sampling has mostly been 180° sampling in Tl-201 SPECT studies of the heart (1-3) but it has also been applied in liver and spleen studies (4). The aim of this work is to compare, on the same patient and same phantom data, 360° slices with those obtained from a limited number of projections (not covering full rotation).

The disadvantage of limited angle sampling in SPECT is that attenuation correction for such studies has not yet been developed and evaluated. Also in such studies it is not possible to average opposite views and in reconstructed images there is a geometrical distortion mainly due to a spatial resolution varying in accordance with the distance from the camera. The system used for tomography consisted of a large-field-of-view gamma camera (GE 400T) with a high-resolution low-energy parallelhole collimator. 64 different views over 360°, 20 sec each, providing sampling for every 5.6° of revolution of the detector, have been stored as 64x64 matrix each in a PDP 11/34 computer. Transverse sectional images have been reconstructed by means of their own software based on filtered backprojection algorithms. This software enables the start to be selected, as well as the last angle and thus makes it possible for all 64 views to be used simulating limited angle sampling in SPECT study with a desired first and last angle. The phantom used in our study consists of four rows each of four empty balls with a diameter of 2.5, 1.8, 1.1 and 0.8 cm placed in a solution of water and cca 100 MBq of ^{99m}Tc. The slices of this phantom are shown on fig. 1, 2, 3 and 4 for 360° sampling, 0°-180° sampling, 90°-270° and 135°-315° sampling, respectively. The object contrast image was better at 90°-270° and 135°-315° slices than at 360° slices. On fig. 5, 0°-180° and 360° slices of the lungs, obtained after i.v. injection of cca 800 MBq of ^{99m}Tc are shown. The geometrical distortion at a limited angle scan is visible. As a conclusion we may say that our comparison, which has been performed on the same patient or phantom data only, indicates that in some SPECT limited angle studies, particularly of the lungs, geometrical distortion can be significant and if a SPECT study is used for lesion sizing or determination of an actual volume, 360° slices should be used, though in some situations limited angle scans have better object contrast images.

1. Coleman, R.E., Jaszczak, R.J. and Cobb, F.R. Comparison of 180° 360° Data Collection in Thallium-201 Imaging Using SPECT. J.Nucl.Med. (1982) 23:655-660.
2. Tamaki, N., Mukai, T., Ishii, Y., et al. Comparative Study of Thallium Emission Myocardial Tomography with 180° and 360° Data Collection. J.Nucl.Med. (1982) 23:661-666.
3. Hoffman,E.J. 180° Compared with 360° Sampling in SPECT. J.Nucl.Med. (1982) 23:745-747.
4. Ott, R.J., Khan, O., Flower, M.A., Kabirai, T., Leach, M.O., Webb, S. and McCready, V.R. A Comparison Between 180° and 360° Data Reconstruction in SPECT of the Liver and Spleen. Eur.J.Nucl.Med. (1983) 8:A3.

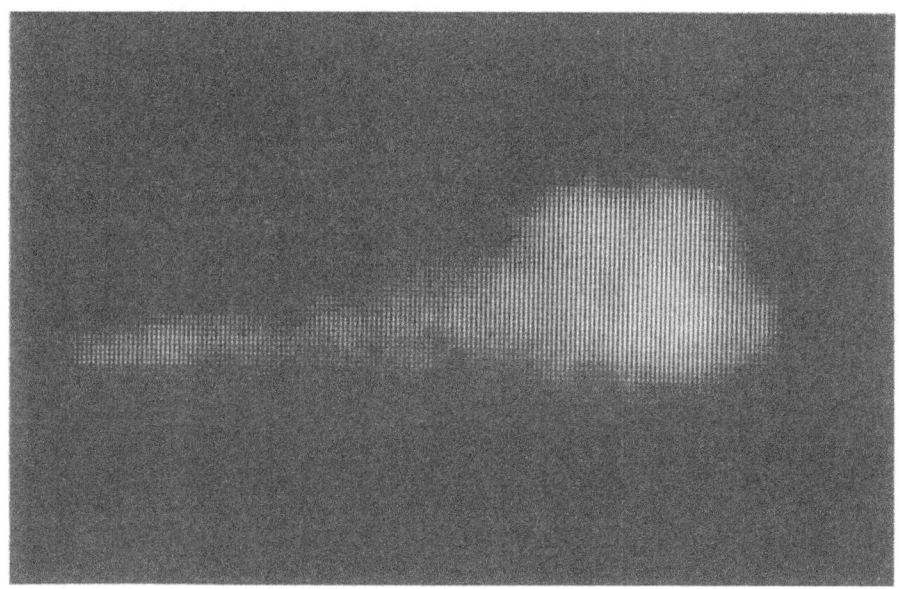

Fig. 1   360° slice of the phantom.

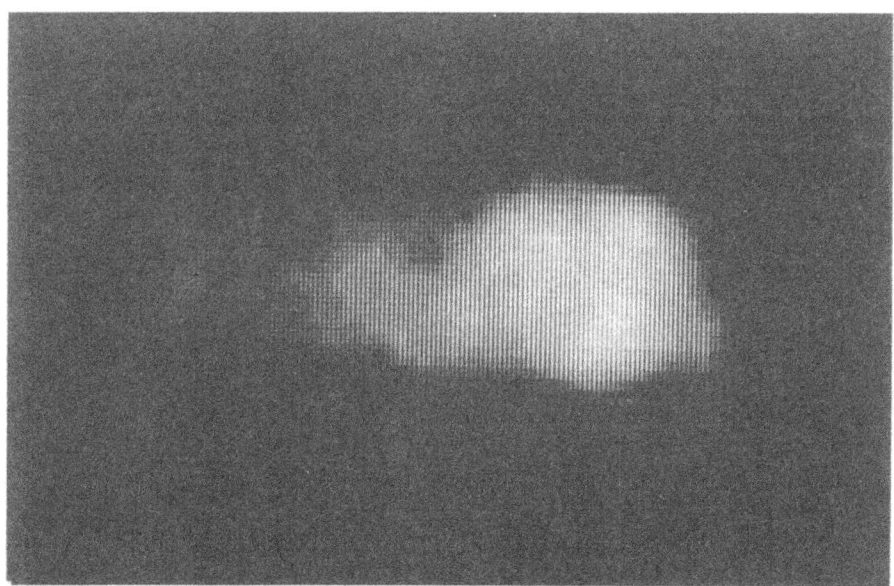

Fig. 2   0°-180° slice of the phantom.

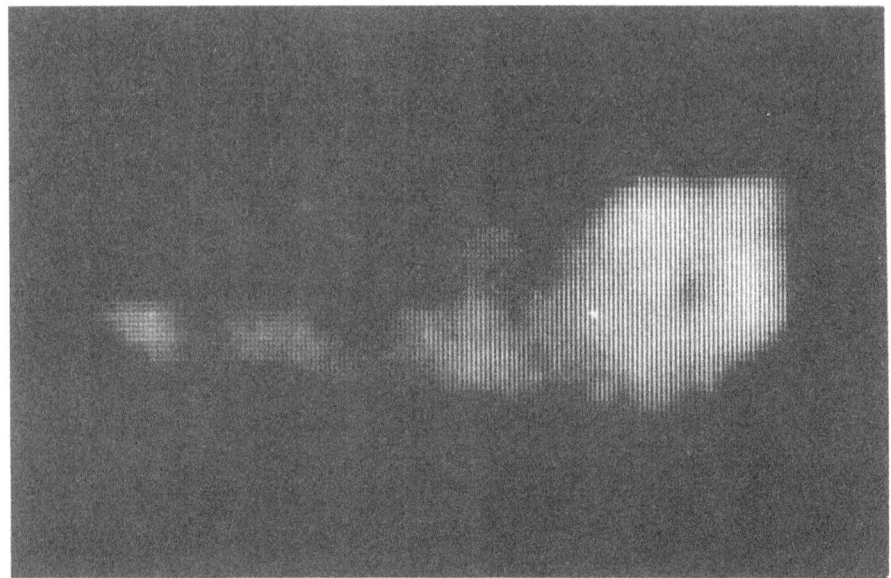

Fig. 3   9°-270° slice of the phantom.

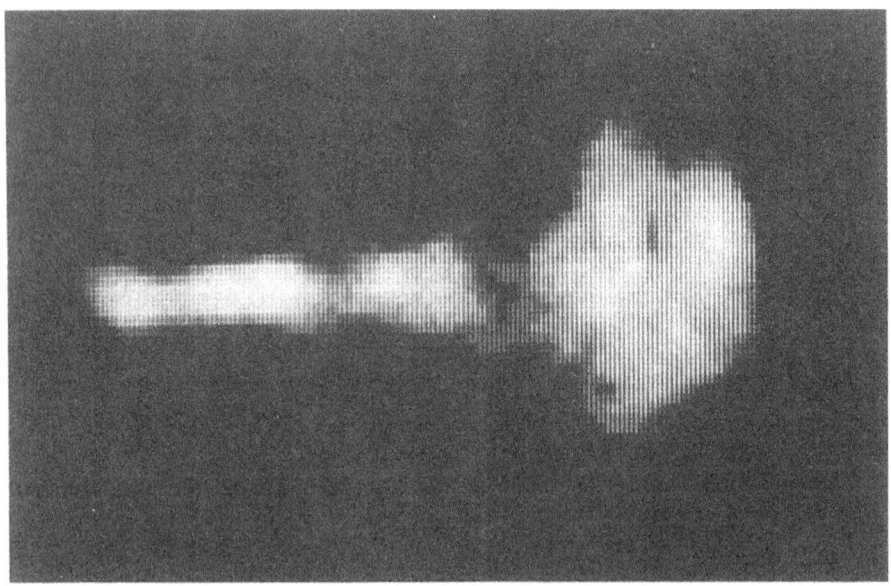

Fig. 4   135°-315° slice of the phantom.

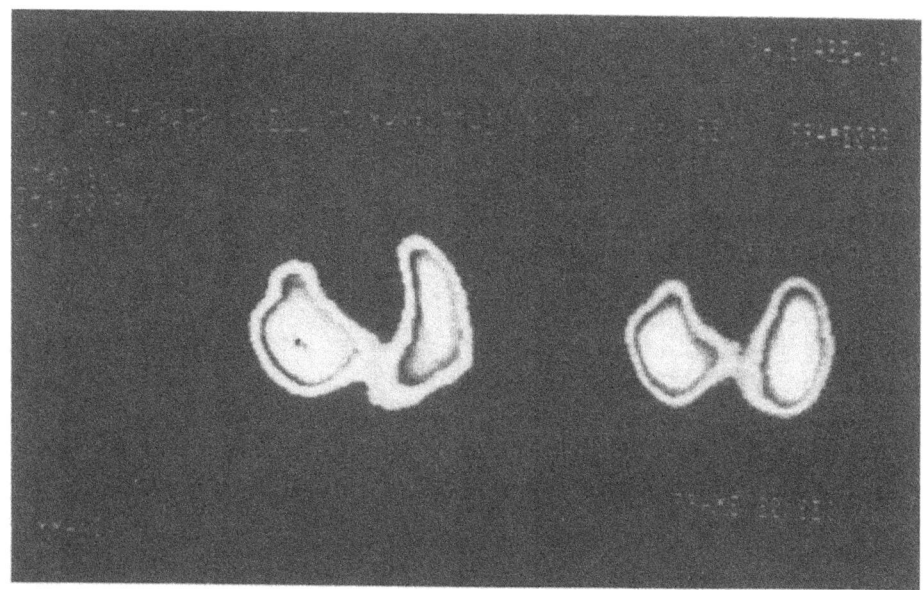

Fig. 5   0°-180° and 360° scan of the lungs.

POSTER SESSION

X-RAY TOMOGRAPHY VS COMPTON SCATTERING IN THE DIAGNOSIS OF PULMONARY DISEASES

Giuseppe Perri*, Barbara Fedeli*, Felicia Zito**, Maurizio Mey**, Riccardo Guzzardi**, Vincenzo Giordano*.

* Istituto di Radiologia dell'Università di Pisa, Italy
**Istituto di Fisiologia Clinica del C.N.R., Pisa, Italy

A comparative study in various pulmonary conditions has been carried out using the methodologies of X-Ray Tomography and Compton Scatter Imaging. This last technique is based on the detection of the photons scattered at 90° by the chest tissues, using a LFOV gamma camera. The radiation source is made up of a laminar beam of photons generated by a twin of 2Ci Ir-192 sources. (1, 2).

The images obtained by the gamma camera represent the density distribution of the irradiated chest section. Twenty patients have been examined with both techniques. Our aim was to assess the applicability and the advantages of Compton Tomography in studying various types of pulmonary involvement.

In short, this new approach allows:

1) to reproduce a selected layer eliminating completely any superimposing shadow. For example, in case of large tubercolomas, Compton Tomography is able to identify and to detect the morphology and the lesion size, at every scanning level, better than conventional X-Ray tomography.
2) to distinguish slight variations of density which are not recognized by chest X-ray or conventional tomography. For example, interlobar effusions poorly revealed by conventional tomography have been clearly identified by the Compton Tomography.

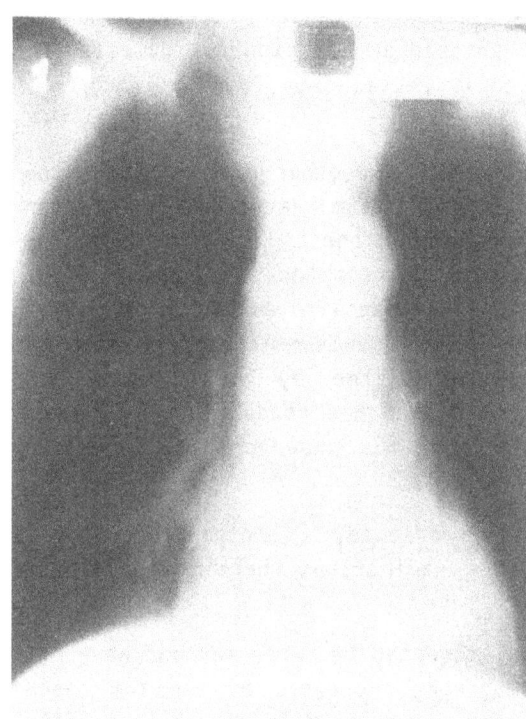

1a

Figs. 1a and 1b.
A pleural interlobar effusion of the right lobe, not detected by conventional X-ray tomography (1a) is clearly revealed by Compton Tomography (1b).

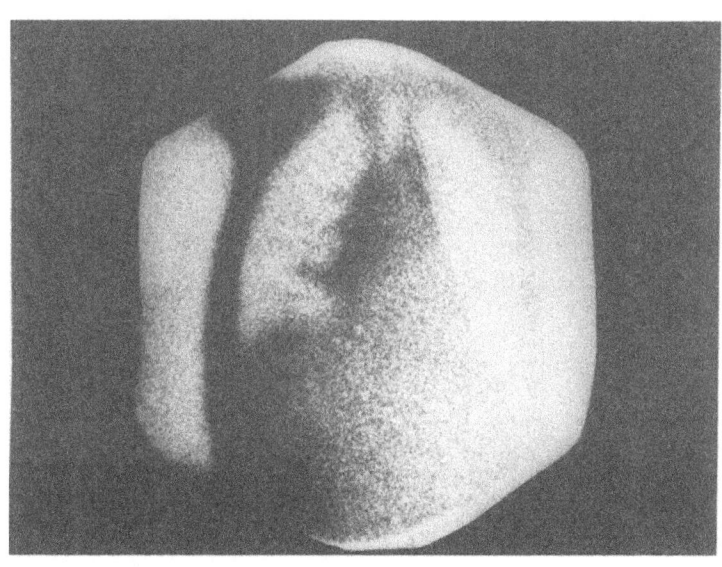

1b

Moreover, Compton Tomography results are more suitable than X-ray tomography in detecting slight increases of the pulmonary density. A case with pleural interlobar effusion not detected by X-ray tomography has been clearly revealed by Compton Tomography (Fig. 1).

These findings were confirmed by another case in which the density increase of the right hilum detected by Compton Tomography has only been revealed by chest X-ray three months later. Moreover, the application of Compton Tomography allows correlation of the hilar density increase with active pathological processes. In some cases the hilum involvement, appreciable by conventional X-ray tomography, was confirmed by Comptom Tomography. In other cases, this technique has revealed an increased density, while the X-ray tomography has shown only an irregular aspect of the hilum.

Judging from our clinical experience, Compton Tomography is not very suited to those chest examinations where the pulmonary density is highly reduced.

Cystic or cavity lesions, revealed by X-ray methods have not been detected by Compton Tomography. However, as for the cases with emphysema, the capability of detecting differences in density should, according to some authors (4), allow the air increase to be shown in relation to the normal pulmonary parenchima in those cases characterized by large lucent lesions.

Acknowledgements: The authors wish to thank Miss Laura Bulleri for her contribution to the preparation of this short paper.

REFERENCES

1) Guzzardi R., Zito M., Mey M.: Compton Tomographic Imaging: Design Aspects and Performance. Diagnostic Imaging in Medicine. (The Hague, Martinus Nijhoff Publishers, 1983 176-193).
2) Pistolesi M., Guzzardi R., Solfanelli S., Mey M., Giuntini C.: Regional Lung Density Imaging by 90° Scattering of External Gamma Camera Ray Source. Proceedings of San Diego Biomedical Symposium 1977, 16: 45-53.
3) Pistolesi M., Solfanelli S., Guzzardi R., Mey M., Giuntini C.: Chest Tomography by Gamma Camera and External Gamma Source. Concise comunication. J.Nucl. Med. 19: 94-97, 1978.
4) Pistolesi M., Miniati M., Solfanelli S., Guzzardi R., Mey M., Giuntini C.: Compton Scattering Tomography: Clinical Application in Various Lung Diseases. J. Nucl. Med. All. Sci. 1981, 25: 182.

POSTER SESSION

SEVEN PINHOLE TOMOGRAPHY OF THE HEART [1]

Max A. Viergever, John W. van Giessen

Department of Mathematics and Informatics
Delft University of Technology, The Netherlands

1. INTRODUCTION

Seven pinhole tomography was introduced as a method of myocardial perfusion imaging by Vogel and coworkers (10). It is a low-cost method because it only requires a simple collimator in addition to a conventional static gamma camera system. Yet seven pinhole imaging has not gained wide appreciation in nuclear cardiology practice. The limited angular sampling of the device was reported to be insufficient to produce images with a quality comparable to those obtained by full angle tomography (7). Also, positioning of the patient relative to the collimator has appeared to be critical for successful reconstructions.

The positioning problem can be reduced by first crudely localizing the heart with the aid of an echometer. A description of the procedure and the results is beyond the scope of this paper, however. We shall confine ourselves to discussing the limited angle problem. Our intention is to show that the quality of the myocardial images greatly depends on the reconstruction algorithm selected, and that the algorithm used so far in seven pinhole tomographic studies is suboptimal.

1. At the symposium, we presented a video registration of our research project on seven pinhole tomography of the heart (9). This article serves to give some of the background of the imaging system and the reconstruction method.

2. IMAGING SYSTEM

The collimator is a lead plate, located 127 mm from the camera crystal, with seven pinholes of 7 mm diameter. The centre of the central pinhole is situated on the optical axis of the system, see Fig. 1. This pinhole has a conical 53° field of view, perpendicular to the crystal face. The six peripheral pinholes are spaced evenly at 63.5 mm from the axis; they have a conical 45° field of view, converging inward at 26.5°. The seven pinhole collimator is used in combination with a wide-field Anger camera. Following intravenous injection of a suitable radionuclide (e.g. ^{201}Tl), this configuration records seven projected images of the radioactivity distribution in the myocardium and its surroundings. The projections are non-overlapping owing to lead septa placed between adjacent pinholes. The pencil-shaped volume simultaneously viewed by the projection sectors through the corresponding pinholes is the reconstruction volume. The camera should be positioned such that the heart falls entirely within this simultaneous field of view.

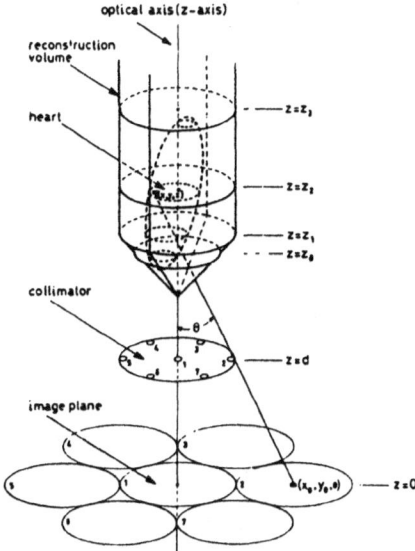

Fig. 1 Schematic representation of the imaging system and the reconstruction volume. Dimensions are given in the text. The division of the reconstruction volume into slices parallel to the detector face, which is characteristic of longitudinal tomography, is also outlined. For simplicity's sake we show here a division into three slices; in the computations eight slices are used.

3. RECONSTRUCTION PROBLEM

The problem to be solved is: given the seven two-dimensional projections and the geometry of the collimator/camera system, estimate the three-dimensional emission distribution of gamma radiation in the reconstruction volume.

The mathematical description of seven pinhole tomography has been derived in (8). The resulting formulation is a set of linear algebraic equations

$$Y = WX, \qquad (1)$$

where Y is a vector containing scaled pixel values, W is a binary-valued projection matrix, and X is a vector of scaled emission intensities of voxels (volume elements in the simultaneous field of view).

The system (1) is more than likely inconsistent owing to noise in the measurements and to simplifying assumptions made in the description of the imaging process. This means that the equations have no exact solution. Hence we introduce an error vector E by

$$E = Y - WX, \qquad (2)$$

and seek for an approximate solution which minimizes the error in some sense. A customary choice is to use the least squares minimum norm criterion, but other optimization criteria have also been applied; see (5) for a survey.

4. RECONSTRUCTION METHODS

The system matrix W is prohibitively large (8232 * 868 entries) for direct pseudo-inversion of Eq. (2) on a minicomputer. The matrix is also sparse, however, having only 2.6 per cent nonzero entries. Iterative techniques make essential use of this sparseness and are therefore more appropriate for seven pinhole tomography than direct methods.

We have compared three algorithms from the class of iterative techniques, viz. the Simultaneous Multiple Angle Reconstruction Technique (SMART) which has been proposed by the designers of the seven pinhole device (6), the Simultaneous Iterative Reconstruction Technique (SIRT) which was introduced by Gilbert (3), and a modified version of Herman's (4) ART3 algorithm which we named ART3H (the acronym ART stands for Algebraic Reconstruction Technique). A description of ART3H is given in (1).

The performance of reconstruction algorithms is highly dependent on the pre-reconstruction processing of the projection data and the postprocessing of the reconstructed intensity distributions. We refer to (2) for details, but mention one important post-reconstruction filter here. This filter, called FIZEVO (FInd ZEro VOxels), searches for all voxels seen by zero-valued pixels. If the intensities of some of these voxels are nonzero, they are set equal to zero except for the voxel with the highest intensity in the ray, the value of which is left unchanged (2).

5. RESULTS

Figure 2 presents reconstructions of a heart phantom with an infarct simulated by a piece of silicone rubber. The ART3H reconstruction is somewhat blurred by the presence of artefacts. Applying FIZEVO to the reconstruction results in a sharp picture, it clearly shows the place where the piece of rubber is positioned. The SIRT algorithm produces an unsharp reconstruction and even smears out the object outside the boundaries of the tomograms (Fig. 2C, slices 1 through 4). Here, FIZEVO is less benificial since it leads to a boundary degradation. The SMART reconstruction is nice and smooth but the resolution is somewhat less than in the ART3H + FIZEVO reconstruction. The effect of FIZEVO upon the SMART reconstruction is very small.

Table 1 gives an indication of the CPU-time needed for the reconstructions and the computer memory required by each algorithm. SIRT is obviously a slow algorithm, using approximately 10 times as much CPU-time as the other two algorithms. ART3H is computationally the fastest, but SMART is only slightly slower. The storage requirements for SIRT and SMART are practically the same. Art3H is the most friendly algorithm for computer storage of the three, using about twice less memory than the others.

Algorithm	CPU-time(s)	Storage (Kb)
ART3H	16	202
ART3H + FIZEVO	17	202
SIRT	175	372
SIRT + FIZEVO	176	372
SMART	19	387
SMART + FIZEVO	20	387

Table 1: CPU-times (HP1000F minicomputer) and storage requirements.

2) The more natural procedure of resetting to zero all voxels contributing to zero-valued pixels leads to severe degradation of the object boundaries.

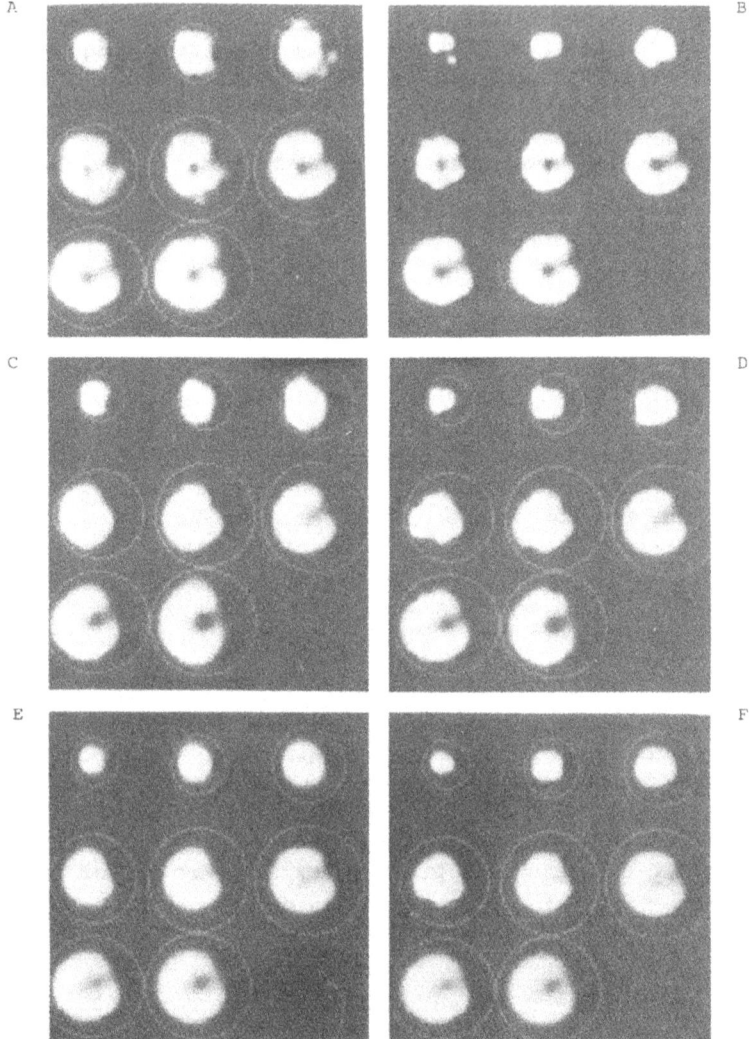

Fig. 2 Reconstructions of a heart phantom with an infarct, simulated by a piece of silicone rubber. The reconstructed tomograms are store from left to right and from top to bottom (the upper left slice is the nearest to the detector). The piece of rubber was positioned on the right hand side of the phantom and extended from the fourth sli through the eighth. A&C&E: reconstructions without FIZEVO (ART3H, SIRT and SMART respectively), B&D&F: as A&C&E with FIZEVO.

6. CONCLUSION

Based on the presented results, as well as on others (2), we conclude that ART3H + FIZEVO is the most suitable technique of reconstruction for seven pinhole imaging. The improved quality of the reconstructions renders it worth while to reconsider the use of seven pinhole tomography as a standard clinical technique for imaging the heart.

REFERENCES

1. Giessen, J.W. van, C.N. de Graaf, M.A. Viergever (1984a). Application of ART3 to seven pinhole tomography, Delft Progr. Rep. $\underline{9}$, 36-48.
2. Giessen, J.W. van, C.N. de Graaf, M.A. Viergever (1984b). Three algorithms for seven pinhole tomography, Delft Progr. Rep. $\underline{9}$, 212-224.
3. Gilbert, P. (1972). Iterative methods for the three-dimensional reconstruction of an object from projections, J. Theor. Biol. $\underline{36}$, 105-117.
4. Herman, G.T. (1975). A relaxation method for reconstructing objects from noisy X-rays, Math. Progr. $\underline{8}$, 1-19.
5. Herman, G.T. (1980). Image reconstruction from projections. The fundamentals of computerized tomography, Academic Press, New York.
6. LeFree, M.T., R.A. Vogel, D.L. Kirch, and P.P. Steele (1981). Seven pinhole tomography - A technical description, J. Nucl. Med. $\underline{22}$, 48-52.
7. Tamaki, N., T. Mukai, Y. Ishii, Y. Yonekura, H. Kambara, C. Kawai, and K. Torizuka (1981). Clinical evaluation of thallium-201 myocardial tomography using a rotating gamma camera: Comparison with seven-pinhole tomography, J. Nucl. Med. $\underline{22}$, 849-855.
8. Viergever, M.A., E. Vreugdenhil, J.W. van Giessen (1983). Mathematical description of seven pinhole tomography. Delft Progr. Rep. $\underline{8}$, 311-321.
9. Viergever, M.A., P.P. van Rijk, J.W. Wassink, N.P.G. Muyen (1984). Seven pinhole tomography of the heart - a work of ART (Video presentation). Audiovisual Centre, Delft University of Technology.
10. Vogel, R.A., D.L. Kirch, M.T. LeFree, and P.P. Steele (1978). A new method of multiplanar emission tomography using a seven pinhole collimator and an Anger scintillation camera, J. Nucl. Med. $\underline{19}$, 648-654.

Poster Session

SPECT COLLIMATION FOR MEDIUM-HIGH ENERGY: INFLUENCE OF SPATIAL
RESOLUTION AND IMAGE CONTRAST WITHIN TRANSVERSE PLANE

Laurence P. Clarke, Amilcare Gentili, Cheng B. Saw,
Peter Kenny, Aldo N. Serafini
University of Miami, Miami, Florida, USA.

1. INTRODUCTION

SPECT has a potentially important role in radioimmunotherapy, where the measurement of the fractional distribution of the labeled antibody in-vivo is required for absorbed dose calculation (1-3). Many of the radionuclides proposed are not ideal for

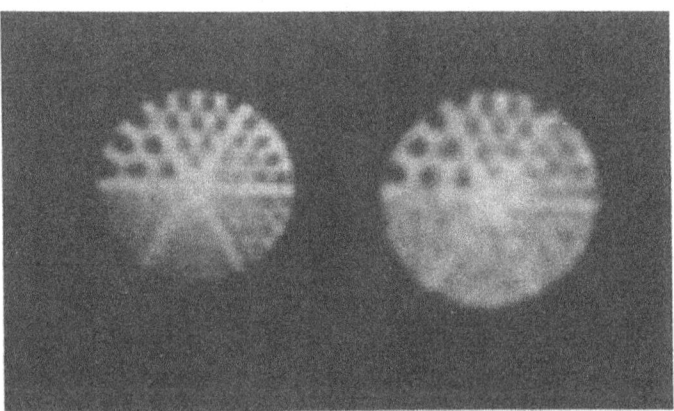

Fig. 1 SPECT phantom (Standard Model, Data Spectrum Corporation, USA). Left: LSMEC using I-131. Right: ultrafine collimator using Tc-99m. Two quadrants of rods 16 and 12.7 mm diameter were resolved in each case. None was resolved for the HSMEC using I-131

Collimator	Diameter	Length	Septa	Theoretical Leakage
HSMEC	3.8	50.8	1.35	<8% (364 keV)
LSMEC	3.4	68.3	1.39	<3% (364 keV)
LSHEC	4.8	102.0	3.3	<10% (511 keV)

Table 1. Collimators dimensions (mm) and leakage through septa.

imaging, since they have medium to high energies, such as I-131 (4) or Br-77. Photon penetration through the collimator degrades the spatial resolution (FWHM, FWTM) in the tomographic plane and slice thickness resolution, resulting in loss of image contrast. An evaluation of two collimators designed for I-131 was performed using a SPECT gamma camera system (Picker Dyna 5, 3/8 inch crystal): (a) a conventional high sensitivity medium energy collimator (HSMEC) employed for renal imaging and (b) a low sensitivity medium energy collimator (LSMEC) designed with thicker septa (table 1). Similar measurements were performed with a low sensitivity high energy collimator (LSHEC) using F-18.

2. RESULT

Table 2 shows a comparison of the line spread function (LSF) measurements performed using I-131. The spatial resolution, in particular the index FWTM was degraded for HSMEC. The planar and SPECT resolution (FWHM, FWTM) for the LSMEC using I-131

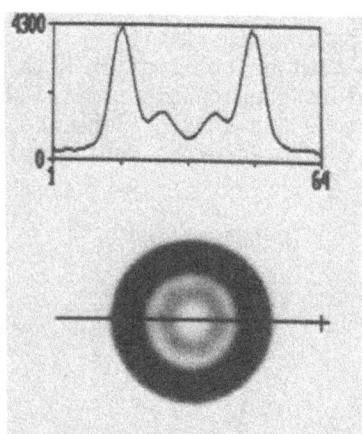 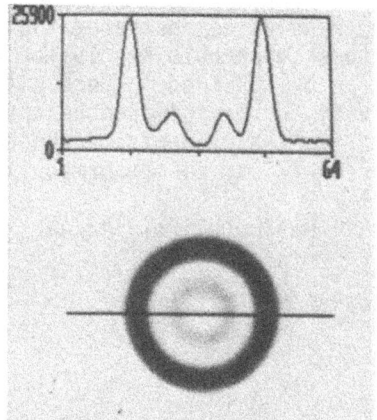

Fig. 2. Transverse images of Ring phantom using I-131. The phantom had four water filled rings (1-4) 5, 10, 15, and 20 cm diameter. Left: HSMEC. Right: LSMEC. The ratio of activity/ml in inner ring 2 to outer ring 4 (A2/A4) was 1:3. IC=(N4-N3)/N3: N4 and N3 are the maximum and mininum counts/pixel in ring 4 and 3.

	HSMEC (I-131)		LSMEC (I-131)		LSHEC (F-18)	
	FWHM	FWTM	FWHM	FWTM	FWHM	FWTM
PLANAR (10 cm)	20.1	48.6	13.3	25.1	14.1	34.4
SPECT Transverse (0 cm)	25.6	45.0	17.0	31.8	22.5	40.1
Sagittal (0 cm)	20.0	39.2	16.9	31.4	19.7	36.0

Table 2. LSF in air using I-131 or F-18.

was comparable to that observed for a ultrafine low energy collimato using Tc-99m (i.e. 15 mm FWHM). This result was further confirmed using a SPECT resolution phantom (fig. 1). The HSMEC resolution was very degraded, and no rods were observed using the SPECT phantom. Measurements performed using a concentric ring (contrast) phantom, shown in Fig. 2 and Table 3, demonstrate the loss of contrast with the HSMEC, partly attributed to septal penetration. The NEMA sensitivity for the HSMEC and LSMEC was 202 and 75 (cpm/µCi I-131) respectively. Comparable resolution was obtained using the LSMEC using F-18 (table 2) with NEMA sensitivity of 64 (cpm/µCi F-18).

3. CONCLUSION

The results demonstrated that using low sensitivity collimators comparable resolution to ultrafine collimation with Tc-99m can be obtained. These collimators should have sufficient sensitivity for radioimmunotherapy imaging and should allow accurate quantitative measurements of antibodies labeled with, for example, I-131 or Br-77, to be performed in vivo.

	Ratio (µCi/ml):A2/A4	IC=(N4-N3)/N3
HSMEC	0:1	3.21
	1:3	2.9
	1:1	1.1
LSMEC	0:1	16.7
	1:3	5.6
	1:1	4.4

Table 3. Image contrast (IC) obtained for I-131 from transverse images of ring phantom. A2 and A4 are the activity/ml in the inner ring 2 and outer ring 4 (Fig. 2).

4. REFERENCES

1. Jaszczak, R.G, Coleman, R.E. and Whitehead, F.R. Physical Factors affecting Quantitative Measurements using Gamma Camera based SPECT. IEEE Trans Nucl Sci NS-28 (1981), 69-78
2. Sfakianakis, G.N, F.H. Deland. Radioimmunodiagnosis and Radioimmunotherapy. J Nucl Med 23(1982), 706-714.
3. Berche, C, J.P. Mach, and J.D. Lambroso et al. Tomoscintigraphy for Detecting Gastrointestinal and Medullary Thyroid Cancer. Br Med J 285(1982) 1447-1451.
4. Clarke, L.P, J.F. Malone, and M. Casey. Quantitative Measurement of Activity of Small Sources Containing Medium Energy Radionuclides. Br J Radiology 55(1982), 125-133.

PART XII POSITRON EMITTERS RADIONUCLIDES, RADIOCHEMISTRY AND BIOTRACERS

Chairman: Alfred P. Wolf (U.S.A.)

CYCLOTRONS AND POSITRON EMITTING RADIOPHARMACEUTICALS

Alfred P. Wolf and Joanna S. Fowler

Chemistry Department, Brookhaven National Laboratory, Upton, NY

INTRODUCTION

Positron Emission Tomography is at the present time in a growth phase with an increasing number of clinical facilities showing interest in the use of PET in routine practice. The consequences of this fact, not only for the technology of PET but also for cyclotron application and radiopharmaceutical production, necessitate a review of what is possible given today's state-of-the-art.

We are now approaching the end of the first decade in which we witnessed the maturing of the three essential components of the PET methodology: radiotracers, positron emission tomographs and tracer kinetic models. As a result, from 1976 to the present, the number of centers acquiring the instrumentation and core team of scientists applying PET to problems in the health sciences has grown exponentially. In the U.S. in 1979, the National Institutes of Health funded the establishment of several regional centers and embarked on a large PET program of its own. All of this was based on the assumption that PET would be able to test a number of important scientific hypotheses in the living human body, that it will provide the means of quantitatively describing disease as well as normal function at the molecular level, and that its use would provide guidance in disease therapy. That PET is already making a contribution in choosing the treatment of certain disease (for example epilepsy, stroke, heart disease) has been recently recognized by the establishment of clinical centers. However, the success of PET as a scientific tool requires not only that investigators proceed beyond the instant gratification provided by a color image but address more difficult issues such as instrument limitations and biochemical and physiological significance of PET measurements. It follows that they use PET to address significant scientific questions.

Basic biomedical research with PET requires a broadly based research team and flexibility in radiotracer production as the demands and interests of the research group changes. This may not be the case in a purely clinical facility where the spectrum of probes is more restricted and depends almost entirely on what are proven compounds with general utility. So, for example, a clinical facility based on using the labeled oxygen moieties O_2, H_2O, CO, and CO_2, labeled deoxyglucose and perhaps a labeled neuroleptic could operate at a limited level with a cyclotron delivering its particles to "black boxes" (a device which is connected directly to the cyclotron target and which can purify a labeled gas or prepare a labeled compound by automated synthesis), and then delivering the needed labeled tracer to a gas bag, or into a gas delivery line or into a multi-injection vial. Such a facility could be operated by technical personnel. It should also be clear under such conditions that the user would be dependent on the manufacturer as a source of "black boxes" for any new useful tracer that might appear. Sufficient flexibility to carry out new synthesis and development in an independent manner bespeaks of a much larger cadre of professionals with a suitable infrastructure.

It is the purpose of this paper to focus on aspects of cyclotron and labeled tracer preparation in light of what is possible today. The references in this paper are not intended to be comprehensive. However, source material and further literature references can be found in these papers. Two books (1,2) have recently been published on positron emission tomography which contain a wealth of material on all aspects of the subject including the subjects addressed in this paper.

Cyclotrons and Radionuclide Production

The cyclotrons currently available are listed in Table I. At the present moment two more manufacturers (Meditron, The Eindhoven, The Netherlands and Shimadzu Co., Japan) are considering supplying machines of the type listed in Table I, however, no concrete plans have as yet been announced, nor is their technical data available.

An elementary description of the technical aspects of cyclotrons is available (3).

Table I
Small Cyclotrons

	Protons, MeV	Deuterons, MeV	Current, μA
JSWBC168	16	8	50
JSWBC1710	17	10	50
MC 16F	17	8.5	50
CGR MeV SUM 325	15	8	50
CGR MeV SUM 370	17	10	50
CTI	11	None	50

JSW - Japan Steel Works, Japan
MC - Scanditronix, Sweden
CGR - CGR Sumitomo, France and Japan
CTI - Computer Technology and Imaging, USA

Two choices can be made with regard to machine type, two particle, i.e. protons and deuterons and one particle proton only. Parenthetically it is worth noting that the earliest machines used <u>full time</u> for medical purposes, those at Hammersmith Hospital, London, Massachusetts General Hospital, Boston, and Washington University, St. Louis were either deuteron only machines or in the case of the Hammersmith machine, deuterons and alpha particles. While a great deal of pioneering work was done with these machines, it became evident that flexibility in research and application required a two particle machine, i.e. protons and deuterons. There are approximately 25 machines of the type listed in Table I in use today. A current listing of cyclotron PET facilities can be found in reference (4). At this writing, the single particle 11 MeV proton only machine has as yet to be installed and tested for general efficacy in a biomedical program. A proton only machine requires the use of enriched stable isotopes for the production of nitrogen-13, oxygen-15 and fluorine-18.

Table II
Positron Emitter Production Reactions Using a Small Cyclotron (p,d)

	Proton Reactions		Deuteron Reactions
Carbon-11	$^{14}N(p,\alpha)^{11}C$	$^{11}B(p,n)^{11}C$	$^{10}B(d,n)^{11}C$
Nitrogen-13	$^{13}C(p,n)^{13}N$	$^{16}O(p,\alpha)^{13}N$	$^{12}C(d,n)^{13}N$
Oxygen-15	$^{15}N(p,n)^{15}O$		$^{14}N(d,n)^{15}O$
Fluorine-18	$^{18}O(p,n)^{18}F$		$^{20}Ne(d,\alpha)^{18}F$

The nuclear reactions which are used to produce the four positron emitters (^{11}C, ^{13}N, ^{15}O, ^{18}F) accounting for over 95% of research with PET today, are listed in Table II. Other useful positron emitters such as gallium-68, bromine-75, strontium-82, and iodine-122 are not covered here since they cannot be effectively prepared using machines of the type listed in Table I.

Let us consider what production levels are possible using these small machines. In order that yield estimates can be made, accurate excitation functions needed to be determined experimentally as a first step in deciding whether or not a particular nuclear reaction were of practical use. Functions for carbon-11 (5) via $^{14}N(p,\alpha)^{11}C$, oxygen-15 (6,7,8) via $^{14}N(d,n)^{15}O$, and $^{15}N(p,n)^{15}O$ and fluorine-18 (9,10,11) via $^{18}O(p,n)^{18}F$ and $^{20}Ne(d,a)^{18}F$ have been published. These references (5-11) give tables or graphs giving thick target saturation yields as a function of particle energy on target. Data from these papers is presented in Tables III-VIII in condensed form and relative only to machines listed in Table I in order to provide a sampling of what practical yields are obtainable, given the energies available. Clearly a "practical yield" is arbitrarily chosen. The choice is based on the minimum time of beam-on-target which provides sufficient radioisotope to effect a synthesis of a needed labeled tracer. Because of its short half-life, carbon-11 production can approach the saturation yield if one bombards for longer than one hour. Twenty microamps was chosen as the beam current since in our experience not a great deal is to be gained by higher beam currents due to the gas density reduction problem (vide infra) which is exacerbated at higher beam currents. It is of course possible with altered target design and a change in beam cross section etc. to go to higher beam currents. Such targets remain to be described in the literature. However, considering what is known and available today, currents between 15 and 30 μA depending on target type are optimal for <u>production runs</u>. A word of caution must be introduced with regard to the last column of the tables. The assumption is made that 100% of the beam hits the target and negligible wall loss occurs due to beam spread. Thus the data should only be used as a guideline since it ignores the aforestated and other possible perturbations. Tables IV and V give typical results for oxygen-15 production via the $^{15}N(p,n)^{15}O$ and $^{14}N(d,n)^{15}O$ reactions. Note that a flowing target using $^{15}N-N_2$ as the target gas is not practical because of the high cost of the stable isotope (cf. Table X). Fluorine-18 is available via the $^{18}O(p,n)^{18}F$ and $^{20}Ne(d,\alpha)^{18}F$ reactions. Here it is impractical to bombard to

Table III
Carbon-11 Yields

$^{14}N_2$ Target		$^{14}N(p,\alpha)^{11}C$		Threshold 2.9 MeV
		$t_{1/2}$ = 20.4 Min		

Energy on Target MeV	Saturation Yield mCi/μA	Yield at 20 μA mCi	Yield at 20 μA 20 Min	Practical Yield $^{11}C(75\%)$
17	184	3680	1840	1380
16	172	3440	1720	1290
15	154	3080	1540	1155
14	135	2700	1350	1012
13	115	2300	1150	862
12	94	1880	940	705
11	77	1540	720	540
10	62	1240	620	465
9	49	980	490	367
8	38	760	380	285
7	22	440	220	165
6	5	100	50	37

Table IV
Oxygen-15

$^{15}N_2$ Target		$^{15}N(p,n)^{15}O$	Threshold 3.5 MeV
	$t_{1/2} = 2.1$ min		
Energy on Target MeV	Saturation Yield mCi/μA	Yield at 20 μA mCi	Practical Yield 20 μA mCi
17	172	3440	1720
16	156	3120	1560
15	140	2800	1400
14	123	2460	1230
13	105	2100	1050
12	86	1720	860
11*	70	1400	700
10	60	1200	600
9	52	1040	520
8	43	860	430
7	29	580	290
6	13	260	130

* A static target with a 0.5 mil foil window will allow ~ 10.7 MeV on target. A thick target assuming no gas density reduction (i.e. 10.7 MeV to 3.5 MeV and requiring a target thickness of 133 mg/cm^3) requires about 580 cc at 20°C for a 2.54 cm internal diameter target.

Table V
Oxygen-15

$^{14}N_2$ Target		$^{14}N(d,n)^{15}O$		Threshold 0
	$t_{1/2} = 2.1$ Min			
Energy on Target MeV	Saturation Yield mCi/μA	Yield 20 μA mCi	Practical Yield 20 μA mCi	1 Min Residence Flowing Target 20 μA
10	88	1760	880	440
9	77	1540	770	385
8	65	1300	650	325
7	53	1060	530	265
6	40	800	400	200

Table VI
Fluorine-18

$^{18}O_2$ Target		$^{18}O(p,n)^{18}F$		Threshold 2.4 MeV
		$t_{1/2}$ = 109.7 min		
Energy on Target MeV	Saturation Yield mCi/µA	Yield at 20 µA mCi	Yield at 20 µA 2 hr	Practical Yield ^{18}F 50%
17	243	4860	2430	1215
16	236	4720	2360	1180
15	226	4520	2260	1130
14	216	4320	2160	1080
11	167	3340	1670	835
10	147	2940	1470	735
9	129	2580	1290	645
8	110	2200	1100	550
7	89	1780	890	445
6	59	1180	590	295

Table VII
Fluorine-18 Via $H_2^{18}O$

$H_2^{18}O$ Target		$^{18}O(p,n)^{18}F$		Threshold 2.4 MeV
		$t_{1/2}$ = 109.7 min		
Energy on Target MeV	Saturation Yield mCi/µA	Yield at 20 µA mCi	Yield at 20 µA 2 hr	Practical Yield ^{18}F 50%
16	184	3680	1840	920
15	176	3520	1760	880
14	168	3360	1680	840
13	159	3180	1090	545
11	130	2600	1300	650
10	115	2300	1150	575
9	101	2020	1010	505
8	86	1720	860	430

near saturation since it would require a beam-on time in excess of 8-10 hrs. In our experience, 1.5 to 2 hrs is optimal although for water targets 1 hr is usually sufficient. The $^{18}O(p,n)^{18}F$ reaction is particularly well suited for the preparation of ^{18}F fluoride ion and the $^{20}Ne(d,\alpha)^{18}F$, Table VIII, is useful for the preparation of $^{18}F\text{-}F_2$. Both targets are simple in construction and use, delivering the needed radionuclide directly at end of bombardment. Problems involving these targets are addressed in the literature (cf. ref 1 and references therein). It should always be kept in mind when considering tables of this sort that windows are required on gas and liquid targets. Thus the maximum energy of any machine is not what is available on target. Examples of how target window thickness affects beam energy on target (energy out) is given in Table IX. Havar, a typical window material, is used as an example. For some liquid and atmospheric pressure gas targets windows as thin as 0.0006 cm can be used. However, with enriched isotopes perhaps 0.00122 cm is the best minimum thickness. When using pressurized targets, thicknesses of 0.00254 cm or greater may be required.

The art of target design and optimization of yield taking all factors into consideration, e.g. cost and complexity of target body, bombardment time necessary in light of quantity of final product required, complexity of chemistry leading to precursor, cost of target material and target material purity (cf. reference 20), and level of expertise needed to produce the product, cannot be addressed in this paper. When considering proton only reactions, target cost cannot be neglected. A list

Table VIII
Fluorine-18

^{20}Ne Target		^{20}Ne(d,α)^{18}F		Threshold 0
		$t_{1/2}$ = 109.7 min		
Energy on Target MeV	Saturation Yield mCi/µA	Yield at 20 µA mCi	Yield at 20 µA 2 hr	Practical Yield ^{18}F 60%
10	69	1380	690	414
9	61	1220	610	366
8	51	1020	510	306
7	40	800	400	240
6	28	560	280	168

of current prices (in the U.S.A.) of enriched isotopes from commercial sources is given in Table X. Boron-11, which is useful for proton only machines, since the carbon-11 yield is higher for the $^{11}B(p,n)^{11}C$ reaction than for the $^{14}N(p,\alpha)^{11}C$ reaction at the same energy, is regrettably not readily available. The cost of a thick target for ^{13}N, ^{15}O and ^{18}F production given 10 MeV on target is given in Table XI. The cost of a water target can be cut to ~ $38.00 (0.5 g) however, even at this price recovery of target material is mandatory. This is readily appreciated given two or more production runs/day throughout the year. By way of comparison the cost of natural abundance nitrogen and neon as target gases is negligible and recovery of target is unnecessary.

One aspect of gases as targets is particularly worthy of mention here and that is the reduction of gas density as the particle beam strikes the gas. This problem, while widely addressed in the literature e.g. ref 12-19, is frequently overlooked when predictions of yield are based on what one measures in a thin target at 1 μA beam current or less. Yields cannot be estimated based on a thin or thick target yield at 1 μA by multiplying by beam current e.g. the 20 μA given in the yield table. Thus a "practical yield" is given where the reduction from theoretical is due to bombardment time, loss by density reduction and losses due to target chemistry. While thick targets can be devised, adjusting for the density reduction loss, pressure and volume are usually a limiting factor.

Table IX
Energy Loss in Havar[a] Target Windows

	Foil Thickness	Protons Energy In	Protons Energy Out	Deuterons Energy In	Deuterons Energy Out
A	0.00122 cm	17	16.8	10	9.5
	0.5 mil	16	15.8	8	7.5
		11	10.7	—	---
B	0.00254 cm	17	16.6	10	9.0
	1.0 mil	16	15.6	8	6.8
		11	10.4	—	---
C	0.0127 cm	17	15.0	10	5.4
	5.0 mil	16	13.9	8	1.3
		11	8.2	—	---

a. Havar composition Co 0.425, Cr 0.20, Fe 0.179, Ni 0.13, W 0.028, Mo 0.02, Mn 0.016

In passing from purely nuclear and physical parameters and the limitations of radionuclide production, one should then consider what is actually occurring in the target during bombardment and how the product radionuclide, whatever its form, is then converted to precursor for organic synthesis or in some cases how it is dealt with when delivered directly (e.g. as in the case of $^{15}O-O_2$ gas etc.). The synthesis of precursors has been reviewed (21) and general aspects of compound synthesis have

Table X
Cost of Stable Isotopes

	Form	Enrichment	1985 Price/g of Isotope
Carbon-13	$^{13}CO_2$	90%	$ 72.40–$89.40
		99%	$ 78.90–$97.50
	$Ba^{13}CO_3$	98+%	$108.00–$133.50
Nitrogen-15	$^{15}N_2$	98+%	$135.00–$166.90
Oxygen-18	$H_2^{18}O$	5–10%	$ 23.80–$29.40
Oxygen-18	$H_2^{18}O$	95%	$ 62.10–$76.80
Oxygen-18	$^{18}O_2$	95%	$118.80–$146.90
Neon-20	Ne	99.95%	$47.30/LITER
Neon	Ne	Nat. Abund.	$ 0.09/LITER
Boron-11	H_3BO_3	98+%	NA

Table XI
Target Cost 1985 (Approximate)

10 MeV Protons on Target

Target	Material	Weight	Isotope Cost
Carbon-13 (^{13}N)	Powder	16mg	$2
Nitrogen-15 (^{15}O)	Gas	680mg	$113
Oxygen-18 (^{18}F)	Gas	821mg	$120
	Water	1g	$77

[Deuterons; Neon (^{18}F) $^{14}N(^{13}N)$: Cost, Negligible]

been addressed (22, cf. also references 1 and 2). A book discussing all aspects of compound synthesis using carbon-11, fluorine-18 and nitrogen-13 has been published (23).

Radiopharmaceutical Development and Application

Progress and some of the pitfalls in the current development and application of radiotracers for PET emphasis on quantitative methods will be described in somewhat greater detail in what follows. Examples will include oxygen-15 tracers (for blood flow, oxygen utilization, and blood volume measurements), and radiotracers for glucose metabolism, neurotransmitter studies, and protein synthesis. The section will be concluded by a short description of some of the newer, developing radiotracers, some of which may provide the basis for the PET methods of the future.

Oxygen-15 Tracers: Oxygen-15 with its 2-minute half-life is readily available on-line in the chemical forms of $[^{15}O]O_2$, $H_2[^{15}O]$, $[^{15}O]CO_2$, $C[^{15}O]$ and $N_2[^{15}O]$. A number of these radiotracers are produced by commercially available black boxes and are therefore ideally suited for clinical application at a hospital based cyclotron. Although no wet chemistry is involved in converting $[^{15}O]O_2$ produced by the target into other radiotracers, quality control of these radiopharmaceuticals is required at frequent intervals to ensure that the black boxes are functioning properly and that radiochemical purity is maintained.

Tracer kinetic models for the use of the oxygen-15 tracers for the measurement of cerebral blood flow and oxygen utilization have been well validated (24-27) and these measurements are frequently used to determine the metabolic status of diseased tissue, for example, in stroke (28) and cerebral malignancy (29). In addition, the use of oxygen-15 has certain advantages in the study of somatosensory stimulation and cognitive tasks. For example, an oxygen-15 study requires only a few minutes of cognitive performance or of stimulation thereby reducing attentional deficits which may occur during longer periods of stimulation (30).

In addition to its use in the study of stroke, cerebral malignancy, PET and oxygen-15 tracers have also recently been applied to the study of regional cerebral blood flow in severe anxiety (31) and in newborn infants at risk (32,33).

Radiotracers and Issues in the Measurement of Brain Glucose Metabolism: The ^{18}FDG method (34) which was based on the ^{14}C-2DG autoradiographic method in animals (35) is now the most frequently used PET method at cyclotron-PET centers around the world. The most widely used method of synthesis is still via electrophilic fluorination using fluorination reagents derived from ^{18}F-labeled elemental fluorine, [^{18}F]F$_2$ (1, and references therein). However, the nucleophilic fluorination reactions (36) which lead to an isomerically pure product (37) in high yields and high specific activity have been described and are being used at an increasing number of institutions. In particular the increase of the reactivity of ^{18}F-fluoride using a crown ether is a noteworthy achievement which should increase the utility of fluoride in other radiotracers as well (38). This is an important development in the potential economical supply of ^{18}FDG from regional cyclotron-PET centers to user groups. ^{11}C-2DG is also being used and offers the possibility of making serial glucose metabolic measurements in a single subject at 2 hour time intervals (39). The frequently raised question of the lumped constant value in normal human brain for ^{11}C-2DG and ^{18}FDG was recently addressed by direct measurement (40). Comparative measurement of lumped constant values in diseased and normal brain tissue was made in vivo recently using sequential PET measurements of glucose transport with 3-0-[^{11}C]methyl glucose and ^{18}FDG (41). The application of the latter technique and the measurement of the LC in other disease states will be important in the widespread utility of the analog method.

A tracer kinetic model for glucose utilization using ^{11}C-labeled glucose was developed nearly a decade ago (42). ^{11}C-Glucose is now available in sufficiently high chemical and radiochemical purity for PET measurements in humans (42-44). Although its rapid metabolism in vivo requires that accurate rapid time-activity tissue and plasma measurements at early times be made, and because of this that a blood volume correction be made, ^{11}C-glucose has an advantage over the use of deoxyglucose analogs such as ^{18}FDG in that it does not require the use of a lumped constant. It is safe to say that unless a purified preparation of ^{11}C-glucose is used and time/activity data from PET is obtained at very early times after an intravenous injection of ^{11}C-glucose and unless a tracer kinetic model is correctly applied, the PET image represents uptake of carbon-11 rather than regional glucose metabolism. This point deserves emphasis in light of a number of reports of PET measurements of "brain glucose metabolism" on subjects who have injested a cocktail of irradiated spinach leaves. Again the lure of the color image, which in this case, falsely claims a relationship to glucose metabolism, seriously compromises the image of PET as a scientific tool.

Radiotracers for Neurotransmitter Studies: The study of the neurotransmitter dopamine has been approached by using labeled antagonists to the dopamine receptor or by using labeled precursors to dopamine. Dopamine itself, (45) unfortunately, does not cross the blood brain barrier. In the first approach labeled butyrophenones, antagonists to the dopamine receptor which cross the blood brain barrier, are the most widely applied. These compounds, the most notable examples of which are spiroperidol and N-methylspiroperidol are highly selective for dopamine receptors in human and baboon (46-48, 51-56) caudate/putamen and are metabolically stable in brain tissue (56). Since the unlabeled molecules contain fluorine, labeling with ^{11}C or ^{18}F does not significantly perturb the biological properties of the labeled drug. Both ^{11}C and ^{18}F N-methylspiroperidol are currently prepared in very high specific activity, (53) an essential requirement in avoiding receptor saturation which can significantly alter time/activity curves and confuse the two different effects of receptor saturation and non-specific binding.

For the ^{11}C-labeled neuroleptics as well as for a large number of other tracers, ^{11}C-methyl iodide has emerged as an essential precursor molecule. Its synthesis has (1 and references therein) recently been streamlined (58). Another dopamine antagonist ^{11}C-raclopride (59) is also prepared via ^{11}C-methyl iodide and used to probe D_2 receptors in vivo (60). Whether in vivo N-[^{11}C]demethylation is a significant metabolic pathway depends on the structure of the molecule and the use of [^{11}C]methyl esters and N-[^{11}C]-methyl compounds must, of course, be devoid of demethylation in the organ of interest within the time course of the study.

While ^{11}C-neuroleptics can be used to study radioligand-receptor interaction for time periods up to 90 minutes, the statistics of measurement at these later time periods rapidly degrade especially in reference areas (such as cerebellum) which are devoid of dopamine receptors. Here ^{18}F-labeled ligands (52, 56) offer a distinct advantage allowing measurements to be made with good statistics for several hours after injection providing high contrast and the measurement of important kinetic parameters. The use of the nucleophilic aromatic substitution reaction represented a breakthrough in the synthesis of ^{18}F-neuroleptics (49-51, 57). A number of models have been proposed to fit the data produced by PET measurement of radioligand-receptor interaction (55, 61,62). However, three factors, high radiotracer specific activity, high quality PET measurements, and plasma input function measurement are essential before attempting a kinetic analysis. In addition, partial volume effects especially with moderate to low resolution PET instruments may significantly change the shape of time/activity curves in small regions of interest which occur in a background of changing radioactivity.

The study of dopamine neurotransmitter systems has also been pursued using ^{18}F-labeled L-DOPA, a precursor to dopamine, which crosses the blood-brain barrier (63). Since fluorine does not naturally occur in L-DOPA, its use as a label represents a potential perturbation in the biological behavior of the molecule. It was found that the substitution of fluorine for hydrogen on position 6 of the DOPA molecule results in the least alteration in the properties of the parent compound (64). Since the multiplicity of labeled molecules produced during normal DOPA metabolism, potentially complicates a PET image, detailed biochemical studies have been and are currently being undertaken to address the interpretation of PET studies in humans using ^{18}F-fluoro-DOPA (65,66). The distribution of ^{18}F after injection of ^{18}F-6-fluoro-DOPA (the fluorine isomer of choice) is predominantly associated with the caudate/putamen a region known to contain high concentration of dopamine and dopamine receptors (67).

The synthesis of ^{18}F-6-fluoro-DOPA has occupied the attention of a number of groups and while a number of sophisticated approaches have been explored, direct fluorination of DOPA with [^{18}F]F$_2$ is currently the method of choice even though the yield is low (68). The synthesis of carbon-11 L-DOPA labeled in the carboxyl group (69) and in the metabolically stable position 3 (70) has also been reported. Asymmetric synthesis has been explored as a route to pure L-amino acids (71). As was the case with ^{18}FDG and ^{18}F-neuroleptics, a demonstrated utility in PET studies generally initiates an increase in development work in the synthesis of a particular radiotracer.

PET Methods for Measuring Regional Brain Protein Synthesis: The measurement of regional brain protein synthesis has been approached using two different radiotracers. In one method, ^{11}C-leucine (^{11}C-carboxyl) is the radiotracer (72). The tracer kinetic model requires the label to be in the ^{11}C-carboxylic acid group of L-leucine (73). In the other method, [^{11}C-methyl]-methionine is the radiotracer and a tracer kinetic model for this tracer was validated using a triple tracer experiment (^{14}C, ^{11}C, and ^{3}H-L-methionine) in baboons (74). At fifty minutes, 50% of the ^{11}C in baboon brain was as ^{11}C-labeled protein (74). Since methionine is well known to participate in transmethylation reactions as well as protein synthesis, the possibility of complications in interpretation of PET data due to ^{11}C-labeled products other than ^{11}C-labeled protein in brain has been recently addressed in rats using tissue extraction and analysis. These studies comparing ^{11}C-leucine and ^{11}C-methionine showed that at 45 minutes after injection, 36% of the label was present as non-protein metabolites with ^{11}C-methionine whereas only 3% of the label was present as non-protein metabolites with ^{11}C-leucine (75). From this study, it was concluded that leucine provides a better measure of brain protein synthesis with PET or autoradiography.

New Radiotracers and Applications for PET: Research and development in PET continues to focus heavily on problems in the neurosciences with a special emphasis on the development of methods for probing neurotransmitter receptor:radioligand interactions. New carbon-11 labeled (76,77) and fluorine-18 (78) labeled radioligands for the opiate receptor have been reported and PET studies have begun. The benzodiazepine receptors (79) and acetylcholine muscarinic receptors (80) are also the object of a number of investigations.

The use of PET to probe in vivo pharmacokinetics has also been explored. Here transport and uptake of drugs across the blood brain barrier and kinetic profiles of uptake and egress have been measured (52, 81-84).

A new area is the development of radiotracers with an affinity for the hypoxic areas of tumors and ischemic areas of heart and brain (85).

In vivo assessment of the metabolic status of tumors continues to be an important problem. Here the tracers of glucose and oxygen metabolism play a major role. In the case of glucose metabolism, glucose metabolic rate parallels degree of malignancy (86). Considerable contrast between tumor and surrounding tissue is obtained with ^{11}C-methionine (87,88). Although the mechanism of trapping of ^{11}C-methionine has not yet been demonstrated, there does appear to be a unidirectional transport of methionine into tumor tissue (89). Another tracer, ^{11}C-putrescine, has been developed to take advantage of the increase in polyamine metabolism associated with rapidly proliferating tissue (90,91). Since uptake in normal brain tissue is very low, a high contrast between tumor and normal brain is obtained in PET studies of human cerebral malignancy with ^{11}C-putrescine.

Yet another area which has shown promise is the use of suicide enzyme inhibitors in conjunction with PET to probe the distribution of enzyme activity in vivo. Feasibility studies with the ^{11}C-labeled suicide inhibitors of monoamine oxidase type A and B (^{11}C-clorgyline and ^{11}C-deprenyl) have shown that this is a potentially fruitful new application for PET (92).

In summary, PET continues to be more critically and creatively applied not only to problems in the neurosciences (93) but to the fields of cardiology as well (94). While there are a great number of tracers being used at cyclotron-PET centers around the world, perhaps three could be categorized as standard in that not only is their use widespread and relatively routine but also they are used in conjunction with a tracer kinetic model. These are the ^{15}O-tracers (95), the deoxyglucose (^{18}FDG and ^{11}C-2DG) (10) and ^{11}C-palmitic acid (96,97). One can expect

Table XII
Requirements for Single (p) or Two Particle (p,d)
Cyclotrons with Proton Energies = 17 MeV

		Description	Cost ($)[a]	Space Requirement
1.	Cyclotron	Machine Only and RF Supply	$7 \times 10^5 - 1.0^6$	20-60 m^2
2.	Cyclotron Operating Peripherals	Control Panel Power Supplies Primary Cooling[b]	Included in (1)	20-40 m^2
3.	Peripherals	Switching Magnets Auto Target Changer Beam Lines Focussing Magnets Black Boxes Gas Delivery System Rabbit System Beam Monitoring System Etc.	Variable Depends on Items $1.0 \times 10^5 - 6 \times 10^5$	Included in (1)
4.	Shielding[c]	Required for all Current Machines. Local Radiation Safety Laws Apply	$2 \times 10^5 - 8 \times 10^5$	1 meter to 2.5 meters of Concrete on all Sides or H$_2$O equivalent
5.	Laboratories	Chemistry Labs Including Shielded Space for Syntheses	---	50-300 m^2

a. Costs are in U. S. Dollars, 1985.
b. Secondary cooling usually supplied by user.
c. Local architects can provide accurate estimates given local radiation safety requirements and local concrete and construction costs. In some local situations, dense concrete is more economical than normal concrete. Building underground can result in savings because wall and floor thicknesses can be reduced.

that in the very near future the neurotransmitter receptor binding radiotracers will also fall into this category since the difficult questions of biochemical validation and modeling are currently being addressed. Thus the number of compounds for which black boxes are an economical investment and can be used without a large professional staff is still limited at present. Their utility is of course the determining factor. The addition of a neuroleptic black box, be it for methylspiroperidol or some other compound, should be realized in the near future.

Economic Considerations

The cost of any installation will clearly depend on local conditions, availability of personnel, and experience in developing an infrastructure for operation of the facility including what is necessary for interpretation of data. Table XII provides some information that can be used by the reader for a crude estimate, in 1985 U.S. dollars of such costs.

There are perhaps two conditions under which cyclotron-PET centers can operate today. What is prevalent at present are centers which combine in most cases large professional staffs, biochemists, chemists, computer specialists, engineers, physicists, and physicians to serve a broadly based research function and in some cases a clinical service function. The second condition which is just now beginning to develop is the purely clinical PET center where technical personnel operate the cyclotrons, black boxes and PET machines providing the physician with a service in his dealing with the disease process in patients in much the same way that CT, NMR or the many types of radioimaging are used in hospitals today. As has already been noted, such centers will, in most cases, be dependent on the university hospitals and research centers for new radiopharmaceuticals.

A cyclotron-PET center in a university hospital or research institute has, in almost all cases, the needed technical and professional services required as backup for a broadly based research program. Included would be adequate computer facilities, machine shops, electronics shops and other mechanical and electrical services. In addition, mathematicians, chemists, biochemists, engineers, and physicians, etc., who are not part of the cyclotron-PET team but who can be consulted as required for any particular need, are convenience adjuncts to the core team. By contrast, a hospital-PET center would not have such an infrastructure and would depend primarily on the manufacturer, consultants and others for help when needed. The cyclotrons noted in Table I can all provide the needed radionuclides with the caveat that the single particle machine, regardless of energy, 11 MeV or higher, <u>requires</u> the use of enriched isotopes for three of the four accessible radionuclides.

A frequently addressed question is the number of individuals needed to support the technical aspects of a cyclotron-PET center. A survey of the cyclotron-PET centers in operation today will show a very wide range in the numbers of professionals and technical staffs involved. To consider the cyclotron as an example, staffing will depend on the factors noted above but also on local law and safety considerations. The currently available machines can be operated by one person and indeed maintained by that person given adequate professional background. However, local radiation safety law and common safety considerations have resulted in at least two individuals being needed in most installations operative today. Given the usual conditions for vacations, illness, etc., a full 8 hour day of operation requires that three individuals be experienced in the operation but not necessarily the maintenance of the machine. The majority of installations have 2 to 5 such personnel usually depending on whether in-house repair and maintenance is done or reliance for repair is placed solely on the manufacturer of the particular machine. There is little point in presenting personnel estimates for labeled tracer research and development as this will vary widely depending on the nature of the institution. Labeled tracers from a hospital clinical service machine, however, could in principal be part of the hospital radiopharmaceutical delivery service. We assume that only hospitals with well developed nuclear medicine services would consider a cyclotron-PET as part of their clinical research and clinical service function. The cyclotron-PET has not as yet developed to the point where its use is as routine as that of a CT device. However, it is our belief that given the uniqueness of the information it provides and the rapid strides being made toward simplicity of design and operation, cyclotron-PET will take its place in the armamentarium of medical practice.

CONCLUSIONS

This paper is not intended as a review of the Cyclotron-PET field. We hope that we have given the reader a conception of what some of the aspects of cyclotron-PET involve, focussing primarily on the cyclotron itself and labeled tracer preparation and application. Accelerators being developed include proton and deuteron linacs and "super conducting" (thus very small) cyclotrons. These have not yet appeared and the demands of cost, maintenance and size will determine whether they replace the conventional cyclotron.

The future looks bright and at the very least it can be stated that cyclotron-PET has given us a tool which can probe human biochemistry and its relation to the normal and pathological state in a manner not possible by any other method existing today. With the rapid advances occurring at present, its function as a research tool will increasingly be complemented with its use in routine clinical service.

ACKNOWLEDGEMENT

This research was carried out at Brookhaven National Laboratory under contract DE-AC02-76CH00016 with the U. S. Department of Energy and supported by its Office of Health and Environmental Research.

REFERENCES

1. Fowler, J.S. and Wolf, A.P. "Positron Emitter Labeled Compounds: Priorities and Problems" in Positron Computed Tomography (M.E. Phelps, J.C. Mazziotta and H. Schelbert, Eds., Raven Press, 1985).

2. Wolf, A.P. and Fowler, J.S. "Positron Emitter Labeled Radiotracers, Chemical Considerations" in Positron Emission Tomography (Alan R. Liss, Inc. Pub., 1985).

3. Wolf, A.P. and Jones, W.B. Cyclotrons for Biomedical Radioisotope Production. Radiochimica Acta 34 (1983) 1-7.

4. Wolf, A.P. and Fowler, J.S. "Small Cyclotrons and the Production of Positron Emitters. Present and Future" in Proceedings of an International Conference on Radiopharmaceuticals and Labelled Compounds, Organized by the IAEA and held in Tokyo, Japan October 22-26, 1984, IAEA Publication CN45/10, 1985.

5. Bida, G.T., Ruth, T.J. and Wolf, A.P. Experimentally Determined Thick Target Yields for the $^{14}N(p,\alpha)^{11}C$ Reaction. Radiochimica Acta 27 (1980) 181-185.

6. Vera Ruiz, H. and Wolf, A.P. Excitation Function for ^{15}O Production Via the $^{14}N(d,n)^{15}O$ Reaction. Radiochimica Acta 24 (1977) 65-67.

7. Sajjad, M., Lambrecht, R.M. and Wolf, A.P. Cyclotron Isotopes and Radiopharmaceuticals. XXXIV. Excitation Function for the $^{15}N(p,n)^{15}O$ Reaction. Radiochimica Acta 36 (1984) 159-162.

8. Sajjad, M., Lambrecht, R.M. and Wolf, A.P. Cyclotron Isotopes and Radiopharmaceuticals. XXXVI. Investigation of Some Excitation Functions for the Preparation of ^{15}O, ^{13}N and ^{11}C. Radiochimica Acta, in press.

9. Nozaki, T., Iwamoto, M., and Ido, T. Yield of ^{18}F for Various Reactions from Oxygen and Neon. International Journal of Applied Radiation and Isotopes 25 (1974) 393-399.

10. Ruth, T.J. and Wolf, A.P. Absolute Cross Sections for the Production of ^{18}F Via the ^{18}O(p,n)^{18}F Reaction. Radiochimica Acta 26 (1979) 21-24.

11. Casella, V., Ido, T., Wolf, A.P., Fowler, J.S., MacGregor, R.R., Ruth, T.J. Anhydrous F-18 Labeled Elemental Fluorine for Radiopharmaceutical Preparation. Journal of Nuclear Medicine 21 (1980) 750-757.

12. Robertson, L.P., White, B.L., and Erdman, K.L. Beam Heating Effects in Gas Targets. Review of Scientific Instruments 32 (1961) 1405.

13. McDaniels, D.K., Berggvist, I., Drake D., and Martin, J.T. Beam Heating in Gas Targets. Nuclear Instruments and Methods 99 (1972) 77-80.

14. Chavet, I., Kanter, M. and Menat, M. Factors Affecting Beam Shape and Quality. Nuclear Instruments and Methods 139 (1976) 47-53.

15. Oselka, M., Gindler, J.E., and Friedman, A.M. Non-Linear Behavior of Gas Targets for Isotope Production. International Journal of Applied Radiation and Isotopes 28 (1977) 804-805.

16. Ruth, T.J. and Wolf, A.P. "Small" Accelerator, Radionuclide and Radiopharmaceutical Production. IEEE Transactions in Nuclear Science NS-26 (1979) 1710-1712.

17. Görres, J., Kettner, K.V., Kräwinkel, H., and Rolfs, C. The Influence of Intense Ion Beams on Gas Target Densities. Nuclear Instruments and Methods 177 (1980) 295-303.

18. Heselius, S.J., Lindblom, P. and Solin, O. Optical Studies of the Influence of an Intense Ion Beam on High-Pressure Gas Targets. International Journal of Applied Radiation and Isotopes 33 (1982) 653-659.

19. Wieland, B.W., Schlyer, D.J. and Wolf, A.P. Charged Particle Penetration in GasTargets Designed for Accelerator Production of Radionuclides Used in Nuclear Medicine. International Journal of Applied Radiation and Isotopes 35, No. 5, (1984) 387-396.

20. Bida, G.T., Ehrenkaufer, R.E., Wolf, A.P., Fowler, J.S., MacGregor, R.R., and Ruth, T.J. The Effect of Target-Gas Purity on the Chemical Form of F-18 During $^{18}F-F_2$ Production Using the Neon/Fluorine Target. Journal of Nuclear Medicine 21 (1980) 758-762.

21. Ferrieri, R.A. and Wolf, A.P. The Chemistry of Positron Emitting Nucleogenic Atoms with Regard to Preparation of Labelled Compounds of Practical Utility. Radiochimica Acta 34 (1983) 69-83.

22. Wolf, A.P. Special Characteristics and Potential for Radiopharmaceuticals for Positron Emission Tomography. Seminars in Nuclear Medicine 11 (1981) 2-12.

23. Fowler, J.S. and Wolf, A.P. "The Synthesis of Carbon-11, Fluorine-18, and Nitrogen-13 Labeled Radiotracers for Biomedical Applications" in Nuclear Science Series, National Academy of Science, National Research Council, Monograph (1982) pp. 1-124.

24. Ter Pogossian, M.M., Eichling, J.O., Davis, D.O., Welch, M.J. and Metzger, M.A. The Determination of Regional Cerebral Blood Flow by Means of Water Labeled with Radioactive Oxygen-15. Radiology 93 (1969) 31-40.

25. Mintun, M.A., Raichle, M.E., Martin, W.R.W. and Herscovitch, P. Brain Oxygen Utilization Measured with O-15 Radiotracers and Positron Emission Tomography. Journal of Nuclear Medicine 25 (1984) 177-187.

26. Herscovitch, P., Markham, J. and Raichle, M.E. Brain Blood Flow Measured with Intravenous $H_2^{15}O$. I. Theory and Error Analysis. Journal of Nuclear Medicine 24 (1983) 782-789.

27. Raichle, M.E., Martin, W.R.W., Herscovitch, P., Mintun, M.A. and Markham, J. Brain Blood Flow Measured with Intravenous $H_2^{15}O$. II. Implementation and Validation. Journal of Nuclear Medicine 24 (1983) 790-798.

28. Ackerman, R.H., Alpert, N.M., Correia, J.A., Finklestein, S., Davis, S.M., Kelley, R.E., Donnan, G.A., D'Alton, J.G. and Tavernas, J.M. Positron Imaging in Ischemic Stroke Disease. Annals of Neurology 15 (1984), S126-S130.

29. Ito, M., Lammertsma, A.A., Wise, R.J.S., Bernardi, S., Frackowiak, R.S.J., Heather, J.D., McKenzie, C.G., Thomas, D.G.T. and Jones, T. Measurement of Regional Cerebral Blood Flow and Oxygen Utilisation in Patients with Cerebral Tumours Using ^{15}O and Positron Emission Tomography: Analytical Techniques and Preliminary Results. Neuroradiology 23 (1982) 63-74.

30. Mazziotta, J.C., Huang, S.-C., Phelps, M.E., Carson, R.E., MacDonald, N.S. and Mahoney, K. A Noninvasive Positron Computed Tomography Technique Using Oxygen-15-Labeled Water for the Evaluation of Neurobehavioral Task Batteries. Journal of Cerebral Blood Flow and Metabolism 5 (1985) 70-78.

31. Reiman, E.M., Raichle, M.E., Butler, F.K., Herscovitch, P. and Robins, E. A Focal Brain Abnormality in Panic Disorder, A Severe Form of Anxiety. Nature 310 (1984) 683-685.

32. Volpe, J.J., Herscovitch, P., Perlman, J.M. and Raichle, M.E. Positron Emission Tomography in the Newborn: Extensive Impairment of Regional Cerebral Blood Flow with Intraventricular Hemorrhage and Hemorrhagic Intracerebral Involvement. Pediatrics 72 (1983) 589-601.

33. Perlman, J.M., Herscovitch, P., Kreusser, K.L., Raichle, M.E. and Volpe, J.J. Positron Emission Tomography in the Newborn: Effect of Seizure on Regional Cerebral Blood Flow in an Asphyxiated Infant. Neurology 35 (1985) 244-247.

34. Reivich, M., Kuhl, D., Wolf, A.P., Greenberg, J., Phelps, M., Ido, T., Casella, V., Hoffman, E., Alavi, A. and Sokoloff, L. The [^{18}F]Fluorodeoxyglucose Method for the Measurement of Local Cerebral Glucose Utilization in Man. Circulation Research 44 (1979) 127-137.

35. Sokoloff, L. Mapping of Local Cerebral Functional Activity by Measurement of Local Cerebral Glucose Utilization with [^{14}C] Deoxyglucose. Brain 102 (1979) 653-668.

36. Tewson, T.J. Synthesis of No-Carrier-Added Fluorine-18 2-Fluoro-2-Deoxy-D-Glucose. Journal of Nuclear Medicine 24 (1983) 718-721.

37. Shiue, C.-Y., Fowler, J.S., Wolf, A.P., Alexoff, D. and MacGregor, R.R. Gas-Liquid Chromatographic Determination of Relative Amounts of 2-Deoxy-2-Fluoro-D-Glucose and 2-Deoxy-2-Fluoro-D-Mannose Synthesized from Various Methods. Journal of Labelled Compounds and Radiopharmaceuticals XXII (1985) 503.

38. Coenen, H.H., Colosimo, M., Schüller, M. and Stöcklin, G. Mild and Effective Aliphatic and Aromatic n.c.a. ^{18}F-Fluorination Using Crown Ether. Journal of Nuclear Medicine 26 (1985) P37, abstract.

39. Reivich, M., Alavi, A., Wolf, A.P., Greenberg, J.H., Fowler, J., Christman, D., MacGregor, R., Jones, S.C., London, J., Shiue, C. and Yonekura, Y. Use of 2-Deoxy-D-[^{11}C]Glucose for the Determination of Local Cerebral Glucose Metabolism in Humans: Variation Within and Between Subjects. Journal of Cerebral Blood Flow and Metabolism 2 (1982) 307-319.

40. Reivich, M., Alavi, A., Wolf, A., Fowler, J., Russell, J., Arnett, C., MacGregor, R.R., Shiue, C.-Y., Atkins, H., Anand, A., Dann, R. and Greenberg, J.H. Glucose Metabolic Rate Kinetic Model Parameter Determination in Humans: The Lumped Constants and Rate Constants for [^{18}F]Fluorodeoxyglucose and [^{11}C]Deoxyglucose. Journal of Cerebral Blood Flow and Metabolism 5 (1985) 179-192.

41. Gjedde, A., Wienhard, K., Heiss, W.-D., Kloster, G., Diemer, N.H., Herholz, K. and Pawlik, G. Comparative Regional Analysis of 2-Fluorodeoxyglucose and Methylglucose Uptake in Brain of Four Stroke Patients. With Special Reference to the Regional Estimation of the Lumped Constant. Journal of Cerebral Blood Flow and Metabolism 5 (1985) 163-178.

42. Ehrin, E., Stone-Elander, S., Nilsson, J.L.G., Bergstrom, M., Blomqvist, G., Brismar, T., Eriksson, L., Greitz, T., Jansson, P.E., Litton, J.-E., Malmborg, P., Ugglas, M. and Widen, L. C-11-Labelled Glucose and its Utilization in Positron-Emission Tomography. Journal of Nuclear Medicine 24 (1983) 326-331.

43. Dence, C.S., Lechner, K.A., Welch, M.J. and Kilbourn, M.R. Remote System for Production of Carbon-11 Labeled glucose Via Photosynthesis. Journal of Labelled Compounds and Radiopharmaceuticals XXI (1984) 743-750.

44. Shiue, C.-Y. and Wolf, A.P. The Synthesis of 1-[^{11}C]-D-Glucose and Related Compounds for the Measurement of Brain Glucose Metabolism. Journal of Labelled Compounds and Radiopharmaceuticals XXII (1985) 171-182.

45. Hoyte, R.M., Lin, S.S., Christman, D.R., Atkins, H.L., Hauser, W. and Wolf, A.P. Organic Radiopharmaceuticals Labeled With Isotopes of Short Half Life. III. ^{18}F-Labeled Phenylalanines. Journal of Nuclear Medicine 12 (1971) 280-286.

46. Kilbourn, M.R., Welch, M.J., Dence, C.S., Tewson, T.J., Saji, H. and Maeda, M. Carrier-Added and No-Carrier-Added Syntheses of [^{18}F]Spiroperidol and [^{18}F]Haloperidol. International Journal of Applied Radiation and Isotopes 35 (1984) 591-598.

47. Welch, M.J., Kilbourn, M.R., Mathias, C.J., Mintun, M.A. and Raichle, M.E. Comparison in Animal Models of ^{18}F-Spiroperidol and ^{18}F-Haloperidol: Potential Agents for Imaging the Dopamine Receptor. Life Science 33 (1983) 1687-1693.

48. Arnett, C.D., Fowler, J.S., Wolf, A.P., Logan, J. and MacGregor, R.R. Mapping Brain Neuroleptic Receptors in the Live Baboon. Biological Psychiatry 19 (1984) 1365.

49. Cacace, F., Speranza, M., Wolf, A.P. and MacGregor, R.R. Nucleophilic Aromatic Substitution Reactions in Polyfluorobenzene Isotopic Exchange Between ^{18}F$^-$ and Polyfluorobenzenes in Dimethylsulfoxide. A Kinetic Study. Journal of Fluorine Chemistry 21 (1982) 145-158.

50. Attina, M., Cacace, F. and Wolf, A.P. Labeled Aryl Fluorides From the Nucleophilic Displacement of Activated Nitro Groups by ^{18}F-F$^-$. Journal of Labelled Compounds and Radiopharmaceuticals XX (1983) 501-514.

51. Shiue, C.-Y., Fowler, J.S., Wolf, A.P., Watanabe, M. and Arnett, C.D. Syntheses and Specific Activity Determinations of No-Carrier-Added (NCA) ^{18}F-Labeled Butyrophenone Neuroleptics - Benperidol, Haloperidol, Spiroperidol, and Pipamperone. Journal of Nuclear Medicine 26 (1985) 181-186.

52. Arnett, C.D., Shiue, C.-Y., Wolf, A.P., Fowler, J.S., Logan, J. and Watanabe M. Comparison of Three ^{18}F-Labeled Butyrophenone Neuroleptic Drugs in the Baboon Using Positron Emission Tomography. Journal of Neurochemistry 44 (1985) 835-844.

53. Burns, H.D., Dannals, R.F., Langström, B., Ravert, H.T., Zemyan, S.E., Duelfer, T., Wong, D.F., Frost, J., Kuhar, M.J. and Wagner, H.N. (3-N-(^{11}C]Methyl)Spiperone, A Ligand Binding to Dopamine Receptors: Radiochemical Synthesis and Biodistribution Studies in Mice. Journal of Nuclear Medicine 25 (1984) 1222-1227.

54. Wagner, H.N., Jr., Burns, H.D., Dannals, R.F., Wong, D.F., Langström, B., Duelfer, T., Frost, J.J., Ravert, H.T., Links, J.M., Rosenbloom, S.B., Lukas, S.E., Dramer, A.V. and Kuhar, M.J. Imaging Dopamine Receptors in the Human Brain by Positron Tomography. Science 221 (1983) 1264-1266.

55. Wong, D.F., Wagner, H.N., Jr., Dannals, R.F., Links, J.M., Frost, J.J., Ravert, H.T., Wilson, A.A., Rosenbaum, A.E., Gjedde, A., Douglass, K.H., Petronis, J.D., Folstein, M.F., Toung, J.K.T., Burns, H.D. and Kuhar, M.J. Effects of Age on Dopamine and Serotonin Receptors Measured by Positron Tomography in the Living Human Brain. Science 226 (1984) 1393-1396.

56. Arnett, C.D., Fowler, J.S., Wolf, A.P., Shiue, C.-Y. and McPherson, D.W. [^{18}F]-N-Methylspiroperidol: The Radioligand of Choice for PETT Studies of the Dopamine Receptor in Human Brain. Life Science 36 (1985) 1359-1366.

57. Shiue, C.-Y., Fowler, J.S., Wolf, A.P., McPherson, D.W., Arnett, C.D. and Zecca, L. No-Carrier-Added (NCA) ^{18}F-Labeled N-Methylspiroperidol - Synthesis and Biodistribution in Mice. Journal of Nuclear Medicine, in press.

58. Dannals, R.F. and Langström, B. A Simple, One-Pot Apparatus for the Production of Carbon-11 Labeled Methyl Iodide. Journal of Nuclear Medicine 26 (1985) P126, abstract.

59. Ehrin, E., Farde, L., De Paulis, T., Eriksson, L., Greitz, T., Johnström, P., Litton, J.-E., Nilsson, J.L.G., Sedvall, G., Stone-Elander, S. and Ögren, S.-O. Preparation of ^{11}C-Labelled Raclopride, a New Potent Dopamine Receptor Antagonist: Preliminary PET Studies of Cerebral Dopamine Receptors in the Monkey. International Journal of Applied Radiation and Isotopes 36 (1985) 269-273.

60. Farde, L., Ehrin, E., Eriksson, L., Greitz, T., Hall, H., Hedström, C.-G., Litton, J.-E. and Sedvall, G. Substituted Benzamides as Ligands for Visualization of Dopamine Receptor Binding in the Human Brain by Positron Emission Tomography. Proceedings of the National Academy of Science USA 82 (1985) 3863-3867.

61. Mintun, M.A., Raichle, M.E., Kilbourn, M.R., Wooten, G.F. and Welch, M.J. A Quantitative Model for the In Vivo Assessment of Drug Binding Sites with Positron Emission Tomography. Annals of Neurology 15 (1984) 217-227.

62. Friedman, A.M., DeJesus, O.T., Revenaugh, B.A. and Dinerstein, R.J. Measurements In Vivo of Parameters of the Dopamine System. Annals of Neurology 15(Suppl) (1984) S66-S76.

63. Garnett, E.S., Firnau, G., Nahmias, C., Sood, S. and Belbeck, L. Blood-Brain Barrier Transport and Cerebral Utilization of Dopa in Living Monkeys. American Journal of Physiology 238 (1980) R318-R327.

64. Firnau, G., Sood, S., Pantel, R. and Garnett, S. Phenol Ionization in Dopa Determines the Site of Methylation by Catechol-O-Methyltransferase. Molecular Pharmacology 19 (1980) 1$\overline{30}$-133.

65. Martin, W.R.W., Boyes, B.E., Leenders, K.L. and Patlak, C.S. A Method for the Quantitative Analysis of 6-Fluorodopa Uptake Data From Positron Emission Tomography. Brain 85, Abstracts, International Society of Cerebral Blood Flow and Metabolism, Lund, Sweden, 1985, p. 204.

66. Garnett, E.S., Nahmias, C., Firnau, G., and Lang, A. DA Metabolism in Parkinson's Disease. Brain 85, Abstracts, International Society of Cerebral Blood Flow and Metabolism, Lund, Sweden, 1985, p. 116.

67. Garnett, E.S., Firnau, G. and Nahmias, C. Dopamine Visualized in Basal Ganglia of Living Man. Nature 305 (1983) 137-138.

68. Firnau, G., Chirakal, R. and Garnett, E.S. Aromatic Radiofluorination with [^{18}F]Fluorine Gas: 6-[^{18}F]Fluoro-L-Dopa. Journal of Nuclear Medicine 25 (1984) 1228-1233.

69. Bolster, J.M., Vaalburg, W., Van Veen, W., Van Dijk, Th., Van Der Molen, H.D., Wynberg, H. and Woldring, M.G. Synthesis of No-Carrier-Added L- and D-[1-^{11}C]-DOPA. International Journal of Applied Radiation and Isotopes 34 (1983) 1650-1652.

70. Halldin, C. and Langström, B. Synthesis of Racemic [3-^{11}C]Phenylalanine and [3-^{11}C]DOPA. International Journal of Applied Radiation and Isotopes 35 (1984) 779-782.

71. Halldin, C. and Langström, B. Asymmetric Synthesis of L-[3-^{11}C]Phynylalanine Using Chiral Hydrogenation Catalysts. International Journal of Applied Radiation and Isotopes 35 (1984) 945-948.

72. Barrio, J.R., Phelps, M.E., Huang, S.C., Keen, R.E. and MacDonald, N.S. 1-(^{11}C)L-Leucine and the Principle of Metabolic Trapping for the Tomographic Measurement of Cerebral Protein Synthesis in Man. Journal of Labelled Compounds and Radiopharmaceuticals XIX (1982) 1271-1272.

73. Smith, C.B., Davidsen, L., Deibler, G., Patlak, C., Pettigrew, K. and Sokoloff, L. A Method for the Determination of Local Rates of Protein Synthesis in Man. Trans. American Society of Neurochemistry 11 (1984) 94.

74. Bustany, P., Henry, J.F., Cabanis, E., Soussaline, F., Crouzel, M. and Comar, D. Incorporation of L-(^{11}C)-Methionine in Brain Proteins Studied by PET in Dementia. Proceedings of the 3rd World Congress of Nuclear Medicine and Biology, II (1982) 2216-2219.

75. Jones, R.M., Cramer, S., Sargent, T. and Budinger, T.F. Brain Protein Synthesis Rates Measured In Vivo Using Methionine and Leucine. Journal of Nuclear Medicine 26 (1985) P168, abstract.

76. Dannals, R.F., Ravert, H.T., Frost, J.J., Wilson, A.A., Burns, H.D. and Wagner, H.N., Jr. Radiosynthesis of an Opiate Receptor Binding Radiotracer: [^{11}C]Carfentanil. International Journal of Applied Radiation and Isotopes 36 (1985) 303-306.

77. Frost, J.J., Wagner, H.N., Jr., Dannals, R.F., Ravert, H.T., Links, J.M., Wilson, A.A., Burns, H.D., Wong, D.F., McPherson, R.W., Rosenbaum, A.E., Kuhar, M.J. and Snyder, S.H. Imaging Opiate Receptors in the Human Brain by Positron Tomography. Journal of Computer Assisted Tomography 9 (1985) 231-236.

78. Pert, C.B., Danks, J.A., Channing, M.A., Eckleman, W.C., Larson, S.M., Bennett, J.M., Burke, T.R. and Rice, K.C. 3-[^{18}F]Acetylcyclofoxy: A Useful Probe for the Visualization of Opiate Receptors in Living Animals. FEBS Letters 177 (1984) 281-286.

79. Samson, Y., Hantraye, P., Baron, J.C., Soussaline, F., Comar, D. and Maziere, M. Kinetics and Displacement of [^{11}C]RO 15-1788, A Benzodiazepine Antagonist, Studied in Human Brain In Vivo by Positron Tomography. European Journal of Pharmacology 110 (1985) 247-251.

80. Vora, M.M., Finn, R.D. and Boothe, T.E. [N-Methyl-^{11}C]-Scopolamine: Synthesis and Distribution in Rat Brain. Journal of Labelled Compounds and Radiopharmaceuticals XX (1983) 1229-1236.

81. Baron, J.C., Comar, D., Crouzel, C., Roeda, D., Mestelan, G., Zarifian, E., Munari, C., Stoffels, C., Bancaud, J., Chodkiewicz, J.P., Loo, H. and Agid. Y. "Brain Regional Pharmacokinetics of ^{11}C-Labeled Diphenylhydantoin and Pimozide in Man" in Positron Emission Tomography of the Brain, (W.-D. Heiss and M.E. Phelps, Eds.), Springer-Verlag Publishers, 1983.

82. Friedman, A.M., DeJesus, O.T., Woolverton, W.L., Van Moffaert, G., Goldberg, L.I., Prasad, A., Barnett, A. and Dinerstein, R.J. Positron Tomography of a Radio-Brominated Analog of the D_1/DA_1 Antagonist, SCH 23390. European Journal of Pharmacology 108 (1985) 327-328.

83. Hartvig, P., Bergström, K., Lindberg, B., Lundberg, P.O., Lundqvist, H., Langström B., Svärd, H. and Rane, A. Kinetics of ^{11}C-Labeled Opiates in the Brain of Rhesus Monkeys. Journal of Pharmacology and Experimental Therapy 230 (1984) 250.

84. Diksic, M., Sako, K., Feindel, W., Kato, A., Yamamoto, Y.L., Farrokhzad, S. and Thompson, C. Pharmacokinetics of Positron-Labeled 1,3-Bis(2-chloroethyl)nitrosourea in Human Brain Tumors Using Positron Emission Tomography. Cancer Research 44 (1984) 3120-3124.

85. Jerabek, P.A., Dischino, D.D., Kilbourn, M.R. and Welch, M.J. Synthesis of a Fluorine-18 Labeled Hypoxic Cell Sensitizer. Journal of Nuclear Medicine 25 (1984) P23, abstract.

86. Di Chiro, G., Brooks, R.A., Patronas, N.J., Bairamian, D., Kornblith, P.L., Smith, B.H., Mansi, L. and Barker, J. Issues in the In Vivo Measurement of Glucose Metabolism of Human Central Nervous System Tumors. Annals of Neurology 15(Suppl) (1984) S-138-S146.

87. Bergström, M., Collins, V.P., Ehrin, E., Ericson, K., Eriksson, L., Greitz, T., Halldin, C., von Holst, H., Langström, B., Lilja, A., Lundqvist, H. and Nagren, K. Discrepancies in Brain Tumor Extent as Shown by Computed Tomography and Positron Emission Tomography Using [^{68}Ga]EDTA, [^{11}C]Glucose, and [^{11}C]Methionine. Journal of Computer Assisted Tomography 7 (1983) 1062-1066.

88. Meyer, G.-J., Schober, O. and Hundeshagen, H. Uptake of ^{11}C-L- and D-Methionine in Brain Tumors. European Journal of Nuclear Medicine 10 (1985) 373-376.

89. Ericson, J., Bergström, M., Lilja, A., Blomqvist, G., Collins, P., Ehrin, E., Eriksson, L., von Holst, H., Johnström, P., Lundqvist, H. and Mosskin, M. (C-11-Methyl)-Methionine and C-11-Glucose in the Diagnosis of Intracranial Tumors. Brain 85, Abstracts, International Society of Cerebral Blood Flow and Metabolism, Lund, Sweden, 1985, p. 425.

90. Volkow, N., Goldman, S.S., Flamm, E.S., Cravioto, H., Wolf, A.P. and Brodie, J.D. Labeled Putrescine as a Probe in Brain Tumors. Science 221 (1983) 673-675.

91. McPherson, D.W., Wolf, A.P., Fowler, J.S., Arnett, C.D., Brodie, J.D. and Volkow, N. Synthesis and Biodistribution of No-Carrier-Added [1-^{11}C]Putrescine. Journal of Nuclear Medicine, in press.

92. MacGregor, R.R., Halldin, C., Fowler, J.S., Wolf, A.P., Arnett, C.D., Langström, B. and Alexoff, D. Selective, Irreversible In Vivo Binding of [^{11}C]Clorgyline and [^{11}C]-L-Deprenyl in Mice: Potential for Measurement of Functional Monoamine Oxidase in Brain Using Positron Emission Tomography. Biochemical Pharmacology, in press.

93. Phelps, M.E. and Mazziotta, J.C. Positron Emission Tomography: Human Brain Function and Biochemistry. Science 228 (1985) 799-809.

94. Goldstein, R.A. Myocardial Metabolic Imaging: A New Diagnostic Era. Journal of Nuclear Medicine 23 (1982) 641-643.

95. Raichle, M.E. Quantitative In Vivo Autoradiography with Positron Emission Tomography. Brain Research Review 1 (1979) 47-68.

96. Weiss, E.S., Hoffman, E.J., Phelps, M.E., et al. External Detection and Visualization of Myocardial Ischemia with ^{11}C-Substrates In Vitro and In Vivo. Circulation Research 39 (1976) 24-32.

97. Schelbert, H.R., Henze, E., Schon, H.R., et al. C-11 Palmitate for the Noninvasive Evaluation of Regional Myocardial Metabolism with Positron Computed Tomography III. In Vivo Demonstration of the Effects of Substrate Availability on Myocardial Metabolism. American Heart Journal 105 (1983) 492-504.

RADIOPHARMACEUTICALS FOR POSITRON TOMOGRAPHY

C. CROUZEL

Service Hospitalier Frédéric Joliot, Commissariat à l'Energie Atomique, Département de Biologie, 91406 Orsay, France.

Over the last fifteen years or so the number of hospital centres using the positron emission tomographic techniques has grown considerably, mainly owing to the appearance of more and more efficient positron cameras.
This trend has led to the development of inorganic and especially organic radiopharmaceuticals which, injected into humans, can be used for metabolic or pharmacokinetic studies or for the measurement of certain physiological parameters (flow, cellular pH, membrane permeability...etc.).
The $\beta+$ emitters most commonly used to date are listed in table 1. Amongst these twelve $\beta+$ radioisotopes a special place is occupied by carbon 11, nitrogen 13 and oxygen 15, being component elements of living matter. Moreover all these $\beta+$ emitters, produced by nuclear transmutation and short-lived (a few minutes to several

Radioisotope	Periode
^{19}Ne	17,4 s
^{11}C	20,4 min
^{13}N	10 min
^{15}O	2,04 min
^{18}F	110 min
^{38}k	7,7 min
^{55}Co	17,5 h
^{62}Cu	9,73 min
^{68}Ga	68 min
^{75}Br	101 min
^{76}Br	16,1 h
^{82}Rb	1,25 min

Table 1 : list of $\beta+$ emitters

hours half-life) are obtained with a high specific activity (amount of radioactivity per unit mass). This means that they can be employed, to label molecules which are at present unusable because of either their high toxicity or their very low concentration in live organisms.

^{11}C, ^{13}N and ^{18}F labelling

Carbon 11 is unquestionably the β + emitter most widely used for labelling purposes.

The synthesis of a new radiopharmaceutical usually takes a few months to a year. Therefore, before any such undertaking is decided on, it should be thorougly ascertained that the new molecule will be suitable for the biochemical or physiological research in view.

This analysis will guide the chemist in the choice of which synthesis method to adopt. DOPA for example can be labelled with carbon 11 on the carbonyl groups or the carbon 3. However a preliminary biochemical study shows that this compound is very quickly decarboxylated and hence the radioactivity followed in the case of carboxyl group labelling would correspond not to the molecule itself but to a metabolite.

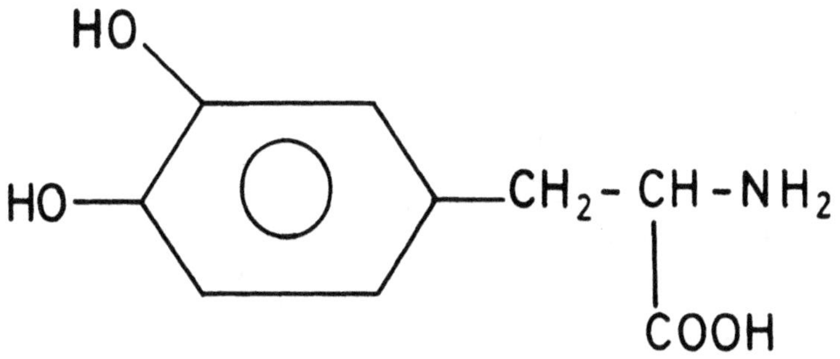

Fig. 1 - DOPA

Similarly the DOPA fluorine-18 labelling position is not without importance. Fluorine 18 may be introduced in the 5 or 6 position. However when ^{18}F-5-fluoro-DOPA is injected intravenously the fluorine atom in position 5 facilitates methylation of the labelled molecule by the liver. O-methyl-fluoro-DOPA is more lipophilic than fluoro-DOPA and passes into the brain much less specifically than ^{18}F-6-fluoro DOPA, which is hardly methylated at all.

Carbon 11 labelling methods often use methylation with ^{11}C-methyl iodide or ^{11}C-formol, and care must be taken to verify that the compound once injected is not demethylated too quickly. A last factor to be borne in mind is that the study in question cannot last longer than three half-lives of the radioelement, i.e. 1 hour for carbon 11.

It may happen that several isotopes are available for the labelling of a given molecule. The choice of which to use will be based on several criteria :
- duration of the study contemplated
- ease of labelling
- whether or not introduction of the isotope will alter the metabolism of the molecule.

An example is that of spiperone.
This neuroleptic may be labelled with ^{18}F, ^{11}C or ^{76}Br.

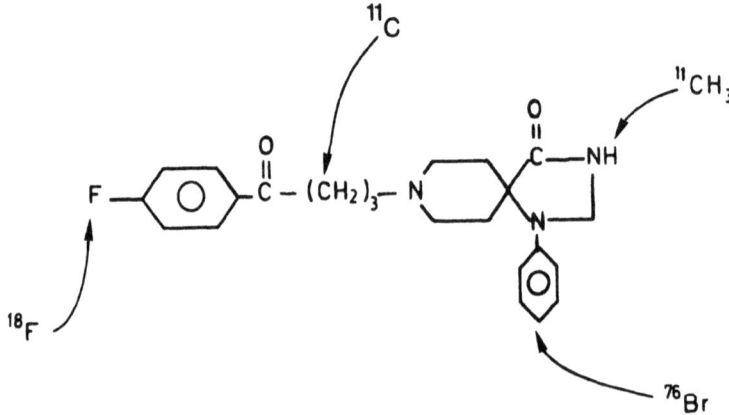

Fig. 2 - Various spiperone labellings

^{18}F seems to be the most logical choice because it leaves the structure of the molecule unchanged, but labelling with high specific activity ^{18}F is difficult technically. Possibilities then are to methylate the compound with $^{11}CH_3$ I or to introduce a radioactive bromine in the paraposition of the phenyl group. These two types of labelling are easier than with ^{18}F but the molecular structure is modified. Before an isotope is chosen it will therefore be necessary to find out what happens to the behaviour of the altered molecule in vivo. In the case of spiperone it seems that the the introduction of a bromine hardly changes the metabolism, whereas that of a methyl group speeds up penetration into the brain (increased lipophilicity) but without affecting the fixation specificity.

Once chosen, the molecule must be labelled. This chapter will only deal with the cases of ^{11}C, ^{13}N and ^{18}F. These isotopes being short-lived the synthesis must not take longer than 2,.5 to 3 times their half-life, i.e. 50 to 60 minutes for carbon 11 for example.

For these fast syntheses the isotope is first converted to a simple, but highly reactive form ; for carbon 11 this will be: $^{11}CH_3I$, $H^{11}CHO$, $^{11}COCl_2$, $(CH_3)_2 - ^{11}CO$, $H^{11}CN$; for nitrogen 13: $^{13}NH_4OH$; for fluorine : $^{18}F-F_2$, $H^{18}F$ or possibly, though less often, $^{18}F-CF_3OF$, $^{18}F-Xe\ F_2$, $^{18}F-NOF$. By the action of these radioactive compounds, known as precursors, on an adequate derivative it is possible to label amino acids, sugars, steroids, fatty acids or drugs. So many labelled molecules have now been obtained that only a few significant examples will be given here.

Amino acids

Amino acids have been labelled either by organic synthesis with ^{11}C and ^{18}F or by biosynthesis with ^{13}N or ^{11}C.
Carbon 11 has been introduced on the carbonyl group by adaptation of the Bücherer-Strecker method, whereby a hydantoin is prepared from KCN and an aldehyde or a ketone and then hydrolysed to give the corresponding amino acid (fig. 3).

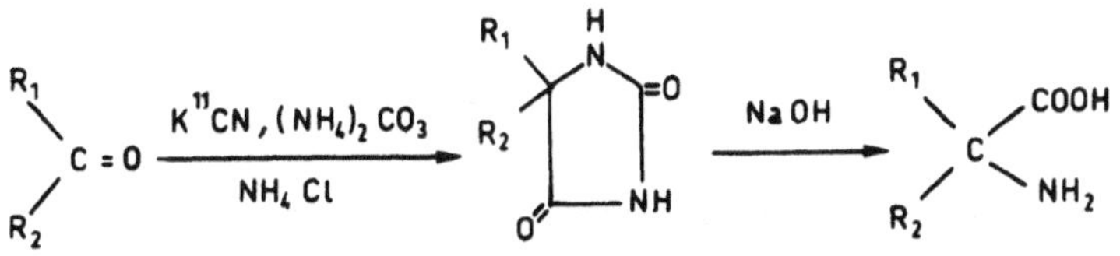

Fig. 3 - Bucherer-strecker synthesis

The first such synthesis to be performed was that of amino cyclo pentane carboxylic acid (ACPC) (1) (Fig. 4).

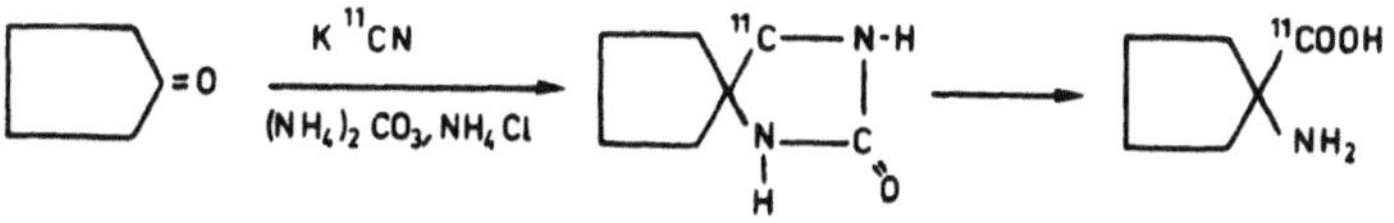

Fig. 4 - ^{11}C-ACPC synthesis

Many amino acids have since been prepared by this method : leucine, valine, tryptophane, phenylalanine and certain cyclic amino acids.

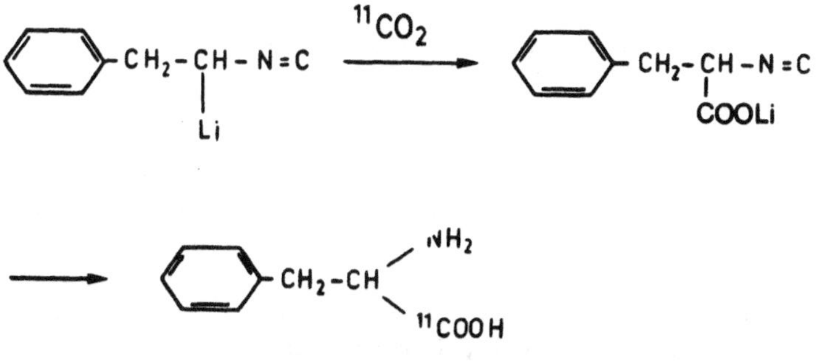

Fig. 5 - Phenylalanine synthesis

The carboxyl group can also be labelled by the action of $^{11}CO_2$ on a lithioisocyanide, a method already used to produce phenylalanine and DOPA (2) (Fig. 5).
A new method reported very recently (3) involves the action of $H^{11}CN$ on an aminosulphite (fig. 6) to give aminonitrile. Hydrolysis then leads to the amino acid :

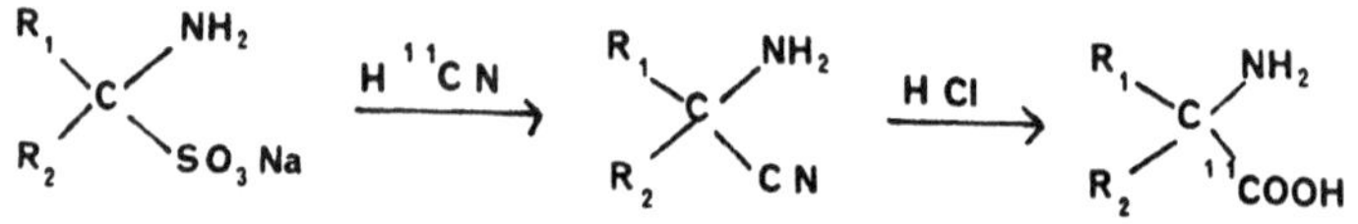

Fig. 6 - Amino acid synthesis from aminosulphite

All these methods supply the DL derivative. The resolution of the 2 isomers calls on chromatographic systems using mobile "chiral" phases. Thus D and L valine have been separated by high performance liquid chromatography and a mobile phase containing: solution of L proline, copper and sodium acetate (4).
Certain amino acids have been methylated with ^{11}C-methyl iodide. Methionine can thus be synthesized by action of $^{11}CH_3I$ on L-homocystein (5) (fig. 7).

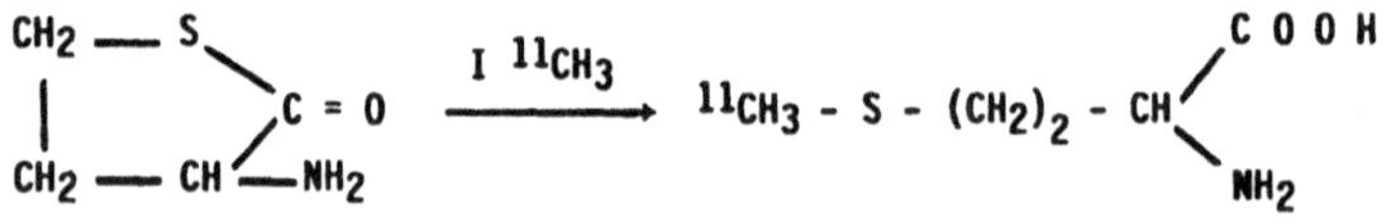

Fig. 7 - Methylation of L-homocystein

Amino acids have also been labelled by biosynthesis on the amino group with ^{13}N-ammonia (6). Whereas the original method called on enzymes in solution. The present trend is more and more towards their fixation on a solid support, which greatly reduces the risk of pyrogenic effects. This enzymatic technique has the advantage of giving only the biologically active isomer and has been used for the preparation of asparagine (fig. 8), glutamine, L-leucine, L-valine, L-alanine, L-methionine.

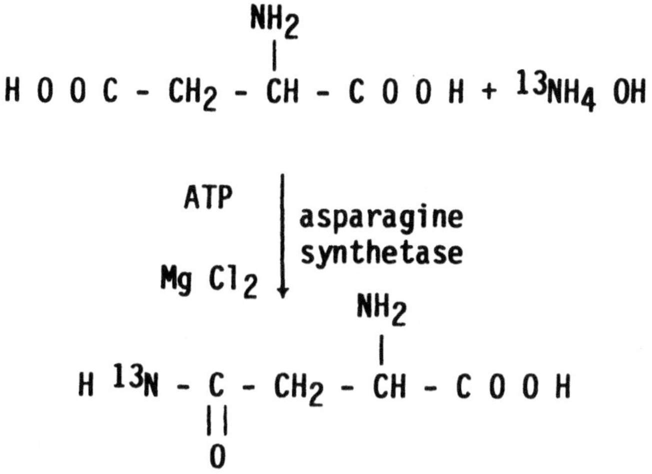

$$HOOC-CH_2-\underset{\underset{NH_2}{|}}{CH}-COOH + {}^{13}NH_4OH$$

$$\xrightarrow[MgCl_2]{ATP \quad | \quad \text{asparagine synthetase}}$$

$$H\,{}^{13}N-\underset{\underset{O}{||}}{C}-CH_2-\underset{\underset{NH_2}{|}}{CH}-COOH$$

Fig. 8 - Enzymatic synthesis of asparagine

Since 1972 certain amino acids have been fluorinated with ^{18}F by the Baltz-Schiemann reaction : an aromatic amine is first diazotized to form an aromatic diazonium tetrafluoroborate, then exchanged with ^{18}F. The ^{18}F-diazonium tetrafluoroborate is decomposed by heat to give the fluorinated compound.
This method has been applied to phenylalanine (7) (fig. 9) and tryptophane.

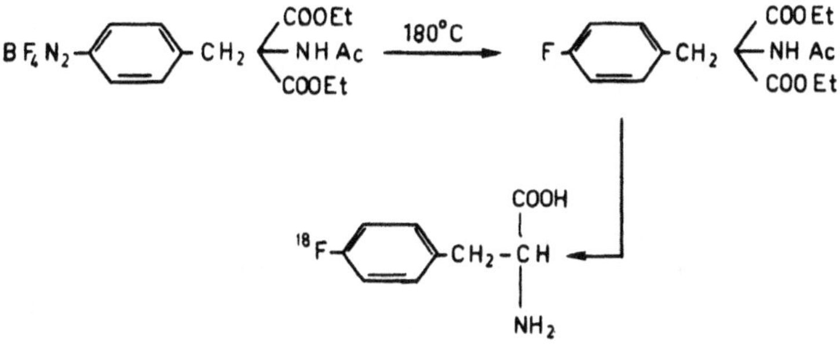

Fig. 9 - ^{18}F-phenylalanine synthesis

Unfortunately the yields and specific activities of the products obtained are low.
An ^{18}F atom may also be introduced into an aromatic nucleus by the use of ^{18}F-Xe F_2. ^{18}F-DOPA has been obtained by this method (8), which gives the L derivative of 6-^{18}F-fluoro-DOPA directly.

Most labelled amino acids have been used in research on the pancreatic function, detection of tumours, protein synthesis.

Sugars

As the main source of energy in the brain the first sugar to be explored in 1971 was glucose labelled biosynthetically with carbon-11 by means of leaves from higher plants. However the incorporation of $^{11}CO_2$ is actually much better if green unicellular algae are used under light in the presence of $^{11}CO_2$ (9).

Being too quickly metabolised this sugar was very soon replaced by deoxyglucose for in vivo metabolism measurements. Labelling was performed with either carbon-11 or fluorine-18, which seems preferable since the build-up in the brain takes 45 minutes to reach a maximum.

The ^{11}C-synthesis takes place by action of $H^{11}CN$ on 1 deoxy-2,3-4,5 di-o-isopropylidene-1-iodo-arabital. The nitrile obtained is hydrogenated (10) (fig. 10).

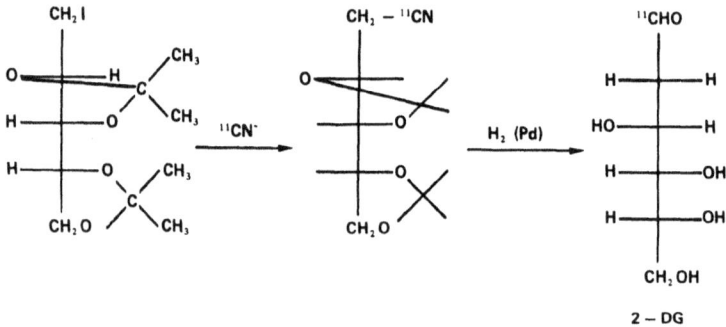

Fig. 10 - Synthesis of ^{11}C-deoxyglucose

^{18}F-labelled deoxyglucose is certainly the most widely used labelled molecule at the present time. It can be synthesized from ^{18}F as F_2 or F^-.

^{18}F-F_2 cannot be obtained carrier-free, which in the case of FDG is not a major disadvantage. The synthesis involves a reaction between ^{18}F in acetyl-hypofluorite form and tri-O-acetyl-glucal, followed by hydrolysis (11) (fig. 11).

This synthesis is only possible with fluorine 18 produced by a cyclotron and its use is therefore restricted. This is why it was necessary to find another method using fluorine in fluoride form, which can be supplied by a cyclotron but also by a reactor. The synthesis proposed takes place by reaction of ^{18}F-tetra ethyl ammonium fluoride on 4,6-benzylidene-1- methylamannopyranoside-2,3 cyclic sulphate (12) (fig. 12). The protection is then removed by boron tris-trifluoroacetate.

Other sugars such as 3-O-methyl-D-glucose, galactose, mannitol, glycerol have also been labelled with ^{18}F or ^{11}C.

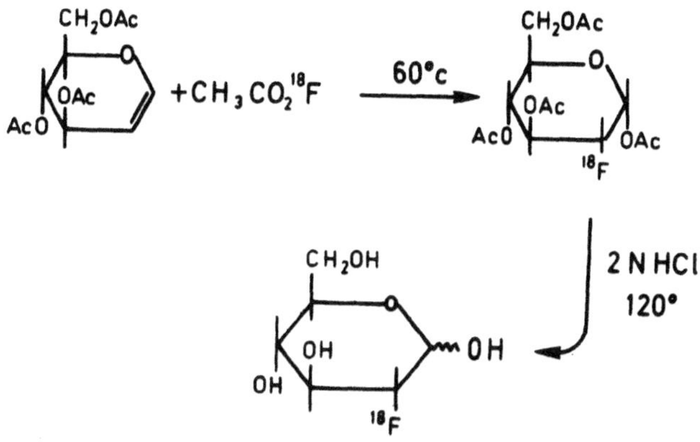

Fig. 11 - Synthesis of ^{18}F-FDG from acetyl hypofluorite

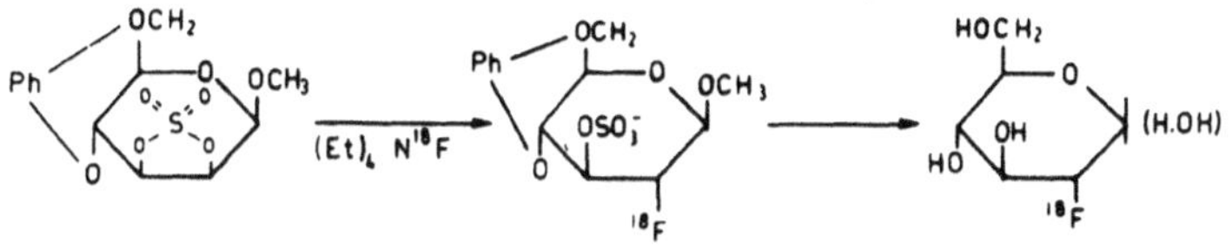

Fig. 12 - Synthesis of ^{18}F-2 FDG from $(Et)_2N^{18}F$

Fatty acids

Labelled fatty acids are useful for heart muscle metabolism studies. The chief example is ^{11}C-palmitic acid, obtained by the action of $^{11}CO_2$ on the corresponding grignard derivative. Although this compound is the most widely used in clinical routine its very fast metabolism is a disadvantage.
Attempts have therefore been made to find ^{11}C or ^{18}F analogues with longer residence times in the heart. Palmitic acid has thus been fluorinated with ^{18}F in the 6 or 7 position (14) and the 7-fluoro acid seems to be better retained.

Steroids

Compounds of this category can only be useful in medicine if obtained with a specific activity of at least 1 Ci per µ-mole. The first attempts at the ^{18}F labelling of hormones such as fluoro-estradiol made use of the Balz-Schiemann reaction, which yielded a low specific activity product (100 mCi/µmole).

Not until 1981 was a method found to prepare ^{11}C-labelled methyl testosterone of high enough specific activity : 1-2 Ci/ mole (15).

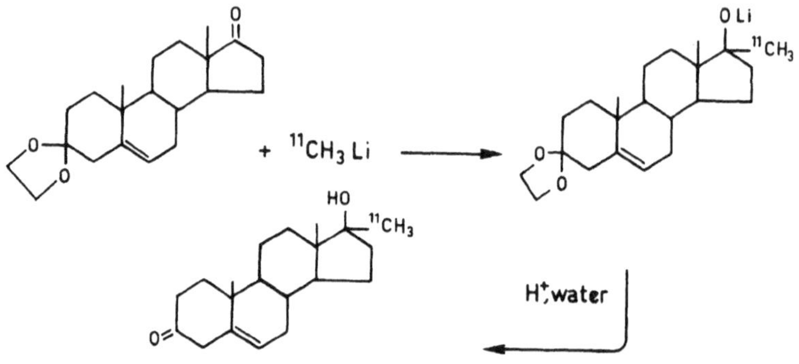

Fig. 13 - Synthesis of ^{11}C-17- methyl testosterone

This synthesis involves action of ^{11}C-methyl lithium on 3,3 ethylene dioxyandrost-5-ene-17 one (fig. 13).

Radiopharmaceuticals for receptor studies

For a long time the brain was one of the organs least explored in nuclear medicine. The possibility of obtaining radiopharmaceuticals able to cross the blood-brain barrier and the availability of instruments to follow in vivo their behaviour in the brain have given a fresh impetus to activities in this field.

Non-traumatic studies of psychiatric illnesses, formerly impossible in live subjects, can now be undertaken. ^{11}C and ^{18}F can be used to obtain high specific activity radiopharmaceuticals of major interest in the study of receptors suspected of involvement in certain diseases of the central nervous system.

Many ligands for both brain and heart receptors have already been obtained and are listed in table II.

Some examples of these radioligand syntheses will be given.

The ligand best suited for the study of brain muscarinic receptors would be quinuclidinyl-benzylate except that its ^{11}C labelling presents difficulties. Methylation of QNB with ^{11}CH$_3$I has been accomplished (16) but its transformation to quaternary ammonium prevents it from crossing the blood-brain barrier. However ^{11}C-MQNB is specific to heart muscarinic receptors (fig. 14).

RO 15 1788 has also been synthesized with ^{11}CH$_3$I for the study of benzodiazepine receptors (fig. 15) (17).

Spiroperidol has been synthesized (18) from H^{11}CN according to the diagram of fig. 16.

Receptor	Labelled ligand
Acetylcholine	MQNB-^{11}C Nicotine-^{11}C
Benzodiazepine	Flunitrazepam-^{11}C Diazepam-^{11}C RO 15 1788-^{11}C
Dopamine	Dopamine-^{11}C DOPA-^{11}C et ^{18}F Benperidol-^{18}F Spiroperidol-^{11}C et ^{18}F Haloperidol-^{18}F Pimozide-^{11}C Chlorpromazine-^{11}C Thioproperazine-^{11}C
Opiate	Etorphine-^{11}C Met-Entephaline-^{11}C Morphine-^{11}C Heroine-^{11}C
α-Noradrenergic	Norepinephrine-^{11}C Epinephrine-^{11}C
β-Noradrenergic	Propranolol-^{11}C Practolol-^{11}C
Serotonine	Serotonine-^{11}C O-Methylbufotenine-^{11}C Ketanserine-^{11}C

Table II : Labelled ligands for in vivo bindings studies

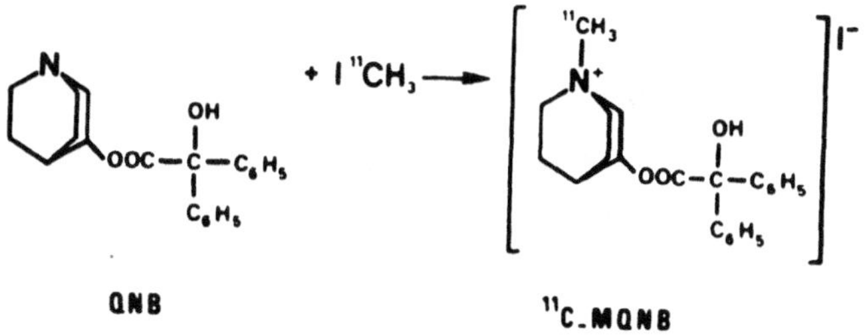

Fig. 14 - ^{11}C-MQNB synthesis

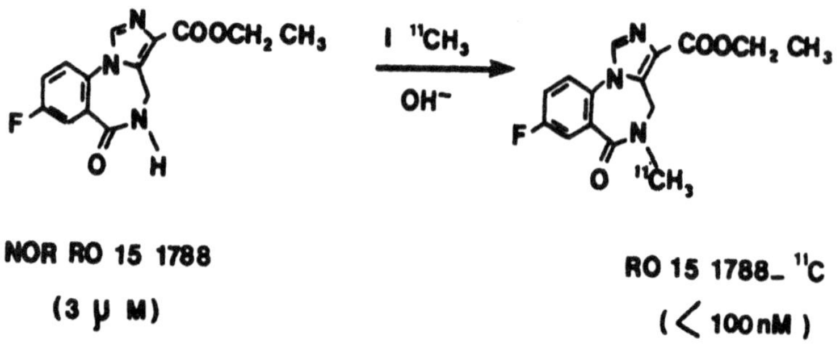

Fig. 15 - ^{11}C-RO 15 1788 Synthesis

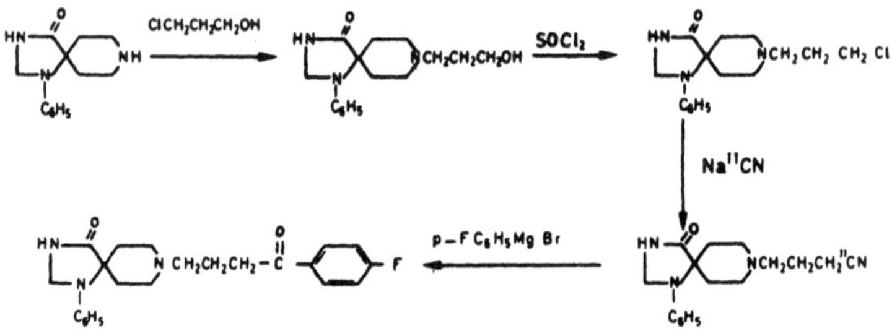

Fig. 16 - ^{11}C-Spiroperidol synthesis

^{11}C-acetone can be used to introduce carbon 11 into the isopropyl group of propranolol (fig. 17) (19).

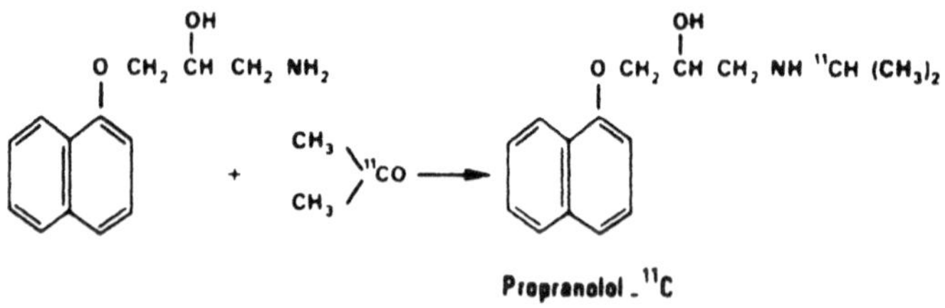

Fig. 17 - ^{11}C-propranolol synthesis

Finally another type of labelling by way of ^{11}C-phosgene leads to ketanserine (fig. 18) (20).

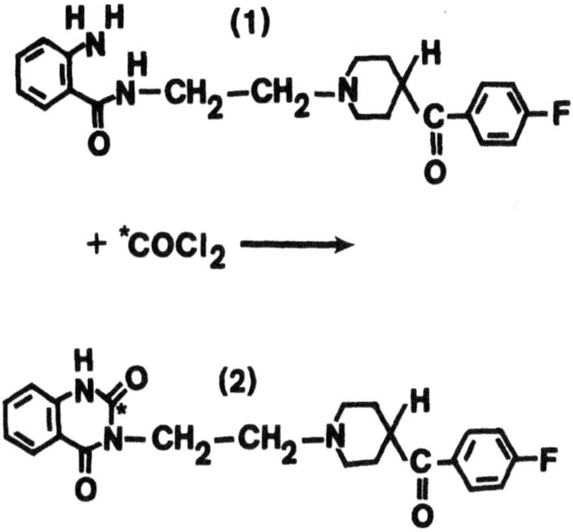

Fig. 18 - ^{11}C-ketanserine synthesis

β + isotopes other than ^{11}C, ^{13}N and ^{18}F

Oxygen 15 having a 2-minutes half-life can only be incorporated in very simple molecules : $^{15}O_2$, $C^{15}O_2$, $C^{15}O$, $H_2^{15}O$, $N_2^{15}O$. This isotope is chiefly used to measure the regional oxygen consumption in the brain.

17.5 h cobalt 55 has served for the labelling of radiopharmaceuticals used for tumour detection : ^{55}Co-bleomycine. Bromine 75 or 76 provides a useful label : its chemistry is simpler than that of fluorine and it is also so small that the molecule on which it is fixed is not denatured. This element has been incorporated in bromocryptine and bromospirosperidol.

While all the isotopes mentioned so far must be prepared on the site of their application some β + emitters, produced in the form of generators, can be used elsewhere.

Examples are ^{62}Zn-^{62}Cu, ^{52}Fe-^{52m}Mn, ^{82}Sr-^{82}Rb, ^{68}Ge-^{68}Ga generators. Of these isotopes ^{68}Ga alone is suitable for incorporation in a radiopharmaceutical : labelling of microspheres for regional blood flow determination or of protein (transferrin) for regional blood volume studies.

Problems raised by the use of β+ emitters : ^{11}C, ^{13}N, ^{18}F.

In the labelling of molecules with ^{11}C, ^{13}N or ^{18}F a number of problems must be solved. These isotopes are so short-lived that to obtain some tens of mCi of injectable product it is necessary to start from high initial radioactivities : a few hundred mCi to 1 Ci. This means working in shielded cells with automated or at least remotely controlled systems. Figure 19 shows such a system (21) in which all operations involved in a synthesis may be performed : activity trapping, heating, cooling, evaporation or addition of a solvent, transfer to a chromatograph injector.

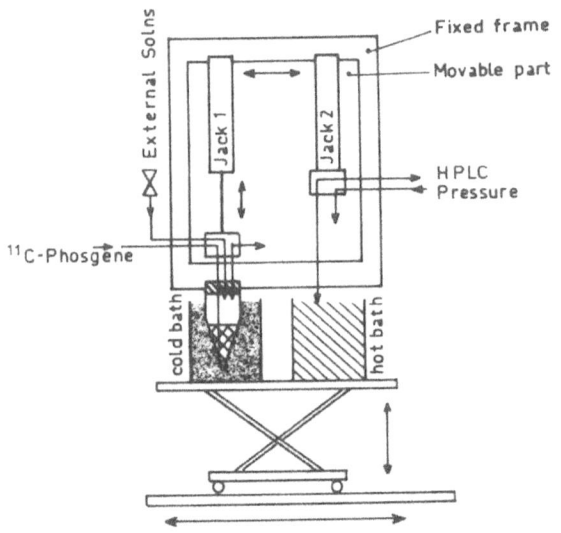

Fig. 19 - Remotely controlled apparatus for ^{11}C-synthesis

The purified radiopharmaceutical must be chemically and radiochemically pure. High performance liquid chromatography (HPLC) is an ideal purification method since it gives a purified and identified product and also its mass and specific activity.
Some restrictions apply however to the eluents used, which must be either directly injectable or highly volatile.
The radiopharmaceutical obtained must be sterile and apyrogenic. For routine use in man an excellent reproducibility of synthesis is necessary.

References

1. Hayes, R.L. et al. Carbonyl labeled ^{11}C-1-aminocyclopentane carboxylic acid, a potential agent for cancer detection. J.N.M. 17 (1976) 748-751.

2. Vaalburg, W. Preparation of carbon-11 labeled phenylalanine and phenylglycine by a new amino acid synthesis. Int. J. Appl. Radiat. Isotopes 27 (1976) 153-157.

3. Kubota, K. Tumor detection with carbon-11 labeled amino-acids. Eur. J. Nucl. Med. 9 (1984) 136-140.

4. Washburn, L.C. et al. Production of L-1-^{11}C valine by HPLC resolution. J. Nucl. Med. 23 (1982) 29-33.

5. Comar, D. et al. Labeling and metabolism of methionine methyl-^{11}C. J. Nucl. Med. 1 (1976) 11.

6. Gelbard, A.S. Biosynthetic methods for incorporating positron emitting radionuclides into compounds of biological interest. J. Lab. Compds Radiopharm. 18 (1981) 933.

7. Goulding, R.W. et al. The preparation of fluorine-18 labeled p-fluorophenylalanine for clinical use. Int. J. Appl. Radiat. Isotopes 23 (1972) 133.

8. Firnau, G. et al. Aromatic fluorination with Xenon-difluoride: L-3,4-dihydroxy-6-fluoro-phenylalanine. Can. J. Chem. 58 (1980) 1449.

9. Ehrin, E. et al. A convenient method for production of ^{11}C labeled glucose. J. Label. Compds Radiopharm. 17 (1980) 453.

10. Shiue, C.Y. et al. The synthesis of 1-^{11}C-2 deoxy-D glucose for measuring regional brain glucose metabolism in vivo. J. Nucl. Med. 19 (1978) 676.

11. Shiue, C.Y. et al. A new improved synthesis of 2-deoxy-2-^{18}F fluoro-D-glucose from ^{18}F labeled acetyl hypofluorite. J. Nucl. Med. 23 (1982) 899.

12. Tewson, T.T. Synthesis of No-carrier-added Fluorine-18 2 Fluoro-2-Deoxy-D Glucose. J. Nucl. Med. 24 (1983) 718.

13. Klein, M.S. et al. External assessment of myocardial metabolism with ^{11}C-palmitate in rabbit heart. Am. J. Physiol. : heart in Physiol. 6 (1980) 451.

14. Berridge, M.S. et al. The preparation of no carrier added fluorine-18 labeled analogue of palmitic acid, 7-^{18}F-palmitic acid for radiopharmaceutical use. J. Label. Compds Radiopharm. 18 (1981) 240.

15. Berger, G. et al. Synthesis of high specific activity of ^{11}C-17- methyl testosterone. Int. J. Appl. Radiat. Isotopes 32 (1981) 811.

16. Mazière, M. et al. ^{11}C-methiodide quinuclidinyl benzylate, a muscarinic antagonist for "in vivo" studies of myocardial muscarinic receptors. J. Radioanal. Chem. 76, 2 (1983) 305.

17. Mazière, M. et al. ^{11}C-RO 15 1788 et ^{11}C flunitrazepam, deux ligands pour l'étude par tomographie par positons des sites de liaison des benzodiazépines. C.R. Acad. Sc. Paris t 296 (1983) 871.

18. Fowler, J.S. et al. ^{11}C spirosperidol : synthesis, specific activity determination and biodistribution in mice. J. Nucl. Med. 23 (1982) 437.

19. Berger, G. et al. Synthesis of ^{11}C-propranolol. J. Radioanal. Chem. 74 (1982) 301.

20. Berridge M. et al. ^{11}C-labelled ketanserine : a selective serotonine S_2 antagonist. J. Label. Compds Radiopharm. XX (1982) 73.

21. Crouzel, C. et al. Remote, semi-automated synthesis of ^{11}C radiopharmaceuticals from ^{11}C phosgene. Int. J. Appl. Radiat. Isotopes 54, 11 (1983) 155P.

DISTRIBUTED MICROPROCESSOR AUTOMATION NETWORK FOR SYNTHESIZING
RADIOTRACERS USED IN POSITRON EMISSION TOMOGRAPHY

Jerome A. G. Russell, David L. Alexoff and Alfred P. Wolf

Chemistry Department, Brookhaven National Laboratory, Upton, NY

INTRODUCTION

This presentation describes the engineering concepts underlying an evolving distributed microprocessor network for automating the routine production synthesis of radiotracers used in Positron Emission Tomography brain studies at the Chemistry Department of the Brookhaven National Laboratory in New York. As an introduction to the distributed system, we will first present a brief overview of the PET method for measuring biological function, and then outline the general procedure for producing a radiotracer. Following this, the paper will then identify the several reasons for our automating the syntheses of these compounds, that is, it will define the major problems which we have encountered in carrying out the syntheses manually. Next, there will be a description of the distributed microprocessor network architecture chose and the rationale for that choice. Finally, we will speculate about how this network may be exploited by ourselves and others to extend the power of the PET method from the large university or National Laboratory to the biomedical research and clinical setting.

An Overview of Positron Emission Tomography

PET (Positron Emission Tomography) has become one of the most important quantitative imaging tools in nuclear medicine, because with PET the clinician and the medical investigator can now <u>measure</u> physiological processes going on in the tissues of living and intact men and animal subjects (1). In particular, using the PET method, scientists are identifying and measuring many of the processes by which the normal and abnormal brain works.

In a nuclear medicine imaging procedure, a radiotracer enters the subject's circulatory system either through an intravenous injection or by inhalation. PET, as does other nuclear medicine techniques, generates images of the spatial distribution of the radiotracer within an organ. But unlike most other nuclear medicine imaging methods, PET quantitates the distribution of the positron-emitting radiotracer. PET produces maps of the brain, for example, that depict the regional concentration of the radiotracer in units of nano curies per gram of tissue, not merely relative densities as a Gamma Camera or SPECT produce.

A radiopharmaceutical becomes a positron-emitting radiotracer by having one of its natural atoms replaced by a radionuclide. The most common of the radionuclides used in PET are ^{15}O, ^{13}N, ^{11}C and ^{18}F whose half-lives are 2.03, 10.3, 20.4 and 109.8 minutes, respectively (2). The short half-lives of these radionuclides offer a great advantage over those of typical radionuclides used in nuclear medicine for studying physiological function because even an initially very active tracer decays away quickly. This characteristic makes it possible to administer a high activity tracer, and then to measure the compound's distribution within the subject's brain tissue using a PET camera, while the counting rates are still high to obtain images of good statistical quality. The exposure to the subject is limited since the radioactivity of the tracer decays away rapidly. In other words, little radioactivity is retained in the tissue after the images have been measured.

In addition to having shorter half lives, the commonly used positron emitting radionuclide labels offer other advantages over the more commonly used isotopes in nuclear medicine. As has been noted, the radionuclides most commonly used as tracers are isotopes of oxygen, nitrogen, carbon and fluorine. Except for fluorine, these can be considered as the elements of life: atoms that are found in living tissue and most nutrients. Compounds including these atoms in their molecules can often participate in biochemical processes. Since living tissue can't distinguish between the normal atom and its isotope a chemist can synthesize a tracer in which the carbon, oxygen, nitrogen or a hydrogen atom is replaced by its positron-emitting isotope. Except for iodine, most radionuclides commonly used in nuclear medicine imaging don't actually participate in the usual metabolic pathways. Technitium and indium are not elements that are accepted by living systems.

But, we named fluorine as one of the useful radionuclides, and one might ask how fluorine fits into this category of atoms involved directly in life processes because, except for its being sequestered in the bones and teeth, this element is strange to most living cells. The answer is that when a chemist replaces a naturally occuring hydrogen atom in a compound with a fluorine atom, the living cell usually accepts the so-labeled molecule in much the same way as it does the natural one.

From the technical viewpoint of quantitative nuclear medicine imaging, the most important advantage that a positron-emitting radionuclide offers over the more commonly used single photon-emitting atom stems from the fate of a positron after it evolves from the decay of the radionuclide. Within a very short time after it has been generated, a positron is annihilated by encountering a nearby electron (a negatron). The masses of these particles are then converted to two photons (gamma rays) of 511 kilo-electron volts each. These photons travel in almost opposite directions to one another, that is their trajectories fall on a common line in space. Since the positron travels only a few millimeters in the tissue before its annihilation, this line passes very near to the point in the tissue at which the positron was generated. One can detect the decay, and hence the tracer activity, along a line by counting the number of times that a coincident-pair of photons are detected along that pathway. The time coincident photon detection of PET identifies <u>electronically</u> the line in space along which the activity decayed. To measure many such lines, one places a ring of coincidence detectors (the PET camera) around the subject's body - in our studies the head - in which tissue the positrons are being generated and annihilated. From an accumulation of the number of many coincident photons that are detected in a given time interval along each of the possible lines-in-space passing through the head, one can compute the two dimensional spatial distribution, a slice, of the radiotracer by applying a mathematical tomographic reconstruction algorithm to the measurements. The algorithms employed to reconstruct PET images are similar to those that reconstruct computed tomography (CT) x-ray images. Both imaging techniques involve reconstructing slice images from a set of planar profiles passing through the body.

In contrast, single photon nuclear medicine imaging such as by gamma cameras or single photon emission tomography (SPECT) achieves this collimation by interposing thick lead plates having parallel channels between the subject being studied and the photon detectors. Only photons traveling down a channel reach the detector. Photons traveling in any other direction are absorbed by the lead and thereby wasted. Accordingly, single photon cameras lack the sensitivity of PET cameras, and as well, their spatial resolution is degraded for objects beyond the collimator plate, that is at different depths in the organ. PET offers greater sensitivity, more uniform quantitative measurement of images, and less exposure to the subject than does any single photon method yet devised.

Major Steps in Producing a Positron-Emitting Radiotracer

The first step in a PET study begins with the bombardment of material in a target vessel by a beam of elementary particles from an accelerator, usually a cyclotron. There follows the transfer of the resulting radionuclide precursor to the synthesis apparatus. Then the radiotracer is synthesized and a sterile, pyrogen free pharmaceutical delivered to the PET. The tracer is administered to the subject and its regional concentration measured by PET. The last step is the interpretation of data on the resulting set of PET quantitative images by the team of scientists and physicians.

The new generation of medical cyclotrons, often called Baby Cyclotrons, are almost completely automated. In contrast to the large control room with a myriad of gauges, meters, and adjustment knobs that we recall from research cyclotron installations, the Baby Cyclotron has only a small panel from which a single technician selects the beam current and particle for the target bombardment. A microprocessor actually tunes the cyclotron and monitors beam, radiofrequency and vacuum parameters without human intervention. After a period of irradiation by the proton or deuteron beam, the original target material will have been converted to the desired precursor radionuclide, that is to ^{15}O, ^{13}N, ^{11}C or ^{18}F.

The atomic species or compound, now highly radioactive, is transferred from the cyclotron shielding vault to the radiotracer synthesis apparatus in the so-called Hot Lab. Whatever the particular configuration of this apparatus may be depends upon the kind of radiotracer to be produced and the particular synthesis procedure to be followed. The operations to be performed, whatever they are specifically, are typically those that are carried out in a chemistry laboratory. Severns and Hawk (3) identify these as LUO (Laboratory Unit Operations). The general categories of LUO's include: manipulation, liquid handling, separation, pulverization, weighing, measurement of physical properties, modifying and controlling the sample environment, using measurements to modify the procedure, conversion of raw data to useful information, and creating records for subsequent retrieval.

LUO's are building-block procedures from which an entire synthesis may be assembled. Once a module procedure works, it can be used repeatedly. For example, moving a liquid between vessels by creating a pressure difference works for a wide variety of vessels and liquids.

At this time, most radiopharmaceutical syntheses are performed manually by remote control, frequently confused with automation, by chemists and technicians.

Since personnel must manipulate highly radioactive materials during the synthesis, a primary consideration is the safeguarding against radiation exposure. The glassware, columns, evaporators, piping, heaters and sensors for a synthesis are assembled within a heavily-shielded lead box for that reason.

Operators open and close valves, or reposition components inside of the box by means of mechanical manipulators while they view the apparatus through a thick leaded glass window. Reagents are added to reaction vessels from syringes mounted outside of the box, and liquids are transferred from one vessel to another within the box by positioning valves to cause a pressure difference to exist between the vessels.

Once the chemical synthesis has been completed, the radiotracer product, now appropriately diluted with saline for administration to the PET subject, is forced through a bank of micropore filters into a sterile collection ampule or syringe. The filters remove organisms and pyrogenetic agents as well. Samples of the product are withdrawn and immediately assayed for chemical purity, absolute activity, and specific activity.

A growing Demand for Radiotracers for PET Studies

The current literature cites over 200 positron-emitting tracers with application to PET studies. Many being used routinely each day in more than sixty PET installations throughout the world (2). Even though the variety of tracers is numerous, the most widely employed today are the analogues of glucose, 2-deoxy-2[^{18}F]fluoro-D-glucose (^{18}FDG) and 2-deoxy-D-[1-^{11}C]glucose (^{11}CDG) for measuring regional tissue glucose metabolic rates (4,5). Also widely used are the compounds of oxygen-15, H_2O, CO, and O_2, for determining regional blood flow, blood volume and oxygen consumption (6). Recently available neuroreceptor binding drugs (7) are being applied to study neurotransmitter-receptor physiology by PET in the continuing effort to understand biochemical processes of normal and abnormal behavior. The demand to produce large quantities of these labeled compounds to support both research and clinical diagnostic program grows each day as the PET method proves its promises. The primary obstacle to extending the PET method from the research and development laboratory where it is now practiced to the setting of the major medical institution is the synthesis of radiotracers. As has been stated, Medical Cyclotrons are now automated and simple to operate. Modern commercially-available PET cameras are easy to operate, and the quantitative image processing of the raw profile data into physiological maps proceeds mostly without human intervention. Only the synthesis of the radiotracers continues to be carried out by chemists and technicians.

The Problems of Manually-Performed Syntheses

Before describing the distributed microprocessor system for automating routine production of radiotracers, let us identify the major problems we intend to solve by that automation.

Since the half-life of the positron-emitting nuclides is short and because the activity of the labeled tracer must be sufficient to obtain high statistical quality PET images, the synthesis must begin with a high activity precursor, and it must proceed rapidly and efficiently. It follows that the problems include working with high activities, working quickly, and working carefully so as not to waste the compound during the synthesis. The high activities present a risk of chronic radiation exposure when one works with the compounds every day.

Even though the syntheses are complex and demand skill, good judgment and vigilance, carrying them out day after day is boring, and boredom promotes human errors. For example, reagent supplies can become exhausted during a synthesis because we forget to check. A procedural step can be neglected, or we can even damage the apparatus by a clumsy movement of the mechanical manipulator. Also, not to be disregarded is the time the technical staff must spend teaching new staff members to perform old syntheses, and to learn new ones themselves.

Clearly, a major problem in routine radiotracer production, as it is mostly managed today, is the waste of professional staff in their performing of robot-like operations. Since all of the steps in a synthesis can be defined in terms of LUO's, and because each LUO can be automated, we believe that the manually performed steps involved in routine syntheses can be replaced by automated physical modules, and that these modules can then be integrated into a totally automated system.

AN AUTOMATED RADIO SYNTHESIS SYSTEM

There are several ways one can automate a complex process such as a radiotracer synthesis. A primitive approach is to hard-wire a set of discrete components to perform a single process. An apparatus resulting from this approach would be much like an American Pinball Game: it would play one game and would require rewiring to change the rules of that game. This style of automation has rarely been applied to radiopharmaceutical synthesis, because it is inherently inflexible, complex and expensive to manufacture. Finding a fault in a pinball machine is a nightmare for an engineer.

To avoid the pitfalls of the hard-wired approach to implementing a process control system, system designers began to apply the mainframe digital computer. The superiority of this concept was, and still is, that with a stored program computer, numerical and logical manipulations to carry out the process can be designed by programming and then implemented on general purpose hardware. Developing and refining a computer-controlled process becomes mostly a software engineering job instead of anelectronics circuitry and mechanical engineering one. A problem encountered in using this kind of automation is the expense of acquiring, operating, and maintaining a mainframe computer. The high expenses were, and still are, spread among several users by timesharing the single computer, but this is achieved at the cost of operating system complexity and increased system response times. Even more important than the expenses, is the reliability of a shared large computer. Since one or more processes are controlled by a single computer and its software, any failure will compromise all of the applications. Computer hardware was costly but no longer a direct consequence of LSI (Large Scale Integration) semiconductor chips.

LSI minicomputers can be economically dedicated to a single process thereby avoiding the complexity of timesharing software and the relative unreliability of electronic circuitry wired from discrete components. LSI chips cost less, operate more reliably, and are usually faster than their discrete component counterparts. In spite of the advantage offered by the procedure-dedicated hardware approach of automation, the minicomputer still requires a multi-tasking operating system and still suffers some degree of the conflicts which plague the timeshared mainframe controller. Nevertheless, the few successful radiotracer synthesis systems that exist today, for example that of (8), employ a single minicomputer as a multitasking controller. As successful and economical as the dedicated minicomputer is, once again, new semiconductor technology, very Large Scale Integration, makes possible an even more modular approach.

Distributed Microprocessor Architecture

Our approach to automation is based on a system architecture that is an extension of the process-dedicated minicomputer: a network of elementary subtask-dedicated microprocessors. In this architecture, individual microprocessors take responsiblity for elementary subtasks. For example, one microprocessor in a network can control and monitor the valves for purging, filling, and emptying a precursor target. That is the limit of its responsibility. This processor receives its command to begin, and the parameters it needs from another microprocessor. It is on the periphery of a network of other processors. The target controller, for example, is connected locally to the valves, and pressure gauges of the target being controlled and it controls the apparatus by executing the program that it holds in its ROM (Read Only Memory). In modern computer vernacular, this ROM program is called firmware in distinction to the terms hardware and software. Another peripheral microprocessor might control the temperature cycling of a reaction vessel, or it could direct a manipulator such as does the Zymark Robot (3,9).

Each task-dedicated module receives commands and data from another module, and in return sends measurements and its task status to other modules. Modules communicate with one another to form an integrated system.

There are three kinds of basic communication linkages over which modules in a distributed intelligence system can exchange information (10). The simplest involves a central microprocessor module having individual data connections to one or more satellite modules - a star pattern. The success of this network depends upon the central module's being able to intercept, interpret and reroute messages to and from the satellites.

A second network communication scheme is one in which every module has a direct line to every other module. In this configuration, command and integration of the network can be vested in either one of the modules or among several. A problem is that each module must include a hardware and software interface for each fellow-processor.

The third communication linkage is the data highway to which each module is attached. The familiar IEEE 488 protocol (11) is an example of a data pathway as is the CAMAC bus. Each microprocessor in a network is attached to the data highway through an interface. A module places a message intended for another module onto the data highway in a packet. The packet includes the destination module's address. The data highway method lends itself to fiber optics, microwave or coaxial cable transmission lines through which message packets may be conducted at very high speeds over a single bit channel.

We have chosen an architecture that combines the first and second network scheme communication linkages. A coordinating microprocessor (IBM PC) exchanges information with task-dedicated peripheral modules (Z-80 STD Bus crates) over individual full-duplex serial input-output cables using either the EIA (Electronics Industries Association) RS-232 or RS-427 protocols, a common way that computers send character codes to terminals. In addition to the link with the IBM PC, a peripheral module is connected directly to the sensors and effectors in the apparatus through STD (Simple to Design) Bus interfacing cards. A peripheral module resides physically near to the apparatus it controls, and the PC is close to the personnel who oversee the synthesis. It is through the PC that the system operator initiates a synthesis and monitors its progress. This configuration minimizes the amount of signal wiring that must be installed in a laboratory because the numerous channels from the microprocessor to the apparatus are short and the EIA RS-232 connections only require double twisted pair cables.

Eventually, when the automated synthesis system is extended to control several syntheses simultaneously, and when the synthesis network exchanges information with the PET scanner and the cyclotron, some kind of PC-to-PC communication linkage must be established. Perhaps the data rates and volumes will require a data highway link, but more likely a serial EIA RS-232 or RS-422 connections among the PCs will still be adequate.

Hardware Engineering

As has been described, the radiotracer synthesis system is a growing network of STD Bus microprocessors clustered about an IBM PC coordinating computer. Our choice of these elements was based on commercial availability, reliability, and simplicity of use. For example, STD Bus Z-80 microprocessor boards and crates are supplied by over 200 companies in the United States, and they are manufactured in high volume for industrial and military applications. The Z-80 microprocessor chip itself is over 10 years old, but is still well supported. As well, several of us know how to program it, and the Z-80 commands are subsets of the more modern 8086, 8088 and 80286 microprocessors, an advantage should we wish to update the peripheral modules. Each Z-80 microprocessor-based peripheral module is housed in a STD Bus mother board crate, and along with the single board computer are the interface boards and power supplies.

Since so many boards are available for interfacing, we have needed to build only a few signal-conditioning circuits. These were engineered to the STD Bus standards, and are installed in the STD Bus crate.

The Z-80 single board microprocessor includes the ROM for the crate program, read-write random access memory (RAM), three timers, and the chips to manage the STD Bus. A typical crate includes the processor and several digital input-output boards such as those manufactured by PROLOG, and an analogue signal interface. A typical peripheral crate includes the following PROLOG (12) digital boards.

7804 Z80 - Single board microprocessor
7504 TRIAC - Optically isolated ac power switches
7301 RS-232 - Serial input-output interface
7602 TTL - Parallel output
7603 TTL - Parallel input
7501 DC - Driver card, open collector power transistors

Incoming analog signals are digitized and placed on the STD Bus by a Data Translation (13) DT-2722, and the Z-80 sends analogue signals to the external apparatus through a DT-2726.

The homemade analogue-conditioning boards convert signals from thermistors or thermocouple probes, from strain gauge bridges, position potentimeters, and from radiation detectors into voltages suitable for being measuring by the DT-2722 analogue-to-digital conversion cards.

One other module must be mentioned in this description of the automation network, it is the Spectracom 8170 (14) synchronized time-of-day master clock and its slaves. This clock broadcasts a time-of-day and date message each second over an independent RS-488 network to several stations throughout the entire cyclotron-PET project. A coordinating PC in the tracer synthesis network reads this clock message through one of its Serial Input Ports.

The IBM PC coordinating processor hardware includes the standard monochome display as well as a TV graphic display. The PC also includes six Serial Input-Output Ports, two 5-1/4" floppy disks and 256 kbytes of RAM.

Software Engineering

The software supporting the distributed microprocessor radiotracer synthesis system is, as is the hardware, modular and task-dedicated. We have carried the concept of modularity beyond the hardware-identifiable levels down into the structure of the subprocedures themselves with the intention that the system, physical and algorithmic, will be assemblies of simple building blocks. In other words, we have attempted to engineer the system in the fashion of a modern structured computer program.

The programs executed by the peripheral microprocessors are written in MOSTEK Z-80 assembly language (15); the IBM PC coordinating processor code is written in Microsoft BASIC (16). As is well known, the advanced BASIC available for a PC does not lend itself to structured programming, but by adhering to a set of Programming Standards (17), we have been able to achieve a well understood structure (18) in all programs. The Standards identify the naming of variables, specify how values are exchanged between procedures and how one allocates specific blocks of line numbers for often-used building block procedures. Also, by adopting a structure of IF-GOTO, ELSE GOTO in the PC BASIC, we have been able to simulate the IF-THEN-ELSE structures of more modern languages. The WHILE-WEND construct of PC BASIC, and its relaxed variable naming restrictions also help in the quest for structure.

Because of its conversational nature, we find that new procedures and programs can be developed more quickly by running them initially in interpretive BASIC than by employing the traditional sequence of EDIT - COMPILE - LINK - RUN while testing and debugging. Once a new program meets its design specifications while executing under interpretive BASIC, it can be compiled (19). The resulting machine code will execute much faster and use less memory storage space than the interpretive version. The IBM PC operates under Microsoft DOS-2.1. There is no operating system in the Z-80s.

Other provisions in the Programming Standards for the project are concerned with data quality. For example, any procedure (or subroutine) that receives a value from another procedure - or from those rare instances of an operator's keyboard entry - tests the range of that datum. A valid numerical value usually falls within an absolute or a relative prescribed range of values. For example, the cyclotron can't develop 200 milliamperes of beam current. An entry requesting that current is rejected. A reaction vessel doesn't hold three liters of a precursor. Strings of numbers must not include letters of the alphabet.

There are other examples of how the programming helps to insure data quality. As an example, a peripheral processor verifies that the analogue signal it sends to a heater controller (or any other device) in the chemistry apparatus, is the intended magnitude. It does this by measuring that signal level through its analogue-to-digital conversion channel. To carry the self-checking concept further, since the electrical signal sent to the heater controller is supposed to raise the temperature of a vessel, the peripheral processor can also monitor that vessel's temperature, just to be sure that the heater and thermistor are working properly. We could cite many other examples of this quality control, but the underlying principle is that the system closes a feedback loop on any process it is controlling whether it be an algorithmic or a physical one.

Each physical module sends the results of its own performance checks and to its task-dedicated controlling module. For example, a peripheral processor tests the electrical continuity between two pins of each of its cable connectors to insure that the plug has been inserted. It measures its own power supply voltages, and tests its own memory and microprocessor chip. These self-checks are a continual background job for the modules. The success or failure of each such test is recorded in the status part of the message sent to the PC, and the PC logs its own status periodically on a disk file.

Several of these algorithmic checking procedures are more complex than the ones we have just described. For example, the gas target handling peripheral processor checks for gas leaks in the vessels and piping by analyzing a series of pressure measurements that have been acquired for a 30 second interval after the target has been filled. None of the pressure data points may fall outside of a predetermined pressure range if the valves have been positioned correctly and no leaks exist.

System Activity Log and Restart Files: Each coodinating PC writes a system status file on a floppy disk every two minutes during a synthesis. The ensemble of these files provide data entries for a detailed log of the process. The most recently recorded file also helps the system or the human operator to restart the synthesis after an abnormal interruption such as from a temporary power failure. The time-annotated log of system states and measurements also are valuable for trouble-shooting the procedures of a synthesis and for refining the control system. When things go wrong, this log makes for a useful postmortem.

Menu Driven Control: The automated system carries on dialogues with the chemistry staff operators through the display screens and keyboard entries at a PC coordinating microprocessor. For example, to begin a synthesis, the operator selects the tracer to be produced, the procedure to be followed, and the conditions under which it is to be performed from a series of plain-language menus. As well, once the process has begun, the operator can monitor the current state of that synthesis by viewing a continually updated schematic representation of the process on the graphics display screen. The operator can also request that specified numeric values describing the process be posted on the text screen.

Communication between the PC and an operator is not limited to menu selection alone. When a manual procedure must be performed in which the operator must participate, such as calibrating a transducer or carrying out certain steps in the synthesis yet to be automated, the system guides the operator through an interactive plain-language prompting protocol. This step-by-step prompting minimizes what an operator must learn about using the system and insures that no part of a procedure is neglected.

Simple Remote Control: A rudimentary manual mode of performing a set of steps is also available to the operator for a backup use when some fault has occured or as a tol for developing a new procedure. In this mode, the coordinating and peripheral microprocessors serve only as a manually operated panel for controlling the valves and other devices in the synthesis apparatus. The screen display indicates the positions of all valves and it also posts any measurements being made by the peripheral processor. While monitoring this display, the operator can control valves and set points by entering appropriate keystrokes at the PC. To install this kind of remote operation costs far less than does building the more conventional hard wired remote controller, and the rudimentary system lends itself more readily to the ultimate automation of the synthesis than does the hard-wired panel. All of the peripheral and communication wiring will already be in place when automation begins.

Alarms: Warning and alarm messages appear on the lowest two rows of the text screen. No other messages appear in that region. To signal the staff that a message has been posted, the PC emits a set of annunciating sounds (the command BEEP in BASIC). In the coming months, we will test the usefulness of a speech synthesis board for the PC. This PC compatible board uses a VOTRAX phoneme chip to generate both voice alarm messages and to "read back"keyboard-entered values as a help to the operator. It is likely that this embellishment provide us with more fun than usefulness.

Application Programs: The application programs that actually direct and monitor the steps in a synthesis are a set of modular procedures. Most of these are simple and involve little mathematical sophistication. For example, the programs in ROM executed by one of the peripheral processors acquire analogue and digital measurements from the chemistry apparatus, control valves and other effecting devices, verify that subsystem is functioning properly (as we have already discusseed), and communicate with the PC coordinating microprocessor. We designed a general purpose peripheral processor that performs this task. It measures 16 (external and internal) analogue signals and 16 digital states, sends to the apparatus 8 analogue signals and 32 digital states. While this continuous measuring and sending is proceeding it also waits for a message to arrive from the coordinating PC over a Serial Input-Output channel. That message instructs the peripheral processor to update the settings of the digital and analogue output signals, and once, the values have been updated, the peripheral processor returns a message to the PC describing the newly-measured output signal values (presumably the latest set) and the most recent sensor measurements from the apparatus being controlled. Whether the peripheral microprocessor controls 32 valves or none, it still executes the same program and must send the same message format. The advantage of having these general purpose modules on the shelf is that a new system or an expansion of an existing one can be implemented in hardware and software in the time necessary to make the electrical connections.

In another version of a peripheral processor, the Z-80 crate subsystem replaces a commercial temperature controller. In this role, its task is to raise a reaction vessel to a predetermined temperature as (measured by a thermistor). To do this the peripheral processor measures the thermistor temperature and controls the electrical power delivered to a heating element. The instantaneous power applied is computed by a PID (Proportional-Integral-Derivative) control algorithm (20). The coefficients in the PID algorithm can be trimmed dynamically by a program to take into account the variety of masses that may need to be heated.

EXPECTATIONS FOR THE SYSTEM

A short-term expectation for this project is that once the synthesis of the basic cerebral metabolic function tracers (FDG, CDG, and the oxygen-15 compounds) has been completely automated, that final obstacle to bringing the PET method into major clinical centers will have been removed. Also, because in building the system to produce these compounds, the basic communications and controls modules will have been defined for synthesizing other positron-emitting pharmaceuticals. By reconfiguring the already-implemented LUOs, the hardware and software task dedicated modules for producing new physiological tracers can be easily integrated into the existing network.

The longer range expectations involve connecting the distributed microprocessor synthesis network to the cyclotron controller and to the PET to form a totally integrated PET research and diagnostic facility. It is a replica of this system that we believe could be installed in a medical-research institution without the need for the highly-specialized staff of chemists and technicians.

Taking advantage of our automated facility, we at BNL will be able to produce large quantities of high-quality radiotracers for both ourselves and for extramural PET studies as well so that regional medical institutions will then be able to measure organ function in subjects with their own PET scanners, using the radiotracers produced at the BNL Center. The precedence and feasibility for such an extra-mural use of BNL radiotracers is well established. For several years, the BNL Chemistry

Department has air transported FDG to the National Institutes of Health, to the University of Pennsylvania, and to Massachusetts General Hospitals. Using a helicopter, we have even delivered CDG to the State University of New York at Stony Brook. For studies involving very short half-life radionuclide tracers, such as oxygen-15 and nitrogen-13, a regional medical institution would refer subjects to the BNL Center for the PET measurements, and then analyze the resulting images at their home laboratory.

The network can easily be installed into a clinical center whose patient care program includes using the PET method as a diagnostic aide and to track the results of therapy. Only those radiotracers of proven clinical usefulness need to be automated by attaching the task-dedicated modules to the supporting network.

SUMMARY

We have proposed a way to minimize the involvement of professional staff members in the routine production of positron-emitting radiotracers by assigning the required operations to automated apparatus controlled by a network of task-dedicated microprocessor modules. The modules are assembled from general purpose microprocessor components and commercially available hardware interfaces. The task-dedication of a microprocessor module is achieved both by virtue of the kinds of sensors and effectors to which it is connected, and by the software procedures it executes.

ACKNOWLEDGEMENT

This research was carried out at Brookhaven National Laboratory under contract DE-AC02-7600016 with the U. S. Department of Energy and supported by its Office of Health and Environmental Research and also supported by the National Institutes of Health Grant NS-15380.

REFERENCES

1. Phelps, M.E. and Mazziotta, J.C. Positron Emission Tomography: Human Brain Function and Biochemistry. Science 228 (1985) 799-809.

2. Wolf, A.P. Special Characteristics and Potential for Radiopharmaceuticals for Positron Emission Tomography. Seminars in Nuclear Medicine 11 (1981) 2-12.

3. Severns, M.L. and Hawk, G.L. "Medical Laboratory Automation Using Robotics" in NATO ASI Series Robotics and Artificial Intelligence, M. Brady, L.A. Gerhardt and H.F. Davidson, Eds. Springer-Verlag (1984) pp. 633-643.

4. Shiue, C.-Y., Salvadori, P.A., Wolf, A.P., Fowler, J.S. and MacGregor, R.R. A New Improved Synthesis of 2-Deoxy-2-[^{18}F]Fluoro-D-Glucose from ^{18}F-Labeled Acetyl Hypofluorite. Journal of Nuclear Medicine 23 (1982) 899-903.

5. MacGregor, R.R., Fowler, J.S., Wolf, A.P., Shiue, C.-Y., Lade, R.E. and Wan, C.N. A Synthesis of 2-Deoxy-D-[1-^{11}C]-Glucose for Regional Metabolism Studies. Journal of Nuclear Medicine 22 (1981) 800-803.

6. Raichle, M.E., Martin, W.R.W., Herscovitch, M. A., et al. Brain Blood Flow Measured with Intravenous $H_2^{15}O$. Journal of Nuclear Medicine 24 (1983) 790-798.

7. Arnett, C.D., Fowler, J.S., Wolf, A.P. and MacGregor, R.R. Specific Binding of [^{11}C]Spiroperidol in Rat Brain In Vivo. Journal of Neurochemistry 40 (1983) 455-459.

8. Iwata, R., Ido, T., Takahashi, T. and Monma, M. Automated Synthesis System for Production of 2-Deoxy-2-[^{18}F]Fluoro-D-Glucose with Computer Control. International Journal of Applied Radiation and Isotopes 35 (1984) 445-454.

9. Zymark Corporation, Hopkinton, MA 01748. Welch, M., et al. demonstrated at 32nd Annual Meeting of the Society of Nuclear Medicine, June 2-5, 1985 in Houston, Texas.

10. Bibbero, R.J. Microprocessors in Instruments and Control. John Wiley and Sons, (1977) pp. 255-257.

11. Clune, T.R. Interfacing for Data Acquisition. Byte 10:2 (1985) 269-282.

12. PRO-LOG Corporation, Monterey, CA 93940. Series 7000 STD Bus Technical Manual (1984).

13. Data Translation, Inc., Marlborough, MA 01752.

14. SPECTRACOM Corporation, East Rochester, NY 14445.

15. Z-80 Programming Manual (1982), Mostek Corporation, Carrollton, TX 75006.

16. BASIC by MICROSOFT, Version 2.10 Personal Computer Reference Library. International Business Machines Corporation (1982) Boca Raton, FL 33432.

17. Nagin, P.A. and Ledgard, H.F. Program Standards, Chapter IV, Hayden Book Co., Inc. (1978) 90-96.

18. Kernighan, B.W. and Planger, P.J. "Structure" in The Elements of Programming Style. McGraw-Hill Book Co. (1974).

19. Basic Compiler for the IBM Personal Computer by Microsoft. IBM Corporation, Boca Raton, FL (1982).

20. Bibbero, R.J. Microprocessors in Instruments and Control. John Wiley and Sons (1977) 157-168.

DESIGN ASPECTS OF INSTALLATION FOR PET RADIOCHEMISTRY

Piero A. Salvadori

C.N.R., Institute of Clinical Physiology, Pisa, Italy

INTRODUCTION

The uniqueness of the information on in vivo metabolism and biochemistry that can be obtained from PET scanning has brought this imaging technique to the attention of the scientific community as one of the most promising tools for the assessment of biological parameters.
Radiochemists on one side, through the production of new radiotracers and the improvement of radiosynthetic techniques, and physicists on the other side through the enhancement of detector performance, have given the physician a tool which, at least in principle, can provide unlimited information.
Continuous improvement in the quality and level of this information has given rise to a continually increasing number of PET installations despite the complexity of their organization and the cost of the required instrumentation.
A PET installation has in fact for many years been a very big commitment for even large resarch institutes and only highly selected scientific environments could afford the price in terms of skilled scientific staff and technical support. The recently increasing interest of industry in this technique plays an important role in the diffusion and increase in the number of PET installations: over many years the complex instrumentation for the production of radiopharmaceuticals, labelled with the appropriate positron emitting radionuclide, had to be home-made. Recently, a high degree of engineering has been reached in the basic components of the production lines of radiopharmaceuticals. It ranges from the cyclotron (in particular small cyclotrons or baby-cyclotrons accelerating protons to 16-17 MeV and deuterons to 8-10 MeV) to the targetry and radiogas processing systems and, very recently, even to automated "black boxes" for the synthesis and purification of radiopharmaceutical products. All these parts

can be bought from different companies with guaranteed performance.

The availability of the components of the PET installation, in particular the radioisotope production and processing units, which are already compatible with each other and logically interfaced, is of primary importance. The first consequence is that systems can be selected for the specific research to be developed. It is also evident that the structure of the installation can be carefully assessed and tailored to this purpose. The result is that these installations provide the best solution for rather small multidisciplinary biomedical institutions or medical centres which , otherwise, would never be able to start a PET project. For obvious reasons the installation of the PET centre inside the medical environment is the most attractive solution as it accomplishes a perfect link between medical facilities and the PET laboratory. However, a discussion of the problems to be solved to put it into practice are relevant, both for achieving the best organization of the site and for handling the safety problems connected with the operation of the cyclotron and radiochemistry facilities. Even if we are dealing with low energy machines, there are still many points which deserve careful evaluation. This paper is thus intended to give some details of the approach which can be used for the installation of a PET centre inside a hospital, focusing on those problems which arise from radiochemistry needs, namely cyclotron and radiopharmaceutical chemistry facilities.

SITE-SELECTION CONSIDERATIONS

It is evident that before considering the constitution of a PET centre it is necessary to have first solved the question: what are we going to study? The direct consequence of the answer to this question in fact decides the structure of the whole installation. If we limit the problem to the centres interested in metabolic studies feasible with the positron-emitting "physiological" radionuclides C-11, O-15, N-13 and F-18, which are the most commonly used in this field, the cyclotron more frequently encountered is the babycyclotron.

In a certain sense this machine represents the baseline of the radioisotope production units for PET centres which are intended to make metabolic studies and bigger cyclotrons are usually considered in those environments where gamma emitting radionuclides are also used or where generators are produced or where time-sharing of the cyclotron is envisaged e.g. for production of radionuclides for multi-centre use or commercial purposes.

The choice of cyclotron size immediately defines a large

number of variables both from the point of view of the site lay-out and from the point of view of radiation-protection. However there are some points which should always be kept in mind:

Logistic: - site accessibility;
- connection to other facilities both medical and non-medical;
- compactness;
- possibility of future site modification and improvement.

Safety: - radiation protection;
- neutron streaming;
- air pollution;
- transfer of radioactive materials.

To assemble all these points into an organic and interconnected structure may require a long time but mistakes in doing so lead to large problems in future exploitation and all factors should be given due consideration. This is particularly true if the installation has to fit into a pre-existing structure.

For more clarity the analysis of the installation of the PET radiochemistry centre may be divided into two parts: first the installation of the cyclotron for radionuclide production and second the installation of the radiochemistry facilities and their connection to the cyclotron.

CYCLOTRON INSTALLATION

The installation of the cyclotron is by far the most difficult problem to be solved: the machine must be adequately shielded to contain the radiation field produced during its operation. The design of this shield, the thickness of which is considerable, requires careful study because it has to be compatible with the normal needs of the maintenance of the machine and, incidentally, for the replacement of damaged parts. Obviously the cyclotron room or vault should be located as close as possible to the radiochemistry facilities to minimize the problem of transferring the activity from the target to the processing facilities. Minimizing the length of the path also means reducing the transit time (especially important with Oxygen-15), radiation hazards and faults in the system as well as improvement of the radiochemical quality of the product.

However the biggest problems of shielding for the cyclotron are its dimensions and its design for the purpose of radiation protection.

If space, costs or technology are not a problem the simplest solution is to overestimate the whole shielding. However, this is not the general case and, especially at present, proper yet safe dimensions for the shielding are usually needed. From this point of view it may be interesting to go through some of the aspects which influence shielding characteristics. Data for this very low energy machine are rare so that some approximation must be proposed.

The design and dimensions of the shielding barriers depend not only on the intensity of the neutron source, but also on the energy spectrum and the angular distribution of neutron emission. The thickness of the shielding is decided by the most energetic neutrons; incidentally, it should be recalled that the dose due to fast neutrons is far more important than that due to both thermal neutrons and gamma rays and, in general, the thickness sufficient to shield the fast neutrons is enough to absorb the other emissions produced during the operation of the cyclotron.

The evaluation of neutron attenuation in the shield is not the only requirement since a careful study of the geometry of the cyclotron vault may reveal the unexpected necessity of additional new shields to contain low energy (thermal and epithermal) scattered neutrons. Indeed very often, the effect of the reflection of primary neutrons as well as that of secondary neutrons represents the most difficult problem in shielding design.

The starting point is the definition of the neutron sources. While the bombardment is on, two main neutron sources are present: i) The electrostatic deflector (source A) used to extract the accelerated beam; and ii) The external target (source B), where the radioisotopes are produced. The values of neutron yields produced by the interaction of protons on copper (1) (Source A) and aluminium (2) (Source B) may be taken as representative of neutron sources, for the evaluation of babycyclotron shielding.

The second important parameter to be considered in the shielding analysis is the angular distribution of the emitted neutrons. In this case it can be approximated by use of a tenfold reduction in beam intensity at 90 degrees from the beamline (2).

This is to account for the generally experienced phenomenon, that neutron production is forward peaked (bombardment direction). Obviously this identifies the most important point of the site's radiation protection.

Finally the mean energy of neutron emission is generally in the few MeV region, and generally in these cases, 10 MeV is not exceeded.

Once the nature and, of course, the positions of the sources have been defined the shielding can be determined by two approaches:
i) using tabulated values of dose transmission vs. thickness at selected values of beam energy of the accelerated particle for materials in standard geometrical conditions (e.g. slab) (2) or
ii) solving the transport equation for the emitted neutrons and considering the actual shape and geometry of the site by the use

of computer codes (3, 4).

According to the environment where the site for the installation is to be located one can choose between these two points. But, in those cases requiring precise prediction the use of computed calculations may be necessary. In fact in this way we can:
  i) take into account the actual geometry of the installation;
  ii) consider the effect of scattered and reflected neutrons;
  iii) take into account radiation produced inside the shields;
  iv) calculate the neutron fluence in almost every point of the installation.

This last point is very important because it is very useful to know the neutron fluence in front of shield openings (doors, pipes, ducts) and to calculate neutron streaming through them.

We should not forget that the cyclotron must have several connections to the power supply room and to the chemistry laboratory.

In the same way we can carry out the evaluation of neutron dose at the entrance maze, usually necessary to protect the entrance from direct fast neutrons, and it is of great importance in deciding the thickness and composition of the neutron shielding door. The computed approach in fact gives the opportunity of estimating the energy distribution of the neutron fluence so that the structure of the door can be improved to ensure the maximum shielding at optimized costs and weights.

The final result of a computed calculation approach is shown in figure 1 and represents the dose at the external surface of an underground vault.

Values have been calculated for a shield thickness of 1 meter of ordinary concrete and a babycyclotron working at maximum proton energy.

Both gamma and neutron doses can be represented; it is evident that the worst situation is, as expected, above the targets (source B), while the neutron emission of source A (the electrostatic deflector) is efficiently shielded by the magnet of the machine. In the example shown the most critical direction, the one at 0 degrees, is completely absorbed by the ground.

RADIOCHEMISTRY FACILITIES

Once the cyclotron site has been defined the problem is how to arrange the remainder of the installation and in particular the chemistry facilities which must be designed according to the research project being undertaken.

In particular, the need to work in a completely shielded environment, which may be quite general for hospital installations, should be stressed. This means providing efficient gamma shielding not only to protect the radiochemistry personnel but also people working nearby, on totally different jobs to radiochemistry. For this purpose special shielded hoods are usually installed which will enable the handling of activities in the Curie range and the dispensing of radiogases both for patient administration and for the production of routine radiopharmacetical compounds.

A possible solution is represented by three separately shielded areas each of them dedicated to a special function.

A possible arrangement of the hoods and of the site for the installation is shown in figure 2.

One of the shielded hoods can work like a black box, that is inaccessible during the operation and can contain the gas processing equipment, which is available remotely controlled, for the purification of radiogas and radioactive precursors piped from the target-holders in the cyclotron vault. According to the following manipulations the radioactive precursors can be transferred to a high activity hot-hood where a master-slave arm is also provided or towards a warm-hood for direct radiocompound handling.

It is clear that the influence of the site geometry on this point is very important. Both radiogases and radiopharmaceuticals may be be delivered directly to the PET room from the shielded hoods e.g. via transfer tubings and a pneumatic rabbit.

A final point to be considered concerns the exhausts from both the cyclotron vault and the radiochemistry hoods which may need to be diluted before being discharged. In any case a stack is usually needed whose height depends on that of the nearest buildings.

CONCLUSIONS

The continuous development of techniques and equipment expressly dedicated to radioisotope production for medical use and, in particular, the improvement the quality of low cost babycyclotron machines and radioactive compound processing units are strongly influencing the diffusion of PET installations.

It is reasonable to imagine that the standardization of technology which has begun between PET users will also be experienced by industry so that the shape of radiochemistry facilities for PET installations will depend more and more on the research projects, reducing shielding problems to routine consideration, but moving the attention toward better selection of procedures, material and new technology.

REFERENCES

1. Patterson, H.W., C.N. Thomas. Accelerator Health Physics. Academic Press, 1973.
2. Radiation Protection Design Guidelines for 0.1-100 MeV Particle Accelerator Facilities. NCRP Report n. 51. Washington, 1977.
3. Engle, W.N. A User manual for ANISN, a one-dimensional Discrete Ordinate Transport Code with anisotropic scattering. USAEC Report K-1693, 1967.
4. Rhoades, W.A., F.R. Mynat. The DOT-111 two-dimensional Discrete Ordinate Code. Report ORNL-TM-4280, 1973.

ACKNOWLEDGEMENT

I am grateful to Dr. T. Spinks for the useful discussion during the preparation of the manuscript.

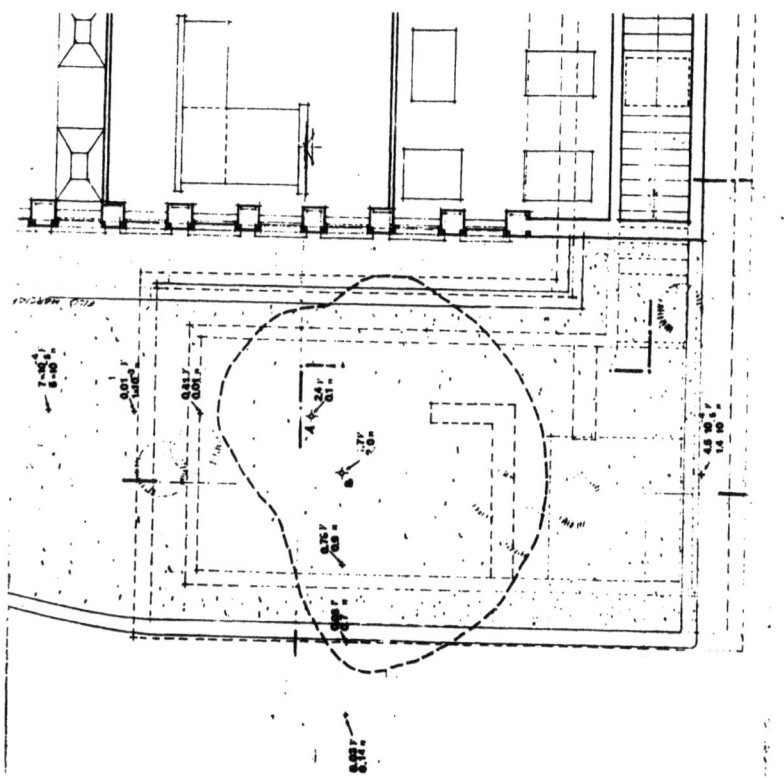

Figure 1a: Gamma and neutron doses calculated via two-dimensional computed calculation for a 50 μA 15MeV proton beam shielded by one meter ordinary concrete (A = machine's deflector; B = external targets). The dotted line represents the 0,5 mRem/h total isodose.

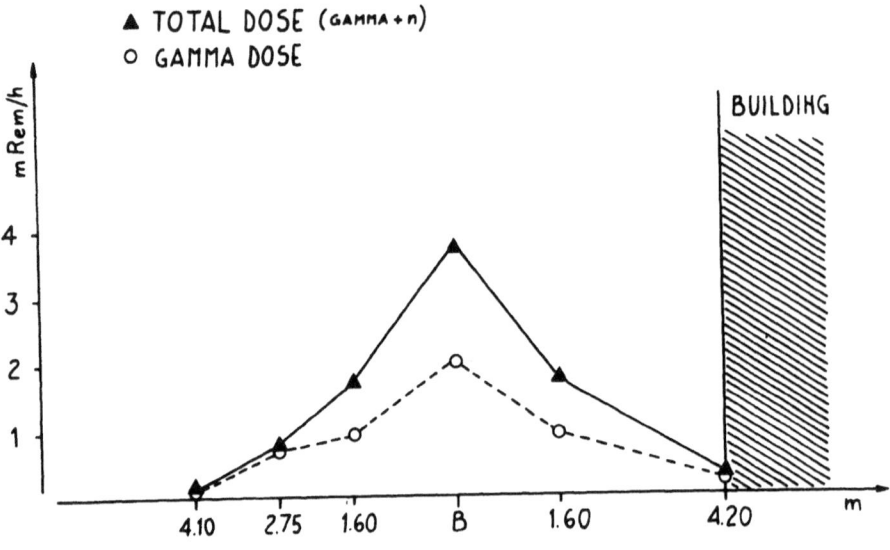

Figure 1b: Radiation dose from the building through source B of figure 1a.

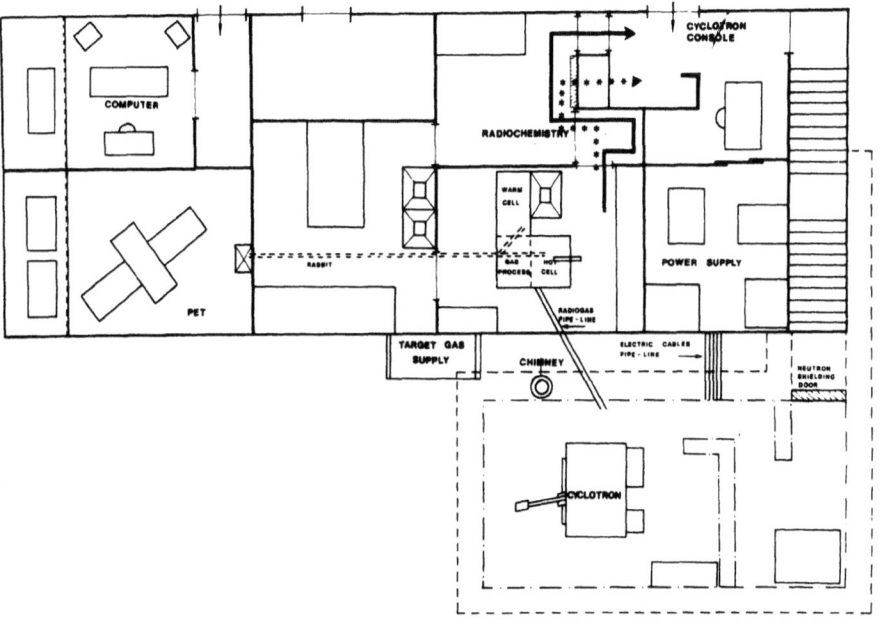

Figure 2: Site arrangement of a PET installation (Pisa, Clinical Physiology Institute).

POSTER SESSION

AN AUTOMATIC LINE FOR THE PRODUCTION OF RADIOPHARMACEUTICALS

E.M. Ferdeghini, P.A. Salvadori, R. Guzzardi and A. Benassi

C.N.R. Clinical Physiology Institute
Via Savi, 8 - PISA - ITALY

INTRODUCTION

After implementing the Positron Emission Tomographic (PET) techniques, the development of an automatic system for the production of the necessary short-lived, positron emitting tracers, has been planned in the C.N.R. Clinical Physiology Institute.

The objective is an "intelligent" machine which performs, in real time, both routine protocols and safety procedures, substituting man in the manipulation of the actuators and the control of the physical variables, leaving, however, the final decisions to the operator.

The automation of the production of radiopharmaceuticals guarantees:
1) the safety of the operator, in consequence of the capability to install the whole line in suitable ambients;
2) the shortening of the intervention times;
3) the optimization of the production methods;
4) the repeatability of the whole process;
5) the increasing of the line productivity.

MATERIALS AND METHODS

The management of the whole system of production and control is assigned to a network of intelligent Peripheral Units (PUs) coordinated by a Central Unit (CU).

The hardware of both the PUs and the CU, built around the

Rockwell International chip 6511, is a flexible support, able to fit different applications fully profiting from the facilities of the chip.

The data storage of the actual status of the chemical line, that is the evolution of the physical variables (temperature, radioactivity, pressure, flow), is assured by the use of up to 52 Kbytes of RAM, plus 8 Kbytes of EPROM, resting on a single eurocard.

A serial-parallel I/O card allows one to interface the computer with a serial videoterminal and to print out data on a parallel printer.

Furthermore, a card for the analog-to-digital conversion of up to 16 analog inputs, selectable via software together with their own gain, has been realized.

The automation of the chemical line, that is the storage and the control of the physical parameters as well as the driving of the actuators, i.e. electrovalves, is strictly committed to the PUs. The CU coordinates the operations of both serial and parallel I/O of the PUs, allowing the use of only one videoterminal and one printer common to all the units (CU included). The CU gives also the timing of the various phases of the line operations.

The system allows the operator to know the actual status of the line, by asking for it through the videoterminal.

Furthermore, in case of unexpected default of the line or exceeding of the overflow limits, the PUs, after having completed the safety operations, allow the previous few minutes story to be plotted on the printer.

CONCLUSIONS

This system, although designed for the production line of ^{18}F-FDG, is suitable for all those lines with analogous characteristics of repetition. Our tested-on-bank prototype confirmed both the high grade of safety for the operator, and good results in the reproducibility of the experiments and production of the tracer.

This work is supported by the C.N.R. Special Program on "Biomedical and Health Engineering".

BIBLIOGRAPHY
1) Ferdeghini E.M., Salvadori P.A., Bellina C.R., Mazzarisi A., Guzzardi R., Benassi A. Proceedings of the AIRP XXIIIrd National Congress, Capri, 77-80 (1983).
2) Iwata R., Ido T., Takahashi T., Monma M. in Int. J. Appl. Radiat. Isotop., 35, No. 6, 445-454 (1984).

PART XIII PHYSIOLOGICAL MEASUREMENTS BY POSITRON EMISSION TOMOGRAPHY

Chairman: Terry Jones (U.K.)

IN VIVO BIOCHEMISTRY, PHYSIOLOGY AND PHARMACOLOGY STUDIES USING POSITRON EMITTING RADIONUCLIDES

Terry Jones

MRC Cyclotron Unit, Hammersmith Hospital, Du Cane Road, London W12 OHS, UK.

The use of positron emitting radioisotopes such as ^{15}O, ^{13}N, ^{11}C and ^{18}F together with positron emission tomography (PET) offers a highly selective and quantitative means for investigating regional tissue biochemistry, physiology and pharmacology. Although short lived, these radioisotopes provide a means for introducing labels into organic molecules such that they can be measured in vivo with radiation detectors placed external to the body. The PET scanner is a detector arrangement whereby transaxial tomographic distributions of tracers through the body can be computed. Attenuation of the recorded signals due to tissue absorption of the emitted photons, can be corrected for such that the tomograms can provide absolute values of the concentration of tracer within tissue.

During the previous panel on positron emitting radionuclides and radiochemistry, it was clear that appreciable advances are being made with respect to the labelling of compounds. Not only is the range of labelled compounds being extended but also a number of technically innovative automatic synthetic processes are being introduced. We shall also hear in a later panel that significant advances are being made to the spatial resolution and sensitivity of the positron emission tomographs themselves. Furthermore, we shall hear how this field is producing new information on focal tissue disease especially in Cardiology and Neurology. Basic biological scientists are beginning to interact with this information since much of it can be expressed quantitatively in scientific units.

The physical and technical restraints for advancing this speciality are covered by many of the papers given at this meeting. It is however important not to lose sight of certain logistical and intellectual problems that also have to be faced in order that new information on focal human disease and its treatment may be forthcoming using PET. Many of these problems are rarely discussed as it is much easier to be concerned with the more physical restraints facing this field. Hence I wish to draw to your attention what are felt to be the additional problems.

Given the tomographic and radiochemistry advances that are being made, to provide clinical scientific information attention has to be paid to:

THE CLINICAL RESEARCH QUESTIONS

This is central to the overall productivity of the work in that not only does this have to be relevant but one has to ensure that only PET can produce the required information.

TRACER MODELS

The goal is to process the recorded data to produce quantitative units of tissue function. Hence tracer models have to be formulated which define the biological fate of the radioisotope. Not only have these to be correct but statistical uncertainties which may be propagated in the computation need to be defined. Furthermore, since the clinical research application of PET involves a multidisciplinary approach, the mathematical tracer modellers should not lose sight of the need for all concerned to understand the model concepts. Relegating this to "black box" mathematical models results in those, who actually use the procedures, being unaware of the importance of the various measurements and the errors that can arise when mistakes are made in either scanning or analysis.

DATA INTERPRETATION

Although the formulated tracer model may be correct for normal biological situations, uncertainties can arise in pathological conditions due to perturbations in tissue structures etc. The chemical resolution of in vivo tracer studies is limited since the data takes the form of regional tissue tracer content and time. It has become clear that to help understand what overall changes have actually occurred in the diseased state, that the results from combinations of tracer procedures greatly enhance interpretation. To solve a jigsaw puzzle, you usually need more than one piece. Also repeat studies, carried out during the evolution of the disease process and its treatment, afford a time dimension which aids biological interpretation. These combined and repeat studies represent a logistical burden and the need for high levels of cooperation between patients, medical doctors and the staff operating and supporting the PET facilities.

DATA ANALYSIS

Although images are used to inspect PET results, these in fact represent arrays of quantitative functional information. A quantitative scrutiny is necessary to define and substantiate changes that may occur from the normal case. The results of this analysis have then to be communicated, in scientific units, to the scientific community at large. Absolute measurements of tissue tracer concentration are restrained by the partial volume effects. The concentration of tracer within a tissue structure is only partially measured if the physical size of that structure is less than twice the scanner's spatial resolution (FWHM). Hence when analysing data from structures smaller than the resolution, consideration has to be given to the reduced recovery of tissue counts. If the physical dimension of the tissue sample is known then some correction can be made for this in the analysis. One useful approach is to ratio scans in which the partial volume effects are common and so cancel out. However, the ratio values will contain uncertainties if the individual data contain a spectra of concentrations below the resolution width. Nevertheless, the ratio does offer a reproducible means for expressing data whereas the individual values will tend to be more vulnerable to poor recovery. A further problem of data analysis is how the units of tissue function are expressed. Tracer procedures are standardly formulated to measure the functional entity in terms of unit tissue volume. However, if a fraction of that physical volume is non functional, eg. due to the presence of dead tissue, then the signal from the functional compartment will be diluted. This will conceal the fact that part of the tissue is working normally. To overcome this, there is a need to provide scans that define tissue viability. In particular, tracers are required which depict cellularity. If these were available, then the functional data could be expressed directly as per unit of viable tissue. Furthermore, such a means for expressing data would help to overcome the partial volume recoverying effects.

THE MULTI DISCIPLINARY PET PROGRAMME

To fully exploit a PET centre as a clinical research facility requires a multi disciplinary approach. The specialists which contribute directly to this field are cyclotron engineers, radiochemists, medical physicists, mathematical modellers, clinician scientists, biochemists, physiologists, pharmacologists, computer programmers and technical staff. The logistics of integrating such diverse specialists are not trivial. To maximise the individual contributions requires consideration to group activity and role playing. Additionally, the central core programme needs to be referred patients and to interact and consult with individuals who reside outside of the PET centre.

New information on human disease is now emerging from the more established PET programmes. It is hoped that this will stimulate the thinking of how to advance therapeutic regimes. To help this transition, it is important that the clinical doctors, who are involved in collecting data, and hence are appreciable of the results from PET, are also actively concerned with patient care. Indeed, the medical involvement needs to be disease and not PET orientated.

The current developments in _in vivo_ NMR spectroscopy is seen as being strongly complementary to the PET field. NMR offers the measurement of biochemicals that are indigenous to the tissues. PET provides a highly sensitive method for selectively studying the transport and accumulation of chemicals within tissues. Analysis of PET data would benefit from an extended interpretation based on corresponding NMR spectroscopy data. Already some PET centres are in the process of installing adjacent _in vivo_ NMR spectrometers.

There is currently much discussion as to whether or not PET will become a routinely used clinical diagnostic procedure. The speciality offers new information on disease which should be of value with regard to the general understanding of disease and its treatment. This is a compelling reason for focusing the power of this speciality into research. However there is interest in introducing PET for routine clinical diagnosis. This has to be recognised especially since the current developments in commercially available equipment are, to some extent, being stimulated by the possible future existence of some routine clinical use of positron emission tomography.

REFERENCES

1. Computed Emission Tomography 1982
    Ed. PJ Ell and BL Holman
    Oxford University Press

2. Research Issues in Positron Emission Tomography 1984
    Suppl to Annals of Neurology 15.

3. Phelps ME, Mazziotta JC, Huang SC 1982
    Study of cerebral function with positron computed tomography
    Journal of Cerebral Blood Flow and Metabolism 2, 113-162

4. Beaney RP 1984
    Positron emission tomography in the study of human tumors
    Seminars in Nuclear Medicine XIV No 4, 324-341.

5. Leenders KL, Gibbs JM, Frackowiak RSJ, Lammertsma AA, Jones T 1984
    Positron emission tomography of the brain: New possibilities for the investigation of human cerebral pathophysiology.
    Progess in Neurobiology 23, 1-38.

6. Proceedings of the Symposium on Regional Myocardial Metabolism by Positron Tomography - Santa Barbara 1984
    Ed Schelbert and Phelps 1985

7. Positron Emission Tomography 1985
    Ed M Reivich, pub Alan R Liss Inc

EVALUATION OF PERFORMANCE AND ACCURACY IN PET

Edward J. Hoffman, Ph.D.

Division of Biophysics, Dept. of Radiological Sciences
UCLA School of Medicine and The Laboratory of Nuclear Medicine
of the Laboratories of Biomedical and Environmental Sciences
University of California, Los Angeles
U.S.A

INTRODUCTION

The performance of PET instrumentation has been evaluated in our laboratory in terms of reproducibility or precision. Measurements were made for current PET systems and simulated by both computer and experimental methods for potential future systems (1). The present and potential future precision of PET systems is on the order of 1-2 % for equilibrium studies, such as FDG metabolism measurements, with a few million counts per image, and better than 10 % for dynamic studies with a few hundred thousand counts per image. To take advantage of this high precision, the instrumental accuracy of PET systems should match or better the precision of the measurements. The major sources of inaccuracy in PET, outside of deficiencies in electronic or computer hardware and software, are poor resolution, nonuniform resolution and scatter. The use of narrow BGO detectors, system designs with adequately large detector ring diameters and properly designed interplane septa provides significant improvement in all of these deficiencies.

The development of test procedures to evaluate the performance and accuracy of PET systems serves two potentially conflicting purposes. The first purpose is to evaluate the device to determine whether or not it will perform the task required of it in the clinic or laboratory. The second purpose is to convince the potential buyer that the system is the best and later, after purchase, that the delivered system does meet the specifications in the purchase agreement. Thus, a person entering the PET field as a user or as a builder must be aware of the potential misrepresentation of performance that a poor set of test procedures can yield.

Evaluation procedures of the second kind have been a continual problem for the purchaser of instrumentation in Nuclear Medicine. For instance, high count rates are required for first pass ejection fraction studies. The measurement in the clinic will be performed in a patient who will produce large amounts of scatter and a scintillation camera will employ a 20 % energy window to reject most of the scatter and perhaps 80 % of the events processed by the camera. Yet the manufacturer may measure and specify the count rate capability with no scatter and an energy window covering the full energy range impinging on the camera. If the buyer is not careful in correctly understanding the specification, he may purchase a camera that does not do the job and have no recourse because it meets the manufacturers specifications.

We have presented studies on the evalution of resolution (2-7), accidental coincidences (8), sensitivity and other parameters (9-12) affecting the accuracy of PET systems. In this work, we will concentrate on two parameters that can cause serious errors in quantitation in PET which have also been measured incorrectly in the evaluation of many PET systems. These parameters are the interplane axial resolution uniformity and the scatter fraction.

UNIFORMITY OF INTERPLANE SLICE THICKNESS IN PET

We have previously shown that there is a very large variation in the interplane resolution of PET systems using standard interplane septa for accidental and scatter rejection (9). The measurements, performed in our laboratory, concentrated on detector pairs and were measured as a function of distance from the center of the Field-of-View (FOV). It was found that there were variations within single planes of as much as a factor of three in the axial resolution and it was demonstrated that this could cause image artefacts and loss of quantitation as well as loss of contrast near the edge of the FOV. In the evaluations of a PET system with detector geometries and septa design similar to those used in our measurements, other investigators reported axial resolution uniformities in total disagreement with our results (13). In a careful reading of their experimental method it was discovered that their method of measurement consisted of stepping a point source axially through the PET system and using the total count rate of the system. This provides and average resolution as a function of distance from the center and has sense of fairness in the measurement, but hides important details from the reader.

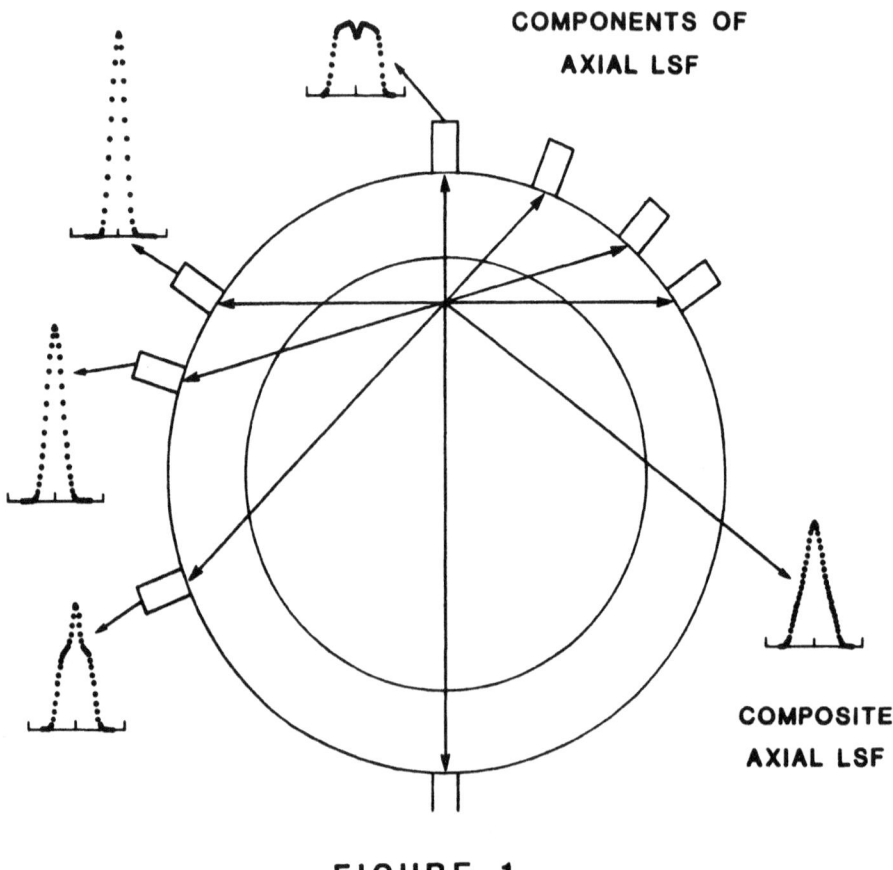

FIGURE 1

The measurement can be understood from a consideration of figure 1. Any point in the FOV is viewed by a number of detectors. The axial Point Spread Function (PSF) for the detector very near the point in figure 1 has a very broad FWHM and the PSF for the two detectors which have the point centered is very narrow. The composite PSF is the average over all the detector pairs.

The attractiveness of the averaged PSF is illustrated in figure 2. The composite PSF for the same system is shown to be very uniform and the apparent slice thickness is always narrower, as much as a factor of 2, than the PSF measured for the individual detector pairs. The composite PSF hides a serious problem of nonuniformity and a source of inconsistent data in the reconstruction. It may not be possible to completely avoid these nonuniformities, but to simply hide them by doing an inappropriate measurement does not help progress in instrumentation in the PET field.

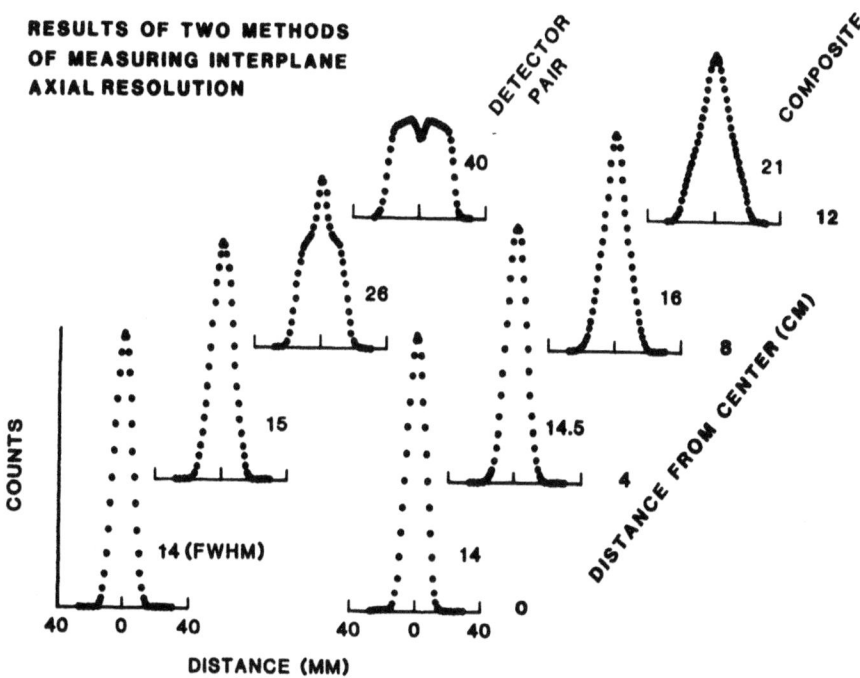

FIGURE 2

SCATTER MEASUREMENT IN PET

The correction for scatter in PET is difficult and may be one of its more intractable sources of error. No method is yet available to measure scatter in an extended activity distribution as can be done with accidental coincidences (8, 14). Therefore, methods of correction are approximate. However, it is possible to get an accurate measure of scatter that can be used to compare the scatter fraction of various PET systems and also be used as a data base for scatter correction (15).

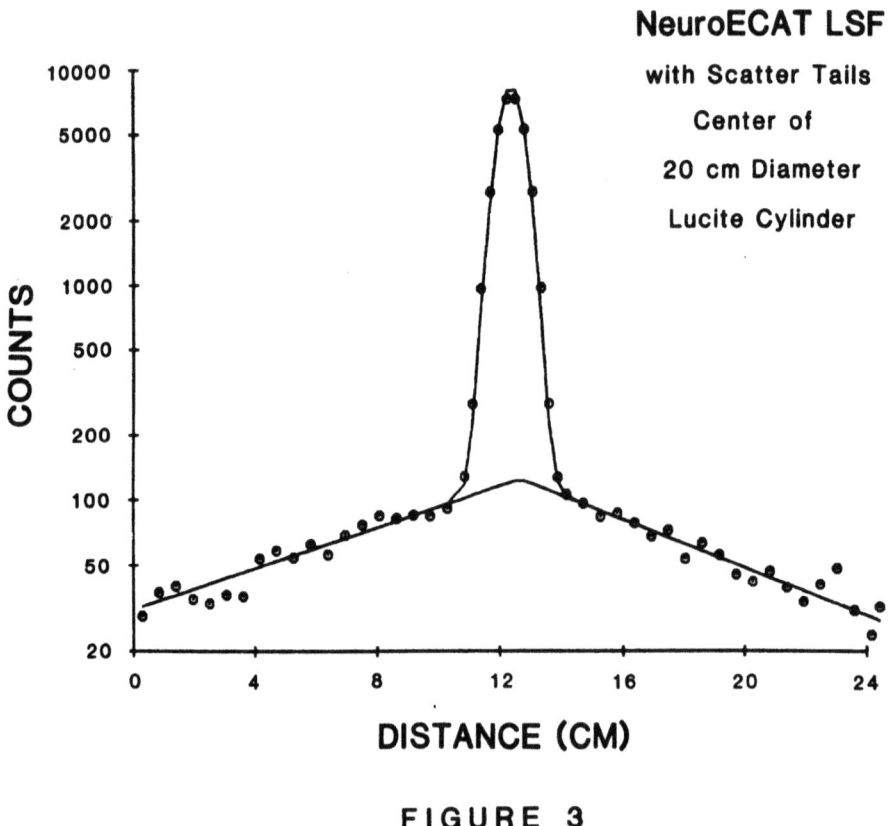

FIGURE 3

Scatter for a typical scattering medium can be measured accurately by using a line source of positron emitter placed in the scattering medium. The scatter is determined from the scan profiles of the PET scan, not the image. In figure 3, a typical scan profile is shown plotted on a log scale versus position in the FOV. The scatter is the tail of activity on each side of the peak. The integral of all the counts outside the physical width of one detector divided by the counts in the integral of the peak area is the scatter fraction. Relative to the peak of the line source, the scatter is less than one percent at any single point but integrated over the FOV, the amount of scatter is significant.

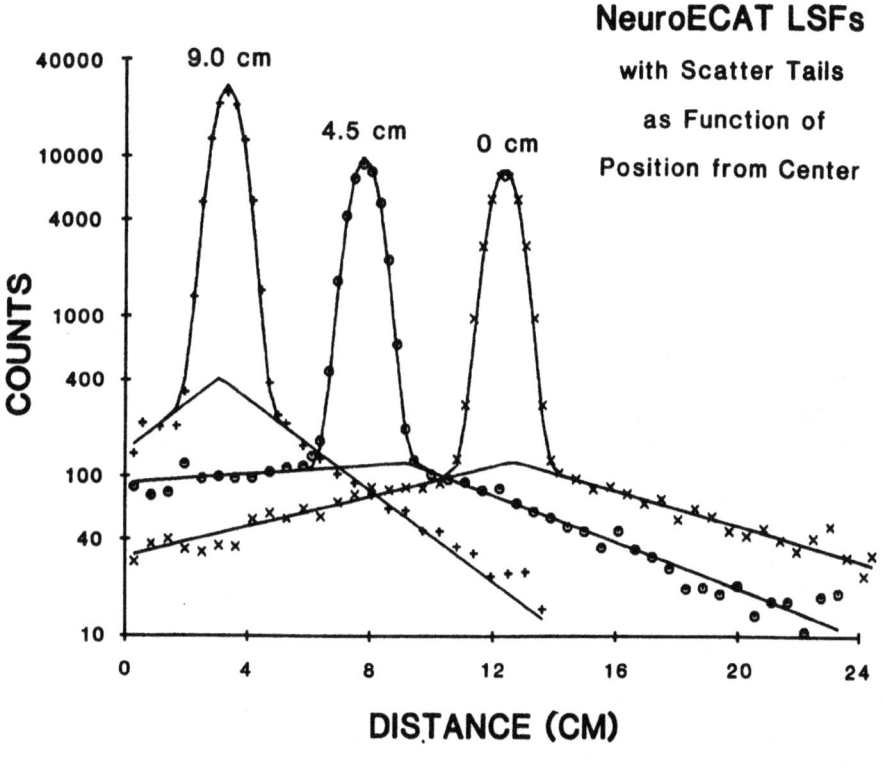

FIGURE 4

In figure 4, the scatter measurement is shown for several positions in the FOV. Unfortunately, the shape of the scatter varies, which makes it impossible to apply a simple deconvolution scheme for an accurate scatter correction. In order to obtain the scatter fraction for the whole object, it is necessary to use a number of these measurements to have a reasonable sampling of the whole object and use a properly weighted average to obtain the scatter fraction equivalent to the scatter for a uniform cylinder of activity. This value can be used for reasonable intercomparison of different PET systems.

FIGURE 5

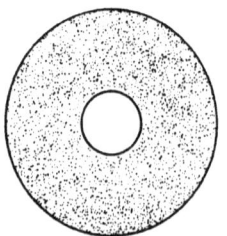

"SCATTER" PHANTOM

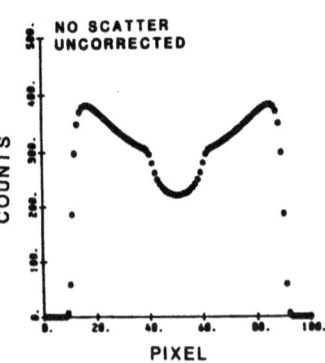

In some evaluations of scatter, the amount of scatter is estimated from activity levels observed in the reconstructed image (16). The usual scatter phantom is shown in figure 5. It is a cylinder of activity with a cold spot in the center with a diameter that is at least three times the resolution width of the PET system. In the measurement of scatter, an image is taken of the phantom and the ratio of the activity in the coldspot to the activity in the surrounding body of the phantom is assumed to be a measure of the scatter fraction of the PET system.

A simulation of this measurement was performed to test its validity. The lower drawing in figure 5 is a scan profile of the data set with no scatter before attenuation correction. Two types of scatter were added to the data profiles: 1) a simple flat scatter distribution equal to 20 % of the true data and 2) a cosine shaped background, peaked in the center, and equal to 10 % of the true data. These profiles are shown in figure 6. The solid line is the data without scatter to illustrate the magnitude of distortion caused by the scatter. The profiles to the right illustrate the effect of attenuation correction.

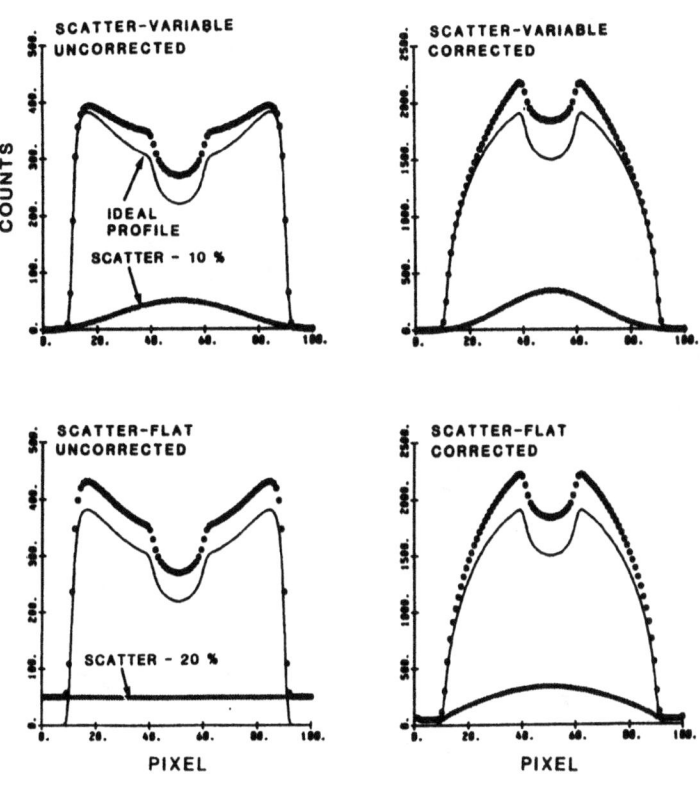

FIGURE 6

Histograms through the center of the reconstructed images are shown in figure 7. The profiles to the left use the correct attenuation coefficient and the results give scatter fractions of 28 % and 17 % for the simulations with 10 % and 20 % scatter, respectively. The profiles on the right employed smaller attenuation coefficients to compensate for scatter, giving 23 % and 12 %, respectively for the same scatter fractions. In neither case did the method give the correct scatter fraction. They measured a number that described the effect of scatter in the center of the FOV, but not what fraction of the accumulated events were due to scatter. The measurement was subject to additional error when there was some spatial distribution to the scatter. In the case of the distributed scatter, the 10 % scatter contribution became 28 % in this measurement. In other words this measurement had very little relationship to evaluating the quantity of interest.

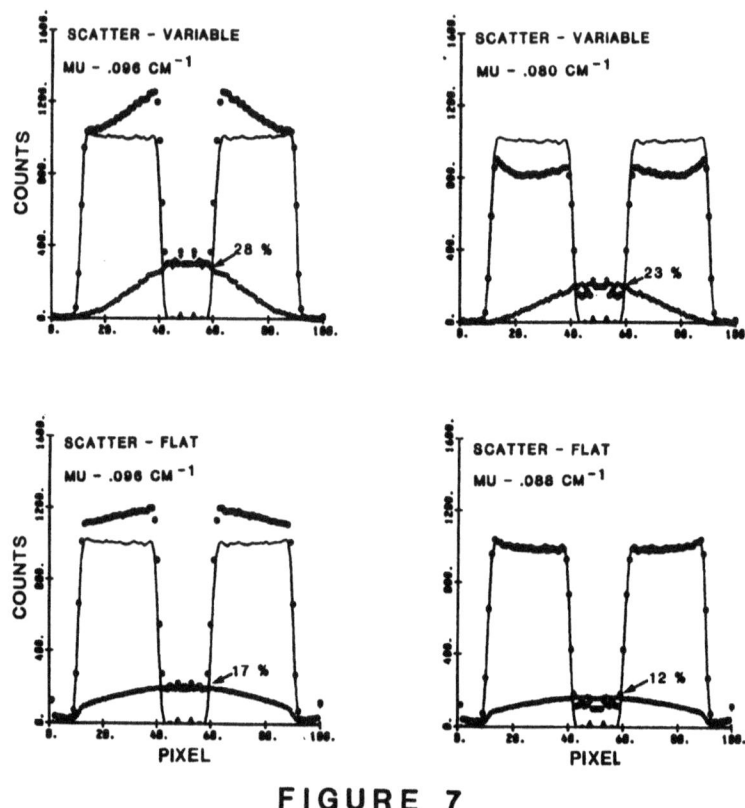

FIGURE 7

DISCUSSION

The temporary advantage to the PET system builder of choosing a misleading method to evaluate his system will probably be outweighed in the long run by eventual loss of reputation. More important is the fact that this type of science is causing a loss of credibility for this field in medical science. It is important to have accurate measures of the performance of PET systems and until these are established, it will be difficult to accurately compare the various systems.

ACKNOWLEDGEMENTS

The author thanks M. Griswold for preparation of the illustrations and A. Ricci and M Dahlbom for technical assistance. This work was supported in part by Department of Energy Contract DE-AM03-76-SF0012, National Institute of Cancer Grant 1-R01-CA33801-02, and National Institutes of Mental Health Grant 1-R01-MH373916-01.

REFERENCES

1. Hoffman EJ, van der Stee M, Ricci AR, Phelps ME: Prospects for Both Precision and Accuracy in Positron Tomography. Ann Neurol 15(Suppl)25:S25-S34, 1984.
2. Hoffman EJ, Barton JB, Phelps ME, Huang SC: New Design Concepts for Quantitative Positron Emission Computed Tomography. Positron Emission Tomography of the Brain. Ed. W.-D. Heiss and M.E. Phelps, Springer-Verlag, New York, Pg. 30-39, 1983.
3. Hoffman EJ, Huang SC, Phelps ME: Quantitation in Positron Emission Computed Tomography: 1. Effect of Object Size. J Comput Assist Tomogr 3:299-308, 1979.
4. Hoffman EJ, Ricci AR, van der Stee LMAM, Phelps ME: ECAT III - Basic Design Considerations. IEEE Trans Nucl Sci NS-30:729-733, 1983.
5. Huang SC, Hoffman EJ, Ricci AR, Phelps ME: Effect of Detector Size and Geometry on Image Signal-to-Noise Ratio in Positron Computed Tomography. Proceedings of workshop on time-of-flight in PET. St. Louis, MO, Pg. 69-74, May 1982, IEEE-CH1791-3182.
6. Mazziotta JC, Phelps ME, Plummer D, Kuhl DE: Quantitation in Positron Emission Computed Tomography: 5. Physical-Anatomical Effects. J Comput Assist Tomogr 5:734-743, 1981.
7. Phelps ME, Huang SC, Hoffman EJ, Plummer D, Carson RE: An Analysis of Signal Amplification Using Small Detectors in Positron Emission Tomography. J Comput Assist Tomogr 6:551-565, 1982.
8. Hoffman EJ, Huang SC, Phelps ME, Kuhl DE: Quantitation in Positron Emission Computed Tomography: 4. Effect of Accidental Coincidences. J Comput Assist Tomogr 5:391-400, 1981.
9. Hoffman EJ, Huang SC, Plummer D, Phelps ME: Quantitation in Positron Emission Computed Tomography: 6. Effect of Nonuniform Resolution. J Comput Assist Tomogr 6:987-999, 1982.
10. Hoffman EJ, Phelps ME, Huang SC: Performance Characteristics of a Multiplane Positron Tomograph Designed for Brain studies. J Nucl Med 24:245-257, 1983.
11. Hoffman EJ, Phelps ME, Huang SC, Kuhl DE, Crabtree MC, Burke M, Burgiss S, Keyser R, Highfill R and Williams C: A New Tomograph for Quantitative Positron Emission Computed Tomography of the Brain. IEEE Trans Nucl Sci NS-28:99-103, 1981.
12. Hoffman EJ, Phelps ME, Huang SC, Plummer D, Kuhl DE: Evaluating the Performance of Multiplane Positron Tomographs Designed for Brain Imaging. IEEE Trans Nucl Sci NS-29:469-473, 1982.

13. Kearfott KJ, Carroll LR: Evaluation of the Performance Characteristics of the PC 4600 Positron Emission Tomograph. J Comput Assist Tomogr 8:502-513, 1984.
14. Williams CW, Crabtree MC, Burgiss SG: Design and Performance Characteristics of a Positron Emission Axial Tomograph--ECAT-II. IEEE Trans Nucl Sci NS-26:619-627, 1979.
15. Bergtrom M, Eriksson L, Bohm C, Blomqvist G, Litton J: Correction for Scattered Radiation in a Ring Detector Positron Camera by Integral Transformation of the Projections. J Comput Assist Tomogr 7:42-50, 1983.
16. Yamamoto M, Ficke DC, Ter-Pogossian MM: Performance Study of PETT VI, a Positron Computed Tomograph with 288 Cesium Fluoride Detectors. IEEE Trans Nucl Sci NS-29:529-533, 1984.

ADVANCED CARDIOLOGICAL APPLICATION OF PET

Oberdan Parodi M.D. and Paolo Camici M.D.

C.N.R. Institute of Clinical Physiology and Istituto di Patologia Medica, University of Pisa, Italy

INTRODUCTION

As recently reported the age-adjusted death rate for coronary artery disease (CAD) in the United States of America was 203 per 100.000 of the population in 1979. In 1981 989.000 americans died of cardiovascular diseases accounting for 51% of all deaths. The above figure was more than twice the mortality for cancer, the second most frequent cause of death. The cost of cardiac care, including cost output due to disability, was estimated to be 64 billion dollars in 1984 (1). These impressive numbers explain the great effort being made in the research of heart disease.

Among all cardiac disorders, ischemic heart disease is the most common cause of morbidity and this justifies the importance of a better understanding of its pathophysiology and early diagnosis.

Myocardial ischemia can be defined as any situation in which the heart muscle is not adequately perfused by coronary flow. This can be due either (a) to a primary reduction of coronary blood flow (spasm, platelet aggregation etc.) or (b) to an imbalance between the blood supply and myocardial energy demand (fixed stenosis etc.).

In the clinical situation myocardial ischemia can be either transient and reversible (i.e. angina pectoris) or prolonged and irreversible (i.e. myocardial infarction). While angina lasts a few minutes and does not cause tissue necrosis, infarction lasts usually more than 20-30 minutes and is associated with permanent tissue damage.

In between these two extremes (i.e. angina and infarction) many situations can be found in which a variable mixture of viable and necrotic tissue coexist (jeopardized myocardium).

Myocardial ischemia is generally a regional phenomenon (involving one of the heart walls) and has different transmural extensions (inner outer myocardial layers). From the pathophysiological point of view the reduction of coronary flow causes a metabolic derangement of myocardial cells which in turn is responsible for an abnormal contractile function.

The main metabolic changes occurring during myocardial ischemia consist of a variable impairment of free fatty acids (FFA) oxidation with a concomitant increase of glucose utilization due to an enhanced anaerobic metabolism (2). The extent and severity of flow reduction and the dependent metabolic abnormalities can cause different degrees of contraction abnormalities, ranging from a reduced wall motion (hypokinesia) to a paradoxical bulging of the ischemic area during systole (dyskinesia).

Thus, the assessment of the presence, location and severity of myocardial ischemia can be derived from the study of regional perfusion, metabolism and function of the heart.

Whilst several techniques exist for the non-invasive assessment of regional myocardial perfusion and contraction in humans, positron emission tomography (PET) is an unique tool for the study of regional myocardial metabolism in man (3).

Potential advantages of PET in the evaluation of CAD

Since the flow abnormalities associated with myocardial ischemia are often spontaneously transient (angina) or partially solved by therapeutical interventions (medical and/or surgical therapy), repeated evaluations of regional myocardial blood flow would allow a better assessment of the patient's clinical state.

The use of very short half life positron emitters and PET allows repeated, non-invasive assessments of regional perfusion in man. Rubidium-82 (Rb) and N13-ammonia (NH_3) are the most interesting flow tracers used with PET (4,5).

Because of its very short half life (78 seconds) Rb renders it possible to assess coronary perfusion repeatedly in the same study. This is particularly useful in those situations where rapid flow changes are expected as in the case of transient ischemic attacks (Figs. 1, 2). In addition, since Rb is obtained from a portable generator (Strontium-82 - Rubidium-82 column), an on line cyclotron is not needed, thus allowing the operator a more independent planning of the studies.

N13-ammonia rapidly clears from the blood and accumulates in the myocardium where it is metabolically trapped with a long retention time. This gives a very favourable target to background ratio with good counting rates and low spill-over fraction from the blood to the myocardial walls. Thus, NH_3 is particularly useful when regional coronary perfusion needs to be accurately determined, as for instance before and after therapeutical interventions (thrombolysis, angioplasty etc.) when the time interval between the different measurements is predictable and sufficiently long (Fig.2).

Nevertheless neither Rb nor NH_3 can be considered as "pure" flow tracers since the uptake of both is influenced by the metabolic state of the heart and their extraction fraction is not linearly related to the flow rates.

Human albumin microspheres labelled with C-11 or Ga-67 may represent the ideal compound for absolute flow measurements with PET (6). However, their use is limited because they require an invasive procedure for the injection and repeated measurements cannot be easily achieved.

The metabolic changes associated with myocardial ischemia in man have been studied in the past mainly by measuring transmyocardial extraction of substrates using the Fick method (7). However this approach is invasive, does not allow the study of regional phenomena and presents several methodological limitations as recently outlined by different authors (8,9).

The recent availability of PET permits the non-invasive assessment of regional myocardial metabolism in man. Different metabolic tracers can be labelled with very short half life (20-110 minutes) positron emitters. In particular, two tracers, F18-2-fluoro-2-deoxyglucose (FDG) and C-11-palmitic acid (PAL), seem to possess the best characteristics for the study of regional myocardial utilization of glucose and FFA in patients.

Assessment of transient ischemia

Following a series of observations in the experimental animal using C14-2-deoxyglucose (10), we have determined myocardial uptake of FDG in patients with exertional angina using PET. The glucose analogue FDG competes with glucose for facilitated transport sites and for phosphorylation by hexokinase in the cell. However, the phosphorylated compound FDG-6-PO$_4$ cannot be further metabolized and is trapped within the cell, allowing the measurement of exogenous glucose uptake in tissue (11). The labelling of deoxyglucose with F-18 (half-life 109.9 minutes) permits the determination of myocardial uptake also relatively late after injection when blood concentration of the tracer is low.

Patients with angiographically proven coronary artery disease and stable angina pectoris (ischemia on exertion) were studied at rest and following exercise induced ischemia (supine bicycle ergometer test within the positron camera). Coronary perfusion was assessed before, during and after the exercise using Rb and PET together with regional myocardial uptake of glucose assessed by FDG (12,13). In fasting patients at rest regional myocardial uptake of FDG was low and matched flow distribution.

The exercise test produced typical electrocardiographic signs of ischemia and pain in all patients. A region of reduced perfusion during exercise was demonstrated for all patients in the Rb tomogram performed during the stress test (Fig. 1,3).
In all patients in whom FDG was injected during the recovery from exercise, when ECG changes and chest pain subsided and coronary perfusion was back to control, tracer uptake in the ischemic area (i.e. the one of abnormal Rb uptake during exercise) was between 1.21 and 2.00 times higher than in non ischemic tissue (Fig. 1,3).

By contrast, when FDG was injected during exercise in the same patients, tracer uptake in the ischemic region was only 0.74 to 0.98 that of normal myocardium (Fig. 3).
Thus the presence and location of transient myocardial ischemia in patients with CAD can be revealed as a positive signal (increased FDG accumulation) if the tracer is injected at the proper time (recovery phase of ischemia).
The explanation of this phenomenon can be found bearing in mind the changes of glucose metabolism occurring during and after myocardial ischemia. Whilst glucose utilization in normal myocardium is low during fasting and low work-load conditions, this can increase when cardiac work is higher independently of insulin action. Glucose utilization in the myocardium is also increased during anoxic or ischemic conditions due to an activation of anaerobic glycolysis at the expenses of both exogenous (plasmatic) and endogenous (glycogen stores) glucose

(2).

Thus during exercise induced ischemia both normal and ischemic areas of the myocardium will increase FDG uptake to a variable extent depending on the amount of myocardial work and flow and the degree of ischemia. This will result in an overall increase of myocardial FDG uptake that will not allow the identification of the ischemic regions as "hot" areas.

In the post-exercise phase glucose utilization will return to the low control levels in the normal muscle, but it will remain elevated in the previously ischemic muscle probably due to repletion of the glycogen stores that were depleted during the ischemic period (14).

For this reason, if FDG injection is properly timed, a high contrast of radioactive content between normal and ischemic myocardium will result, thus allowing the identification of the ischemic segments as hot areas (Fig. 1,3).

The 16-carbon-chain fatty acid palmitate (PAL) labelled with C-11 (half life 20.3 minutes) has been proposed as a potential tracer for the study of regional myocardial fatty acid metabolism in man using PET (15). The labelling of palmitate with C-11 does not interfere with the biochemical and physiological properties of the native compound.

Two major metabolic pathways can be entered by PAL once the tracer has diffused into the myocardial cell. On the one hand PAL can be transported inside mitochondria via the carnitine shuttle and oxidized to CO_2 for energy production; on the other hand PAL can be stored in the triglyceride pool in the cytosol (Fig. 4). In a series of different animal studies, Schon et al. (15-16) used PAL to assess regional myocardial fatty acid metabolism in normal and ischemic myocardium. In the open chest dog with normal hemodynamics, PAL rapidly clears from the blood after its injection and it accumulates in myocardial tissue.

The washout of the tracer from the myocardium was assessed by repeated tomograms of the heart using PET (Fig. 5). A typical biphasic tissue activity curve was observed under controlled conditions. The first rapid phase, with a half-life of about 2.7 minutes, mainly reflects palmitate oxidation and is accompanied by 11-CO_2 production (Fig. 6). The late phase, with a half life of about 180 minutes mainly represents storage of palmitate in the triglyceride pool. The slope of the rapid phase is linearly correlated with myocardial oxygen consumption and is steeper when myocardial oxygen consumption is high than when myocardial oxygen consumption and cardiac work are low (16).

During myocardial ischemia a different behaviour of PAL both in terms of oxidation and intermediate storage in endogenous lipid pools was observed. Delays in regional clearance of C-11 activity from the myocardium are consistent with a decline in free fatty acid oxidation and a disproportionately greater fraction of C-11 activity into the intracellular lipid stores. Differences in regional PAL uptake and washout-rates assessed by regional analysis of PET acquisition may allow distinction between ischemic and normo-oxigenated myocardium (15-16) (Fig. 6). Because of the very high extraction fraction with the first pass, C-11 PAL uptake is largely affected by the flow rates. For this reason, it does not appear to be the ideal metabolic tracer when coronary flow is markedly impaired, such as during transient coronary occlusion (spasm). PAL may find an useful application when flow is not markedly impaired and beta-oxidation declines (demand-induced ischemia) (Fig. 6).

Evaluation of myocardial infarction

Evaluation of the extent of myocardial infarction in vivo has become increasingly important because prognosis is affected by infarct size and because reversibly injured myocardium may recover after interventions implemented during the early phase of the insult.

Assessment of myocardial perfusion and wall motion in the early evolution of infarction cannot predict the outcome of the involved segments. Tissue viability can be assessed by tracers that accumulate into myocardial cells (positive spot) with residual, although abnormal metabolism. Experimental and clinical studies show that FDG accumulation in myocardial segments undergoing infarction may anticipate a functional recovery of these areas (17-18). This seems particularly important in an area where revascularization of ischemic-necrotic myocardium is made possible by surgical (aorto-coronary by-pass) or pharmacological (intracoronary thrombolysis) interventions. A comparison of FDG and PAL indicates that the former better predicts the evolution of areas undergoing infarction. Although PAL has been proposed for in vivo quantification of infarction (19) we do not see any further improvement in comparison to the use of flow tracers (NH_3) combined with PET. Flow studies with NH_3 and PET have recently contributed to the clinical characterization and understanding of the subendocardial infarction (20). These techniques have provided new insights into the conventional electrocardiographic interpretation of this syndrome.

Conclusions and future perspectives

Although PET is a recent and evolving technique, and the results obtained up to now must be considered as preliminary and not conclusive, its introduction in clinical research offers new possibilities for the study of the pathophysiology of cardiac diseases. The major problems still limiting a reliable quantification of measurable parameters are at present both technical and theoretical: a) tracer kinetics models are still over-simplifications of the actual biochemical processes; they do not apply to dynamic conditions, in which a steady-state is not achieved or kinetics are too long with respect to positron half-lives or too short with respect to PET sampling; b) the transport rates and metabolic utilization of natural substrates relative to the labelled analogues (referred to as the lumped constant, e.g. between glucose and F-18 fluorodeoxyglucose) can be altered by pathological conditions and are still uncertain in normal patients; c) the low resolution of the present instrumentation and the related partial volume effect still represent important error sources in quantitative analysis of PET images. This is due to the unpredictable cross-talk contamination between the cavity and the myocardial wall and to the underestimation of tracer content in myocardial structures, whose thickness falls below the instrument resolution (21). The above problems prevent accurate measurements of input function and tissue tracer concentrations; d) the heart motion and the uncertain definition of cardiac contours (a $C^{15}O$ blood pool should always be performed as a reference to myocardial wall boundaries) may be responsible for artefacts and misinterpretations of tomographic images.

A new generation of positron scanners will soon be available allowing faster and more efficient data acquisition together with a greatly improved spatial resolution. This technical improvement will in turn allow a more reliable quantification of the measured parameters thus solving some of the problems encountered in tracer kinetics.

Finally, the medical users should realize that this sophisticated technique is not a very expensive imaging device, but a powerful tool which may answer important clinical problems if properly formulated.

Acknowledgments

The Authors wish to thank Drs. Heinrich R. Schelbert and Terry Jones who generously contributed their time and data in positron computed tomography. The Authors also thank Mrs. Daniela Banti for her skillful secretarial assistance in preparing this manuscript.

REFERENCES

1) Kannel W.B., Doyle J.T., Ostfeld A.M., Jenkins C.D., Kuller L., Podell R.N., Stamler J.. Optimal resources for primary prevention of atherosclerotic diseases. Circulation 70 (1984) 157A-205A.
2) Neely J.R. and Morgan H.E.. Relationship between carbohydrate and lipid metabolism and the energy balance of heart muscle. Annual Reviews of Physiology 36 (1974) 413-459.
3) Phelps M.E.. Emission computed tomography. Seminary of Nuclear Medicine 7 (1977) 337-344.
4) Selwyn A.P., Allan R.M., L'Abbate A., Horlock P., Camici P., Clark J., O'Brien H.A., Grant P.M.. Relation between regional myocardial uptake of Rubidium-82 and perfusion: absolute reduction of cation uptake in ischemia. American Journal of Cardiology 50 (1982) 112-121.
5) Schelbert H.R., Phelps M.E., Hoffman E., Huang S.C., Selin C., Kuhl D.E.. Regional myocardial perfusion assessed with N-13 labeled ammonia and positron emission computerized axial tomography. American Journal of Cardiology 43 (1979) 209-218.
6) Wilson R.A., Shea M.J., De Landsheere C.M., Turton D., Brady F., Deanfield J.E., Selwyn A.P.. Validation of quantitation of regional myocardial blood flow in vivo with C11-labeled human albumin microspheres and positron emission tomography. Circulation 70 (1984) 717-723.
7) Most A.S., Gorlin R., Stuart Soeldner J.. Glucose extraction by the human myocardium during pacing stress. Circulation 45 (1972) 92-96.

8) Gertz E.W., Wisneski J.A., Neese R., Bristow D., Searle G., Hanlon J.T.. Myocardial lactate metabolism: evidence of lactate release during net chemical extraction in man. Circulation 63 (1981) 1273-1279.
9) Brachfeld N.. Characterization of the ischemic process by regional metabolism. American Journal of Cardiology 37 (1976) 467-473.
10) L'Abbate A., Camici P., Trivella M.G., Pelosi G., Taddei L., Valli G., Placidi G.F.. Uneven myocardial glucose utilization as determined by regional C14-deoxyglucose uptake. Journal of Nuclear Medicine & Allied Sciences 23 (1979) 167-172.
11) Phelps M.E., Hoffman E.J., Selin C.E., Huang S.C., Schelbert H.R., Kuhl D.E.. Investigation of (F18)-2-fluoro-2-deoxyglucose for the measurement of myocardial glucose metabolism. Journal of Nuclear Medicine 19 (1978) 1311-1319.
12) Camici P., Kaski J.C., Shea M.J., Selwyn A.P., Jones T., Maseri A.. Increased myocardial glucose utilization in exertional angina. Circulation 68 (1983) III-324.
13) Camici P., Kaski J.C., Shea M.J., Lammertsma A.A., Aranjo L., Jones T.. Selective increase of glucose utilisation in the postischemic myocardium of patients with stable angina. In Hammersmith Cardiology Workshop Series, vol. 2 (Raven Press, New York, 1985) 81-85.
14) Camici P., Bailey I.A.. time course of myocardial glycogen repletion following acute transient ischemia. Circulation 70 (1984) II-85.
15) Schon H.R., Schelbert H.R., Robinson G., Najafi A., Huang S.C., Hansen H., Barrio J., Kuhl D.E., Phelps M.E.. C-11 labeled palmitic acid for the noninvasive evaluation of regional myocardial fatty acid metabolism with positron-computed tomography. I. Kinetics of C-11 palmitic acid in normal myocardium. American Heart Journal 103 (1982) 532-547.
16) Schon H.R., Schelbert H.R., Robinson G., Najafi A., Hansen H., Huang H., Barrio J., Phelps M.E.. C-11 labeled palmitic acid for the noninvasive evaluation of regional myocardial fatty acid metabolism with positron-computed tomography. II. Kinetics of C-11 palmitic acid in acutely ischemic myocardium. American Heart Journal 103 (1982) 548-561.
17) Schwaiger M., Hansen H.W., Sochor M., Parodi O., Yeatman L.A., Ellison D.J., Selin C., Grover M., Schelbert H.R.. Delayed recovery of regional glucose metabolism in reperfused canine myocardium demonstrated by positron-CT. Journal of the

American College of Cardiology 3, vol. 2 (1984) 574.
18) Marshall R.C., Tillish J.H., Phelps M.E., Huang S.C., Carson R., Henze E., Schelbert H.R.. Identification and differentiation of resting myocardial ischemia and infarction in man while positron computed tomography, F18-labeled-fluorodeoxyglucose and N13-ammonia. Circulation 67 (1983) 766-774.
19) Weiss E.S., Ahmed S.A., Welch M.J., Williamson J.R., Ter-Pogossian M.M., Sobel B.E.. Quantification of infarction in cross sections of canine myocardium in vivo positron emission transaxial tomography and ^{11}C-palmitate. Circulation 55 (1977) 66-73.
20) Parodi O., Schwaiger M., Krivokapich J., Schelbert H.R.. Regional myocardial blood flow and wall motion study in patients with designated acute "subendocardial infarction". Journal of the American College of Cardiology 3, vol. 2 (1984) 552.
21) Parodi O., Schelbert H.R., Schwaiger M., Hansen H., Selin C., Hoffman E.J.. Cardiac emission computed tomography: underestimation of regional tracer concentrations due to wall motion abnormalities. Journal of Computer Assisted Tomography 6, vol.8 (1984) 1083-1092.

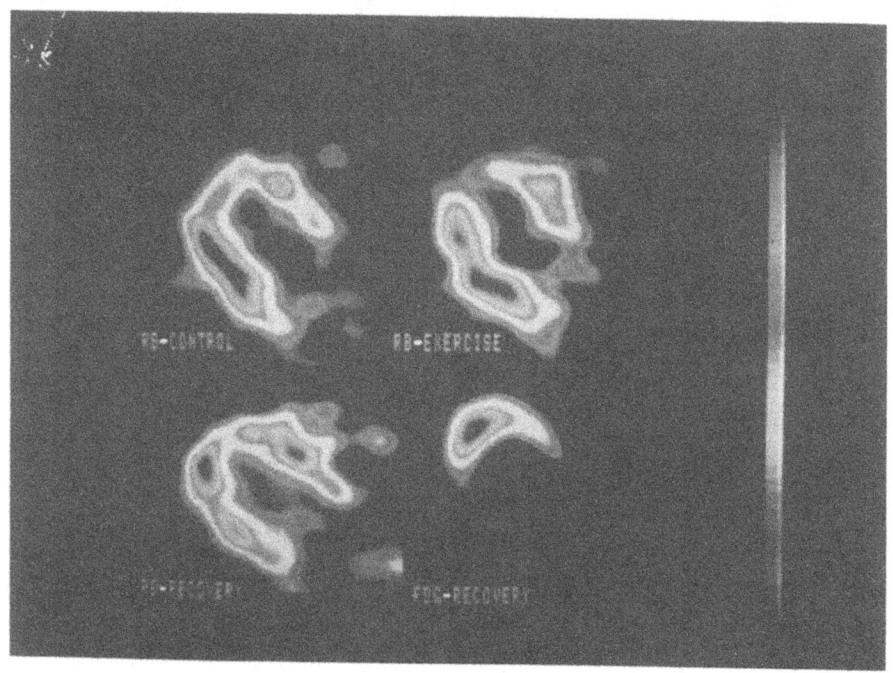

Figure 1 - Positron computed tomographic images of Rb and FDG uptake in the left ventricle of a patient with exertional angina. Each image is a transaxial slice of the heart (1.8 cm thick). In each image the LV free wall is in the 6 to 10 o'clock position, the anterior wall and septum are in the 10 to 3 o'clock position, and the remaining open area is the plane of the mitral valve. The Rb scan at rest (top left) shows a reduced cation uptake in the anterior wall of the left ventricle, corresponding to an old infarction. The same region becomes acutely ischemic during exercise as shown by the Rb scan recorded during the exercise test (top right). Seven minutes after exercise the Rb scan (bottom left) is comparable to the control. FDG was injected 9 minutes after the end of the exercise when all the signs of ischemia subsided. The area of transient ischemia is positively outlined on the FDG scan (bottom right), that was recorded 60 minutes after tracer injection, as a region of increased FDG uptake. The uptake in the anterior wall (ischemic area) is 1.77 times higher than in non-ischemic tissue.

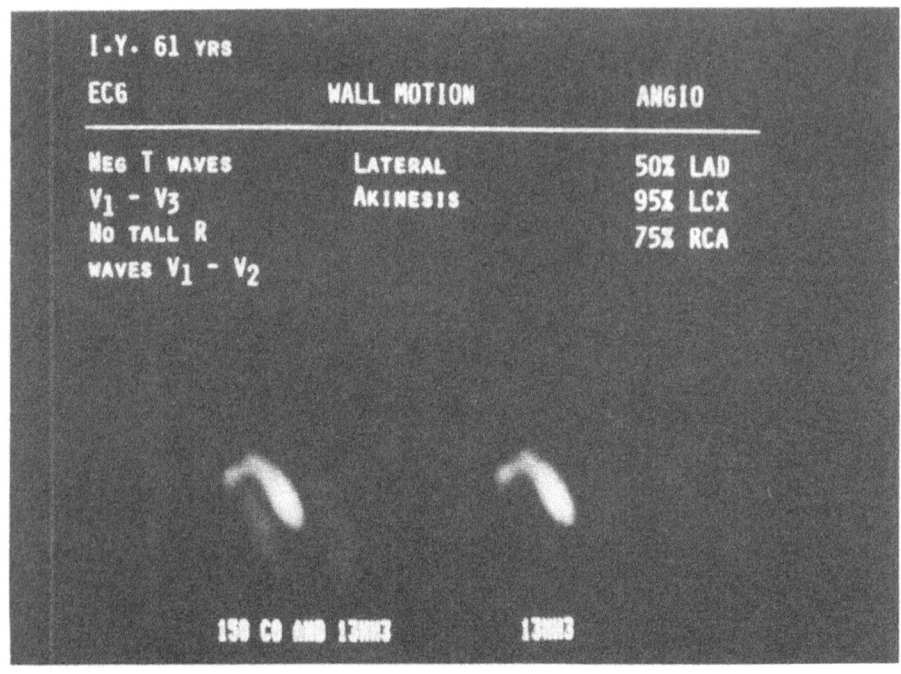

Figure 2 - Combined flow and blood pool studies with N-13 Ammonia and O-15 carbon monoxide in a patient with acute subendocardial infarction. The superimposition of the perfusion image (green) to the blood pool image (red) permits the identification of the necrotic area and its extension. PET data are correlated with electrocardiographic, angiographic and wall motion findings.

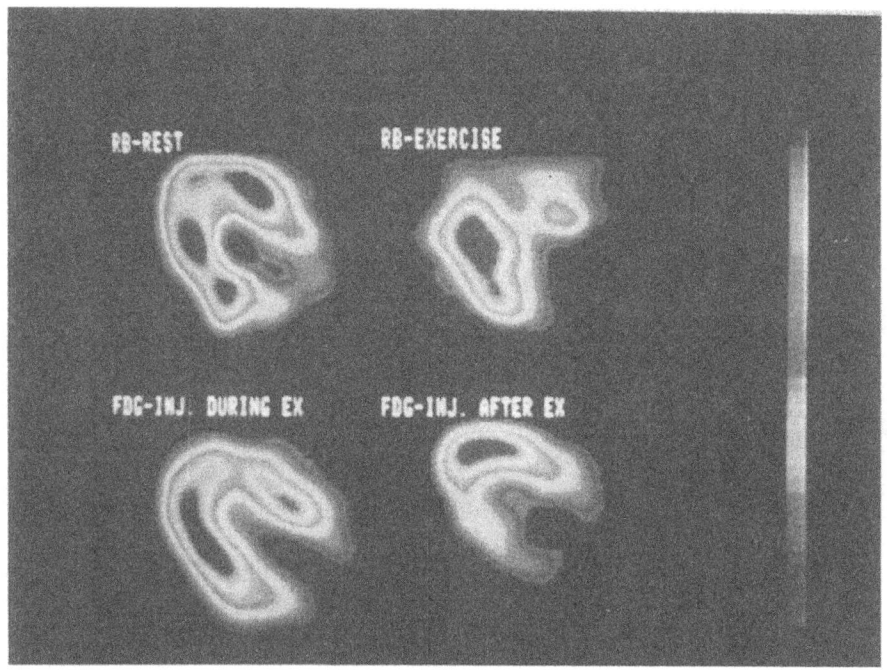

Figure 3 - Positron computed tomographic images of Rb and FDG uptake in the left ventricle of a patient with exertional angina. The Rb scan at rest (top left) shows a homogenous cation uptake in all myocardial walls. The Rb scan recorded during exercise (top right) shows a severely reduced cation uptake in the anterior left ventricle wall. When FDG was injected during the exercise, tracer uptake in normal myocardium was 1.29 that of the ischemic region. When the exercise test was repeated and FDG injected after 8 minutes of recovery (when all the signs of ischemia subsided and the Rb scan was back to normal), the ischemic region was positively outlined from normal myocardium (bottom right), the uptake in the anterior wall being 2.00 times higher than in the non-ischemic muscle. For figure orientation see legend to figure 1.

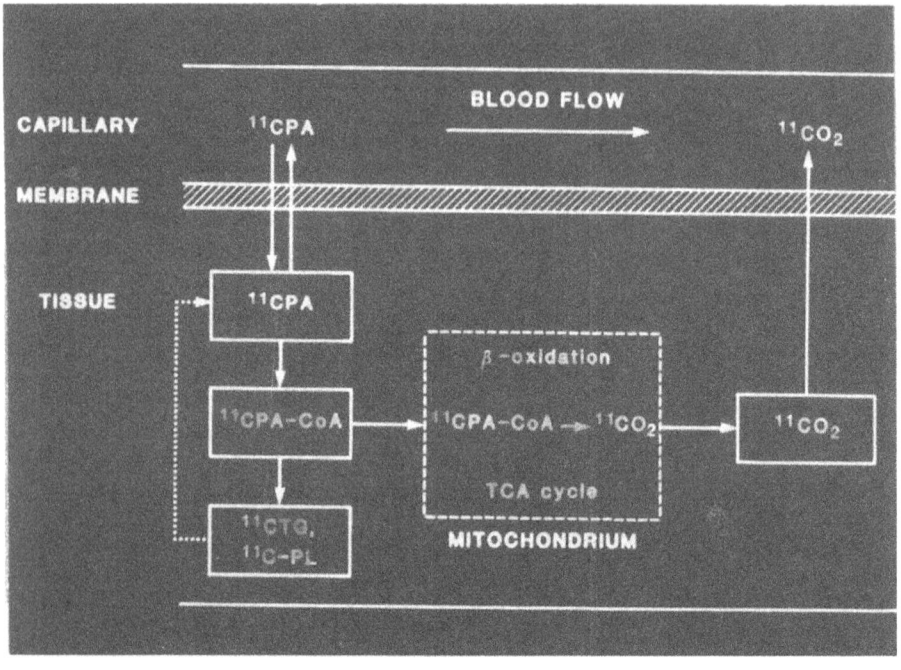

Figure 4 - Block diagram of C-11 PAL (11C PA) kinetics in the myocardium. Once extracted from the blood, C-11 PAL appears to enter two pools with different turnover rates that represent oxidation (dashed box) and esterification (left lower corner, 11C TG, 11C-PL), as the two major metabolic pathways of FFA. C-11 CO_2 (11CO_2), the end product of PAL oxidation, is rapidly cleared from the cells. The relative size of these two pools accounts for different washout slopes recorded by PET, when cardiac work or substrate availability change.

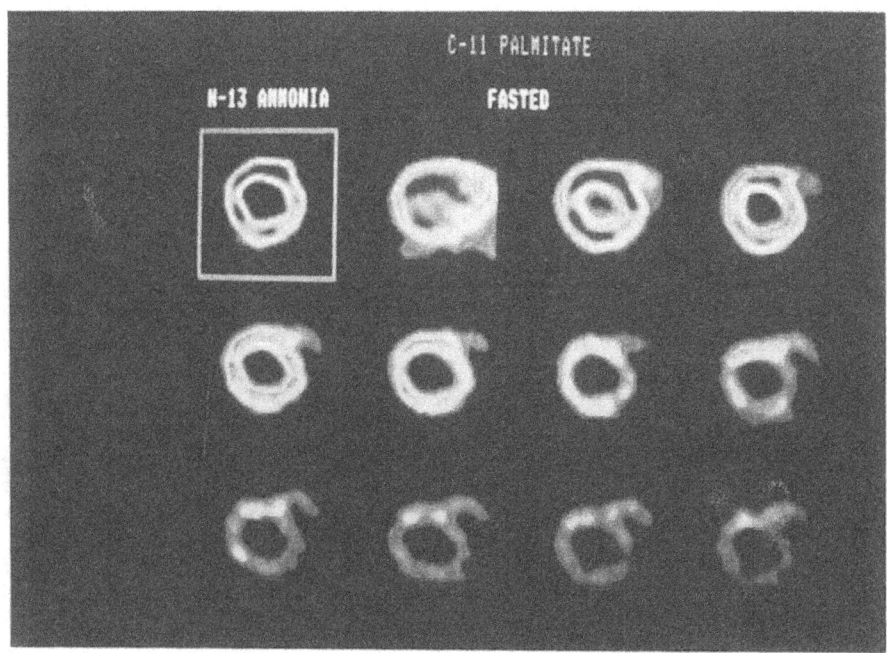

Figure 5 - Sequential 90-second cross-sectional images of myocardial C-11 PAL uptake and washout after its intravenous injection. The flow distribution recorded at the same cross-section with N-13 Ammonia is shown in the square. The initial 90 second image shows both intramyocardial and blood pool activity. After C-11 activity is cleared from the blood, the myocardium is well visualized and shows homogenous PAL distribution. Note that myocardial activity quickly declines (fourth image) because a larger fraction of extracted PAL undergoes oxidation and the product of its oxidation, C-11 CO_2, is cleared from the cells.

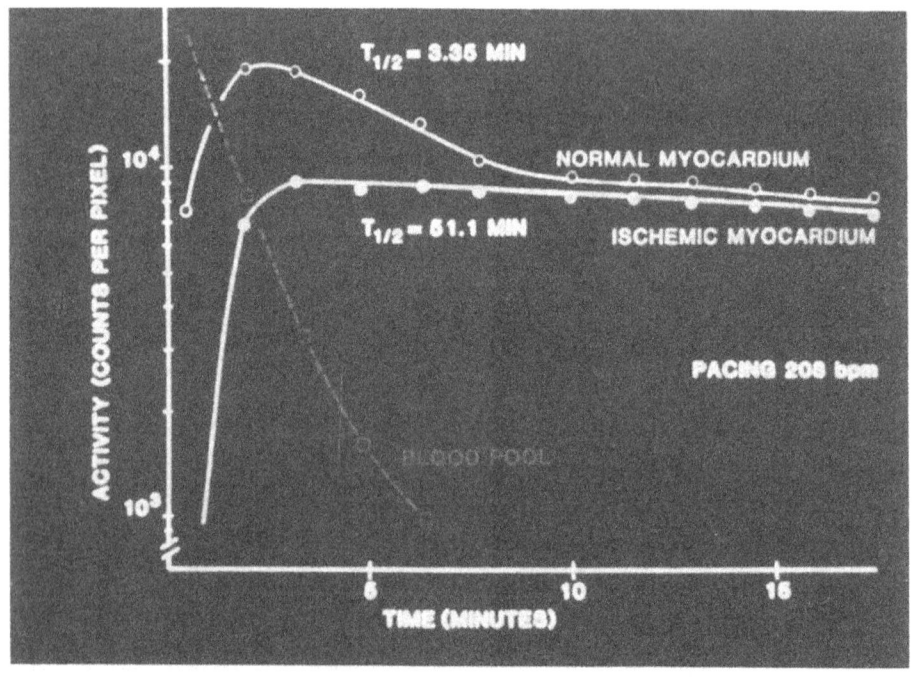

Figure 6 - Time-activity curves of C-11 palmitate uptake and washout obtained in experimental ischemia (stenosis + atrial pacing) by positron emission tomography and regional analysis of sequential scintigrams. Normal perfused myocardium is characterized by a rapid tracer accumulation and biexponential tracer clearance (early phase T 1/2 = 3.35 min, green line). Ischemic myocardium is characterized by a lower C-11 accumulation and a very slow washout rate (early and late phases are not distinguishable, T 1/2 = 51.1 min, yellow line). Blood pool activity quickly declines (red line), allowing good visualization of intramyocardial C-11 activity.

PET IN NEUROLOGY: AN OUTLINE OF PROBLEMS, RECENT ACQUISITIONS AND FUTURE PERSPECTIVES.

G.L. Lenzi and C. Fieschi

Dipartimento di Scienze Neurologiche - Università di Roma "La Sapienza"

The impact of computerized neuro-imaging in the neurological sciences has been so dramatic that our approach to the individual patient has changed completely since C.T. scan availability. Further changes may be expected from the recently born positron emission tomography (PET) in particular if the exploitation of this technique is performed in close relationship with physiopathological questions and clinical problems.

Moreover, the potentials and the obvious interest of PET, particularly in neurology, yield a series of problems that have to be faced without excessive fears or restraints.

Our problem is certainly the amount and the quality of the information.

Every new issue of the most diffused neurological journals contains at least one report obtained with PET, and specialized journals have also appeared. Thus, the "average" neurologist is confronted with a large bulk of information and data, sometimes incomprehensible because mainly technological or methodological and other times strikingly suited to the working hypothesis.

The evident increase in our knowledge is thus challenged by a parallel increase in "entropy" of the knowledge itself, and the usual cooperation between basic sciences and clinical neurology is, in the field of Positron Emission Tomography, less active than before and this gap seems to be increasing at a dangerous rate.

In fact, Positron Emission Tomography requires a close collaboration between clinicians, physicists, engineers, biochemists and physiologists, plus the availability of economical and technological facilities that become prohibitive in particular when working with short-lived positron emitters.

Let us consider a new-born PET Center, strictly devoted to neurological research. The techniques and the models for measuring cerebral blood flow and metabolism (for oxygen and glucose) are available.

We may therefore study how Cockayne's Syndrome affects basic cerebral metabolism and publish the very first report on it. Is this science, however ?

The struggle scientists must face, first to obtain a grant, then to justify the grant obtained and to request further grants, is reflecting itself in a decreasing attention towards the pitfalls of the methodology. Emission Tomography tends to be used as a black-box, leaving to a few the boring task of looking into it.

Basic aspects such as the real soundness of the models, the reproducibility of the values in the same patient at short and long terms, the possibility of applying the models to pathological conditions, the effects of aging, of attention, of sensory stimuli, and so on, all deserve closer scrutiny.

Let me quote one example: the Crossed Cerebellar Diaschisis. This phenomenon has been described by BARON et al (1), by LENZI et al (2,3), by MARTIN and RAICHLE (4), by CELESIA et al. (5) and by KUSHNER et al. (6). That means that nearly all the mayor PET centers in the world have studied this phenomenon: Orsay, London, S. Louis, Philadelphia, Madison. In all the patients studied by these groups, and with a mean decrease of 15-20% in cerebral blood flow and metabolism, no cerebellar sign or symptom has been reported. In certain patients, the asymmetry reached 40% for CBF, 25% for metabolism, with still no cerebellar deficit. Is our brain able to carry out the same performances working

30% below its normal energy standards? It is difficult to believe in such a large redundancy.

In our recent studies with single photon emission tomography (SPECT), we have been able to demonstrate the phenomenon of the Crossed Cerebellar Diaschisis in patients presenting minor or reversible ischemic neurological events, in whom SPECT with I-123-HIPDM demonstrated a decrease of regional blood flow in the territory of the middle cerebral artery because of occlusion of the internal carotid artery (7).

In some patients, we observed the disappearance of the Crossed Cerebellar Diaschisis after the EC-IC by-pass surgery, as well as its reappearance a few months later, always without any cerebellar sign or symptom.

The phenomenon of the "diaschisis" may be in some way related to the recently challenged "sleeping beauty" or "penumbra" concept (8).

The relationship between CT scan results and the extent of flow and metabolism impairments is constantly poor. In addition, not unfrequently we may see patients with small CT scan lesions and severe neurological deficit and vice-versa.

What is known about the relationship between cerebral metabolic rates and function?

The field is still unclear.

Let us summarize here the problems and questions that may be raised in reviewing PET results on the more diffuse biological phenomenon: aging.

Morphological, cellular and subcellular changes occur in the aged human brain.

In particular, the aging brain shows a progressive and parallel decline in both cerebral blood flow (CBF) and metabolism, be it glucose (CMRGlu) or oxygen utilization (CMRO2).

In fact CBF and metabolism reductions are only apparent because the energy supply to the remaining functioning neurons remains quantitatively unchanged.

Moreover, in old people, these data are largely dependent on the control subjects selected for the study.

Furthermore, other factors interfering with the energetic balance of the brain must be taken into account, such as:
a) reduction of the respiratory function; b) reduction of

the capability of the red cells to transport oxygen; c) thickening of the vessel's wall with narrowing of the lumen; d) slower time-course of some enzymatic activities.

Altogether these events increase the cerebral arteriovenous oxygen difference. This increase is utilized by the nervous tissue in order to maintain a nearly constant metabolic level despite the decrease of CBF.

By means of the increased nutrient's extraction the nervous tissue maintains the balance between energy supply and demand.

Additionally, the physiological increase of the nutrient's ER narrows the brain reserve capabilities. At this point, if a new pathological event occurs, the threshold is diminished and neurological signs and symptoms can occur more easily.

The rise in the nutrient's ER thus represents one of the factors that possibly increases the incidence of cerebral ischemic events in old age.

Therefore, while stressing that the aged brain is not an ischemic brain, cerebral ischemia is nevertheless more frequent during old age because of the decreased strategic reserve which allows the possibility of increasing the extraction of the fundamental nutrients (glucose and oxygen).

The breakdown of the physiological equilibrium between function, metabolism and cerebral blood flow occurs when the decrease of supply greatly exceeds the regional or global demands.

In any event, a decreased supply (i.e. reduced regional CBF) does not constantly represent a pathological condition.

Thus, the largest bulk of PET data indicates that CMR for glucose and oxygen decreases with aging (9-10-11-12). The decrease of CMRGlc appears larger than that of oxygen, possibly because of impairment of glucose metabolic pathways or because of utilization of other substrates.

significant CMRGlc decrease with aging. Rapaport et al. (14) and Pantano et al (12) stress the effect of the global volume decrease of the brain, resulting in an artifactual CMRGlc reduction.

Moreover, the possible reduction of CMR and CBF in aging could be completely irrelevant. In fact, what is the

Pet in Neurology

correlation between CM Rates and superior neurological functions ?

METTER et al (16) have studied the pattern of metabolic activation following a sensorial stimulus. In young people, the activation spread to many more cortical regions than in the older volunteers.

Is the aged brain more selective?

Is the young brain a squanderer?

Is the mean age of the patients less important than the mean age of the authors?

In conclusion, the brain offers us modes of measurement signals which we still are unable to understand because they do not "fit" into our previous patterns of knowledge. It is therefore possible that our interpretation of other phenomena and changes in cerebral blood flow and metabolism visualized with Positron Emission Tomography may be greatly biased by our own scientific "natural history".

References

1. Baron J.C., Bousser M.G., Comar D.and P. Castaigne. "Crossed cerebellar diaschisis" in human supratentorial infarction. Trans. Am. Neurol. Assoc. 105 (1980)459-461.
2. Lenzi G.L., Frackowiak R.S.J. and T. Jones. Regional cerebral blood flow (CBF), oxygen utilization (CMRO2) and oxygen extraction ratio (OER) in acute hemispheric stroke. Journal of Cerebral Blood Flow and Metabol., Suppl.1 (1981) S504-505.
3. Lenzi G.L., Frackowiak R.S.J.and T. Jones. Ccrebral oxygen metabolism and blood flow in human cerebral ischemic infarction. Journal Cerebral Blood Flow and Metabol. 2 (1982) 321-335.
4. Martin W.R.W. and M.E. Raichle . Cerebellar blood flow and metabolism in cerebral hemisphere infarction.: Ann. Neurol.14 (1983)168-176.
5. Celesia G.G., Poleyb R.E., Holden J.E., Nickes R.J., Koeppe R.A. and S.I. Gatley. Determination of regional cerebral blood flow in patients with cerebral infarction. Use of fluoromethane labeled with Fluorine 18 and positron emission tomography. Arch. Neurol. 41 (1984) 262-267.
6. Kushner M., Alavi A., Reivich M., Dann R., Burke A. and G. Robinson: Contralateral cerebellar hypometabolism following cerebral insult: a positron emission tomographic study. Ann. Neurol. 15 (1984) 425-434.
7. Fazio F., Lenzi G.L., Gerundini P., Collice M., Gilardi M.C., Taddei G., Delmaschio A., Piacentini G.F., Colombo R., Kung H. F. and M. Blau. Tomographic assessment of reginal cerebral perfusion using intravenous HIPDM and a rotating gamma-camera. Journal of Comp. Assist. Tom. (1984) (in press).
8. Lassen N.A. and S. Vorstrup. Ischemic Penumbra Results in Incomplete Infarction: Is the Sleeping Beauty Dead? Stroke Letters to the Editor.Vol. 15, 4 (1984) 755.
9. Frackowiak R.S., Lenzi G.L., Jones T. and J.D. Heather.Quantitative measurement of regional cerebral blood flow and oxygen metabolism in man using 15-0 and positron emission tomography: theory, procedure and normal values. Journal Comput. Tomogr. 4 (1980) 727-736.

10. Lenzi G.L., Frackowiak R.S.J., Jones T., Heather J.D., Lammertsma A.A., Rhodes C.G. and C. Pozzilli. CMRO2 and CBF by oxygen-15 inhalation technique. Europ Neurol. 20 (1981) 285-290.
11. Kuhl D.E., Metter E.J., Riege W.A. and M.E. Phelps. Effects of human aging on patients of local cerebral glucose utilization determined by the18FDG fluorode oxyglucose method. Journal of Cereb. Blood and Metabol. 2 (1982a) 163-171.
12. Pantano P., Baron J.C., Lebrun-Grandiè P., Duquesnay N., Bousser M.G., and D. Comar. Regional cerebral blood flow and oxygen consumption in human aging. Stroke (in press)
13. Rapoport S.I., Duara R., Horwitz B., Kessler R.M., Sokoloff L., Ingvar D.H., Grady C. and N. Cutler. Brain Aging in 40 healthy men: rCMRGlu and correlated functional activity in various brain regions in the resting state. Journal of Cereb. Blood Flow and Metabol. 3 (Suppl. 1) (1983) S484-S485.
14. de Leon m.J., Ferris S.H., George A.E., Reisberg B., Christman D.R., Kricheff I.I. and A.P. Wolf. Computed tomography and positron emission transaxial tomography evaluations of normal aging and Alzheimer's disease. Journal of Cereb. Blood Flow and Metabol. 3 (1983) 391-394.
15. Hawkins R.A., Mazziotta J.C., Phelps M.E., Huang S.C., Kuhl D.E., Carson R.E., Metter E.J. and W.H. Riege. Journal of Cereb. Blood Flow and Metabol. 3 (1983) 250-253.
16. Metter E.J., Riege W.H., Kuhl D.E. and M.E. Phelps. Differences in regioonal glucose metabolic intercorrelations with aging. Journal of Cereb. Blood Flow and Metabol. 3 (1983) S482-483.

SIMULTANEOUS DETERMINATION OF CEREBRAL BLOOD FLOW AND PARTITION COEFFICIENT WITH A FREELY DIFFUSABLE TRACER

Aldo Rescigno[*+], Richard M. Lambrecht[+], Charles C. Duncan[*],
C.-Y. Shiue[+], and Laura R. Ment[#]

[*]Section of Neurosurgery, [#]Department of Neurology,
 Yale University School of Medicine, New Haven, CT
[+]Chemistry Department,
 Brookhaven National Laboratory, Upton, NY 11973

Cerebral blood flow (CBF) measurements with freely diffusable tracers have depended upon separate partition coefficients (lambda) for grey and white matter. Furthermore, certain tracers have been considered inadequate in species with very high CBF as the lambda diminishes at high flow rates. Similarly, the relation of CBF in normal and pathological circumstances related to the reliability of the measurement remains poorly understood.

As we have shown (1), the cerebral blood concentration $C_b(t)$ of a tracer can be described by the differential equation

(1) $$dC_b(t)/dt + f/L \cdot C_b(t) = f \cdot C_a(t)$$

where $C_a(t)$ is the concentration of the tracer in the arterial blood, f is the CBF, and L is defined by

$$L = C_b(t)/C_v(t),$$

with $C_v(t)$ the concentration of the tracer in the venous blood. This equation is rather general because it is equivalent to equation

(2) $$dC_b(t)/dt = f \cdot [C_a(t) - C_v(t)],$$

representing the conservation of the tracer.

Note that L defined above is not in general a constant; it is constant in particular when the system is at a steady state, because in this case both $C_b(t)$ and $C_v(t)$ are constant. Under this condition L coincides with the partition coefficient lambda as defined by most authors (2).

By utilizing a Harvard Infusion Pump driven by a Servo Amplifier (3), we were able to produce a linearly increasing arterial concentration

$$(3) \quad C_a(t) = S \cdot (t-t_0)$$

of the freely diffusable tracer, ^{18}F-4-fluoroantipyrine (^{18}FAP), in the baboon, and at the same time we measured the concentration $C_b(t)$ of the tracer in different parts of the brain with a Positron Emission Tomograph (PET).

If f and L are constant at least in the interval from t_0 to t, then equation 1 can be integrated and with condition 3 it becomes

$$(4) \quad C_b(t) = SL \cdot (t-t_0-L/f) + $$
$$+ [C_b(t_0)+SL^2/f] \cdot \exp[-f/L \cdot (t-t_0)],$$

where $C_b(t_0)$ is the value of $C_b(t)$ at time t_0.

After a short interval of time, usually of the order of a few minutes, the exponential term in the expression above becomes negligible, and we have simply

$$(5) \quad C_b(t) = SL \cdot (t-t_0-L/f),$$

i.e. the equation of a straight line of slope SL and intersecting the time-axis at the point $t=t_0+L/f$.

As shown by equation 3, S is by definition the slope of $C_a(t)$ versus t; therefore the partition coefficient L is the slope of $C_b(t)$ divided by the slope of $C_a(t)$. Once L is known, the value of f can be computed from L/f.

The following table shows the relative errors made by computing C_b with equation 5 instead of 4, i.e. by ignoring the exponential term in equation 4:

ft/L	dC_b/C_b
1.0	1.000
1.2	0.601
1.4	0.381
1.6	0.252
1.8	0.171
2.0	0.119
2.4	0.061
2.8	0.033
3.2	0.018
3.6	0.010

With typical values of $f = 0.3$ min^{-1} and $L = 1$, the error in C_b is approximately 6% after 8 minutes.

With the PET, the acquisition time of a typical experiment is of the order of two minutes, therefore the tracer activity is not measured as a continuous function of time, but rather by discrete intervals; instead of the instantaneous value $C_b(t)$, its average value

$$1/(t_2-t_1) \cdot \int_{t_1}^{t_2} C_b(u)\,du$$

over the interval t_1, t_2 is measured. As long as $C_b(t)$ is a linear function, no error is made by taking the above average value as the value of function $C_b(t)$ at the center of the time interval t_1, t_2; in other words if t is large enough we have exactly

$$1/(t_2-t_1) \cdot \int_{t_1}^{t_2} C_b(u)\,du = C_b[(t_2-t_1)/2].$$

So far we have indicated by $C_a(t)$ and $C_b(t)$ the concentration of the tracer if it had an infinite life, or after correction for its radioactive decay; what the tomograph actually measures in the interval t_1, t_2 is

$$1/(t_2-t_1) \cdot \int_{t_1}^{t_2} e^{-kt} C_b(t)\,dt,$$

where k is the disintegration constant; this value is then corrected for the radioactive decay of the nuclide at the middle of the time interval. After this last correction and ignoring the exponential term of equation 4 the integral above becomes

$$SL/(kt_m) \cdot [(t_1-L/f-t_0+1/k)\exp(+kt_m/2) -$$

$$- (t_2-L/f-t_0+1/k)\exp(-kt_m/2)]$$

where

$$t_m = t_2-t_1$$

is the acquisition time interval. With ^{18}F (half life = 109.7 min, $k = 6.32 \cdot 10^{-3}$ min^{-1}) and in the typical experimental conditions, i.e. by making $t_1 > 5$ min and $t_2-t_1 = 2$ min, this expression differs from the theoretical value of $C_b(t)$ at time $(t_1+t_2)/2$ by much less than one percent.

When using isotopes with a much shorter half life, or when experimenting with a different input function, the above error may not be negligible at all and a different correction may be necessary, as outlined in a previous paper (4).

Suppose that $C_b(t)$ has been measured, after the exponential term has become negligible, at two different times t_1 and t_2, and call A and B the values found (see fig.1):

t	$C_b(t)$
t_1	A
t_2	B

The slope of the straight line extrapolating $C_b(t)$ is given by

$$SL = (B-A)/(t_2-t_1);$$

the intercept D of this straight line with the t-axis is

$$D = (t_1 B - t_2 A)/(B-A),$$

with

$$D = t_0 + L/f;$$

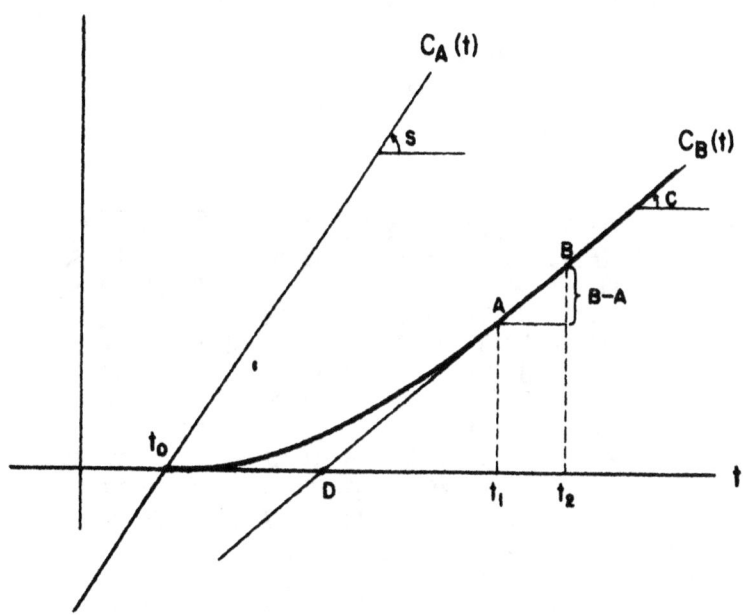

Figure 1.

thence

$$L = 1/S \cdot (B-A)/(t_2-t_1)$$

and

$$f = 1/S \cdot (B-A)/(t_2-t_1) \cdot 1/(D-t_0).$$

Taking the total differentials of the last two expressions,

(6) $dL/L = (t_2-D)/(t_2-t_1) \cdot dB/B -$

$- (t_1-D)/(t_2-t_1) \cdot dA/A - dS/S$

(7) $df/f = (t_2-D)/(t_2-t_1) \cdot [1-(t_1-D)/(D-t_0)] \cdot dB/B -$

$- (t_1-D)/(t_2-t_1) \cdot [1-(t_2-D)/(D-t_0)] \cdot dA/A +$

$+ t_0/(D-t_0) \cdot dt_0/t_0 - dS/S.$

These two equations show how the errors in the measurements of A, B, D, S and t_0 propagate in the computation of L and f; of course all equations above ignore infinitesimals of any order higher than one, therefore these results are valid only for small errors.

Figure 2 shows the values of L computed for a particular region of the brain of a baboon, and fig.3 shows the corresponding values of f, in ml.min^{-1} per 100 gr of tissue.

```
64 66 69 71 73 75 77 79 79 79 79 78 79 81 82 81 77
64 69 73 76 79 81 82 83 83 83 82 82 82 83 84 83 80
62 69 75 80 83 84 85 85 85 85 84 84 84 84 85 84 80
60 68 75 81 85 87 87 86 86 85 85 84 84 84 84 82 78
60 68 76 82 86 88 87 86 84 84 83 83 83 82 81 78 74
63 71 79 85 88 88 87 85 83 82 81 81 81 80 77 74 69
69 77 84 89 91 90 88 85 83 81 80 80 79 77 75 70 65
76 84 91 94 95 94 91 87 84 82 81 80 79 77 74 69 62
82 90 96 99 99 98 94 91 88 85 84 82 81 79 75 70 62
85 94 99 99 99 99 98 95 92 89 87 85 83 81 77 71 63
84 93 99 99 99 99 99 98 95 92 90 87 85 82 78 72 63
75 88 96 99 99 99 99 99 97 94 90 88 84 81 77 70 61
72 80 88 94 97 98 98 97 95 92 88 85 81 77 72 65 56
62 70 78 85 89 91 92 91 90 87 83 79 75 70 64 57 48
52 59 66 73 77 80 82 82 81 79 76 71 66 60 54 47 39
40 46 53 59 64 67 69 70 70 68 65 61 56 50 44 37 30
```

FIGURE 2
Values of L $.10^2$

```
24 32 39 42 39 34 30 28 29 32 37 40 35 27 21 17 15
27 31 32 32 31 30 29 28 28 30 32 33 30 25 20 17 14
41 36 32 30 29 29 29 29 30 31 31 30 28 24 20 17 15
   50 35 30 29 30 32 34 36 37 35 32 29 25 21 18 15
   59 37 31 30 33 38 46 53 54 47 39 33 28 24 20 17
   43 32 30 31 36 48 71       82 56 41 34 29 25 20
34 28 26 26 29 36 52 96          78 52 41 36 32 26
22 21 21 23 26 32 45 75          72 49 40 37 34 30
19 18 19 20 22 26 34 47 64 73 63 48 37 32 29 27 25
18 17 18 18 20 23 27 33 38 41 39 33 28 25 22 21 19
18 17 17 18 19 21 23 26 29 30 29 27 24 21 19 17 15
19 18 17 17 18 19 21 23 25 26 25 23 21 19 16 14 12
21 19 18 18 18 19 21 22 23 23 23 21 19 17 15 13 11
25 21 19 18 19 20 21 22 22 22 21 19 18 15 13 11  9
37 28 23 21 21 21 21 21 21 19 18 17 15 13 11  9  7
   79 36 27 25 24 23 21 19 17 15 14 12 10  8  7  6
```

FIGURE 3
Values of f in ml.min^{-1} per 100 gr of tissue

The iso-lines of these figures connect points of equal L.
The values shown are computed using equation 5, i.e. by ignoring the exponential term in equation 4; to give an idea of the precision obtained we can analyze a particular pixel, say the one in the row and column shown by the small arrows in figures 2 and 3. The following table summarizes the results.

	Measured value	Error due to exp. term
A	2245.44	1.8%
B	2712.04	.88%

L = 0.997; f = 17.65 ml.min^{-1}/100 gr

Equations 6 and 7 become

$$dL/L = 5.8\, dB/B - 4.8\, dA/A - dS/S,$$

$$df/f = -9.0\, dB/B + 10.0\, dA/A - dS/S + 4.9\, dt_0/t_0;$$

they show that the error in f is about twice as large as the error in L, that the errors caused by A and by B act in opposite directions and could partly compensate each other, and finally that the determination of the time t_0 of the beginning of the ramp injection is critical in the computation of f.

We return now to equation 1, valid if L and f are constant at least for $t > t_0$; in particular the assumption that L is constant implies a rapid equilibration of the tracer between brain and venous blood, i.e. it requires that the region of the brain under observation behaves like a single perfect compartment. We can now drop this restriction and substitute it with the much broader assumption that the tracer is transferred from the arterial blood to the brain through an unspecified number of linear compartments. We can therefore write the set of differential equations

$$dC_a/dt = -K_a C_a(t)$$

$$dC_b/dt = -K_b C_b(t) + \Sigma_j k_{jb} X_j(t) + k_{ab} C_a(t),$$

$$dX_j/dt = -K_j X_j(t) + \Sigma_l k_{lj} X_l(t) + k_{aj} C_a(t),$$

$$j = 1, 2, \ldots$$

where the $X_j(t)$ are the state variables of the intermediate compartments between arterial blood and brain, the small k's are transfer rates between compartments, and the capital K's are turnover rates of compartments.

With the standard methods of compartmental analysis (5) and assuming for convenience that all compartments are empty at time 0, the above equations reduce to the integral equation

(8) $$C_b(t) = \int_0^t g(t-u) C_a(u) du.$$

Define now the moments

$$A_i = \int_0^\infty t^i/i! \cdot C_a(t) dt,$$

$$B_i = \int_0^\infty t^i/i! \cdot C_b(t) dt,$$

$$G_i = \int_0^\infty t^i/i! \cdot g(t) dt,$$

for $i = 0, 1, 2, \ldots$; multiply both terms of equation 8 by $t^i/i! \cdot dt$ and integrate from 0 to ∞; after a few transformations we obtain

(9) $\qquad B_0 = G_0 A_0,$

(10) $\qquad B_1 = G_0 A_1 + G_1 A_0,$

(11) $\qquad B_2 = G_0 A_2 + G_1 A_1 + G_2 A_0,$

and so forth. From these equations, if the moments of $C_a(t)$ and $C_b(t)$ are measured, the moments of $g(t)$ can be computed, pixel by pixel.

To clarify the physical meaning of these moments, write

$$B_0 = 1/K_b \cdot \int_0^\infty K_b C_b(t)dt,$$

where $1/K_b$ is the transit time through compartment $\underline{b}$, while

$$\int_0^\infty K_b C_b(t)dt,$$

is the total number of tracer particles that leave this compartment; therefore B_0 is the total expected time spent in this compartment by a tracer particle. The same can be said of A_0, so that from equation 9,

$$G_0 = B_0/A_0$$

is the ratio of those times, a quantity called weight of the transfer from $\underline{a}$, the compartment of the arterial blood, to $\underline{b}$, the compartment of the particular section of the brain under observation (6).

Dividing equation 10 by equation 9,

$$B_1/B_0 = A_1/A_0 + G_1/G_0;$$

but

$$B_1/B_0 = \int_0^\infty t \cdot C_b(t)dt / \int_0^\infty C_b(t)dt$$

is the expected time a tracer particle leaves compartment $\underline{b}$, and

$$A_1/A_0 = \int_0^\infty t \cdot C_a(t)dt / \int_0^\infty C_a(t)dt$$

is the expected time it leaves compartment $\underline{a}$, therefore G_1/G_0 is the transfer time from $\underline{a}$ to $\underline{b}$ (5).

Similarly from equation 11 we obtain

$$B_2/B_0 = A_2/A_0 + G_1/G_0 \cdot A_1/A_0 + G_2/G_0,$$

where the ratio G_2/G_0 is the second moment of the transfer time from $\underline{a}$ to $\underline{b}$ (7).

The next step consists in mapping separately the values of G_0, G_1/G_0, G_2/G_0, and so forth. The map of G_0 shows the distribution of the weight, a quantity strictly related to the bioavailability. The map of G_1/G_0 shows the distribution of the transfer time; the smaller this time is, the faster the arterial blood reaches that region of the brain. The map of G_2/G_0 shows the distribution of the variance of the transfer time; the closer this value is to $(G_1/G_0)^2$, the better that region of the brain approximates a single compartment; a value of G_2/G_0 much smaller than $(G_1/G_0)^2$ indicates that the blood is supplied to that region of the brain by several compartments in series; larger values of G_2/G_0 reveal the presence of parallel compartments.

Aknowledgment: Research carried out at Brookhaven National Laboratory under contract DE-AC02-76CH00016 with the U. S. Department of Energy and supported by its Office of Health and Environmental Research. Research at Yale University was supported by NIH Grant No. R01-NS-16802.

References

1. C.C.Duncan, R.M.Lambrecht, A.Rescigno, C.Y.Shiue, G.W.Bennett and L.R.Ment, The Ramp Injection of Radiotracers for Blood Flow Measurements by Emission Tomography. Phys.Med.Biol. 28(1983)963-972.
2. S.S.Kety. The Theory and Applications of the Exchange of Inert Gas at the Lungs and Tissues. Pharmacological Reviews 3(1951)1-41.
3. R.M.Lambrecht, G.W.Bennett, C.C.Duncan, L.W.Ducote. Method and Apparatus for Injection of a Substance into the Blood Stream of a Subject. U.S.Patent 4,409,966. October 18, 1983.
4. A.Rescigno, R.M.Lambrecht and C.C.Duncan, Stochastic Modelling of Physiologic Processes with Radiotracers and Positron Emission Tomography; in Applications of Physics to Medicine and Biology (Alberi, Bajzer and Baxa, editors). Pages 303-318. World Scientific Publ.Co., Singapore, 1983.
5. A.Rescigno and G.Segre. Drug and Tracer Kinetics. Blaisdell, Waltham, Mass., 1964.
6. A.Rescigno. On Transfer Times in Tracer Experiments. J.Theor. Biol. 39(1973)9-27.
7. A.Rescigno and L.D.Michels. On Dispersion in Tracer Experiments. J.Theor.Biol. 41(1973)451-460.

DISCUSSION SUMMARY

PANEL ON
PHYSIOLOGICAL   MEASUREMENTS   BY   POSITRON   EMISSION   TOMOGRAPHY

Todd Pokropek asked for the meaning of "High Chemical Resolution in NMR/MRI". Jones answered that current developments in In Vivo NMR spectroscopy indicate the possibility for simultaneously detecting a range of biochemicals that are indigenous to the tissue (Shulman et al. J Clin Invest 1984, 74 1127 - 1131).

As for the possibilities of developing a "cerebral exercise test" for patients with carotid artery stenosis (Adelstein), it has been shown that the cerebral tissue volume in these patients increases in order to maintain baseline values of cerebral blood flow. As the disease advances, the vessels appear to become maximally dilated (Gibbs et al. Lancet 1984, 310-314). One cerebral exercise that has been used is the test of cerebral vessel reactivity to increased arterial pCO_2. Mendelow et al. (to be published 12th Int Symp of CBF & Met, Sweden 1985) have shown that patients with carotid artery stenosis are less able to increase their CBF when inhaling CO_2 compared to normals. This non reactivity has shown to be reversible following endarterectomy and EC-IC bypass (Jones). Adelstein raised the question on how it could be possible to distinguish between diseases that reduce the number of receptor sites from those that change receptor affinity. The direct way of doing this would be to plot a tissue uptake curve for the labelled ligand against the concentration of free non-superficial bound ligand. This would involve each individual being subjected to a number of separate administrations of tracers (Jones).

POSTER SESSION

COMPUTERIZED MILLIMETRIC MAPPING OF MYOCARDIAL
BLOOD FLOW AND METABOLISM

C. Paoli[1], R. Porinelli[1], M.G. Trivella[2], R. Bellazzini[3]
M. Massai[3], M. Dalle Vacche[2], G. Pelosi[2], A. L'Abbate[2]
[1] IBM Scientific Center, Pisa, Italy.
[2] C.N.R. Institute of Clinical Physiology, Pisa, Italy.
[3] Institute of Physics, University of Pisa, and INFN, Italy.

1. INTRODUCTION

Radioactive microsphere technique is a well established and widely employed method for measuring myocardial blood flow distribution. The conventional well-counting technique allows several flow measurements by the use of different isotopes, but has a limited spatial resolution, which is related to the number and specific activity of microspheres and to the size of tissue specimen (1,2).
On the contrary, autoradiographic technique offers a much higher resolution, but it is unable to discriminate between isotopes of different energies.
The present study is intended to document the possibility of discriminating between two particulate radioactive tracers in order to obtain two flow maps with high spatial resolution, as well as the possibility of a comparison of blood flow distribution with a corresponding metabolic map.

2. MATERIALS AND METHODS

This evaluation was performed on open chest anesthetized mongrel dogs. Two types of microspheres, labeled with different isotopes previously tested to produce spots of different sizes on autoradiographs, were injected into the Left Atrium in different haemodynamic conditions. In order to obtain absolute values of regional myocardial blood flow, simultaneously to microsphere injection, a reference blood sample was withdrawn from a peripheral artery at a constant pump rate.

At the same time as the second microspheres injection, 5mCi of 3H-deoxy-glucose were given intravenously.
Twenty minutes later, the animal was killed by an overdose of anesthetic. The heart was excised, put in a cardboard box full of cellulose as support and immediately frozen by immersion in liquid Nitrogen. Three vertical radioactive markers were positioned at three corners of the box, one anteriorly and two posteriorly, in order to have reference points for the correct alignment of autoradiographic images. Subsequently each heart was cut in one centimeter thick transverse sections.

3. AUTORADIOGRAPHY and DIGITAL IMAGES ACQUISITION

From each transverse section, 15-20 consecutive microslices, 40µ thick, were obtained by means of a LKB microtome kept at -20°C. After dehydratation, microslices were mounted on a radiographic film and exposed for 2-3 weeks.
Reference blood samples obtained during each injection of microspheres were counted in a gamma-counter, in order to obtain counts per ml/min of blood flow. Then, samples of 0.1 ml of blood containing different amounts of radioactivity were smeared on a plastic rigid sheet and exposed on a radiographic film.
Two microslices are used to obtain by means of a special designed Multiwire Proportional Chamber digital images of the regional myocardial uptake of 3H-deoxy-glucose (3); this instrument has a resolution of 700μ. To digitize autoradiographs of microspheres, an optical scanner, having a response of 256 levels of grey and a spatial resolution varying from 12.5µ to 400µ, is employed.
For this work a resolution of 100µ on both X and Y directions is used. An area of 80 by 80 millimeters is digitized, so that each digital image produced has a dimension of 800 by 800 pixels (8 bits per pixel).

4. COMPUTER PROCESSING

To process and analyze the digital images, a specific software package has been developed; this package uses the IBM-7350 as image processing system, taking advantage of its internal special computational capabilities (4,5).
To describe how the package works the symbolic concept of "section process" must be introduced. A "section process" is the sequence of operations necessary to process all the digital images of a section. The operations involved in a "section process" can be grouped into steps.
The two steps of a "section process" are the following:

1) Images Processing
2) Images Analysis

4.1 Images Processing

Digital images relative to the deoxy-glucose uptake are processed in order to remove the noise introduced by the Multiwire Proportional Chamber and then enlarged to obtain an image of the same size as the digital image of microspheres; this digital image (J) represents the metabolic map (Fig. 1).

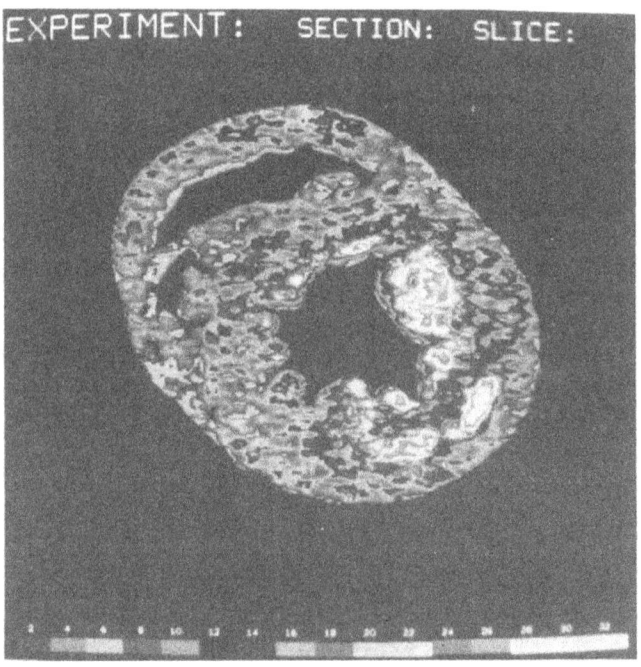

Fig. 1. Deoxy-glucose uptake distribution map.

During digitization (optical scanner or multiwire proportional chamber), due to the fact that manual operations are required, alignment error between slices, may happen. To remove these possible errors the positions of the three markers on the digital image of the first slice of the selected section are taken as references. Then all digital images of the section are translated, if necessary, by means of an interactive procedure, in order to overlap their markers to the references ones.

The first operation performed on the input digital image of microspheres (A) is to separate the microspheres from the background, the result of this operation is the generation of a binary image (B), which is characterized by pixels with a value of 255 for the microspheres and 0 for the background. The image (B) is processed by means of a 7 by 7 smoothing filter and a thresholding operation; a binary digital image (C), containing microspheres of

one type only (big microspheres), is produced (pixels of value 1 for the microspheres, pixels of value 0 for the background).
By adding images (B) and (C) pixel by pixel and performing a thresholding operation on the result, a binary digital image (D), containing microspheres of the second type only (small microspheres), is produced (pixels of value 1 for the microspheres, pixels of value 0 for the background). Both images (C and D) are processed by means of a sequence of smoothing filters and thresholding operations; the purpose of this process is to produce two new binary digital images (E and F) where all the microspheres have the shape of a standard square (7 pixels of side). These binary images are histogrammed, the total number of pixels with value 1 is divided by the standard square area's value; the resulting value represents the number of microspheres present on the image.

The procedure described in this paragraph is applied to all the section's input digital images, obtaining two series of images (E and F). All the images of each series are summed pixel by pixel to generate two images (G and H) representing the section distribution maps of the two types of microspheres: an example of (G) image is shown in Fig.2.

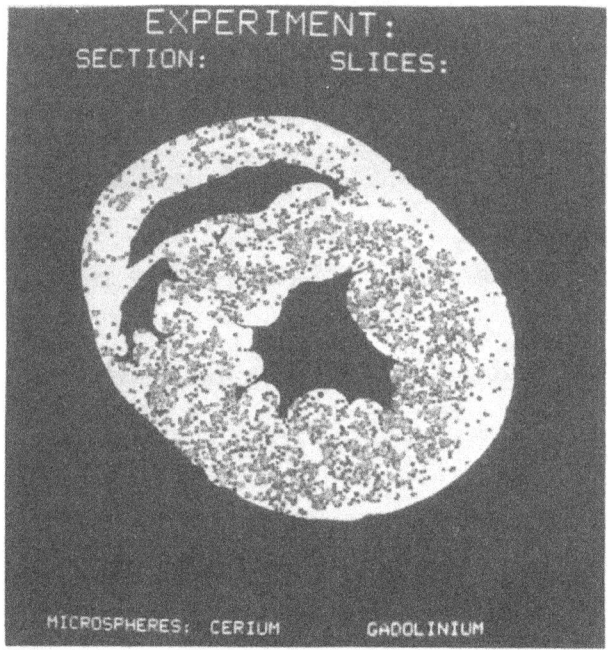

Fig. 2. Microspheres distribution map.

A similar procedure has also been used to count the microspheres contained in the autoradiography of blood smears in order to obtain a correlation between the radioactivity per unit of volume and the

number of microspheres of each type per unit of volume; in this way it is possible to compute absolute blood flow values.
Images (G) (H) and (J) can be displayed in colors to evaluate the microspheres's distribution maps and metabolism.

4.2 Images Analysis

Images (G, H and J) can be analyzed separately or in a comparative way to evaluate the blood flow and deoxy-glucose uptake in different areas. The analysis can be performed separately on the two ventricles; image splitting is performed by means of an interactive procedure.
After the splitting the interactive procedure allows the division of the selected ventricle in a number of wedges (from 8 to 36). An example of blood flow analysis, performed on the left ventricle, is presented in Fig. 3.

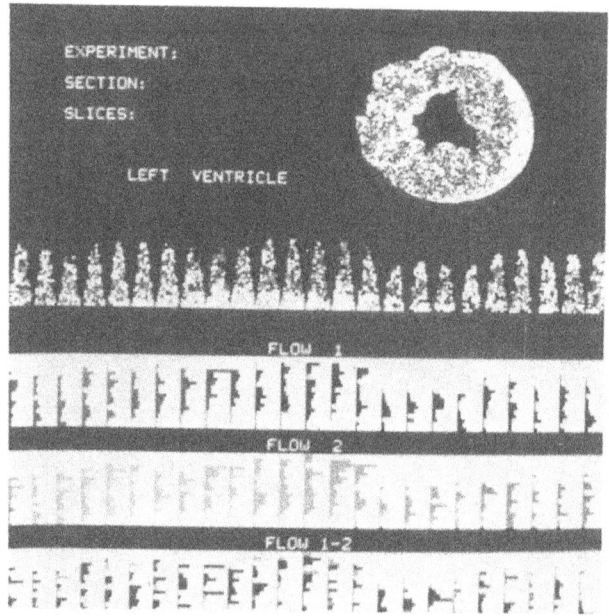

Fig. 3. Blood flow analysis on the left ventricle.

5. CONCLUSIONS

The physiological interest of high spatial resolution tracer mapping is obvious, especially if applied to the simultaneous study of regional perfusion and metabolism, in order to detect their

possible spatial heterogeneity in the heart as well in other organs.
Finally, since tomographic nuclear techniques are becoming available today for clinical studies of organ perfusion and metabolism, experimental techniques like the one described here could be of great interest for basic research in this field.

6. REFERENCES

1. Domenech RJ, Hoffman JIE, Noble MIM, Saunders KB, Henson JR, Subijanto S. Total and Regional Coronary Blood Flow Measured by Radioactive Microspheres in Conscious and Anesthetized Dogs. Circ Res 25:581-95. 1969.
2. Buckberg GD, Luck JC, Payne DB, Hoffman JIE, Archie JP, Fixler DE. Some sources of error in measuring regional blood flow with radioactive microspheres. Journal of Applied Physiology 4:598-604. 1971.
3. Bellazzini R, Del Guerra A, Massai M, Spandre' G, Ragadini M and Tonelli G. A MWPC with a cathode coupled delay-line read-out for DNA repair studies Nucl. Instr. Meth. 190:627-638. 1981.
4. IBM Corporation. IBM-7350 Host Basic User Subroutines. IBM Corporation (SH19-6298). 1983.
5. Rosenfeld A, Kak AC. Digital Picture Processing. New York: Academic Press. 1976.

PART XIV STATE-OF-THE-ART AND FUTURE TRENDS IN PET INSTRUMENTATION

Chairman: Riccardo Guzzardi (Italy)

ADVANCED INSTRUMENTATION FOR POSITRON EMISSION TOMOGRAPHY

S.E. Derenzo and T.F. Budinger

Lawrence Berkeley Laboratory
and Donner Laboratory
Berkeley, CA
U.S.A.

ABSTRACT

This paper summarizes the physical processes and medical science goals that underly modern instrumentation design for Positron Emission Tomography. The paper discusses design factors such as detector material, crystal-phototube coupling, shielding geometry, sampling motion, electronics design, time-of-flight, and the interrelationships with quantitative accuracy, spatial resolution, temporal resolution, maximum data rates, and cost.

1 INTRODUCTION

Positron Emission Tomography (PET) serves a unique and important role in medical research because it permits the non-invasive, quantitative study of biological processes as they occur using minute quantities of tracer material. This tracer can be in ionic form, such as 75-second ^{82}Rb, which is rapidly taken up by active heart muscle, or in molecular form, such as 20-min ^{11}C-palmitic acid, which is taken up and oxidized by active heart muscle. Similarly, 108-min ^{18}F-deoxyglucose is taken up by active brain tissue. The physiological processes involved include:

1) Labeled compounds are usually administered by intravenous injection or by inhalation of a radioactive gas. Rapid injections (< 5 sec) are essential when the processes to be studied are also rapid.

2) After passing through the lungs and heart chambers, the tracer is delivered by the arteries to the various tissues in proportion to the blood flow that they receive from the heart. The activity delivered to each organ depends not only on the amount administered, but also on the fraction of cardiac output received and the amount extracted from the lungs during passage of the tracer from the right to the left heart.

3) The tracer is extracted by the tissues through diffusion, active transport or selective binding.

4) The label may undergo several fates, depending on the biochemical processes in the tissue– The tracer may be (i) trapped in its original form, or (ii) diffuse back into the circulation (washout), or (iii) be metabolized and the products either trapped or washed out.

The function of PET instrumentation is the measurement of positron tracer concentration in well-defined volumes as a function of time. Depending on the nature of the tracer and the biochemical processes that it undergoes, compartment models are fit to these data to yield information about tissue extraction, metabolic rate constants, blood volumes, and blood flow. See reference (1) for a review of physiological modeling of PET data.

Section 2 below considers the physical processes that occur during PET and the special advantages of PET for 3-D tomographic imaging.

Section 3 discusses the instrumentation design factors that affect quantitative accuracy, temporal resolution, and spatial resolution.

Section 4 discusses design tradeoffs as well as some recently developed high resolution state-of-the-art tomographs.

2 PHYSICAL CONSIDERATIONS

2.1 PHYSICAL PROCESSES IN PET

The ability of PET instrumentation to measure tracer concentrations is strongly influenced by the physical processes involved in positron emission, the detection of the annihilation photons, and the tomographic reconstruction, which we summarize below in 11 steps:

1) The nucleus decays with the emission of a positron (e^+) and a neutrino (ν). The positrons have a spread of energies from zero to a maximum energy which varies from 0.64 MeV for ^{18}F to 3.35 MeV for ^{82}Rb.

2) The positron looses most of its kinetic energy in the tissue as it travels a few mm from the point of emission to the point of annihilation with a nearby electron (2-4).

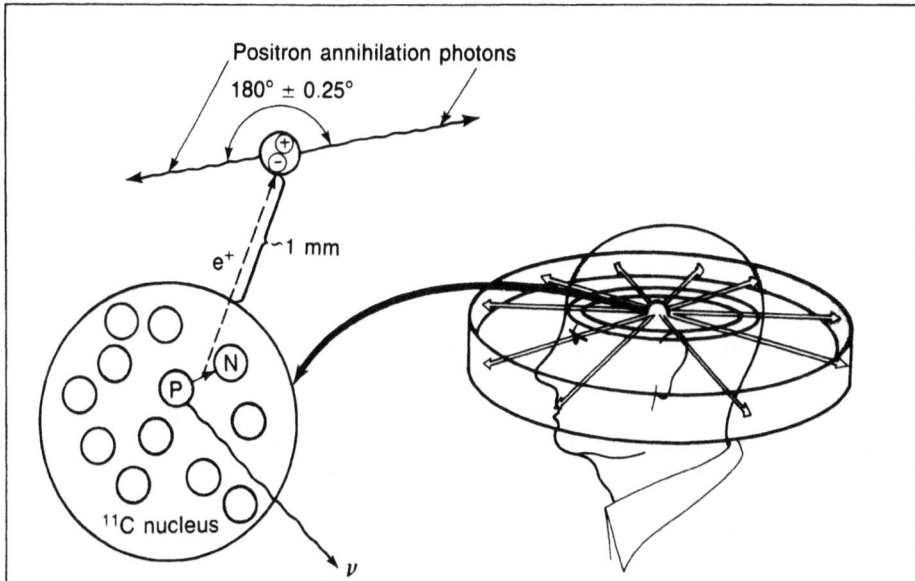

Figure 1: A positron emitted by nuclear decay stops in tissue and annihilates with a nearby electron, producing two 511 keV annihilation photons that fly off in nearly opposite directions.

3) If the positron were able to loose all of its kinetic energy before annihilation, the two 511 keV annihilation photons would be emitted in exactly opposite directions. However, the positron has a residual energy of typically 10 eV, and this causes the angle between the photon pair to have a Gaussian distribution with a full-width at half-maximum (FWHM) of 0.50° (5).

4) A 511 keV photon will travel an average of 10 cm in water before interacting by Compton scattering. This process reduces its energy and randomly changes its direction, effectively loosing all image information. Since the human head or chest is approximately two interaction lengths thick, the probability that both annihilation photons leave the body unscattered is only about 20%. This represents a significant loss of events and requires large correction factors. Also, a small but significant fraction of the annihilation photons scatter "in the plane" of the tomograph and are detected as prompt (non-random) coincidences. These result in a heterogeneous background that extends beyond the subject over the entire imaging field.

5) The annihilation photons can interact in the scintillator in two ways— (i) by photoelectric effect, whereby the entire 511 keV is given to a recoil electron, or (ii) by Compton scattering, where only a portion of the full energy is given to a recoil electron and the photon is reduced in energy and scattered into a new (random) angle. For BGO the probability of a photoelectric event is about 50% for the first interaction. For BaF_2 this probability is about

25%. A successful event requires that both annihilation photons pass the pulse height requirements in both opposing detectors (6,7).

6) The recoil electrons produce ionization and excited atomic electrons in the scintillation crystal. Some of the excited electrons return to their ground states by the emission of scintillation light. The luminous efficiency (number of scintillation photons per keV loss) and the speed of emission vary from crystal to crystal (8).

7) Light in the scintillator can be trapped by total internal reflection, absorbed by internal impurities and imperfections, absorbed by external reflectors, or collected by the photodetector. The collection efficiency is the fraction of light that reaches the photodetector (9).

8) The photodetector converts collected scintillation light to a useful electrical pulse. The quantum efficiency is the probability that an incident photon will produce a photoelectron in the photodetector. The photomultiplier tube has an internal gain of typically 1 million and a single photoelectron produces a pulse several nsec wide and many mV high.

9) Electronic circuits determine whenever two opposing crystals have detected photons within a short time interval (5 to 20 nsec, depending on the detector material) and store the addresses of the crystals involved. For the time-of-flight mode, the differential time of arrival is also recorded.

10) Before tomographic reconstruction, the data must be corrected for (i) the loss of events due to attenuation in the tissue, (ii) accidental background events (random coincident detections of unrelated annihilation photons), (iii) scattered background events (coincident detections of photon pairs from the same positron but one or both have scattered), and (iv) the loss of events due to deadtime in the detectors and electronics.

11) The tomographic reconstruction usually involves filtering the parallel-ray projections either by convolution or frequency filtering and then back-projecting to form the image array. Alternate procedures involve iterative methods of estimating the true distribution such as maximum likelihood or least squares techniques.

Note that 4 different efficiencies appear in these steps:
–detection efficiency (in step 5)
–luminous efficiency (in step 6)
–light collection efficiency (in step 7)
–quantum efficiency (in step 8)

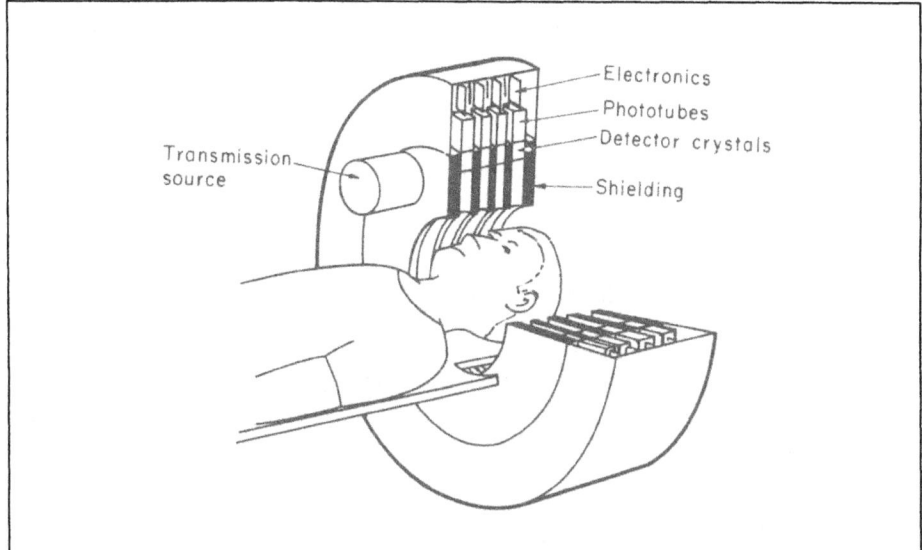

Figure 2: Modern tomograph design using several rings of small crystals that encircle the patient.

2.2 ADVANTAGES OF PET FOR TOMOGRAPHIC IMAGING

Almost all modern positron tomographs use several rings of small crystals that encircle the patient (Figure 2), and utilize the following advantages of PET for tomographic imaging:

1) The total number of coincident events between each detector pair is a measure of all the positron activity along the line between them.

2) The principle of electronic collimation allows small crystals to achieve very good spatial resolution with good sensitivity.

3) The spatial resolution is best at the center of the imaging field, far from material bodies. (In single-gamma imaging, the resolution is best at the front face of the collimator).

4) The sensitivity and spatial resolution are very uniform within the patient port (usually one-half the diameter of the detector ring).

5) Tissue attenuation corrections are straightforward because the attenuation between any two crystals can be measured with an external source and this correction directly applied to the tracer emission data before tomographic reconstruction.

6) Using the difference of arrival time of the coincident photons, the position of the annihilation point along the line between the detector pair can be estimated and this information improves the statistical accuracy (but not the spatial resolution).

Note that PET cannot determine the chemical form of the tracer – metabolic processes must be inferred from the change in measured tracer concentration as a function of time.

3 TOMOGRAPH DESIGN FACTORS

The goal of all tomograph designs is the accurate and rapid measurement of tracer concentration in sharply-defined volume elements in an organ such as the brain or the heart. This requires temporal resolution, spatial resolution, and the quantitative measurement of activity concentration, as discussed below.

3.1 QUANTITATIVE ACCURACY–STATISTICAL FACTORS

Statistical accuracy in the reconstructed image depends on the number of coincident events that can be collected within the available time. This is determined both by the available positron activity and the sensitivity of the tomograph in events per second per radionuclide activity in the imaging field. In addition, some detector materials provide time-of-flight information, which reduces statistical fluctuations in the reconstructed image. The system sensitivity depends on the following 4 factors:

1) Solid angle coverage: Multiple rings of detectors that encircle the patient provide the best acceptance solid angle for the annihilation photons. Utilization of the cross-ring coincidences is very important in realizing the full available solid angle.

2) Axial coverage: Multiple detector rings also serve to cover a larger volume of tissue, thus providing a higher event rate for a given amount of administered tracer activity.

3) Detector Material (Table 1): Except for applications requiring very high light output, BGO has replaced NaI(Tl) in non-time-of-flight PET instrumentation. BGO has the highest density and the highest atomic number of any detector material, and as a result is best able to totally absorb 511 keV photons efficiently in small crystals.

A new material, gadolinium orthosilicate (GSO), was reported in 1982 (10) and has speed advantages over BGO but a lower detection efficiency. Its use is under investigation and is planned for several tomographs (11).

Table 1. DETECTOR MATERIALS FOR PET

Material	NaI(Tl)	CsF	BGO[a]	GSO[b]	BaF$_2$
Density (gm/cm^3)	3.67	4.61	7.13	6.71	4.8
Atomic Numbers	11,53	55,9	83,32,8	64,16,8	56,9
Emission wavelength (nm)	410	390	480	430	310;225
Index of refraction	1.85	1.48	2.15	1.9	1.56
Hygroscopic	YES	VERY	NO	NO	NO
Photoelectrons per 511 keV	3,000	200	400	600	800;200
Scintillation decay time (nsec)	230	2.5	300	60	620;0.8
Photoelectrons/ns (peak rate)	13	60	1.3	11	1.3;250

[a]bismuth germanate, $Bi_4Ge_3O_{12}$
[b]gadolinium orthosilicate (Cerium activated), $Gd_2SiO_5(Ce)$

BaF$_2$ has replaced CsF for time-of-flight positron instrumentation. In 1982 a very fast (800 psec) scintillation component was discovered, making BaF$_2$ the highest speed inorganic scintillator known (12). BaF$_2$ is not hygroscopic (unlike CsF) and the crystals do not have to be sealed in bulky cans, which improves the detection efficiency.

For any detector material, the detection efficiency depends on the detector material, size, and pulse height thresholds used (6,7).

4) Time-of-flight information: Modern BaF$_2$ detectors have excellent timing resolution (typically 400 psec FWHM) and are able to measure the arrival time difference between the two photons and determine the annihilation point with an uncertainty of 6 cm FWHM. In conventional tomography, the annihilation point is only known to lie somewhere along the line between the two coincident detectors. The time-of-flight information is able to reduce the rms statistical uncertainty in the reconstructed image by the ratio of the distance across the emitting region to the time-of-flight uncertainty times twice the speed of light (15 cm per nsec) (13-15). For example, for a time-of-flight uncertainty of 6 cm and a 24 cm diam emission region, the time-of-flight information reduces the statistical uncertainty by a factor of 2 which corresponds to a four-fold decrease in the imaging time.

3.2 QUANTITATIVE ACCURACY–SYSTEMATIC FACTORS

PET data are subject to 6 major systematic errors:

1) attenuation of the annihilation photons in the tissue

2) partial volume effects due to limited axial resolution

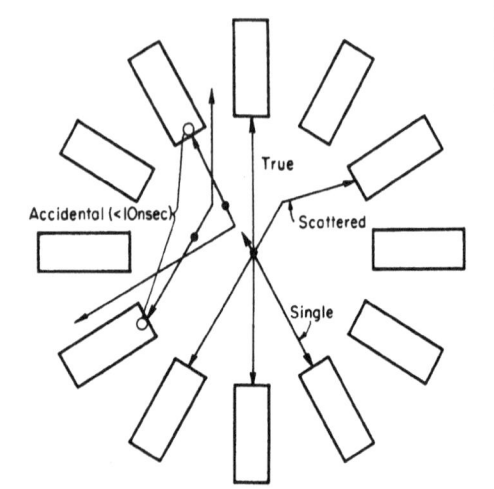

Figure 3: Types of Positron Annihilation Events–
True events are coincident detections of unscattered photon pairs from the same e^+.
Scattered events are coincident detections of photon pairs from the same e^+ where one or both have scattered.
Accidental events are unrelated photons detected in coincidence by chance.

3) smearing due to limited in-plane resolution (16)

4) background events due to accidental coincidences (17,18)

5) background events due to prompt scatter (18-21)

6) losses due to deadtime in the detectors and electronic circuits

The two types of events leading to background types 4) and 5) are illustrated in Figure 3.

3.3 TEMPORAL RESOLUTION

The ability to measure the tracer concentration with good temporal resolution (i.e. in a series of rapid time sequence images) requires the collection of a large number of events during the study, which requires good detection efficiency, low deadtime, high maximum data rates, and a minimum of detector motion. Note the ability to fit compartment model rate constants to PET data depends primarily on the total number of events collected in the study and the temporal resolution. The number of events in each time sequence image is of less importance.

3.4 SPATIAL RESOLUTION

Quantitation within regions of size D requires combined system spatial resolution with $FWHM \leq D/2$. Eight components of the system resolution are discussed below:

Table 2. POSITRON RANGES IN WATER

Isotope	^{18}F	^{11}C	^{68}Ga	^{82}Rb
Maximum Energy	0.64 MeV	0.96 MeV	1.90 MeV	3.35 MeV
PSF FWHM[a]	0.13 mm	0.13 mm	0.31 mm	0.42 mm
PSF rms[b]	0.23 mm	0.39 mm	1.2 mm	2.6 mm
Diameter(75%)	1.2 mm	2.1 mm	5.4 mm	12.4 mm

[a]Full width at half maximum of projected point spread function
[b]Root-mean-square deviation from center of projected point spread function
[c]Diameter of circle containing 75% of the projected annihilations

1) The positron range distribution is sharply peaked and has narrow FWHM and standard deviation values (Table 2). However, most of the annihilations occur in the extensive tails of the distribution, as evidenced by the diameter of the circle that contains 75% of the projected annihilation points (2-4).

2) The deviations from 180° have a nearly Gaussian distribution with a FWHM of 0.50° (5). This contributes 1.3 mm FWHM for a 60 cm diam detector ring.

3) The geometrical component of the detector resolution (at the center of the imaging port) is approximately equal to one-half of the detector width (22-24).

4) Annihilation photons from off-axis sources can penetrate one or more detectors before interacting and this results in a radial elongation of the PSF at the edge of the field (25,26).

5) Compton scattering of the annihilation photons in the detectors can result in a mis-identification of the detector of first interaction. This can be reduced by (i) coupling each scintillator to its individual photodetector and requiring single detector interactions only (22), or (ii) placing shielding material between the detectors, but this reduces the detection efficiency, especially for off-angle rays (6,23,24).

6) For detectors of width W, the geometrical resolution of W/2 discussed in part 3) above will not be realized in the reconstructed image unless the tomographic sampling distance is W/4 or finer throughout the image region. A stationary circular array has a sampling distance of W/2. The most frequently employed method of improving the sampling is by the "wobble" motion- rotating the detector array about a small circle centered at the system axis (27-30). A sampling distance of W/4 can also be achieved with only two mechanical positions by using the "clam" motion (31).

7) reconstruction filter frequency roll-off should be determined by the system resolution, not by statistical fluctuations

8) the effects of organ and tracer motion are reduced by gating for cardiac imaging and rapid sequence imaging for fast dynamic processes

4 TOMOGRAPH DESIGN FACTORS

4.1 CRYSTAL-PHOTOTUBE COUPLING

One of the most fundamental limits to detector resolution is that available phototubes are larger than the crystals we wish to use. Below we summarize many of the efforts to couple small crystals to larger phototubes:

1) Several groups over the years have coupled phototubes to a larger number of smaller crystals so that the light may be split between several phototubes. The light ratio is then used to identify which crystal is scintillating (32-35).

2) Several positron detectors (starting with the Anger positron camera) use the large light output of NaI(Tl) so that signals from several phototubes coupled to a single large crystal of NaI(Tl) can be used to determine the location of the scintillation point (36,37).

3) In another approach a grid of wires is mounted between one or more scintillation crystals and the photocathode of a photomultiplier tube. After the appearance of a photomultiplier pulse, portions of the grid are selectively pulsed to alter the electron trajectories near the adjacent photocathode. The scintillating crystal can thus be identified because the phototube output pulse will only be affected when the associated portion of the grid is pulsed (38-41).

4) Some effort has been directed toward developing phototubes with multiple electron multipliers and anodes, to eliminate some of the glass walls between phototubes, but this approach is presently limited to crystals 6 mm or larger. (42-45).

5) A most promising recent approach uses a photomultiplier combined with solid state photodetectors. A group of crystals is coupled to a relatively large photomultiplier tube which determines the timing for the group. The solid-state photodetectors are coupled individually to each crystal to determine the identity of the scintillating crystal. HgI_2, (46-48) silicon photodiodes (22,49,50), silicon avalanche photodiodes (51-54), and small low-gain phototubes (41) have been suggested for the crystal identifier.

4.2 TRADEOFFS IN TOMOGRAPH DESIGN

1) Patient port size:- A head tomograph has a smaller patient port than a whole-body tomograph (30 cm vs 50 cm diam) and a smaller detector ring (60 cm vs 100 cm diam). This results in increased sensitivity, lower cost (fewer detectors) and improved spatial resolution because the angulation error is less. The primary advantage of the body tomograph is that it can image the human thorax and abdomen.

2) Shielding gap thickness, S: A large shielding gap enhances the sensitivity because the image event rate varies as S^2. However, increasing S increases the scatter backgrounds (which vary as S^3), and increases the accidental backgrounds (which vary as S^4). For single ring systems, the shielding gap defines the slice thickness. For multiple ring systems, the relationship between axial resolution, sensitivity, and backgrounds is more involved as it depends on the design of the inter-ring shielding.

3) Shielding depth: Given a patient port size and shielding gap thickness, it is possible to select a shielding depth that minimizes the statistical fluctuations in the reconstructed image. A smaller shielding depth reduces the detector diameter and enhances the sensitivity for image-forming events, but also increases the number of scattered and random background events. A greater shielding depth reduces these backgrounds but also reduces the image-forming events. An analysis of these tradeoffs is treated in reference (18).

4) Positron isotopes and compounds: As shown in table 2, some of the positron-emitting isotopes (such as ^{18}F) have less blurring due to positron range and are preferred whenever high spatial resolution is important. Isotopes with a short half life and advantageous biodistribution are also preferred because a large amount of tracer activity can be used for a given radiation dose to the patient, and this provides good counting statistics.

5) Time-of-flight vs conventional tomography : BaF_2 provides very good timing resolution which results in low accidental backgrounds, very high maximum event rates, and information on the location of the point of annihilation which reduces the statistical fluctuations in the reconstructed image. However, this advantage is partially offset by the reduced detection efficiency and a greater difficulty in using small crystals for good spatial resolution. BGO provides the ability to use smaller crystals and phototubes and simplifies the electronics and data storage.

6) Number of detectors: The use of many small detectors aids in reducing the overall system deadtime and in improving spatial resolution. However, the cost of the tomograph is related to the number of detectors.

7) Circuit deadtime: The use of many parallel circuits increases the cost of the electronics but can provide very high data rates, even when using BGO, which is relatively slow.

8) The reconstruction algorithm: By using a reconstruction filter that maintains the higher spatial frequencies (within the limits of the overall system spatial resolution), quantitation within well-defined volume elements is improved. Reducing the amplitude of these higher frequencies decreases the apparent noise in the reconstructed images and is frequently used when the tomographic reconstruction is to be viewed as an image.

9) Sampling motion: The use of a detector sampling motion improves the image quality and quantitation by more densely sampling the image space. However, this motion conflicts with requirements for high temporal resolution, particularly for gated cardiac imaging. Although the most common sampling motion is the circular "wobble", the "clam" motion involves only two positions and can be performed even for gated cardiac studies.

See references (11,44,55-59) for more complete discussions of these factors in tomograph design.

4.3 ADVANCED TOMOGRAPHS

Table 3 describes some modern positron tomographs with <7 mm resolution.

See references (60-62) for descriptions of positron tomographs using time-of-flight information.

Table 3. COMPARISON OF POSITRON TOMOGRAPHS WITH SPATIAL RESOLUTIONS FINER THAN 7 mm FWHM

Institution References	MGH Boston (63-66)	NIRS Japan (67,68)	CTI Knoxville (69)	LBL Berkeley (70)	Univ Penn (71,72)
Detector Material	BGO	BGO	BGO	BGO	NaI(Tl)
Number of Rings	1	1	1-4	1	1
Number of Crystals	360	128	512[a]	600	6
Detector Ring Diam (cm)	46	26.5	100	60	85[b]
Patient Port Diam (cm)	28	13.5	65	30	50
Crystal Width (mm)	4	4	5.6	3	–
Crystal C-C Spacing (mm)	4.0	6.5	6.1	3.15	–
In-plane Resolution (mm)[c]	4.8	3	5	2.6	6.5
Axial Resolution (mm)	10	5	18	5	13

[a]per ring
[b]hexagonal
[c]FWHM of reconstructed point spread function near center of system

5 CONCLUSIONS

1) Positron Emission Tomography measures regional biochemical processes (and is complementary to X-ray CT and Magnetic Resonance Imaging).

2) The choices of detector material, crystal-photomultiplier coupling, sampling motion, and shielding geometry have a significant effect on spatial resolution, temporal resolution, and the ability to accurately measure tracer concentration.

3) Multilayer tomograph designs are important in being able to collect more information for a given administered activity.

4) PET instrumentation has evolved in two distinct directions: (a) the use of very small BGO or GSO crystals for high spatial resolution (<5mm FWHM) conventional tomography or (b) the use of BaF_2 with good timing resolution (<500 psec FWHM) for time-of-flight tomography.

5) Efforts are underway throughout the world to improve the timing resolution of BGO and GSO systems, and to improve the spatial resolution of BaF_2 systems.

ACKNOWLEDGEMENTS

We thank R. Huesman and J. Cahoon for helpful discussions.

This work was supported in part by the Director, Office of Energy Research, Office of Health and Environmental Research of the U.S. Department of Energy, under Contract No. DE-AC03-76SF00098, and in part by the National Institutes of Health, National Heart, Lung, and Blood Institute under grant No. P01 HL25840.

Reference to a company or product name does not imply approval or recommendation of the product by the University of California or the U.S. Department of Energy to the exclusion of others that may be suitable.

REFERENCES

1. Budinger TF, Huesman RH, Knittel B, Friedland R, and Derenzo SE: Physiological modeling of dynamic measurements of metabolism using positron emission tomography. In *The Metabolism of the Human Brain Studied with Positron Emission Tomography,* T. Greitz, Ed, Raven Press, New York, pp 165-183, 1984

2. Cho ZH, Chan JK, Eriksson L, et al: Positron ranges obtained from biomedically important positron-emitting radionuclides. *J Nucl Med* 16: 1174-1176, 1975

3. Phelps ME, Hoffman EJ, Huang SC, et al: Effect of positron range on spatial resolution. *J Nucl Med* 16: 649-652, 1975

4. Derenzo, SE: Precision measurement of annihilation point spread distributions for medically important positron emitters. In: *Positron Annihilation,* Hasiguti RR and Fujiwara K, eds, pp 819-823, The Japan Institute of Metals, Sendai, Japan, 1979

5. Colombino P, Fiscella B, Trossi L: Study of positronium in water and ice from 22 to -144 °C by annihilation quantum measurements. *Nuovo Cimento* 38: 707-723, 1965

6. Derenzo SE: Monte Carlo calculations of the detection efficiency of arrays of NaI(Tl), BGO, CsF, Ge, and plastic detectors for 511 keV photons. *IEEE Trans Nucl Sci* NS-28: 131-136, 1981

7. Derenzo SE: Comparison of detector materials for time-of-flight positron tomography. *Proceedings of the International Workshop on Time-of-Flight Positron Tomography,* Thomas LJ and Ter-Pogossian MM, eds. pp 63-68, IEEE Computer Society Cat No 82CH1791-3, 1982.

8. Birks JB: *The Theory and Practice of Scintillation Counting* Pergamon Press, Oxford, England, 1964, pp 473-474

9. Derenzo SE and Riles J: Monte Carlo calculations of the optical coupling between bismuth germanate crystals and photomultiplier tubes. *IEEE Trans Nucl Sci* NS-29: 191-195, 1982

10. Takagi K, and Fukazawa T: Cerium activated Gd_2SiO_5 single crystal scintillator. *Appl Phys Lett* 42: 43-45, 1983

11. Eriksson L, Bohm C, Kesselberg M, et al: A high resolution positron camera. In *The Metabolism of the Human Brain Studied with Positron Emission Tomography,* Greitz T, ed, Raven Press, New York, 1985, pp 13-20

12. Gariod R, Allemand R, Cormoreche E, et al: The LETI positron tomograph architecture and time of flight improvements. *Workshop on Time-of-Flight Tomography,* IEEE Catalog No 82CH1719-3, 1982.

13. Snyder DL, Thomas LJ and Ter-Pogossian MM: A mathematical model for positron-emission tomography systems having time-of-flight measurements. *IEEE Trans Nucl Sci* NS-28: 3575-3583, 1981

14. Tomitani T and Tanaka E: Image reconstruction and noise evaluation in photon time-of-flight assisted positron emission tomography. *IEEE Trans Nucl Sci* NS-28: 4582-4589, 1981

15. Snyder DL: Some noise comparisons of data-collection arrays for emission tomography-systems having time-of-flight measurements. *IEEE Trans Nucl Sci* NS-29: 1029-1033, 1982

16. Hoffman EJ, Huang SC, and Phelps ME: Quantitation in positron emission tomography: 1. Effect of object size. *J Comput Assist Tomogr* 3: 299-308, 1979

17. Burnham CA, Alpert NM, Hoop B, Jr., et al: Correction of positron scintigrams for degradation due to random coincidences. *J Nucl Med* 18: 604 (Abstract), 1977

18. Derenzo SE: Method for optimizing side shielding in positron emission tomographs and for comparing detector materials. *J Nucl Med* 21: 971-977, 1980

19. Wong WH and Adler S: Characterization of the scattered radiation fraction in PET or SPECT cameras with a novel phantom design. *IEEE Trans Nucl Sci* NS-32: 831-834, 1985

20. Bergström M, Eriksson L, Bohm C, Blomqvist G and Litton J: Correction for scattered radiation in a ring detector positron camera by integral transformation of the projections. *J Comput Assist Tomogr* 7: 42-50, 1982

21. Bruno MF, Huesman RH, Derenzo SE, and Budinger TF: Characterization of Compton Scattering in Emission Tomography. *J Nucl Med*, 25: P14, 1984

22. Derenzo SE: Initial characterization of a BGO-silicon photodiode detector for high resolution PET. *IEEE Trans Nucl Sci* NS-31(1): 620-626, 1984

23. Holmes TJ and Ficke DC: Analysis of positron-emission tomography scintillation-detectors with wedge faces and inter-crystal septa. *IEEE Trans Nucl Sci* NS-32: 826-830, 1985

24. Kesselberg M, Bohm C, Litton JE, et al: Design considerations of small crystal positron camera systems. *IEEE Trans Nucl Sci* NS-32: 907-911, 1985

25. Derenzo SE, Budinger TF, Cahoon JL, Greenberg WL, Huesman RH, and Vuletich T: The Donner 280-crystal high resolution positron tomograph. *IEEE Trans Nucl Sci* NS-26: 2790-2793, 1979

26. Eriksson L, Bohm C, Kesselberg M, et al: A four ring positron camera system for emission tomography of the brain. *IEEE Trans Nucl Sci* NS-29: 539-543, 1982

27. Bohm C, Eriksson L, Bergström M, et al: A computer assisted ring detector positron camera system for reconstruction tomography of the brain. *IEEE Trans Nucl Sci* NS-25: 624-637, 1978

28. Brooks RA, Sank VJ, Talbert AJ, et al: Sampling requirements and detector motion for positron emission tomography. *IEEE Trans Nucl Sci* NS-26: 2760-2763, 1979

29. Herman GT: The mathematics of wobbling a ring of positron annihilation detectors. *IEEE Trans Nucl Sci* NS-26: 2756-2759, 1979

30. Colsher JG and Muehllehner G: Effects of wobbling motion on image quality in positron tomography. *IEEE Trans Nucl Sci* NS-28: 90-93, 1981

31. Huesman RH, Derenzo SE and Budinger TF: A two-position sampling scheme for positron emission tomography. In *Nuclear Medicine and Biology*, Raynaud C, ed., Pergammon Press, New York, Vol I, pp 542-545, 1983.

32. Burnham CA and Brownell GL: A multi-crystal positron camera. *IEEE Trans Nucl Sci* NS-19(3): 201-205, 1972

33. Burnham C, Bradshaw J, Kaufman D, et al: Application of a one dimensional scintillation camera in a positron tomographic ring detector. *IEEE Trans Nucl Sci* NS-29(1): 461-464, 1982

34. Takami K, Ishimatsu K, Hayashi T, et al: Design considerations for a continuously rotating positron computed tomograph. *IEEE Trans Nucl Sci* NS-29: 534-538, 1982

35. Ricci A, Hoffman E, Phelps M, et al: Investigation of a technique for providing a pseudo-continuous detector ring for positron tomography. *IEEE Trans Nucl Sci* NS-29: 452-456, 1982

36. Anger HO: Survey of radioisotope cameras. *ISA Trans* 5: 311-334, 1966

37. Muehllehner G, Colsher JG, and Lewitt RM: A hexagonal bar positron camera: problems and solutions. *IEEE Trans Nucl Sci* NS-30: 652-660, 1983

38. Charpak G: The localization of the position of light impact on the photocathode of a photomultiplier. *Nucl Instr Meth* 48: 151-153, 1967

39. Charpak G: Retardation effects due to the localized application of electric fields on the photocathode of a photomultiplier. *Nucl Instr Meth* 51: 125-128, 1967

40. Boutot JP and Pietri G: Photomultiplier control by a clamping cross-bar grid. *IEEE Trans Nucl Sci* NS-19(3): 101-106, 1972

41. Yamashita Y, Uchida H, Yamashita T and Hayashi T: Recent development in detectors for high spatial resolution positron CT. *IEEE Trans Nucl Sci* NS-31, 424- 428, 1984

42. Murayama H, Nohara N, Tanaka E, et al: A quad BGO detector and its timing and positioning discrimination for positron computed tomography. *Nucl Instr Meth* 192: 501-511, 1982

43. Uchida H, Yamashita Y, Yamashita T, et al: Advantageous use of new dual rectangular photomultiplier for positron CT. *IEEE Trans Nucl Sci* NS-30: 451-454, 1983

44. Okajima K, Ueda K, Takami K, et al: Performance study of the whole-body, multilayer positron computed tomograph –PCTW–II–. *IEEE Trans Nucl Sci* NS-32: 902-906, 1985

45. Kume H, Suzuki S, Takeuchi J, et al: Newly developed photomultiplier tubes with position sensitivity capability. *IEEE Trans Nucl Sci* NS-32: 448-452, 1985

46. Barton JB, Hoffman EJ, Iwanczyk JS, et al: A high-resolution detection system for positron tomography. *IEEE Trans Nucl Sci* NS-30: 671-675, 1983

47. Groom DE: Silicon photodiode detection of bismuth germanate scintillation light, *Nucl Instr Meth*, 219: 141-148, 1984

48. Iwanczyk JS, Barton JB, Dabrowski AJ, et al: A novel radiation detector consisting of an HgI_2 photodetector coupled to a scintillator. *IEEE Trans Nucl Sci* NS-30: 363-367, 1983

49. Derenzo SE: Gamma-ray spectroscopy using small, cooled bismuth germanate scintillators and silicon photodiodes. *Nucl Instr Meth*, 219: 117-122, 1984

50. Derenzo SE, Budinger TF, and Huesman RH: Detectors for high resolution dynamic PET. In *The Metabolism of the Human Brain Studied with Positron Emission Tomography*, T. Greitz, Ed, Raven Press, New York, pp 21-31, 1984

51. Entine E, Reiff G, Squillante M, et al: Scintillation detectors using large area silicon avalanche photodiodes. *IEEE Trans Nucl Sci* NS-30: 431-435, 1983

52. Lecomte R, Schmitt D, Lightstone AW, et al: Performance characteristics of BGO-silicon avalanche photodetectors for PET. *IEEE Trans Nucl Sci* NS-32: 482-486, 1985

53. Dahlbom M, Mandelkern MA, Hoffman EJ, et al: Hybrid mercuric iodide (HgI_2) – gadolinium orthosilicate (GSO) detector for PET. *IEEE Trans Nucl Sci* NS-32: 533-537, 1985

54. Squillante MR, Reiff G, and Entine G: Recent advances in large area avalanche photodiodes. *IEEE Trans Nucl Sci* NS-32: 563-566

55. Uemura K, Kanno I, Miura S, et al: High resolution positron tomograph: HEADTOME III: system description and preliminary report on the performances. In *The Metabolism of the Human Brain Studied with Positron Emission Tomography*, Greitz T, ed, Raven Press, New York, 1985, pp 47-56

56. Brooks RA, Friauf WS, Sank VJ, et al: Initial evaluation of a high resolution positron emission tomograph. In *The Metabolism of the Human Brain Studied with Positron Emission Tomography*, Greitz T, ed, Raven Press, New York, 1985, pp 57-68

57. Hoffman EJ, van der Stee M, Ricci AR, et al: System features that are determinate in precision and accuracy in positron emission tomographs. In *The Metabolism of the Human Brain Studied with Positron Emission Tomography*, Greitz T, ed, Raven Press, New York, 1985, pp 69-84

58. Brooks RA, Sank VJ, Friauf WS, Leighton SB, Cascio HE and DiChiro G: Design considerations for positron emission tomography. *IEEE Trans Biomed Eng* BME-28: No 2, 158-177, 1981

59. Budinger TF, Derenzo SE, Huesman RH and Cahoon JL: Medical criteria for the design of a dynamic positron tomograph for heart studies. *IEEE Trans Nucl Sci* NS-29: 488-492, 1982

60. Ter-Pogossian MM, Mullani NA, Ficke DC, et al: Photon time-of-flight-assisted positron emission tomography. *J Comput Assist Tomogr* 5: 227-239, 1981

61. Mullani NA, Gaeta J, Yerian K, et al: Dynamic imaging with high resolution time-of-flight PET camera - TOFPET I. *IEEE Trans Nucl Sci* NS-31: 609-613, 1984

62. Soussaline F, Comar D, Allemand R, et al: New developments in positron emission tomography instrumentation using the time-of-flight information. In *The Metabolism of the Human Brain Studied with Positron Emission Tomography*, Greitz T, ed, Raven Press, New York, 1985, pp 1-12

63. Burnham CA, Bradshaw J, Kaufman D, et al: A stationary positron emission ring tomograph using BGO detector and analog readout. *IEEE Trans Nucl Sci* NS-31(1): 632-636, 1984

64. Brownell GL, Burnham CA and Chesler DA: High resolution tomograph using analog coding. In *The Metabolism of the Human Brain Studied with Positron Emission Tomography*, Greitz T, ed, Raven Press, New York, 1985, pp 13-20

65. Stearns CW, Chesler DA, Kirsch JE, et al: Quantitative imaging with the MGH analog ring positron tomograph. *IEEE Trans Nucl Sci* NS-32: 898-901, 1985

66. Burnham CA, Bradshaw J, Kaufman D, et al: Design of cylindrical shaped scintillation camera for positron tomographs. *IEEE Trans Nucl Sci* NS-32: 889-893, 1985

67. Nohara N, Tanaka E, and Tomitani T: Analytical study of performance of high resolution positron emission computed tomographs for animal study. *IEEE Trans Nucl Sci* NS-32: 818-821, 1985

68. Tomitani T, Nohara N, Morayama H, et al: Development of a high resolution positron CT for animal studies. *IEEE Trans Nucl Sci* NS-32: 822-825, 1985
69. Computer Technology and Imaging, Inc. Knoxville, Tennessee, MODEL PT 931 ECAT Scanner System Description.
70. Derenzo SE, Huesman RH, Budinger FT, Cahoon JL, and Vuletich T: High resolution positron emission tomography using 3 mm wide bismuth germanate crystals. (in preparation) 1985
71. Karp JS and Muehllehner G: Performance of a position-sensitive scintillation detector. *Phys Med Biol* 1985 (in press)
72. Muehllehner G and Karp JS: A positron camera using position sensitive detectors: PENN-PET. (submitted for publication) 1985

SIGNAL TO NOISE IMPROVEMENT IN PET USING BGO

Edward J. Hoffman, Ph.D.

Division of Biophysics, Dept. of Radiological Sciences
UCLA School of Medicine and The Laboratory of Nuclear Medicine
of the Laboratories of Biomedical and Environmental Sciences
University of California, Los Angeles

INTRODUCTION

Improvement in resolution in nuclear medicine has generally been at a cost in system sensitivity, due to requirements of collimator design. In PET, the collimator is eliminated and resolution is limited, primarily, by properties of the detector. The high energy of annihilation photons cause difficulty in localizing events in narrow detectors. The primary problem is scatter of photons from primary to neighboring detectors. This may lead to, rejection of events, if two detectors register the photon, or misplacement of events if only secondary detectors register events. It is possible to compensate for lower intrinsic detection efficiency by using deeper detectors. But, it is not possible to use wider detectors and still obtain high resolution. BGO provides a remedy for these difficulties because of its very high fraction of photoelectric absorption in interacting with 511 keV photons and its high physical density. The probability that first interactions with BGO detectors will be photoelectric is three times that of such detectors as NaI(Tl), BaF_2 and CsF (ca. 42 % of the first interaction). In these detectors, the probability that scattered photons will be absorbed within a thin primary detector is very poor, because in addition to lower photoelectric cross-sections, their densities are also almost a factor of two lower than BGO.

The properties of BGO allow fabrication of PET systems with closely packed, very narrow detectors (3-6 mm), that suffer very little loss in either sensitivity or resolution. Detectors as small as 3 mm wide still retain almost 75 percent of their intrinsic efficiency. The noise in a PET image is a function of the total number of counts (i.e. noise) per image can be identical to a the number of counts (i.e.noise) per image can be identcal to a system built with larger detectors, and the small detectors will selectively increase the strength of the signal in its higher frequency components (1-3). In structured images this allows very high local signal to noise ratios in high resolution images, while images of uniform distributions of activity will have the same signal to noise properties as systems with large detectors.

In this chapter, I will present several key pieces of experimental data that demonstrate the physical properties that make BGO superior to the detectors composed of lower atomic number atoms.

INTERDETECTOR SCATTER AND CROSSTALK

The major weakness of the low Z detector in PET is its inability to fully absorb the 511 keV annihilation photon in a narrow detector. The problem is demonstrated in figures 1 and 2, which show the energy spectra of two types of interdetector scatter that can lead to loss of data or mispositioning. The first type of scatter is one in which enough energy is deposited in both detectors to trigger both timing discriminators. In this case the system has an ambiguous piece of data (a triple coincidence), since the true crystal of the first interaction cannot be distinguished from the second crystal. The usual system response is to reject the event, causing a loss in efficiency of the system. Figure 1 shows the true coincidence spectrum for a line source centered between two BaF_2 crystals (5.6 X 29 X 45 mm deep), and the triple coincidence spectrum in the adjacent crystal.

The second type of scatter is the most prevalent. It is forward angle scatter in which very little energy is deposited on first interaction and the gamma-ray is detected in a second crystal. If the energy threshold on the PET system is about 100 keV, photons with energies of 411 to 511 keV after scatter will not be detected as triple coincidences. This corresponds to gamma-rays that are scattered at angles from 0 to 41 degrees. In long narrow crystals a large fraction of these scatters will enter neighboring crystals. The magnitude of the scatter can be appreciated from figure 2, which shows the same geometry and true coincidence spectrum as figure 1 and the coincidence spectrum in the adjacent crystal with the triple coincidences subtracted. In a PET system, these events are not recognized as scattered and are simply recorded as part of the data. This leads to a loss in

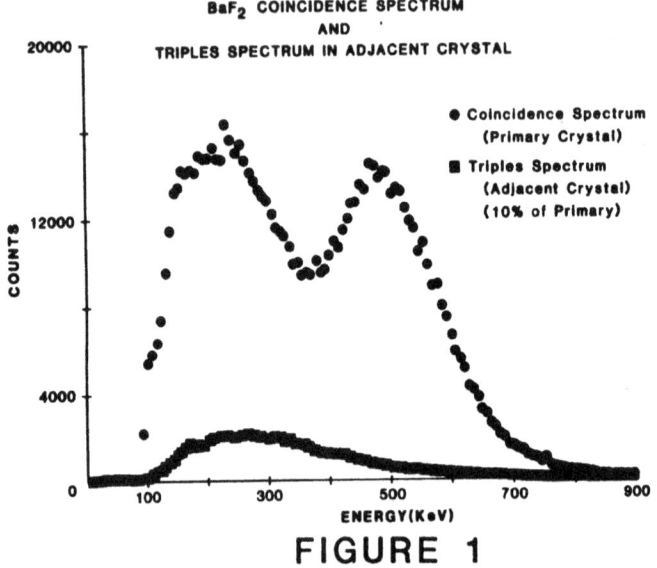

FIGURE 1

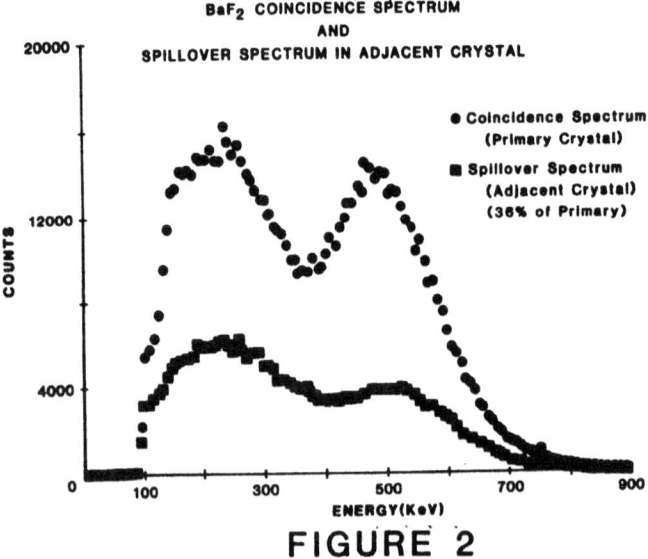

FIGURE 2

resolution at the FWHM for off center events in circular PET designs and loss at the FWTM at all positions in the system. In the crystal adjacent to the neighboring crystal, the total spillover was still 40 % of that in the neighboring crystal. In the measurement, there were multiple crystals only on one side of the line source. In a PET system the interdetector crosstalk and scatter will be compounded by contributions on both sides of the source.

An identical set of measurements were performed for 5.6 X 29 X 30 mm deep BGO crystals with the exception that the BGO measurement was performed with multiple BGO detectors on both sides of the line source. The results of these measurements are shown in figures 3 and 4. The most striking feature of these measurements is the large fraction of the events in the photopeak in the true coincidence spectrum. The fraction of cross talk and

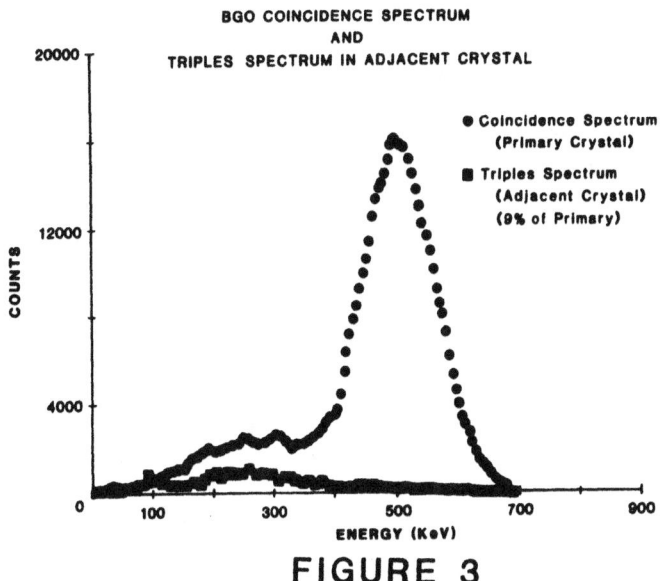

FIGURE 3

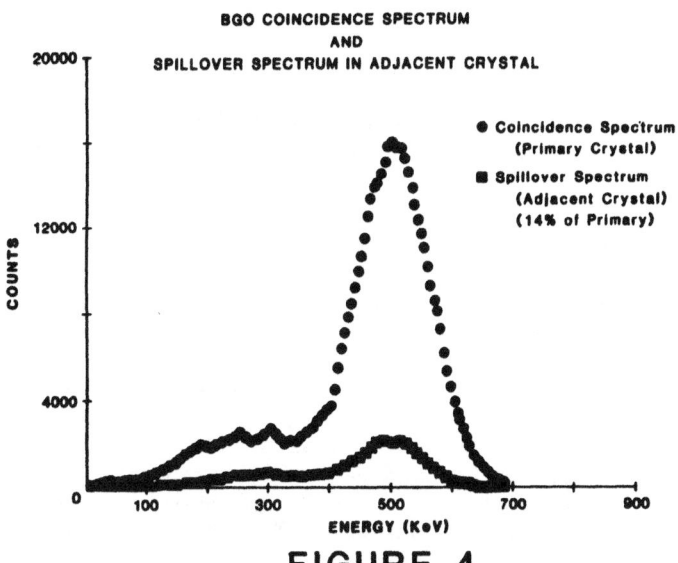

FIGURE 4

scatter is a little misleading in comparison to the BaF_2 results. It should be remembered that this measurement was done in a scatter environment resembling a PET system and does represent what will be seen in such a system. Also in the BGO measurement, virtually all the scatter and crosstalk was confined to only the adjacent crystal and very few events were recorded in the next crystal.

The use of lead or tungsten septa between neighboring BaF_2 crystals has been suggested as a remedy for cross talk in PET systems. It should be remembered that the efficiency of a PET system is proportional to the square of the solid angle of the detectors. Since two photons are detected per event, the product of the probability of detection of both photons defines the efficiency. If 1 or 2 mm lead or tungsten septa are used with the BaF_2 crystals tested here, the system efficiency loss would be approximately 26 or 43 %, respectively. In addition the effectiveness of such shielding is questionable. In the spectra shown in figures 2 and 4, the shape of the scatter and primary coincidence spectra are essentially the same, indicating that the scattered photon is very nearly 511 keV, probably in the 400 to 500 keV range that would be prevalent for the 100 keV discriminator threshold discussed above. The half value layer for tungsten and lead at 400 to 500 keV is 2 to 3 and 3 to 4 mm, respectively. Therefore the penetration of 1 mm septa would be very high even though the septa are struck at an angle. The half value layer tables are given for narrow beam geometry and ignores the fact that many of the photons are scattered forward and still strike the neighboring detector.

RESOLUTION

The scatter between crystals is also important in determing the intrinsic resolution characteristics of a PET system. The LSFs in figure 5 show a comparison between the BGO crystals and the BaF_2 crystals. The coaxial measurement is for detectors directly opposite each other across the diameter of the PET system. The 15° off axis measurement is equivalent to detectors that are off center and tilted a full 30° relative to each others. In a 100 (80) cm diameter PET system they would be viewing data at 15 (12) cm from the center. In comparing the coaxial LSFs, it is seen that the FWHMs are identical while the FWTM is somewhat poorer for the BaF_2. The off axis BaF_2 LSF is significantly worse in both the FWHM and FWTM. The off axis FWHM is 60 % larger than axial FWHM for BaF_2, which would generally be considered too large a variation in resolution. It will probably be necessary to employ wider crystals in a practical PET system that uses BaF_2 to find a reasonable compromise between resolution and efficiency.

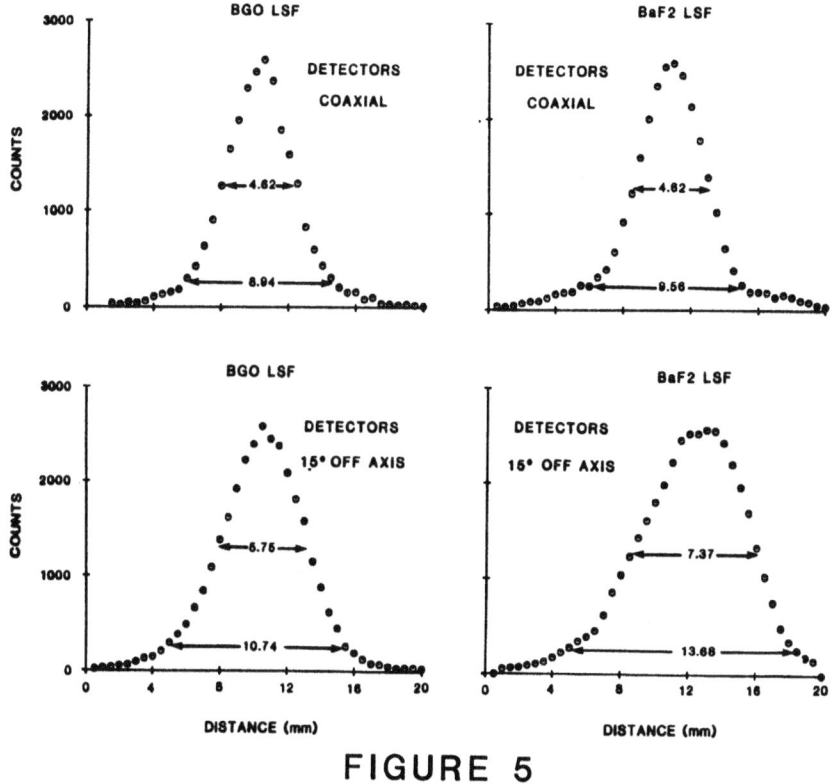

FIGURE 5

DISCUSSION

It is obvious that BGO is the current choice for PET systems that are attepting the highest possible intrinsic resolution. A number of PET designers are using the high speed of the BaF_2 to measure the approximate position of the annihilation event along the line between the coincident detectors and using this information to reduce the noise in the image (see chapter by Allemand). If the BaF_2 is too narrow, the improvement in noise will only compensate for the loss in efficiency of the narrow detector. The loss can easily be a factor of two for detectors of the size used in our measurements. If the detectors are larger, the efficiency will be improved at the expense of resolution. In recent work (1-3) we have shown the high signal to noise characteristics of very high intrinsic resolution. In cases in which the images are limited by statistics, spatial averaging will allow reduction in the noise in the image at some cost in resolution. The cost in resolution is surprisingly small and the system is also capable of very high resolution studies when adequate count densities are available. A visual demonstration of this property is given in figure 6. In this figure a data set was

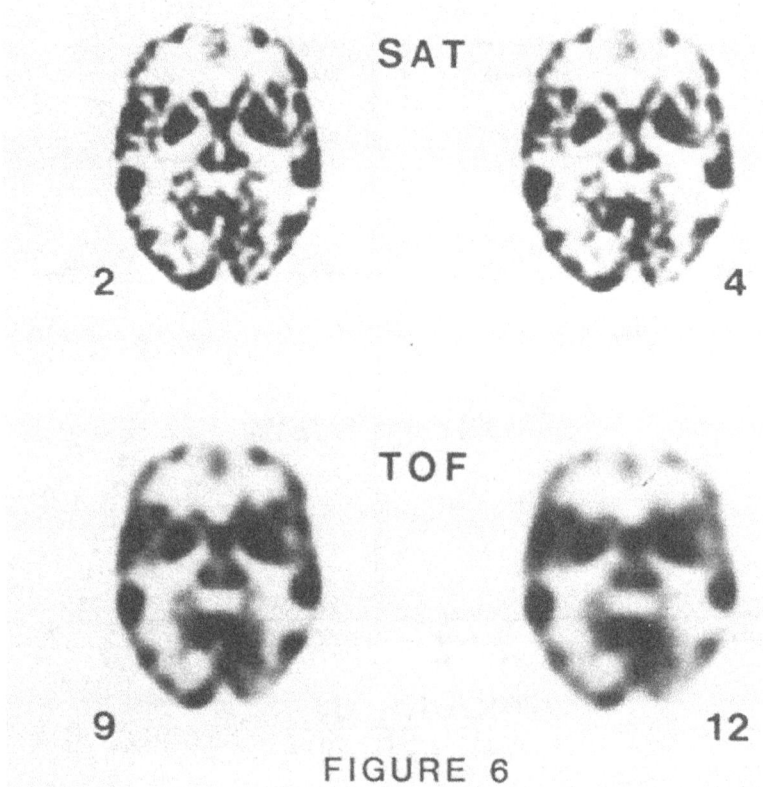

FIGURE 6

created from the digitized image of an actual brain slice, the data were blurred with the intrinsic resolution indicated in millimeters on the figure, and noise equivalent to one million counts was added to the data for the upper images and noise equivalent to 20 million counts added to the lower image. The 20 million counts but lower resolution is equivalent to what a very good time of flight system might produce and the one million count images is what a high resolution system can produce. The slightly noisier but more detailed high resolution images would certainly seem to be the most useful images.

ACKNOWLEDGEMENTS

The author thanks M. Griswold for preparation of the illustrations and A. Ricci and M Dahlbom for technical assistance. This work was supported in part by Department of Energy Contract DE-AM03-76-SF0012, National Institute of Cancer Grant 1-R01-CA33801-02, and National Institutes of Mental Health Grant 1-R01-MH373916-01.

REFERENCES

1. Hoffman EJ, van der Stee M, Ricci AR, Phelps ME: Prospects for Both Precision and Accuracy in Positron Tomography. Ann Neurol 15(Suppl)25:S25-S34, 1984.
2. Huang SC, Hoffman EJ, Ricci AR, Phelps ME: Effect of Detector Size and Geometry on Image Signal-to-Noise Ratio in Positron Computed Tomography. Proceedings of workshop on time-of-flight in PET. St. Louis, MO, Pg. 69-74, May 1982, IEEE-CH1791-3182.
3. Phelps ME, Huang SC, Hoffman EJ, Plummer D, Carson RE: An Analysis of Signal Amplification Using Small Detectors in Positron Emission Tomography. J Comput Assist Tomogr 6:551-565, 1982.

THE ECAT: A RECENT SOLUTION TO HIGH EFFICIENCY, HIGH RESOLUTION TOMOGRAPHY

Ronald Nutt and Michael Crabtree

Computer Technology and Imaging, Inc., Knoxville, Tn, U.S.A.

The CTI Model PT 911 ECAT* positron emission tomograph is of the latest state-of-the-art design. The ECAT includes a totally automated gantry and patient bed, an electronic processing sub-system an array processor, a display processor and a VAX central processing computer. The gantry rotates, wobbles and can be automatically positioned with respect to the patient. The gantry includes up to four image plane slices with 512 individual detectors per slice or a total of 2048 detectors. The detector aperture can be automatically adjusted to optimize the transaxial resolution. The timing coincidence and position information word is generated in a microprocessor controlled electronics sub-system located on the detector ring. The front-end electronics can operate at a maximum rate of 2 million events per second per ring or a total of 8 million events per second for the system. The maximum data rate for the system is established by the rate that the list data can be stored on the data disks. The maximum data rate is 220,000 events per second for each ring for a total system data rate of 880,000 events per second. The transaxial resolution of the PT 911 ECAT detector is established by the 5.6 mm wide BGO crystals. The continuous wobble capability permits adequate sampling frequency to eliminate possible artifacts. The resolution in the axial dimension is established by the 30 mm height of the crystal. The overall efficiency is established by the 30 x 30 x 5.6 mm crystals closely packed in a one meter diameter ring. The array processor allows the image to be corrected, filtered and back projected within one minute. The display processor coupled with the unique ECAT software allows the operator to manipulate the 512 x 512 pixel image with maximum convenience.

---

* ECAT is a Registered Trademark of Computer Technology and Imaging, Inc.

INTRODUCTION

The ECAT Scanner is a Positron Emission Tomography (PET) scanning system consisting of all the components required for acquisition and processing of PET data including:

1. Physical Scanning Unit
2. Data Acquisition Unit
3. Data Processing Unit
4. Software

The ECAT Scanner is capable of producing reconstructed cross-sectional images of isotope activity which have been properly calibrated and corrected for the physical factors associated with PET. The system is a state-of-the-art design with high spatial resolution and detection efficiency, and is designed to perform static, dynamic, and gated imaging. The data acquisition and processing system is designed to streamline the use of the scanner for routine scanning protocols (high throughput). The software system provides substantial flexibility and is fully documented to allow investigators to develop and implement new algorithms for data acquisition and post-processing.

Fundamental Features

Our basic design configuration as outlined below offers the following fundamental advantages:

1. Superior image resolution in both transaxial and axial dimension
2. High sensitivity
3. Excellent uniformity of response
4. High signal-to-noise (S/N) ratio and image quality
5. High throughput rate
6. Excellent data storage capability
7. Automatic control on gantry, patient couch, and other mechanical motions
8. Analytical software packages
9. Operational, processing

Whole Body System

The ECAT has a large detector diameter and patient FOV to image equally well the torso and brain of the adult human body. The patient opening is large enough to permit rotation and tilting of the detector plane for optimized perpendicular imaging of the long axis of a torso organ (i.e. heart).

Smallest Scintillator Width

Crystal width used in the ECAT is the smallest crystal PET system commercially available. This allows the ECAT to have the highest intrinsic resolution which guarantees the best resolution and image quality (S/N).

Signal Amplification Technique

The signal amplification technique (SAT) used together with the smallest crystal width gives the ECAT a fundamental advantage over other PET designs (1). Previously spatial reconstructed resolution was extracted to the limit on intrinsic resolution but at the expense a third power degradation in image quality. Two improvements can be realized from the SAT principles. First, improvements in tomographic resolution by amplifying the signal and not noise components can be realized. Second, in low statistical imaging situations, S/N can be improved by lowering the convolution filter cut-off frequency.

List Mode Data Acquisition
The list mode data stream give maximum flexibility for analyzing data. This technique allows not only standard images to be reconstructed but also the capability to add gating inputs (e.g. physiologically synced routes) to partition the data. This data may be partioned in an infinite number of ways, reconstructed, and analyzed to make maximum use of the once acquired data.

PHYSICAL SCANNING UNIT

Configuration
The gantry is designed for whole body imaging of the adult human with a diameter at the shoulder of 50.3 cm (97.5% norm). Each detector ring is made up of 16 detector buckets (modules) arranged in a circular geometry. A detector bucket contains the detector channels and associated front-end electronics. The ECAT can be configured with 1 to 4 detector rings producing one to seven image planes. The unique modular design makes possible fast maintenance replacement, as well as cost effective upgrades to both increase the number of detector rings and to facilitate future detector upgrades protecting against technological obsolescence.

Detector Package
The crystal type used in the ECAT detector is Bismuth Germanate (BGO). These scintillator crystals are reliable, field-proven, and commercially available from a number of manufacturers at reproducible specifications. The 5.6 mm crystal width offers very high intrinsic resolution. The package containing dual detector assemblies (BGO/PMT) has been designed for very high precision alignment and minimal radial gapping. These packages allow rapid, cost-effective maintenance replacement, as well as the capability to upgrade with future detector enhancements.

1. Scintillator Type: Bismuth Germanate (BGO)
2. Size: 5.6 mm wide x 30.0 mm high x 30.0 mm deep
3. Number/Ring: 512
4. Type of PMTs: Hammamatsu R-1635, 10 mm diameter tube
5. Number PMTs/Crystal: 1/1

Geometry
1. Circular ring geometry
2. Detector Separation
   (a) Ring diameter : 100 cm diameter
   (b) In-plane (center-to-center) : 6.1 mm
   (c) Axial spacing (center-to-center) : 36 mm
3. Number of Detector Rings: 1, 2, 3, or 4 rings and 1, 3, 5, or 7 image planes which are field upgradeable.
4. Patient Opening: 65 cm diameter
5. Transverse Field-of-View (FOV): Operator selectable and electronically adjustable to either 50 cm or 20 cm diameter image FOV. This capability to electronically limit the FOV to 20 cm limits noise components and speeds up image processing when imaging the brain.
6. Axial FOV: Detectors are 30 mm in the axial direction and are separated by 36 mm center-to-center. Total axial FOV therefore varies between 1.8 cm to 13.8 cm for the 1 to 4 detector ring systems.

Gantry and Patient Couch Motions

The ECAT gantry is designed to maximize the cross-sectional imaging of non-axially oriented organs, especially the heart. For this important feature we chose to rotate and tilt the gantry (and its detectors) in order to properly align with the main axis of an patient organ.

1. Gantry Rotation: +/- 30 degrees
2. Gantry Tilt: + 30 degrees, - 90 degrees.
3. Detector Wobble: 2 detector diameter, 12.2 mm at 1 rev/sec speed incrementally encoded to 1024 positions.
4. Detector Rotation: +/- 15 degrees
5. Rotating Phantom Holder: 360 degree rotation monitored by 1024 point incremental encoder.
6. Horizontal Patient Couch Motion: 137 cm distance in 1 mm steps.
7. Vertical Patient Couch Motion: 30 cm distance in 1 mm steps.
8. Patient Couch Repositioning Method: A low power laser provides a line of red light for convenient and accurate positioning of the patient with the center of the detector array. Both computer control and operator pushbutton control are provided with positive encoding to ensure accurate and repeatable positioning in 1 mm increments. Position is continually displayed for the operator.
9. Computer Control : Distributed microprocessor architecture is used independently to control and monitor all mechanical motions of the gantry and patient couch. Both operator pushbutton and computer inputs are accepted for the motions.
10. Encoding of Positions : Positive encoding is incorporated in all mechanical motions to emphasize precision and repeatability using computer readable 1024 position absolute encoders.

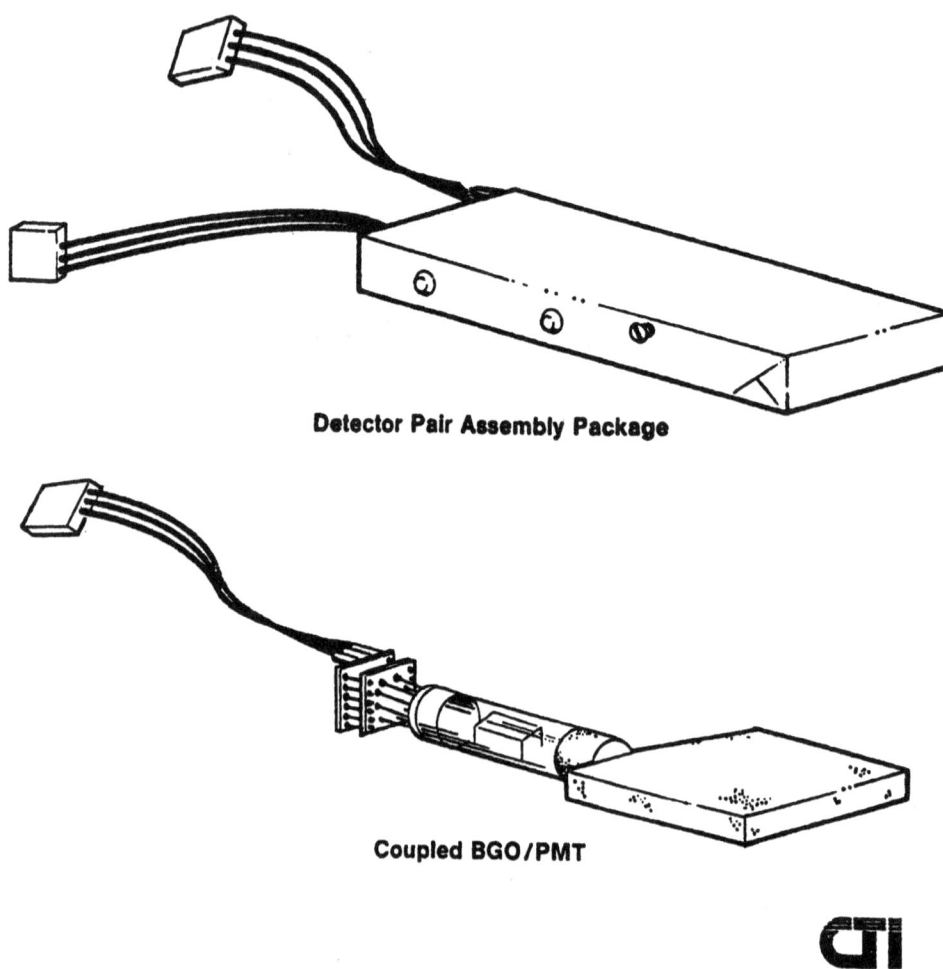

Figure 1

Shielding: Interplane

Removable and customer selectable interplane septa are used to reduce the detector solid angle for activity outside the image plane. The standard interplane septa are triangularly shaped lead with 0.4 mm aluminum sheath and 1.5 mm stainless core with a thickness of 6 mm at detector face down to 1.5 mm at patient opening. Extending from the detector face to the patient opening, the septa is 17 cm long.

Shielding: Adjustable Axial Resolution

A desirable feature in PET imaging is the ability to modify the scanning slice thickness dependent on the requirements of a particular study. Electrically operated side shielding plates will allow the operator to selectably change the slice thickness of the one and two plane ECAT Scanners from the nominal 18 mm to 5 mm FWHM. This adjustment is easily performed under pushbutton control and an absolute encoded position is fed back to the computer.

Other Shielding

Internal to the gantry cover and surrounding the detectors is additional lead shielding to reduce detected activity outside of the field of view. Front and rear plates shield the detectors from radiation originating outside the planes of interest.

Detector Sampling Modes

The imaging unit has two scanning resolutions using stationary and wobble sampling modes. High resolution studies are obtained with a 2 detector diameter (12.2 mm) wobble motion and operator selectable 4/8 position binary to improve the spatial sampling. The stationary mode relies on the intrinsic detector resolution (4.2 mm FWHM) and detector sampling density (6.1 mm).

Rotating Phantom Source Holder

A rotating phantom holder internal to the gantry is provided. This rotating holder has a very accurate 1024 point incremental position encoder. Various external phantom sources can be manually mounted to this holder to perform several important tasks.

DATA ACQUISITION SYSTEM

The data acquisition system was designed with the requirement to maximize front-end acquisition speed, maximize system throughput, minimize cost, limit the exponentially increasing complexity of coincidence logic required in previous PET designs, utilize list mode data acquisition technique for flexible reprocessing of raw data (especially with physiological inputs for gating), and distribute processing for larger and faster collection of data. Another major requirement was modularity and flexibility of design in order to allow upgradability and protection from technological obsolescence.

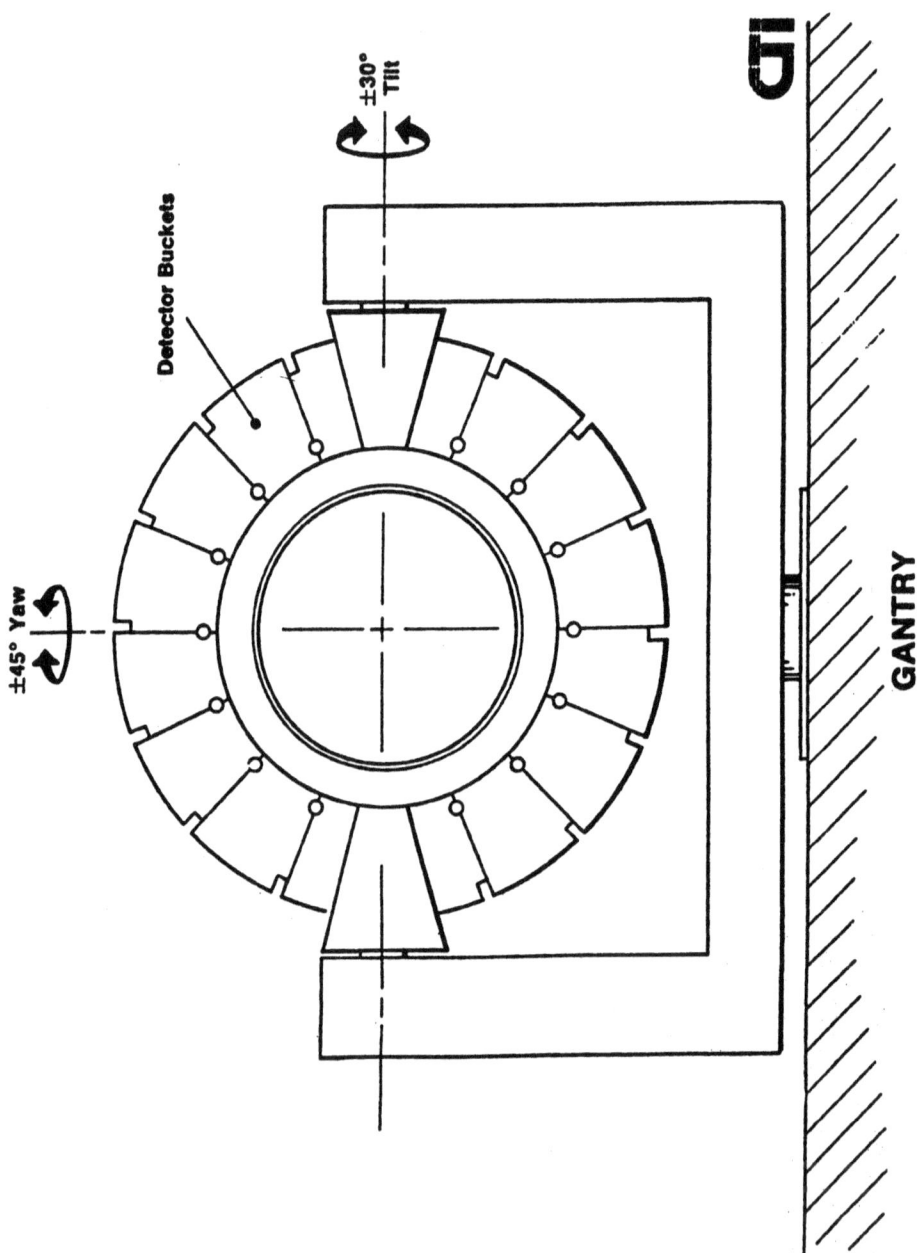

Figure 2

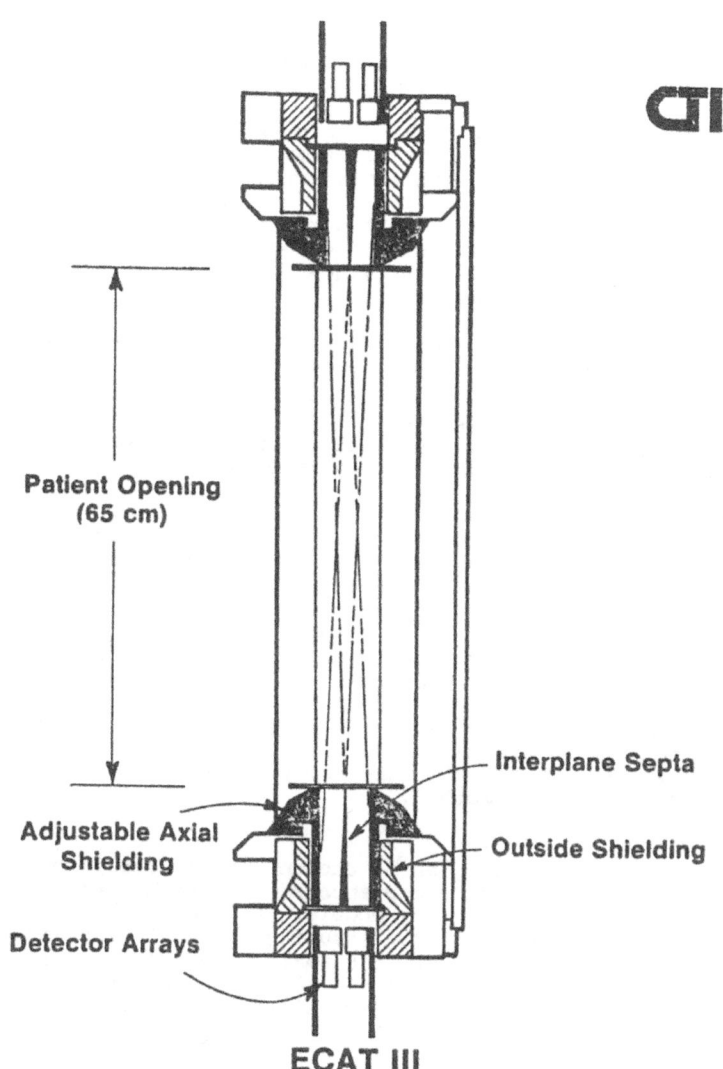

ECAT III
SCANNING UNIT SHIELDING CROSS SECTION

Figure 3

Data Acquisition Electronics

The data acquisition front-end is sub-divided into 16 modules per ring. Detector module electronics (located in the physical scanning unit) includes analog-to-digital signal conversion, digital time encoding electronics, and microprocessor driven detector controller. The detector module's primary function is to process single gamma events. The ECAT Scanner has over 65 distributed processors controlling only data acquisition and raw data storage.

Individual detector signals (analog electron pulses) are passed through specially designed, hybridized amplifier and constant fraction timing discriminator. A gamma-ray event is converted to a digital signal which is processed by the time encoder logic. An event is thus translated into a 14-bit word with event time and detector number and pipelined to the coincidence processor. All 16 detector modules operate in this manner and the output is a list of digitally encoded, gamma-ray events.

Also secondary functions of the detector module includes: sampling the singles countrate (for both diagnostic information and calculated correction for accidentals), enabling/inhibiting detector output (for temporary "noisy" or intermittent detectors), adjusting detector energy thresholds, and diagnostic testing (by simulating an event completely through the system).

Coincidence Processing

True coincidences are detected in the coincidence processor by digitally comparing the time that an event occurred in one module with the time that events occurred in other modules. Once a coincidence line-of-response (LOR) has been detected, a word describing the LOR is formed and written sequentially in list mode format to a data storage disk for processing later. Randoms are detected in the same way as true coincidences. That is, a delayed time window forms accidental coincidences and a detected LOR random word is also written sequentially in list mode data stream. Multiple or triple coincidences are similarly detected and routed into the list mode data stream where operator selectable software control will determine the correction method.

Selectable FOV

The field-of-view (FOV) can be chosen electronically by selecting the detector coincidence acceptance range. Rather than one module looking at seven (7) opposing modules, this can be limited to five (5) or three (3) modules thus reducing the FOV. The advantage of this is to allow focusing in on a smaller FOV of interest and thus eliminating extraneous information. Also, limiting the FOV improves the image processing speed and capability by a factor of 4 or more.

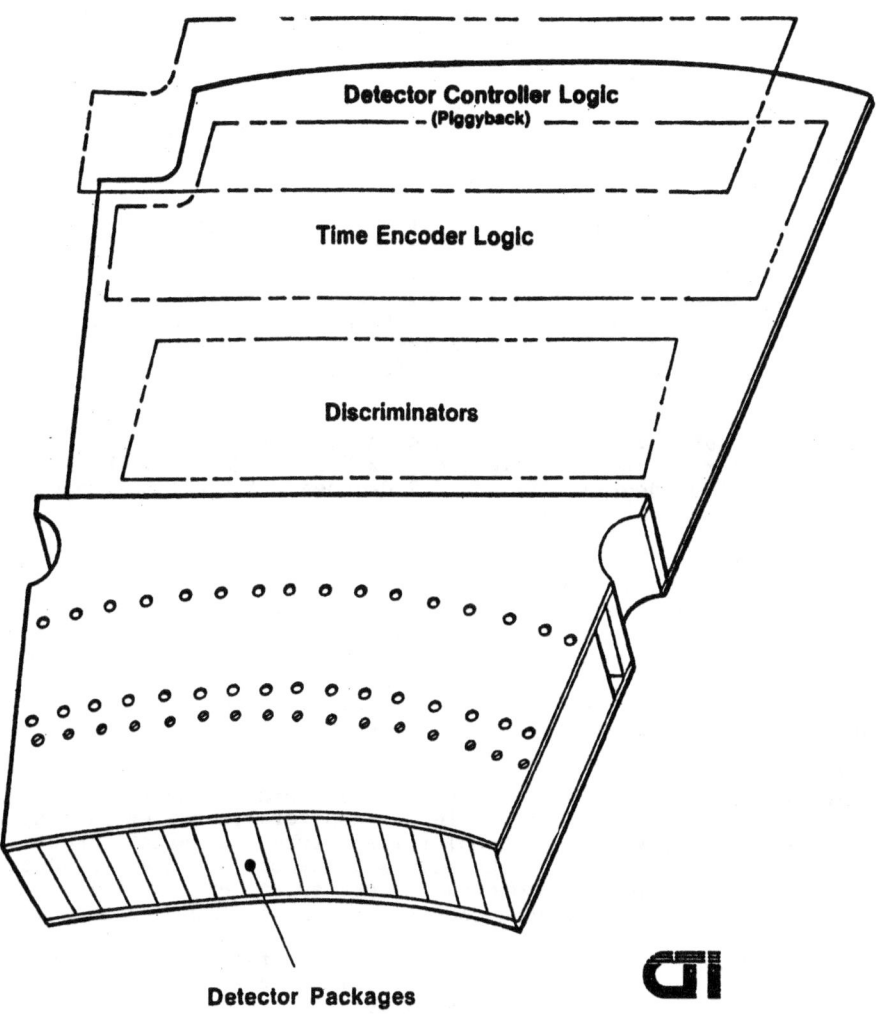

Figure 4

List Mode Data

The list mode data stream gives maximum flexibility for analyzing data. This technique allows not only standard images to be reconstructed but also the capability to add gating inputs (physiologically synced routes) to partition the data. This data may be partioned in an infinite number of ways, reconstructed, and analyzed to make maximum use of the once acquired data.

List Mode Data Stream

The front-end list mode data stream is composed of 14-bit single event words containing event time and detector number information. These words are loaded in parallel into the coincidence processor which generates coincidence LOR pairs and types. The coincidence processed list mode data stream is composed of three types of 32-bit words: the coincidence event word, the physiological input gating word, and the gantry (wobble) position word. Timing information is inserted synchronously at 500 microsecond intervals via the physiological input gating and gantry position words.

Sampling

The LOR data is acquired in a fan beam and further projected into a sort matrix with dimensions of 512 X 88. Therefore the angular sampling is 180 degrees/256 or 0.7 degrees and the linear spatial sampling is 50 cm/176 or 2.8 mm.

Raw Data Storage

The list mode data acquisition is fundamental to two PET scanning modes, dynamic and physiological input gating. Two memory systems maximize the countrate and storage capacity. First, a double-buffered dual-ported memory with a 16 KWord capacity for each detector plane derandomizes the input. Second, the list mode raw data on a PT 911/02 is standardly stored on large Winchester disks giving a maximum dynamic raw data storage of 240 million LOR events.

Deadtime

Electronic deadtime resulting in true coincident count losses are caused by paralyzable and non-paralyzable operation of the detector crystal, photomultiplier tube, constant fraction discriminator, coincidence latches, and memory storage. Deadtime losses result in both uncounted coincidences and multiple (3 or more single events) coincidence counts from the following sources:

1. Deadtime for Singles - There is a fixed 2.5 microsecond deadtime per detector channel which fixes the singles deadtime. This results in a 3% deadtime for 50,000 true coincidence events/ second and 10% deadtime for 100,000 true coincidence events/second.

Display Processor

The display processor (Gould/DeAnza FD 5000) will be a 512 x 512 pixel image processor with 12 bits of memory/pixel and 4 bits overlay/pixel. The complete display system also includes a 17" high resolution monochrome monitor, a 19" high resolution RGB color monitor (optional), and interactive cursors controls via trackball.

Control Console

The control console is the operator's interface to the system. It contains a command video terminal (VT 220) used in system interaction, printing terminal, an image display monitor, and a cursor control interface device (trackball), and line printer.

Archival Data Storage

Raw data (list mode non-processed LOR coincidence events and physiological inputs) as well as patient image data (sorted projection and a reconstructed image data) may be archived for immediate or long term storage on magnetic media peripherals. The standard RA80 Winchester (121 MB) and the RL02 removable disk (10 MB) provide immediate access to almost 600 images. Additional storage capacity is available in low cost media storage via magnetic tape transport or laser (write once) disks.

Data Processing Speed: Sorting

When the list mode data acquisition mode is used, data processing can be a real time speed limitation. The ECAT's solution to this problem is a distributed architecture and fast array processors. List mode data can be read from the raw data storage Winchesters and sorted into projection sinograms at the rate of 30 microseconds per event or over 33,000 events/second. The A/P's large memory capacity, 2 MB (this can be optionally expanded to 8 MB) can standardly sort up to twelve 88 X 512 sinograms at one time. In a typical imaging situation with high resolution wobble sampling or physiological gating, a standard PT 911/02 can simultaneously sort data into all three images with either a 4 bin wobble sampling or 4 gates per image at a rate of over 33,000 events/second without losing pace with the list mode data acquired. If greater dynamic realtime sorting capability is needed, the array processor memory can be expanded to simultaneously sort 44 images in any number of combinations of images, wobble binning, and physiological gating.

Data Processing Speed: Reconstruction

Reconstruction speed is primarily a functon of the input data volume and final reconstruction matrix. With the array processor, the standard ECAT station scan projection sinogram (88 x 512) is reconstructed into an image matrix (256 x 256) in approximately 40 seconds. Using the optional electronic FOV reduction, a 128 x 128 image is reconstructed in approximately 15 seconds.

2. Deadtime for Coincidences - Six coincidences per 240 nanoseconds per detector plane (a maximum of 25 million events per second per plane) can be processed in list mode to the Winchester disks. A derandomizing buffer, 16 KW per plane, allows high burst rates to be processed. The average data throughput per plane is limited by the 220,000 events/second average disk write time. Average data throughput for a four plane system is 880,000 events/second.

Deadtime corrections are made by first counting the multiple or triple coincidences in the list mode data and then employing a correction algorithm based on the multiple rate (2).

DATA PROCESSING SYSTEM

Distributed processing is the key to maximizing speed for simultaneous data collection, image reconstruction, and analysis. A single computer cannot expeditiously process the large amounts of data in multiplane tomographs and that is why the ECAT VAX-11/730 functions primarily as a "traffic cop" regulating the operations. A four plane ECAT has almost 80 distributed processors controlling data acquisition, raw data storage, array processing, display processing, host controller/user interface, and mechanical motion control.

Control Processor

The main control processor will minimally be a VAX 11/730 (32-bit addressing architecture) with 1MB of main memory, RA80 (121 MB) Winchester disk and RL02 (10 MS) removaable disk. This host processor operating in the VMS operating system environment, will remain relatively idle as it routes jobs to the various ECAT distributed subsystems, controls operator interaction, and directs input/output operations. A majority of the computing time will be available for background tasks (i.e, program development, image analysis, network communication with other computers). If the user envisions a large number of background tasks, a computer upgrade to the VAX-11/750 or VAX-11/780, may be considered as an option.

Array Processor

A specialized array processor (CD&A MSP 3000) is standard for the large image analyzing function. The array processor, a special pipeline oriented processor is used to speed up arithmatic operation (sorting LOR events into a projection sinogram and reconstructing images) at a 5.0 MFLOP (million floating point operations per second) rate.

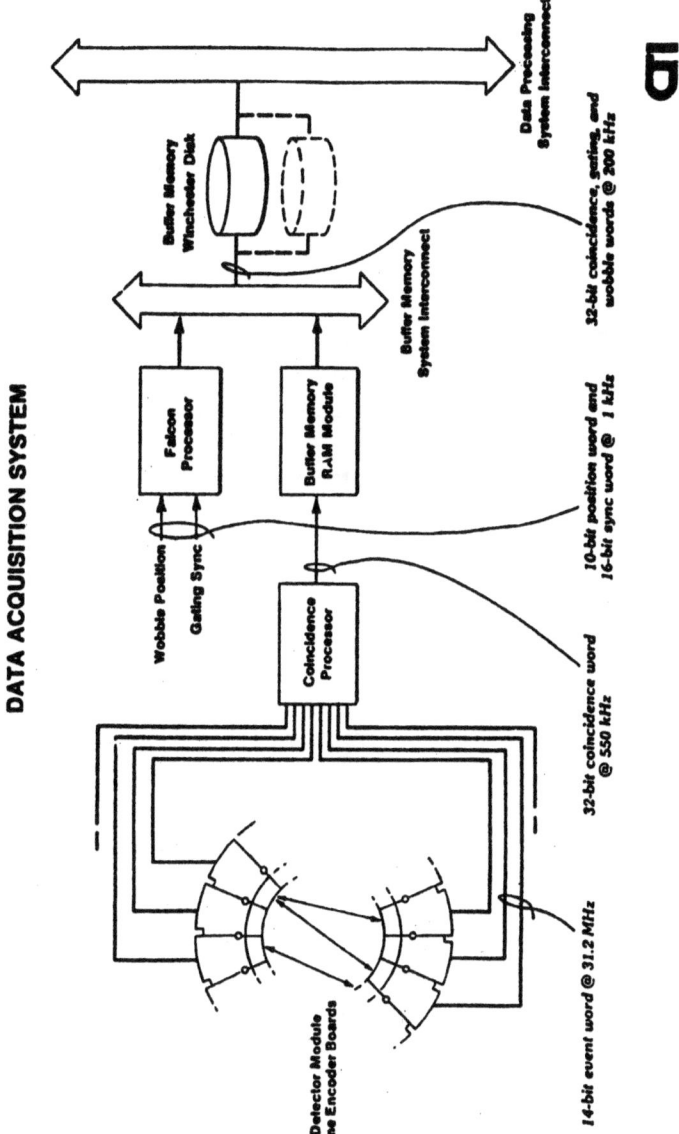

Figure 5

ECAT III SCANNER PROCESSING SYSTEM OVERVIEW

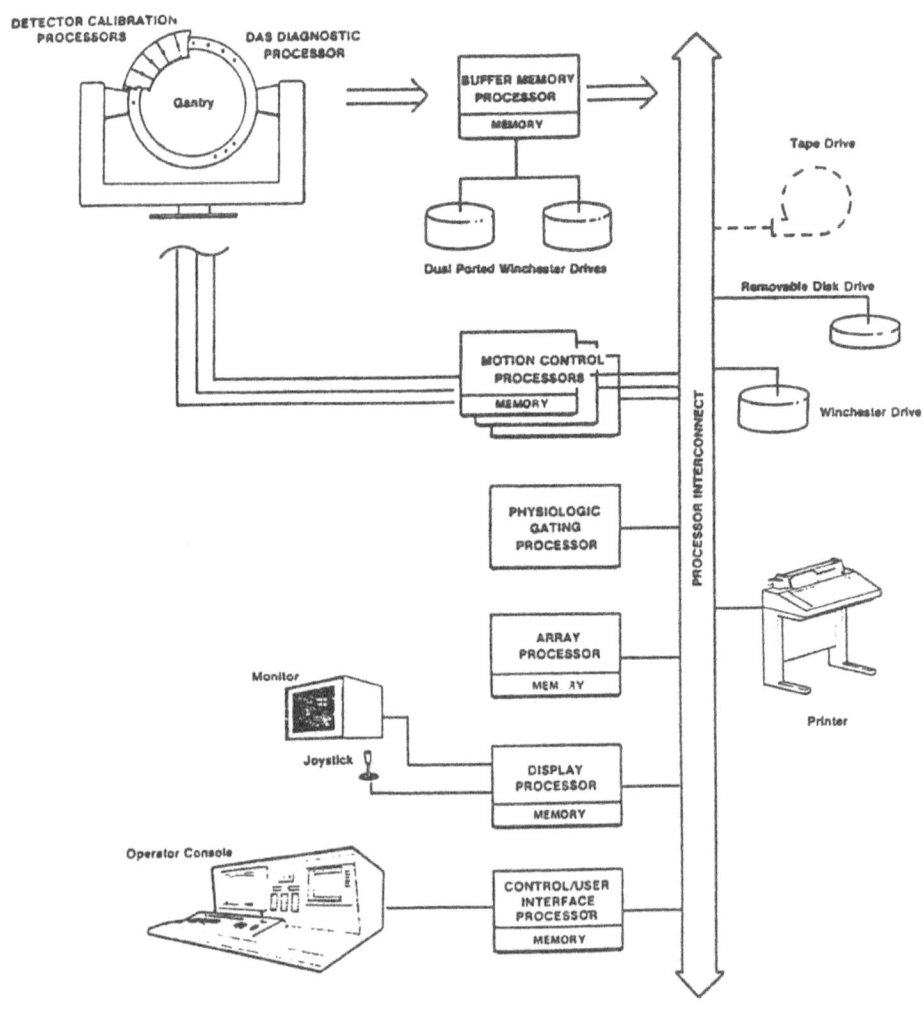

Figure 6

SOFTWARE

The ECAT Software is user-friendly based on PET imaging techniques proven at 17 installed ECAT and NeuroECAT Scanner sites and over 40 man-years of ECAT software design experience. Fundamental to the design is a set of primitive operations that appear in a fixed question and answer menu format to the technician operator but are infinitely usable to the experienced scientist in either single execution or chained multiple operation. The basic programs of the ECAT can be run simultaneously under the VAX/VMS operating system and/or under the VAL/CLONE (Command Language On Line Execution) system interpreter: Data Acquisition, Image Reconstruction, Image Processing, Application Packages, Utility Functions, User-Generated Software, and Diagnostic Software.

Data Aquisition

(1) Patient Scanning
(2) Detector Calibration (Normalization)
(3) Count Rate Monitor

Image Reconstruction

(1) Corrections for Attenuation
    (a) Calculated
    (b) Measured
    (c) Hybrid
    (d) User generated
(2) Correction for Deadtime
(3) Correction for Randoms (Accidentals)
(4) Correction for Scatter
(5) Choice of Filters
(6) Image scaling
(7) Smoothing
(8) Reconstructed Image Position and Size

Image Processing (Manipulation)

Image analysis is the most used feature and includes the following fundamental processing of tomographic and rectilinear images:

(1) Image Display
(2) Windowing
(3) Histograms
(4) Region of Interest (ROI)
(5) Time Activity Curves
(6) Image Listing

Application Packages

(1) Free Fatty Acid Metabolism
(2) Glucose Metabolism
(3) Cerebral Blood Flow
(4) Cerebral Blood Volume
(5) Oxygen Extraction Ratio

Utility

(1) Patient Scan Archival Storage/Retreval
(2) Patient Scan Editing
(3) System Default Parameters Editing

Diagnostic Software

(1) System diagnostics
(2) Component diagnotics

PRELIMINARY PERFORMANCE CHARACTERISTICS

CTI is conservative regarding specifications due to our commitment of designing and manufacturing equipment which meets and exceeds published specs and because the specifications in PET scanners are the subject of discussion in accuracy and interpretation.

Resolution

Resolution and its uniformity across the FOV are physical functions of detector width, the stopping power of the detector material, the spatial sampling frequency, and the reconstruction filter cut-off frequency. Considering all of the factors, the PT 911 exceeds minimum requirements of for static, dynamic, or gated (heart) imaging.

Initial measurements of transaxial reconstructed spatial resolution with a 2 mm diameter line source in air and a RAMP filter have superior results of 4.6 mm FWHM in the high resolution mode and 7.2 mm FWHM in the low resolution mode. The axial resolution (slice thickness) of the Model PT 911/02 is continuously variable from 5.0 to 18.0 mm FWHM. Resolution uniformity has not been measured to date but the Derenzo and Hoffman brain phantoms (See Figures 7 & 8) gives strong credibility to the uniformity of response.

Sensitivity

Sensitivity in PET has been typically quoted for total coincidence events (true, scatter, and accidental events) in a 20 cm diameter cylindrical phantom with a uniform distribution of positron activity in units of counts/second per microCurie/milliliter. We believe the emphasis should be placed on image quality and quantitation and thus efficiency should include true and scattered events but exclude accidental (or random) events. The preliminary efficiency of the PT 911/01 ECAT is 50,000 counts/second per microcuries/milliliter.

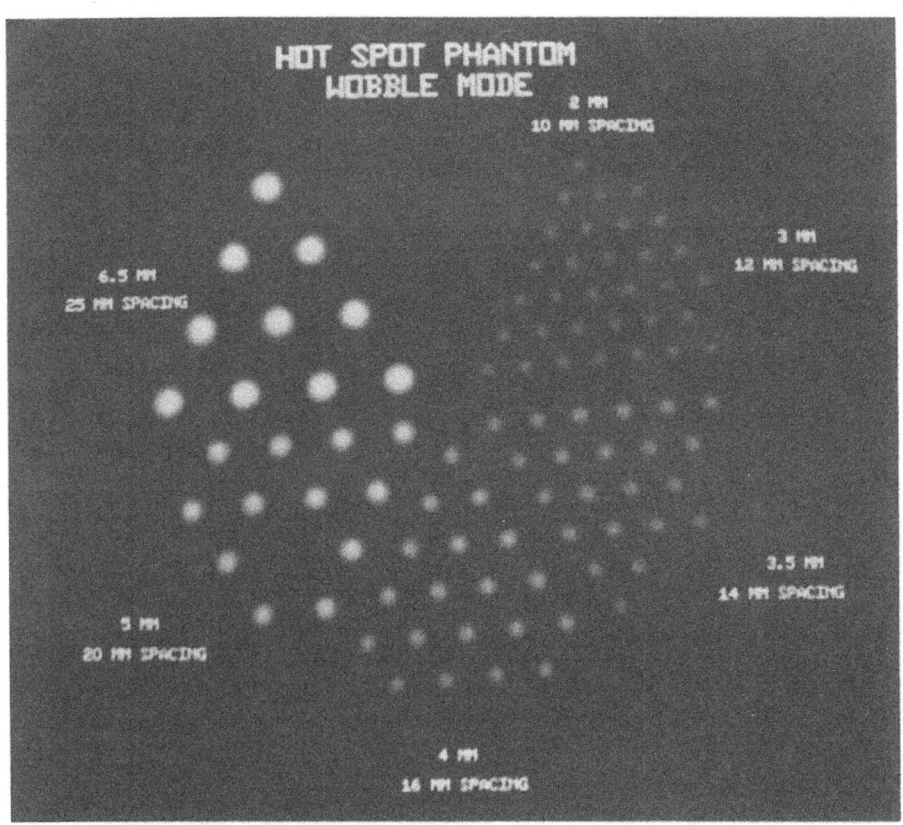

Figure 7 - A high resolution PT 911 ECAT image (4 position wobble sampling and 4.6 mm FWHM reconstructed spatial resolution) image of the Derenzo type phantom with 16 million events. The 20 cm diameter cyclinder has line sources 6 mm, 5 mm, 4 mm, 3.5 mm, 3 mm, and 2 mm spaced respectively with 25 mm, 20 mm, 16 mm, 14 mm, 12 mm, and 10 mm separation.

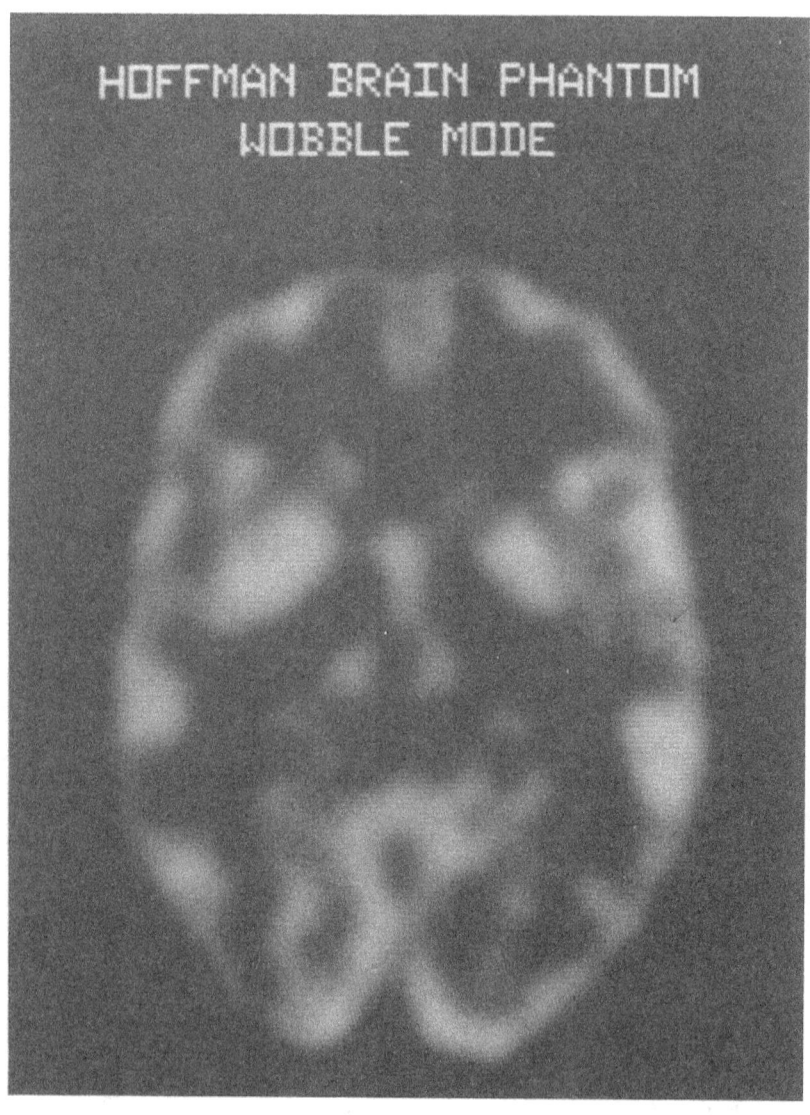

Figure 8 - A high resolution PT 911 ECAT image of the Hoffman brain phantom.

ACKNOWLEDGMENTS

The authors thank Dr. E. J. Hoffman, Michael Casey, Larry Byars and Dr. M. E. Phelps for technical assistance, J. Schall for illustration preparation and L. Glover for manuscript preparation.

REFERENCES

1. Phelps, M.E., Huang S.C., Hoffman, E.J., et al: An Analysis of Signal Amplification using Small Detectors in Positron Emission Tomography. J. Comput Assist Tomogr 6: 551-565, 1982.

2. Hoffman E.J., et al: Performance Evaluation of a Positron Tomograph Designed for Brain Imaging. J. Nucl Med 24: 245-257, 1983.

TIME-OF-FLIGHT POSITRON EMISSION TOMOGRAPHY (T.O.F. P.E.T.)

R. ALLEMAND

CEA - CENG LETI/MCTE - 85 X 38041 GRENOBLE CEDEX FRANCE

1 INTRODUCTION

Positron emission tomography (P.E.T.) consists in yielding images representing the spatial and temporal distribution of specific molecules labelled with positron emitting radionuclides (^{11}C, ^{13}N, ^{15}O, ^{18}F...). The goal of PET is to study organ physiology by detecting, in vivo, biochemical processes.

The basic concept of positron imaging consists in detecting the annihilation radiation limited to a transverse plane of the subject and reconstructing from these data the activity distribution image.

In the conventional method, each event is detected by measuring the time coincidence between the two 511 KeV annihilation photons emitted 180° apart with two opposing detectors. Thus, the position of each event is located on a straight line joining the detectors. In the reconstruction process, this means that each event is back-projected on the whole size of the image matrix.

Time-of-flight (T.O.F.) concept (1) (2) (3) consists in measuring the time difference between the arrivals of the two photons on the two detectors operating in coincidence. For this method, a very fast time measurement should be obtained since a time interval of 1 nsec. corresponds to a position variation of the point source of 15 cm. In measuring the time distribution of the events with far greater accuracy than the transit time of a photon through an object, the gaussian spatial distribution of the events may be used. Therefore, in the T.O.F. reconstruction process, each event is back-projected on a length which is only a fraction of the image matrix resulting in a better signal-to-noise ratio than in the conventional technique. This statement represents the basic difference between the two methods (3) (4) (5).

2 T.O.F. TOMOGRAPHIC IMAGING CHARACTERISTICS

An imaging device can be characterized by three main parameters : the spatial resolution, the temporal resolution and the sensitivity.

The physical limitation of the spatial resolution is about two millimeters, due to the non-collinearity of the two 511 KeV γ rays and the positron range inside the tissue. State of the art P.E.T. devices provide images with a spatial resolution of 5 to 10 millimeters. Great efforts are presently being made in order to improve that characteristic.

The temporal resolution is a second important parameter for positron imaging. The random coincidence rate is proportional to the coincidence time. For dynamic studies with short life radionuclides, the random coincidence rate can reach the same level as the true events in conventional P.E.T.. This leads to an image contrast degradation and to an error of quantitative activity measurements.

The sensitivity is the third major parameter of positron imaging. It is essential to detect the largest possible fraction of the events escaping from the organ in order to minimize the radiation dose to the patient.

2.1. Advantages of T.O.F. P.E.T.

2.1.1. Sensitivity

The advantage of signal-to-noise ratio improvement with T.O.F. technique has been extensively reviewed in published works (4) (5) (7). This advantage can be expressed in defining a sensitivity gain which is the ratio of the number of counts needed to obtain the same signal-to-noise ratio by T.O.F. or by conventional methods. For a typical time resolution of 500 psec. the sensitivity gain varies from 2 to 4, depending on the size of the object. That sensitivity gain definition is somewhat formal as it establishes the comparison between two identical devices as a function of the only time resolution parameter. It is clear that a real sensitivity comparison must take into account (as it will be seen later) other parameters and particularly the detection efficiency. The only goal of the sensitivity gain G expression is to quantify the signal-to-noise ratio improvement due to the T.O.F. method.

These considerations can be summarized by the following relation (11) :

$$G = \frac{2D}{C \Delta t}$$

where C is the speed of light $(3.10^{10} cm/s^{-1})$, D is the diameter of the object and Δt is the timing accuracy in seconds.

2.1.2. Counting rate capability

Coincidence event rate represents only a low percentage of the total counting rate due to the important contribution of scattered radiation and accidental coincidences in the total number of detected events. This means that high counting rates ($\sim 10^5$ c/s) are obtained at the level of each detection probe in dynamic studies with short life radionuclides. For example, 50 to 60 mCi of O^{15} can be currently administrated, because the ^{15}O half life is only 2 minutes. No significant saturation effect due to pile-up of light in the crystal is observed with T.O.F. P.E.T. because of the very short light emission of the scintillators, well appropriate for T.O.F. (8) (10).

2.1.3. Response to the random coincidences

Random coincidence rate is proportional to the coincidence time. In the conventional method, the coincidence time is determined by the dead time of the detectors (about 8 to 10nsec. for BGO crystals), while in the T.O.F. technique, the only limitation is given by the size of the object to be imaged (usually 3 nsec.) (5) (6) (8).

2.1.4. Further advantages

As each event is back-projected on only a part of the image matrix, the angular sampling condition for T.O.F. technique does not need such a large number of directions of projections as in conventional method. The practical result is that no angular motion is needed for T.O.F. P.E.T. device (12) (13).

Furthermore, the good rejection of random coincidences in T.O.F. P.E.T. allows a more intense transmission source to be used than for conventional devices. It can be used either to obtain a better transmission measurements accuracy or to obtain a shorter time exposure (11) (13).

2.2. Limitations of first generation T.O.F. P.E.T.

The label of "first generation" is devoted to T.O.F. P.E.T device using Cesium Fluoride (CsF) crystals as detection scintillator (6) (7) (8).

The two main criticisms (11) concern the spatial resolution and the sensitivity. These two points merit some comment.

2.2.1. Spatial resolution

The lack of commercially available small and fast photomultipliers was a major drawback in the first generation T.O.F. P.E.T. for achieving a spatial resolution competitive with conventional P.E.T. A typical resolution of 12 mm (FWHM) was obtained with the first generation T.O.F. P.E.T. using cylindrical CsF crystals and 1"1/8 in diameter fast phototubes. Several attempts have been made to overcome this technological limitation. These are reviewed in this paper in the second generation T.O.F. P.E.T. description.

2.2.2. Sensitivity

As mentioned above, the sensitivity gain expression given by T.O.F. technique does not take into account the detection efficiency parameter.

Table 1 gives the physical characteristics of different scintillators. For the first generation T.O.F. P.E.T. using CsF crystals the coincidence detection efficiency is significantly lower than for conventional P.E.T. using BGO scintillators, but this efficiency loss is compensated by the sensitivity gain which, for a typical time resolution of 500 psec, varies from 2 to 4, depending on the size of the organ.

3 - THE SECOND GENERATION T.O.F. P.E.T. PHYSICAL AND TECHNOLOGICAL CONCEPTS

Efforts have been made by different groups in order to improve the quality of T.O.F. P.E.T. images. The technological developments have been focused on the two critical parameters which are the detection efficiency and the spatial resolution.

3.1. Detection efficiency

Barium fluoride (BaF2) was suggested (6) (9) (10) in 1982 to be used as a new scintillator for T.O.F. P.E.T. designs. The light emission slow component (decay time $\sim$ 600 nsec.) was already well-known and this crystal had been used as a conventional scintillator in applications where a non hygroscopic material is needed. The U.V. light emission fast component from high purity crystals was recently found (6) (10) and this new property raised   great interest for fast timing measurements and particularly in the field of high energy physics and positron imaging.

Table 1 summarizes the main properties of the most interesting materials. BaF2 clearly appears to be a much more suitable scintillator for T.O.F. P.E.T. than CsF. It exhibits a better packing fraction (non hygroscopic material), a higher detection efficiency, a faster timing, and its lower price is also worth mentioning. Nevertheless, it must also be noticed that a quartz window is required for the photomultiplier tube (PMT) as the light emission is located in the UV region (220 nm), and this results in an increasing of the PMT cost.

Table 1 : Main properties of scintillation materials for P.E.T.

	BGO	CsF	BaF2	
			fast**	slow
Density	7.1	4.6	4.9	
Linear attenuation coeff. at 511 KeV (cm^{-1})	0.9	0.42	0.44	
Scintillation decay time (nsec.)	300	2.5	0.8	630
Relative scintillation output	1	0.9	0.6	2.5
Wavelength emission (nm)	480	390	225	330
Hygroscopic	NO	YES	NO	
Detection efficiency*	0.77	0.50	0.60	

* Derenzo numbers : for a 20 x 20 x 40 mm^3 deep detector including packing fraction parameter (14)

** The two numbers correspond to the fast and slow light emission components

A factor of merit (FM) has been defined (14)

$$FM = \frac{\text{coincidence efficiency}}{\text{time resolution}}$$

where the (γ,γ) coincidence efficiency is the square of the single photon efficiency and where the time resolution roughly varies in the inverse ratio of sensitivity. Based on that FM definition, BaF2 has about twice the value of CsF.

In the last two years different companies have made strong efforts to develop BaF2 because of its great potential for high energy physics, and its technology and characteristics are now well controlled. Thus, curiously, the first aim of T.O.F P.E.T. imaging will take advantage of the new developments linked to the high energy physics market.

3.2. Spatial resolution

Technological efforts have been carried out by manufacturers of photomultiplier tubes (PMTs) in order to optimize the T.O.F. P.E.T. spatial resolution with BaF2 crystals. The first approach was to mount a quartz window on a fast photomultiplier tube of 1"1/8 in diameter (Hamamatsu R 1398 PMT) and more recently, a small and fast phototube (Hamamatsu R 2076 PMT) was developed. This exhibits a good trade-off between the size (3/4" in diameter) and the time response ($\sim$ 500 psec. FWHM with a 4 cm long BaF2 crystal).

Furthermore, several approaches have been investigated by different research groups in the two last years to improve the spatial resolution. All these efforts consist in coupling more than one crystal on each PMT and in proposing a localization method able to determine the triggered crystal.

Mullani's group (15) suggests to couple two different crystals (one CsF and one BaF2) on each 3/4" diameter PMT and the light decay time difference between the two crystals is used to find out the position.

Ter Pogossian's group has studied a modular structure made of eight BaF2 crystals optically coupled to 5 PMT (3/4" in diameter). The geometrical arrangement allows the impinged crystal to be determined by coincidence (or anticoincidence) measurements between two PMTs.

A third approach has been investigated by LETI group (13) (16) in taking advantage of the slow component of BaF2. The principle of the method is shown in fig. 1. Each PMT is optically coupled to two crystals. A pulse signal is triggered

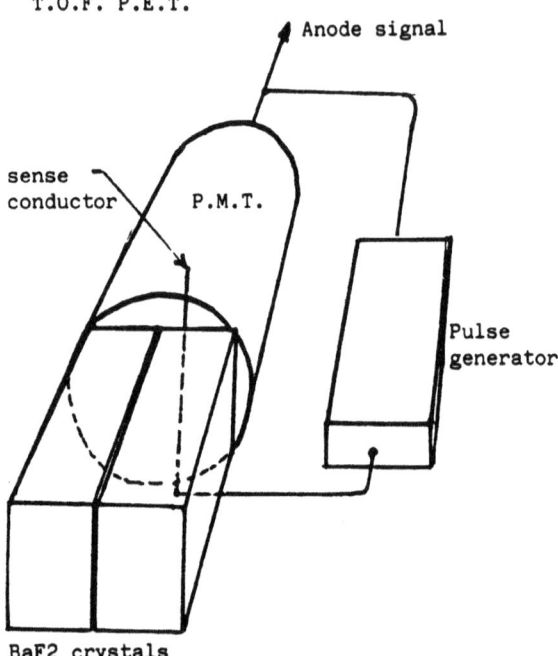

Figure 1 : Identification system for high spatial resolution T.O.F. P.E.T.

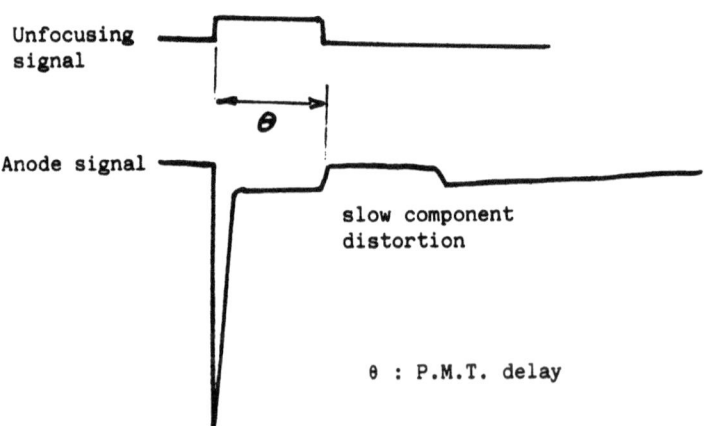

by the anode signal fast component and is applied at the level of the photocathode through an appropriate conductor. The electrical field generated by the pulse unfocuses the photoelectron collection on the first dynode, and therefore a modification of the slow component shape is observed. The conductor positionning and the pulse amplitude are determined to have an unfocusing effect only under one of the two crystals, making thus the position determination. Very good results have been obtained with the two types of PMT mentioned above and this solution can be now used for the design of a complete machine. In a further step, this approach could be advanced by incorporating the sense conductor inside the PMT itself.

From the results of these new developments, it follows that the spatial resolution of the second generation T.O.F. P.E.T. will be strongly increased without involving a significant degradation of time resolution. Based on the laboratory experimental results, the expected values for a complete device are as follows:

- with 3/4" PMT = . spatial resolution : 5 - 6 mm
              . time resolution : $\sim$ 550 psec.
- with 1"1/8 PMT = . spatial resolution : 7 - 8 mm
              . time resolution : $\sim$ 500 psec.

These values are related to a transverse plane. It is important to notice that longitudinal resolution is much lower in all the devices (conventional or T.O.F.). That aspect needs to be pointed out because it can be the source of errors regarding some fundamental characteristics such as the sensitivity, the partial volume effects, etc... A positron image represents the activity distribution in each volume element (voxel) ; thus, in order to characterize a P.E.T. device, it is essential to normalize the physical performance by introducing the "voxel" notion.

4 SECOND GENERATION T.O.F. P.E.T. DESIGN

The label of "second generation" is related to high spatial resolution devices using BaF2 crystals.

Based on the above-mentioned new developments, detailed designs have been carried out by different groups and now the realization of the first prototypes begins. The spatial resolution value, which is usually announced, varies from 5 to 6 mm for brain devices to 7 to 8 mm for whole body machines. In both cases, the time resolution is typically around 500 psec. The sensitivity values can change in a rather large ratio depending on several technical choices of the design:

ring diameter, slice thickness, shielding dimensions between slices and between crystals, scintillator packing fraction... Furthermore, great efforts have been made to improve the reconstruction procedures (17) (18) and to make the operating conditions and maintenance easier:
- optimization of the hardware configuration of the data collection
- faster processing system
- implementation of software

5 - CONCLUSION

An important new step has been made in the performance of the time-of-flight positron imaging over the last two years. It has been proved that a high spatial resolution can be obtained with the T.O.F. technique. It has also been shown that the overall sensitivity (taking into account the sensitivity gain and BaF2 detection characteristics) is quite close to that of conventional methods.

On the other hand, the basic advantages related to the high counting rate capability, the random coincidence rejection, etc... do, of course, remain.

It is probably safe to assume that significant improvements can be expected if new technological efforts are made. Unfortunately, P.E.T. is a complex and expensive tool which up to now, has only been used in reasearch groups (about 50 centers in the world). The justification of new technical developments will be quite clear when this modality is considered in the assessment of diseases and in clinical diagnostic applications.

REFERENCES

1. G.L. Brownell, C.A. Burnham and al. New development in scintigraphy and the application of cyclotron produced positron emitters. Medical Radioisotope scintigraphy - Vol 1 - Proceedings of a Symposium - Salzburg August 6-15, 1968
2. W.L. Dunn. Time-of-flight localization of positron emitting isotopes. Thesis in physics - Vanderbilt University- Nashville Tenessee, 1975
3. R. Allemand, C. Gresset, J. Vacher. Potential advantages of a Cesium fluoride scintillator for a time-of-flight positron camera. J. Nucl. Med. 21 (2) 153, 155 - 1980
4. R. Campagnolo, Ph. Garderet, J. Vacher. Tomographie par émetteurs de positrons avec mesure de temps de vol. Colloque international sur le traitement du signal - Nice - Mai 1979
5. R. Allemand, R. Campagnolo, Ph. Garderet, R. Gariod, C. Gresset, C. Janin, M. Laval, R. Odru, E. Tournier, J. Vacher. A new time-of-flight method for positron computed tomography. U.S.A. France Seminar on biomedical image processing. St Pierre de Chartreuse (France) - May, 26 1980
6. M. Laval, R. Gariod, R. Allemand, E. Cormorèche, M. Moszynski. The "LETI" positron tomograph architecture and time-of-flight improvements. Workshop on time-of-flight tomography - May, 17-19 1982. Washington University - St Louis - Mo
7. M.M. Ter Pogossian, N.A. Mullani, D.C. Ficke, S. Murkham, D.L. Snyder. Photon time-of-flight assisted positron emission tomography. J. Comput. Assist. Tomogr. 5 (2) 227-239, 1981
8. M.M. Ter Pogossian, D.C. Ficke, M. Yamamoto, J.T. Hood. Design characteristics and preliminary testing of super PET 1. Workshop on time-of-flight tomography, May 17-19, 1982. Washington University - St Louis - Mo
9. M. Laval, M. Moszynski, R. Allemand, E. Cormorèche, P. Guinet, R. Odru and J. Vacher. BaF2 inorganic scintillator for subnanosecond timing - Nucl. Instr. and Meth.
10. J. Vacher, R. Allemand, M. Laval, M. Moszynski and R. Odru. New development on detection and fast timing on the time-of-flight LETI device. Workshop on time-of-flight tomography, May 17-19, 1982. Washington University - St Louis - Mo
11. T.F. Budinger. Time-of-flight positron emission tomography. Status relative to conventional P.E.T. J. of Nucl. Med. Vol 24 (1) - 73-78, 1983
12. E. Tanaka. Line-writing data acquisition and signal-to-noise ratio in time-of-flight positron emission tomography. Workshop on time-of-flight tomography May 17-19 1982. Washington University - St Louis - Mo
13. R. Allemand, JL. Lecomte. Methodology of positron emission tomography. An european workshop sponsored by EEC. London March 1984

14. S.E. Derenzo. Comparison of detector materials for time-of-flight positron tomography. Workshop on time-of-flight tomography - May 17-19 1982. p 63-69 - Washington University St louis Mo
15. W.H. Wong, N. Mullani and al. Characteristics of small barium fluoride scintillator for high intrinsic resolution time-of-flight positron emission tomography.
16. R. Allemand and al. Nouvelles perspectives technologiques pour la tomographie à positons par temps de vol. Symposium Liège 15-16 avril 1983.
17. D.C. Ficke and al. Recent developments in image reconstruction using a time-of-flight assisted positron emission tomography. IEEE Transactions on nuclear science, 1983, vol NS-31, Nb 1, p 605-609
18. D.G. Politte and D.L. Snyder. Results of a comparative study for a reconstruction procedure for producing improved estimates of radioactivity distributions in time-of-flight tomography. IEEE transactions on nuclear science, 1984, Vol. NS-31, Nb 1, p 614-620.

POTENTIAL IMPROVEMENTS IN INSTRUMENTATION FOR PET

Stephen E. Derenzo

Lawrence Berkeley Laboratory
and Donner Laboratory
Berkeley, CA 94720
U.S.A.

ABSTRACT

This paper discusses the potential for improved detectors in Positron Emission Tomography (PET) and explores the ultimate limits that might be achieved in the areas of spatial resolution, sensitivity, and maximum imaging rates. It is shown that if an ultra-fast, high efficiency scintillator and a thin, low-noise, position-sensitive photodetector were available, a multi-layer time-of-flight tomograph would be possible with a 10 cm axial field of view, a 3-dimensional spatial resolution of 2 mm fwhm, and >700,000 prompt unscattered coincidences per sec for 1 μCi per cm^3 in a 20 cm diam cylinder of water.

1 IMPROVED DETECTORS

1.1 SCINTILLATION CRYSTALS

Table 1 lists properties of three detector materials commonly used in positron tomographs, NaI(Tl), BaF_2, and bismuth germanate (BGO). NaI(Tl) has the best photon yield and pulse height resolution, BaF_2 has the best timing resolution, and BGO has the best detection efficiency. An "ideal detector" with the best properties of all three has not yet been found. However, the scintillation properties of three important heavy inorganic crystals have been discovered rather recently: BaF_2 in 1971 (1), BGO in 1973 (2), the fast component of BaF_2 in 1982 (3,4), and GSO in 1982 (5). Further efforts in this direction are essential if the potentials of PET are to be fully realized.

TABLE 1. PROPERTIES OF SCINTILLATION MATERIALS
FOR POSITRON EMISSION TOMOGRAPHY

Material	NaI(Tl)	BaF$_2$	BGO	"Ideal Detector"
Density (gm/cm^3)	3.67	4.8	7.13	>7
Atomic numbers	11,53	56,9	83,32,8	>80
Index of refraction	1.85	1.56	2.15	$\simeq 2^a$
Hygroscopic?	YES	NO	NO	NO
Photoelectron yield (511 keV)	2,500	800;200	300	>1,000^b
Scintillation decay time (nsec)	230	620;0.8	300	<1
Photoelectrons/nsec (peak rate)	11	1.3;250	1	>1,000
Time resolution (fwhm nsec)	1.5	0.2	5	<0.2
Energy resolution (% fwhm)	7	20	10	<8
INTERACTION PROBABILITIES FOR 511 keV PHOTONS:				
Photoelectric (cm^{-1})	0.060	0.085	0.393	>0.4
Compton (cm^{-1})	0.268	0.353	0.510	>0.5
Total (cm^{-1})	0.328	0.438	0.903	>0.9
Photoelectric fraction^c	0.183	0.194	0.435	>0.4

^{a}A high index is chosen to define a photon "escape cone" that can be used to determine the position of interaction in 3 dimensions (see section 2.1 below).
^{b}Efficient coupling to a phototube (20% quantum efficiency) or escape cone coupling to a solid state photodetector (80% quantum efficiency)
^{c}Ratio of photoelectric/total, or the probability of full photoelectric absorption on the first interaction

1.2 SOLID STATE DETECTORS

While germanium detectors have been suggested for the detection of annihilation photons in positron emission tomography (6,7), it is not possible to use their excellent pulse height resolution because their photopeak detection efficiency is extremely low. For example, there is only a 5% probability that an incident 511 keV photon will deposit all its energy in a 5 mm x 5 mm x 30 mm deep germanium crystal (8). The detection efficiency can be significantly improved (to over 50%) by using a low pulse height threshold, but the efficiency is still well below that of the heavy element scintillators. Both HgI$_2$ and CdTe have good detection efficiency due to their high atomic numbers and densities but have not yet been developed to the point where thousands of detectors can be used in large tomographs. The development of such heavy element semiconductors (9,10), would provide an attractive alternative to the scintillator detector by eliminating the photomultiplier coupling problem and by providing better pulse height resolution than scintillation detectors.

1.3 COMBINED PHOTOTUBE- SOLID STATE READOUT

One promising approach uses a photomultiplier combined with solid state photodetectors. A group of crystals is coupled to a relatively large photomultiplier tube which determines the timing for the group. The solid-state photodetectors are coupled individually to each crystal to determine the identity of the scintillating crystal. HgI_2 (11-13), silicon photodiodes (14-16), silicon avalanche photodiodes (17-20), and small low-gain phototubes (21) have been suggested for the crystal identifier. This method is good for very small crystals, since the noise of solid state photodetectors decreases with decreasing area, and the signal is nearly independent of crystal size. In addition, it permits the rejection of multiple-crystal interactions that degrade spatial resolution.

This approach has been demonstrated using a 3 mm wide BGO crystal in coincidence with two 3 mm wide BGO crystals coupled to a common 14 mm PMT and individually coupled to silicon photodiodes. The signal to noise ratio was adequate for the identification of the individual crystals on an event-by-event basis and the measured detector pair resolution was 2.0 mm fwhm (14,15). A multi-layer positron tomograph design using this technology is sketched in Figures 1 and 2.

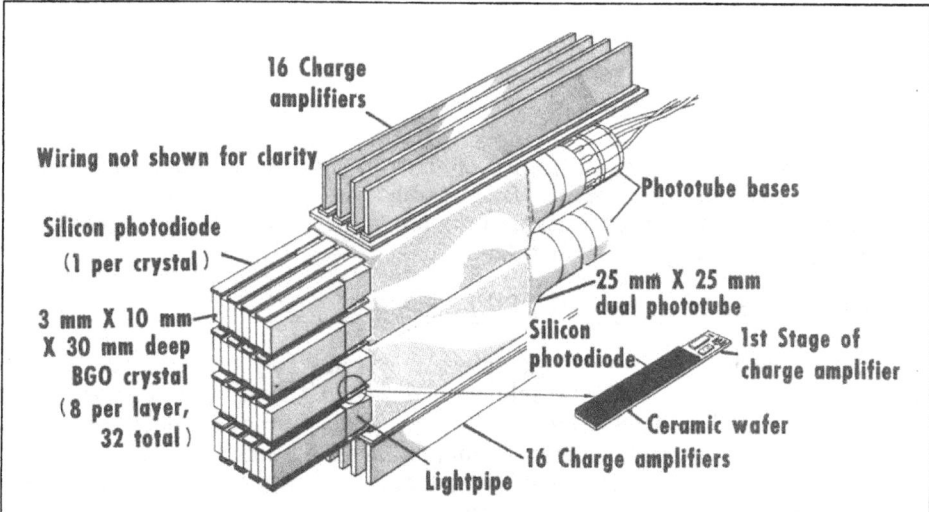

Figure 1: Multi-ring detector array where groups of 8 crystals are coupled to a common phototube for timing information and coupled individually to silicon photodiodes for the identification of the crystal of interaction. Square phototube (Hamamatsu R1548) has two independent electron multipliers and first stage of charge amplifier is mounted near photodiode.

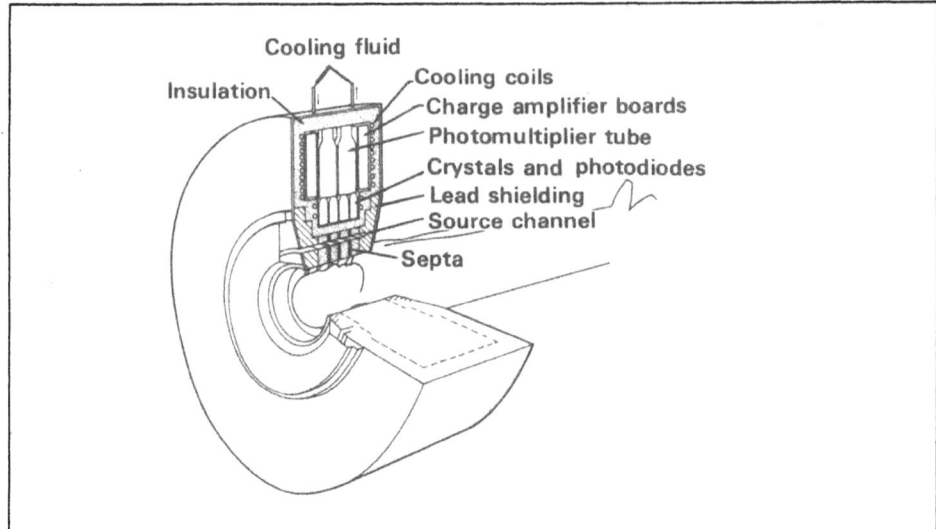

Figure 2: Cooled tomograph gantry for keeping silicon photodiodes and charge amplifiers at a reduced temperature (typically -30C°).

2 ULTIMATE LIMITS

To explore the ultimate limits of instrumentation in positron emission tomography, in the next section we introduce an ideal detector module, and then use it in the following sections to explore the ultimate spatial resolution, sensitivity, and maximum event rates.

2.1 A HIGH-RESOLUTION DETECTOR MODULE

Many recent high resolution detector systems rely on large numbers of small crystals for good spatial resolution (22-24). Although a spatial resolution of 2.5 mm fwhm has been achieved this way (22), a practical detector system with a spatial resolution finer than 1 mm may involve a smaller number of larger detectors that are able to measure the location of the recoil electron tracks from which all the scintillation photons originate. In the case of photoelectric absorption on the first interaction (which for 511 keV photons happens 44% of the time for BGO and 19% for BaF_2) all the light originates from a short (<1 mm long) recoil electron. In the case of multiple interactions (one or more Compton scatters followed by photoelectric absorption) the center of intensity of a pattern of recoil electron tracks would be measured.

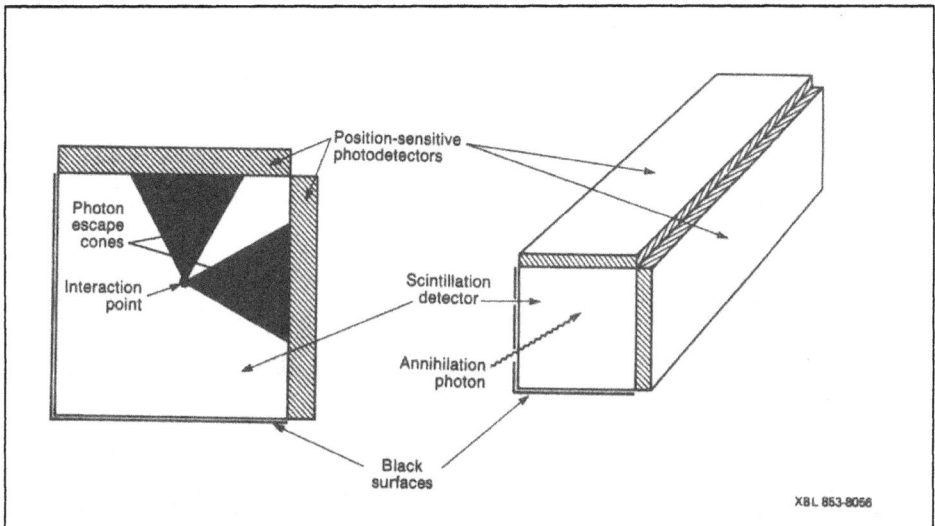

Figure 3: Detector module consisting of a rectangular scintillation crystal and photodetectors capable of determining the location of the interaction point within the crystal.

One scheme for this detector module is a scintillator block coupled to position-sensitive photodetectors on two orthogonal sides (Figure 3). The ideal photodetector for this application would be thin, have high quantum efficiency, be able to amplify photoelectrons internally with sufficient signal-to-noise that individual photons can be detected, and be able to determine position of the center of intensity of the arriving photons. Position sensitive silicon avalanche photodiodes or multi-anode phototubes may evolve to serve this function (20,25,26). The other sides of the crystal would be painted black so that any photon that does not reach a photodetector surface is absorbed. Photons reaching a photodetector surface outside an "escape cone" are internally reflected and absorbed on the other surfaces. Also, some photons within the escape cone are Fresnel reflected and absorbed. While this scheme collects only a small fraction of the available photons (see below), the collected fraction consists of photons that have spread the least in space and time. The opening angle θ_o for the escape cone is given by $sin(\theta_o) = n_2/n_1$, where n_1 is the index of refraction of the scintillator and n_2 is the index of refraction of the external window. For a heavy oxide crystal ($n_1 = 2$) and a glass window ($n_2 = 1.5$) between the scintillator and the photodetector, $\theta_o = 48.6°$. As determined by Monte Carlo calculation, 16% of the photons reach the photodetector (27).

Another potential candidate for this detector is a heavy element semiconductor with a 2-dimensional position sensitive readout (similar to the germanium gamma camera). If the electrons and holes have different drift velocity, the 3rd coordinate can be determined by measuring the pulse shape. Although subnanosecond timing has been achieved for germanium detectors (7,28), the detection efficiency and timing resolution of scintillators such as BaF_2 is significantly better, and we will restrict our considerations below to scintillation detectors.

If the ideal scintillation detector of table 1 and a thin, high-gain imaging photodetector were available, we could expect the following properties:

1) energy resolution: 8% fwhm, based on the statistical fluctuations of 1000 photoelectrons.

2) spatial resolution: less than 0.5 mm fwhm in x,y, and z, based on the fluctuations in the center of gravity of 1000 photoelectrons in an escape cone with a spread of 10 mm fwhm. If the interaction is close to the edge of the crystal, part of the escape cone is cut off, resulting in a non-linear response. It is expected that the correction factor can be measured and tabulated, and applied during data taking.

3) timing resolution: The number of photoelectrons and the decay time is similar to that of plastic detectors or BaF_2, which have achieved an annihilation pair coincidence timing resolution of 200 psec fwhm (4).

4) depth of interaction: By measuring the depth of interaction, the parallax error due to off-axis penetration can be essentially eliminated. In addition, the time-of-flight information can be corrected for the flight time of the scintillation photons in the crystal.

In the following sections we summarize the principal limits of PET instrumentation, given the scintillation detector module just described.

2.2 SPATIAL RESOLUTION

There are 7 primary contributions to spatial resolution in PET.

1) In positron emission, the positrons are emitted with a range of energies from zero to a maximum which varies from 640 keV for ^{18}F to 3350 keV for ^{82}Rb. Due to the non-linear relationship between energy and range for subrelativistic charged particles (such as positrons below 200 keV), a significant fraction of the emitted positrons travel less than 1 mm in tissue. The resulting distribution has a central spike that preserves some of the high spatial frequency information and permits the deconvolution of the range broadening effects, but with some noise amplification (29).

2) Because the positron and electron are not at rest in the laboratory frame when they annihilate, they are not emitted at exactly 180° and have a Gaussian distribution with 0.5° fwhm (30). Unfortunately, such distributions are difficult to deconvolve because of the loss of information at the higher spatial frequencies. As a result, the random deviations from 180° emission is the most fundamental limit to spatial resolution in PET.

3) Detector Resolution, 4) Parallax error and 5) Sampling: By using a detector that can measure the location of the scintillation flash in 3-dimensions with good spatial resolution (< 1 mm fwhm), contributions from parallax error for off-axis rays, and limited linear sampling density are greatly reduced.

6) The high resolution imaging detector module mentioned above can only measure the center of energy deposition. In the case of a single photoelectric absorption interaction, the full energy is deposited in a small region along a short (<1 mm long) recoil electron track. In the case of one or more Compton scatters followed by photoelectric absorption the energy is deposited at several points several mm apart. Thus the distribution of measured positions consists of a sharp central spike flanked by tails that extend on each side by approximately one attenuation length (31,32). As with the positron range blurring, the multiple interaction blurring can be deconvolved with some amplification in statistical noise.

7) The motion of the head can be kept to within 1 mm during a ≤ 1 min imaging time in favorable cases. The motion of the heart is far greater and a blur of 2 mm is possible even when gating for both the beating of the heart and the motion of breathing.

TABLE 2. SUMMARY OF CONTRIBUTIONS TO SPATIAL RESOLUTION (fwhm)

FACTOR	HEAD[a]	HEART[b]
β^+ range	< 1 mm	< 1 mm
angulation error	1.3 mm	2 mm
detector resolution	< 1 mm	< 1 mm
off-axis penetration	< 1 mm	< 1 mm
sampling[c]	0 mm	0 mm
scatter in detectors	<1 mm	<1 mm
organ motion	<1 mm (fast scan)	2 mm (double gate)
TOTAL	2 mm	4 mm

[a] Detector ring diameter 60 cm
[b] Detector ring diameter 100 cm
[c] assuming continuous sampling

2.3 AXIAL RESOLUTION VS IN-PLANE RESOLUTION

Generally, different imaging planes are defined with trans-axial lead or tungsten shields and the design tradeoff between shielding gap and counting sensitivity results in an axial resolution that is 2 to 4 times coarser than the in-plane resolution. Using a detector module able to measure the point of interaction in all three spatial coordinates, the tomograph axial resolution could be as fine as the in-plane resolution. The proper utilization of the resulting out-of-plane rays will require a true 3-dimensional reconstruction algorithm able to use all the rays in an equatorial belt, resulting in a large number of image planes. For example, if the detector spatial resolution is 2 mm fwhm in all 3 dimensions and the volume to be imaged is 25 cm x 25 cm in the plane and 10 cm in axial thickness, then the reconstructed image set of 1 mm^3 pixels would consist of 100 transverse sections each consisting of a 256 x 256 array. Using a single video display, it is possible to view an image plane at any selected position, angular orientation, and thickness.

2.4 SENSITIVITY, SHIELDING APERTURE, AND SCATTER REJECTION

The greatest geometrical acceptance is achieved when the detector rings have greater axial extent than the organ to be imaged, and when the trans-axial shielding permits the detectors to record the full angular range of possible cross-plane coincidences. Two problems arise: 1) the geometrical acceptance of prompt scatter and random backgrounds (which are both non-collinear) is also large, and 2) reconstruction of data from a limited equatorial band is necessary. To address the first problem, we have used the methods of reference (33) to calculate the optimum shielding depth and determine the sensitivity and maximum event rates for a 10 cm shielding gap (Table 3). This wide shielding aperture provides an excellent imaging event rate but also introduces a large fraction of prompt scattered events. A pulse height resolution of 8% fwhm permits the rejection of pulses below 450 keV, but this corresponds to an in-plane angle cut-off of 30°, which has a limited ability to reject prompt scatters. Reducing the angle cut off to 5° would require a threshold of 509 keV, which is only possible using the best semiconductor detectors. The practical solution to this problem requires the accurate computation and subtraction of the prompt scatter background.

TABLE 3. POTENTIAL SENSITIVITY AND EVENT RATES

TOMOGRAPH PARAMETERS:	
Patient port diam P	30 cm
Shielding gap S	10 cm
Detection efficiency	70%
Coincidence window	3 nsec
Activity	1 µCi per cm³ in a 20 cm cylinder of water

RESULTS OF SHIELDING DEPTH OPTIMIZATION	
Optimum shielding depth T	25 cm
Detector ring diameter (P+2T)	80 cm
Image event rate[a]	710,000 per sec
Random event rate[b]	550,000 per sec
Prompt scatter rate[c]	780,000 per sec
Total event rate	2,040,000 per sec
Effective event rate Q[d]	307,000 per sec

[a]Unscattered annihilation photon pair detected in coincidence. Only these events are collinear and can contribute to the image.
[b]Background due to unrelated photons detected in time coincidence by chance.
[c]Background due to annihilation photon pair detected in coincidence but one or both have scattered.
[d]Event rate needed in an ideal tomograph (no background events) for the same signal-to-noise ratio in the reconstructed image.

2.5 TIME-OF-FLIGHT

For a detector with a timing resolution that can localize the point of annihilation (along the line between the detector pairs) to a spatial accuracy (fwhm) of d, and for an emission distribution of effective diameter D, the time-of-flight information reduces the uncertainty in the reconstructed image and enhances the effective sensitivity by the factor D/d (34-38). The ideal time-of-flight scintillator would have a high single interaction photopeak efficiency (>60%), produce a large number of photons (>1000) in a short time (<1 nsec), and be able to measure the depth of interaction to compensate for the difference in velocity between the annihilation photon and the scintillation photons. The timing resolution should be better than 200 psec fwhm, which has been obtained with thin plastic scintillators (4). If D=18 cm (human head) and d=3 cm (200 psec), then $D/d=6$. This factor would increase the effective event rate described in the previous section to 1.8×10^6 non-time-of-flight events/sec for 1 µCi/cm³. This sensitivity advantage is so large that the existence of the "ideal detector" would make time-of-flight a compelling consideration in all tomograph designs.

2.6 RANDOMS REJECTION AND MAXIMUM RATES

Even with arbitrarily good timing resolution, it is not possible to reject random events if their time-of-flight difference places them within the emission region. Thus the effective coincidence window for randoms acceptance is the electronic timing window or the size of the emission region, whichever is larger. For a quantitative analysis, see Ref. (39), where it is shown that in time-of-flight positron tomography, the statistical uncertainty in both the reconstructed true and random events is proportional to the detector timing resolution, and that the ratio is independent of the timing resolution. In table 3, we have used a coincidence window of 2 nsec, which corresponds to a 30 cm diam emission region. We see in this table that the randoms event rate is only slightly less than the image event rate, so 700,000 image events per sec represents a practical rate limit.

The maximum event rate is also a function of the detector deadtime and the number of detectors that are in the system. A large number of detectors operating in parallel permit a high maximum data rate. Electronics deadtime is not a fundamental limit, as many parallel circuits can be used.

3 CONCLUSIONS

The ultimate limits of PET instrumentation have not been realized because of the lack of: 1) an ultra-fast, high efficiency scintillator and 2) a thin photodetector with good timing and position accuracies. If these were available, then a multi-layer time-of-flight tomograph would be possible with a 10 cm axial field of view, a 3-dimensional spatial resolution of 2 mm fwhm, and >700,000 prompt unscattered coincidences per sec for 1 μCi per cm^3 in a 20 cm diam cylinder of water.

ACKNOWLEDGEMENTS

I thank T. Budinger and R. Huesman for helpful discussions.

This work was supported in part by the Director, Office of Energy Research, Office of Health and Environmental Research of the U.S. Department of Energy, under Contract No. DE-AC03-76SF00098, and in part by the National Institutes of Health, National Heart, Lung, and Blood Institute under grant No. P01 HL25840.

Reference to a company or product name does not imply approval or recommendation of the product by the University of California or the U.S. Department of Energy to the exclusion of others that may be suitable.

REFERENCES

1. Farukhi MR and Swinehart CF: Barium fluoride as a gamma ray and charged particle detector. *IEEE Trans Nucl Sci* NS-18(1): 200-204, 1971

2. Weber MJ and Monchamp RR: Luminescence of $Bi_4Ge_3O_{12}$: spectral and decay properties. *J Appl Phys* 44: 5495-5499, 1973

3. Gariod R, Allemand R, Cormoreche E, et al: The "LETI" positron tomograph architecture and time of flight improvements. *Workshop on Time-of-Flight Tomography*, IEEE Catalog No 82CH1719-3, 1982.

4. Laval M, Moszynski M, Allemand R, et al: Barium fluoride: inorganic scintillator for subnanosecond timing. *Nucl Instr Meth* 206: 169-176, 1983

5. Takagi K, and Fukazawa T: Cerium activated Gd_2SiO_5 single crystal scintillator. *Appl Phys Lett* 42: 43-45, 1983

6. Kaufman L, Williams S, Hosier K, et al: An evaluation of semiconductor detectors for positron tomography. *IEEE Trans Nucl Sci* NS-26: 648, 1979

7. Kaufman L, Ewins J, Rowan W, et al: Semiconductor gamma cameras in nuclear medicine. *IEEE Trans Nucl Sci* NS-27: 1073-1079, 1980

8. Derenzo SE: Comparison of detector materials for time-of-flight positron tomography. *Proceedings of the International Workshop on Time-of-Flight Positron Tomography*, Thomas LJ and Ter-Pogossian MM, eds. pp 63-68, IEEE Computer Society Cat No 82CH1791-3, 1982.

9. Armantrout GA, Swierkowski SP, Sherohman JW, and Yee JH: What can be expected from high-Z semiconductor detectors? *IEEE Trans Nucl Sci* NS-24: 121-125, 1977

10. Ortendahl D, Kaufman L, Hosier K, et al: Operating characteristics of small position-sensitive mercuric iodide detectors. *IEEE Trans Nucl Sci* NS-29: 784-788, 1982

11. Barton JB, Hoffman EJ, Iwanczyk JS, et al: A high-resolution detection system for positron tomography. *IEEE Trans Nucl Sci* NS-30: 671-675, 1983

12. Groom DE: Silicon photodiode detection of bismuth germanate scintillation light, *Nucl Instr Meth*, 219: 141-148, 1984

13. Iwanczyk JS, Barton JB, Dabrowski AJ, et al: A novel radiation detector consisting of an HgI_2 photodetector coupled to a scintillator. *IEEE Trans Nucl Sci* NS-30: 363-367, 1983

14. Derenzo SE: Initial characterization of a BGO-silicon photodiode detector for high resolution PET. *IEEE Trans Nucl Sci* NS-31: 620-626, 1984

15. Derenzo SE: Gamma-ray spectroscopy using small, cooled bismuth germanate scintillators and silicon photodiodes. *Nucl Instr Meth*, 219: 117-122, 1984

16. Derenzo SE, Budinger TF, and Huesman RH: Detectors for high resolution dynamic PET. In *The Metabolism of the Human Brain Studied with Positron Emission Tomography,* T. Greitz, Ed, Raven Press, New York, pp 21-31, 1985

17. Entine E, Reiff G, Squillante M, et al: Scintillation detectors using large area silicon avalanche photodiodes. *IEEE Trans Nucl Sci* **NS-30**: 431-435, 1983

18. Lecomte R, Schmitt D, Lightstone AW, et al: Performance characteristics of BGO-silicon avalanche photodetectors for PET. *IEEE Trans Nucl Sci* **NS-32**: 482-486, 1985

19. Dahlbom M, Mandelkern MA, Hoffman EJ, et al: Hybrid mercuric iodide (HgI_2) – gadolinium orthosilicate (GSO) detector for PET. *IEEE Trans Nucl Sci* **NS-32**: 533-537, 1985

20. Squillante MR, Reiff G, and Entine G: Recent advances in large area avalanche photodiodes. *IEEE Trans Nucl Sci* **NS-32**: 563-566

21. Yamashita Y, Uchida H, Yamashita T and Hayashi T: Recent development in detectors for high spatial resolution positron CT. *IEEE Trans Nucl Sci* **NS-31**: 424- 428, 1984

22. Derenzo SE, Huesman RH, Budinger FT, Cahoon JL, and Vuletich T: High resolution positron emission tomography using 3 mm wide bismuth germanate crystals, 1985 (in preparation)

23. Computer Technology and Imaging, Inc. Knoxville, Tennessee, MODEL PT 931 ECAT Scanner System Description.

24. Burnham CA, Bradshaw J, Kaufman D, et al: Design of cylindrical shaped scintillation camera for positron tomographs. *IEEE Trans Nucl Sci* **NS-32**: 889-893, 1985

25. Timothy JG: Electronic readout systems for microchannel plates. *IEEE Trans Nucl Sci* **NS-32**: 427-432, 1985

26. Kume H, Suzuki S, Takeuchi J, et al: Newly developed photomultiplier tubes with position sensitivity capability. *IEEE Trans Nucl Sci* **NS-32**: 448-452, 1985

27. Derenzo SE and Riles J: Monte Carlo calculations of the optical coupling between bismuth germanate crystals and photomultiplier tubes. *IEEE Trans Nucl Sci* **NS-29**: 191-195, 1982

28. Bengtson B and Moszynski M: Subnanosecond timing with planar Ge(Li) detectors. *Nucl Instr Meth* **100**: 293, 1972

29. Derenzo SE: Mathematical removal of positron range blurring in high resolution tomography, 1986 (in preparation).

30. Colombino P, Fiscella B, Trossi L: Study of positronium in water and ice from 22 to -144 °C by annihilation quantum measurements. *Nuovo Cimento* **38**: 707-723, 1965

31. Anger HO: Survey of radioisotope cameras. *ISA Trans* **5**: 311-334, 1966

32. Parker RP: Degradation of spatial resolution in gamma cameras employing sodium iodide or germanium detectors. *Phys Med Biol* **15**: 493-502, 1970

33. Derenzo SE: Method for optimizing side shielding in positron emission tomographs and for comparing detector materials. *J Nucl Med* **21**: 971-977, 1980

34. Budinger TF, Derenzo SE, Greenberg WL, Gullberg GT, and Huesman RH: Quantitative potentials of dynamic emission computed tomography. *J Nucl Med* **19**: 309-315, 1978

35. Allemand R, Gresset C, and Vacher J: Potential advantages of a Cesium Fluoride scintillator for a time-of-flight positron camera. *J Nucl Med* **21**: 153-155, 1980

36. Snyder DL, Thomas LJ and Ter-Pogossian MM: A mathematical model for positron-emission tomography systems having time-of-flight measurements. *IEEE Trans Nucl Sci* **NS-28**: 3575-3583, 1981

37. Snyder DL: Some noise comparisons of data-collection arrays for emission tomography-systems having time-of-flight measurements. *IEEE Trans Nucl Sci* **NS-29**: 1029-1033, 1982

38. Tomitani T and Tanaka E: Image reconstruction and noise evaluation in photon time-of-flight assisted positron emission tomography. *IEEE Trans Nucl Sci* **NS-28**: 4582-4589, 1981

39. Holmes TJ, Ficke DC, and Snyder DL: Modeling of accidental coincidences in both conventional and time-of-flight positron-emission tomography. *IEEE Trans Nucl Sci* **NS-31**: 627-631, 1984

DISCUSSION SUMMARY

PANEL ON STATE-OF-THE-ART AND FUTURE TRENDS IN PET INSTRUMENTATION

The most important points raised during the panel were on design problems and perspectives in tomograph design.

As for the limitation, T. Jones asked why the means of removing the scatter fraction with respect to optimizing the future systems were not mentioned. R. Allemand answered that he restricted his talk to the hardware limitation and to the removal of scatter fraction as a data analysis problem. Jones asked for the statistical problems of using Anger logic with BGO for the few quanta relative to NaI. S. Derenzo answered that Burnham and Brownell's design (IEEE Trans Nucl Sci NS - 29: 461-466, 1982) is able to provide efficient light transfer from the narrow BGO crystals to the phototubes, using total internal reflection in the crystal. In addition, the lightpipe is chosen to allow the light to spread over the number of phototubes that provides the best spatial resolution. The result is a good spatial resolution in spite of the smaller number of photons. Then it was asked (R. Guzzardi) if the SAT approach in dynamic studies would mean optimizing each image for the filter function with different total number of counts. E. Hoffmann's answer was negative. T. Jones commented that, in order to narrow the slice thickness, lead shielding to cover some of the BGOs is used. This is a poor use of the crystal which represents much of the cost of the scanner (Jones). M. Crabtree replied that the ECAT III was designed for a variety of applications and requirements in the heart and brain. These requirements ranged from viewing a single organ (i.e. the heart) at one scanning position (the heart is 12 cm long) to very fine slice thickness at one or two slices. Under present-day technology the best alternative for the above requirements is collimation (or side shielding plates). The ECAT III side shielding plates continuously vary slice thickness by reducing detector area and efficiency. S. Derenzo asked M. Crabtree what his coincidence timing window was. The answer was: with 30-35% phr, FWHM is 8nsec and with a current setting of time window at 24nsec FWTM is 20nsec. R. Guzzardi asked which kind of set-up was used by Siemens for measuring efficiency. Van Oortmarssen replied that a point source in the air at 25 cm distance was used. At R. Guzzardi's second question to Van Oortmarssen on the eventuality of putting on the market a system suitable for 2-D reconstruction,

SPECT and PET Imaging, the answer was positive.

As a general conclusion, the participants agreed on the future expectancy of significant improvements both in timing perfomance of BGO and in spatial resolution for BaF2.

POSTER SESSION

COMPARISON OF RESOLUTION AND CROSSTALK AMONG DETECTORS USED IN POSITRON EMISSION TOMOGRAPHY

Anthony R. Ricci, Magnus Dahlbom, and Edward J. Hoffman

Division of Biophysics, Dept. of Radiological Sciences,
UCLA School of Medicine and The Laboratory of Nuclear Medicine
of the Laboratories of Biomedical and Environmental Sciences,
University of California, Los Angeles.

INTRODUCTION

This chapter concerns a work in progress in which we are evaluating the detailed physical properties of various detector systems employed in PET. These detectors, which are Barium Fluoride (BaF_2), Gadolinium Orthosilicate (GSO) and Bismuth Germanate (BGO), were configured on the UCLA Tomographic Simulator (1) as a small section of a PET system with appropiate distances and shielding. The basic test detector size is a 29 mm high by 5.6 mm wide by 45 mm deep (30 mm for BGO) detector, similar in size to ones used in some commercial PET systems (2). The system diameter is 100 cm.

In this work we were primarily interested in comparing the resolution and amount of interdetector crosstalk among nearest neighbor detectors. The primary experimental configuration is illustrated in figure 1. Since the photomultipliers (PMTs) were much wider than the detectors, they were coupled to the crystals in an orthogonal staggered pattern as indicated in the figure. The signals from PMTs 1, 2 and 3 were ORed together for timing with PMT 4 and separate address signals were routed to the coincidence latch to identify in which detectors the interactions took place. This arrangement allows the simultaneous measurement of resolution and interdetector crosstalk with correction of the data for accidental coincidences.

Examples of these measurements are given in figures 2-4. In these figures, the circles show the prompt coincidences between detectors 2 and 4. The X's indicate the region in which the line

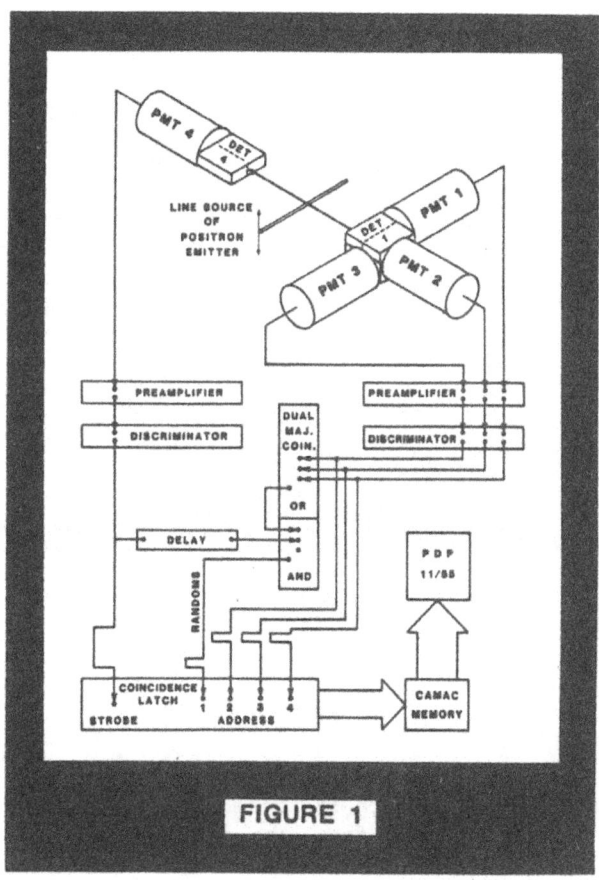

FIGURE 1

source is physically over the adjacent detector, yet the coincidence is between detectors 2 and 4. This is clearly mispositioned and is probably due to a scatter between detector 2 and either detector 1 or 3. However, not enough energy is deposited in one detector for the event to be recorded as a triple coincidence. The triangles and squares are triple coincidences involving detectors 2 and 1 and 2 and 3, respectively.

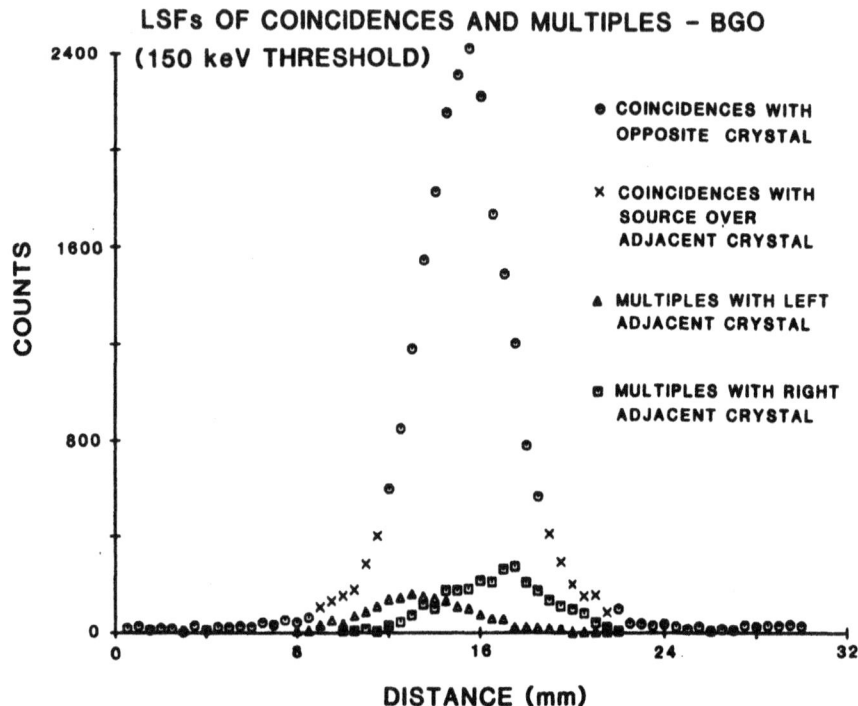

FIGURE 2

Data were also obtained with the detectors tilted 15 degrees to simulate data taken 15 cm from the center of a circular PET system with a 100 cm diameter. Resolution values measured for the case when the detectors are coaxial are 4.6 mm FWHM and 8.9 mm FWTM for BGO; while those for BaF_2 are 4.6 mm FWHM and 9.6 mm FWTM. However, data acquired with the detectors 15 degrees off axis showed the resolutions to be 5.8 mm FWHM and 10.7 mm FWTM for BGO; while BaF_2 measured 7.4 mm FWHM and 13.7 mm FWTM.

In order to clarify these properties of detectors as a function of energy threshold, energy spectra were obtained for the various types of events. The spectra were taken with a line source centered between detectors 2 and 4. Event mispositioning data derived from these spectra are shown in Table 1 for each of the detector materials. Multiples, or triples, are those mispositionings where events are recorded in two adjacent crystals in coincidence with the opposite crystal; e.g., both detectors 1 and 2 in coincidence with detector 4. Spillover includes those mispositioning of events recorded as a coincidence between detectors 1 or 3 and detector 4, instead of the true coincidence between detectors 2 and 4.

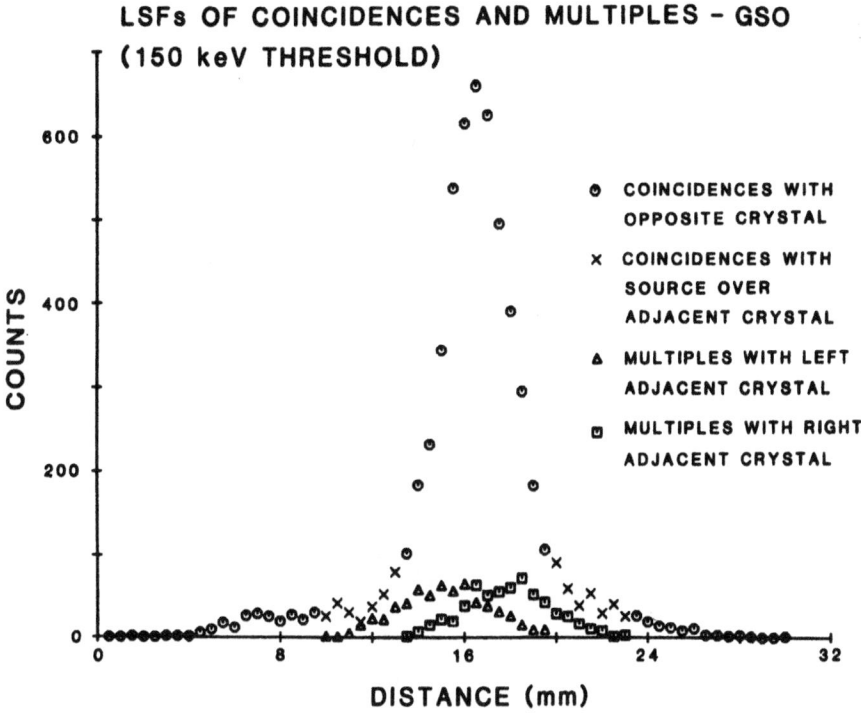

FIGURE 3

DISCUSSION

A primary factor in resolution and efficiency in PET is the ability of detector materials to absorb 511 keV annihilation photons in a single crystal. The fraction of events that fall into photopeaks, generally provides a good measure of the localizing ability of a detector. It is difficult to accurately measure photofractions because scatter from surroundings will add events to low energy portions of spectra. With the arrangement shown in figure 1, we are able to effectively collimate the 511 keV photon flux and remove most of the scatter from adjacent crystals by measuring triple coincidences, which can be subtracted from the coincidence spectra. In this arrangement, we found photofractions of 88 % for BGO, 56 % for GSO and 44 % for BaF_2. Because of poor resolution, the BaF_2 photofraction is overestimated. In addition, for BaF_2 and to lesser extent GSO, energy thresholds are eliminating a significant number of events, which are either not detected or scattered into neighboring crystals.

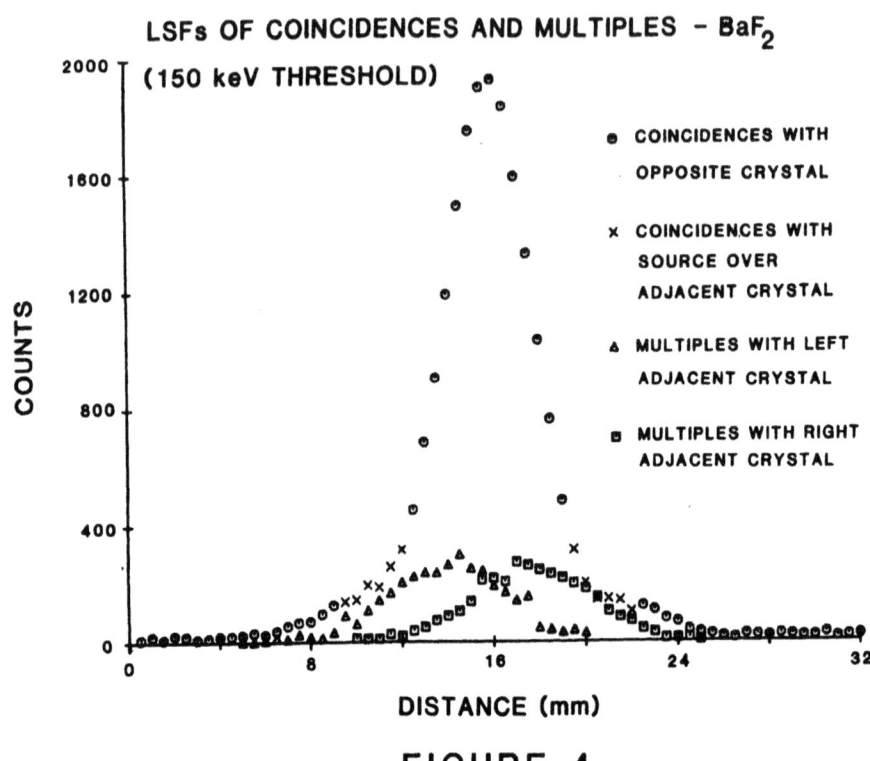

FIGURE 4

TABLE 1: EVENT MISPOSITIONING FOR PET DETECTORS

	BGO		GSO		BaF$_2$	
Threshold [keV]	Multiples* [%]	Errors** [%]	Multiples [%]	Errors [%]	Multiples [%]	Errors [%]
100			14.0	26.4		
150	9.4	14.4	11.3	22.6	20.0	33.1
200	4.9	10.5	5.6	16.1		
250	1.3	6.1	1.8	11.0		
300			0.2	7.4		
350	0.0	5.2				

* Two adjacent crystals in coincidence with opposite crystal
** Sum of multiples and spillover

The measurements in figures 2 thru 4 evaluate the ability of these detectors to localize events. There are two types of mispositioning events that can degrade resolution or efficiency. First, gamma-rays can scatter from one crystal to another, depositing enough energy in each crystal to be detected. In this case the event can be be rejected, arbitrarily assigned to a crystal or half an event assigned to each crystal. Second, gamma-rays can scatter at a forward angle, leaving very little energy in the first crystal and interacting in a neighboring crystal. In this case the first interaction may not be detected and the event will be assigned to the second crystal. Since a 30 degree scatter will deposit only 60 keV of energy in the first crystal, the first interaction can frequently be near noise levels and be difficult to detect with good timing information to establish a coincidence relationship. Generally, these events will be assigned to the wrong crystal. These events are represented by X's for adjacent crystals in figures 2 thru 4 and are referred to as spillover in the table.

As expected, mispositionings increase as we go from BGO to GSO to BaF_2. A misleading measure of localization for detectors is the FWHM of pairs of coaxial detectors. As described above, the FWHM is identical for BGO and BaF_2 for coaxial detectors, yet for a small rotation as might be seen at 15 cm from center of the FOV of a whole body PET system, there is about a 3 mm increase in FWHM for BaF_2 as compared to 1 mm for the BGO. In addition, FWTMs are significantly worse for BaF_2. Crosstalk between detectors 1 and 3 (figure 1) was negligible for BGO and GSO, but was 40 % of the multiples level for BaF_2. This means positioning errors are equal to at least 40 % of correctly positioned events.

We will refine our measurements in the future, but from these preliminary results, we anticipate that it will be very difficult to match resolution capabilities of BGO with BaF_2 in PET. Refinements in measurements include using PMTs with fused silicate windows instead of UV transparent glass to obtain better energy and timing resolution with BaF_2, using 3 crystals on each side, and packing crystals between additional crystals of the same material instead of lead to obtain a better simulation of scatter environment of a PET system.

ACKNOWLEDGEMENTS

The authors thank M. Griswold for assistance in preparation of the illustrations. This work was supported in part by Department of Energy Contract DE-AM03-76-SF0012, National Institute of Cancer Grant 1-R01-CA33801-02, and National Institutes of Mental Health Grant 1-R01-MH373916-01.

PART XV GENERAL REMARKS

Chairman: S. James Adelstein (U.S.A.)

COMPARATIVE ASSESSMENT OF IMAGING

S. J. Adelstein

Department of Radiology
Harvard Medical School
Boston, Ma, U.S.A.

The recent development of several imaging technologies raises questions as to how they are to be utilized in clinical practice. Foremost among these is the selection of the proper test for individual patients. Practising physicians and their radiologist colleagues used to know which test or tests (if any) are necessary to reveal the state of the patient's health and to guide his decisions with regard to treatment. When two or more tests can be used to provide equivalent information those who order and interpret these tests should know the relative merits of each (1).

In evaluating diagnostic tests a number of attributes may be examined. First, the technical merit of the test can be determined and compared with the technical merit of similar tests; this is particularly true in the field of imaging modalities where technical criteria have been carefully elaborated. Second, it is possible to compare the accuracy of diagnostic tests in terms of their sensitivity, specificity, and predictive outcome. Third, one can attempt to determine the extent to which test outcomes influence physician behavior and, indirectly, patient care; in the comparison of the test and no-test situations, one could try to compare the behavior of physicians with and without the information that the test provides. Fourth, the influence of the test on health outcome can be assessed; these outcomes are usually expressed in terms of morbidity, mortality, and quality of life. Fifth, the cost-effectiveness of the procedure can be compared to other procedures or to the no-test scenario; cost-effectiveness calculations are usually expressed in terms such as cost per case found, cost per death averted, or cost per hospital day avoided.

Each step of this process is susceptible to errors of commission, omission, and interpretation. I shall attempt to demonstrate some of the difficulties that can be found at the various stages elaborated above.

COMPARING TECHNICAL MERIT

In nuclear medicine we have seen an enormous improvement in technology, both in instrumentation and in radio-pharmaceuticals, dating from 1954 to the present. In the case of liver scanning for the detection of metastatic malignancy, there has been a revolutionary change both in the instruments and radio-indicators employed. This improvement can be summarized quantitatively by a figure-of-merit (FOM) that incorporates factors relating to the fidelity of the instrument (measured in terms of resolution and sensitivity), the number of photons available from the radionuclide incorporated into the liver, and the radiation dose received by critical organs. Table 1 shows a comparison of two techniques in which the figure of merit is raised significantly (a factor of 25) by alterations in the radiopharmaceutical (^{131}I to ^{99m}Tc) and the instrument (3" scanner to Anger camera). Despite these changes the sensitivities and specificities are virtually the same.

A similar observation has been made in the employment of ultrasound for abdominal abscesses. Real-time scanning was introduced to improve the man/machine interface by selecting the most appropriate imaging planes for inspection. When real-time scanning was compared with B-mode scanning, no significant difference in sensitivity or specificity could be found (2).

In both these examples, improvements in technology have not been translated into more accurate diagnosis. Thus, although such improvements (e.g. fidelity of images, contrast, etc) must be documented they do not by themselves signify diagnostic success.

Table 1 Effect of Changes in Figure of Merit on True Positive (TP) and False Positive (FP) Ratios

Year	Radiopharmaceutical	Instrument	Figure of Merit	Test Indices TP	FP
1954	^{131}I-Rose Bengal	3" scanner	7	.94	.37
1972	^{99m}Tc-Sulfur Colloid	Anger camera	172	.90	.37

ACCURACY AND PREDICTIVE VALUE

The Data Base

A good data base for absolute or relative measures of accuracy and predictive value is very difficult to obtain. Very often a single investigator or institution will attempt to collect sufficient data to determine the sensitivity and specificity of a diagnostic test and then, in some instances, to obtain predictive value from these data. A number of hazards have been identified with studies of this type (3). First, there may be biases in work-up and the establishment of truth. Second, instrumentation technique, data collection, and follow-up may be inadequate. Third, instabilities in the prevalence and spectrum of disease may flaw any attempt to establish predictive outcome.

The Liver Scan

Some of these problems can be illustrated by the study of 650 sequential liver scans taken at the Peter Bent Brigham Hospital in Boston (Figure 1) (4). Of the 429 patients with abnormal liver scans in this group, 61 percent (263) had histological diagnosis made by biopsy, surgical exploration, or autopsy; however, of the 221 normal scans, only 37 percent (81) had a histological diagnosis. Because the decision to obtain histological data was determined to some degree by the outcome of the test, the population from which the sensitivity and specificity of the liver scans were determined was not an unbiased one. This type of bias occurs frequently with retrospective analyses and is one reason for preferring prospective studies, in which the definitive standard for the diagnosis end point is selected independently of test outcomes. From the histological examinations (see Figure 2: "Results of Further Examination of the Liver"), the sensitivity of the liver scan in this group of patients was 90 percent and its specificity 63 percent (false-positive value of 37 percent).

Use of these sensitivity and specificity data to calculate the predictive value of the liver scan 1) in a particular patient requires knowledge of the prior probability of disease in that patient. This is notoriously difficult to obtain because the prevalence of disease in an entire population can be used only as a first approximation of the value for a particular patient. Even then, this population prevalence may be biased because it depends so heavily on the referral patterns and the behavior of referring physicians. For the liver scan data, the prevalence of disease was determined using both histological and follow-up data at 18 months (see Figure 1, line marked "Clinical Decision:). With this figure of 64 percent, the probability that a patient with an abnormal scan will have liver disease is 90 percent and the probability that a patient with a normal scan will be free of disease is 86 percent.

CT of the Head

An alternative and preferable manner for collecting data to evaluate a particular test is exemplified by a prospective cooperative study involving several medical centers. Under the best of circumstances, such studies are expensive and require considerable planning and expertise to achieve unbiased results within a reasonable period. A study by the National Cancer Institute on computerized tomography and radionuclide scanning in the diagnosis of cerebral tumors illustrates some of the problems with prospective studies.

At the time the study was started, computerized tomography of the brain was on the border between an emerging and a new technology, and five institutions were selected for this comparative study. The institutions were comparable in terms of their technical capabilities for CT scanning, and it was assumed that they were comparable in terms of their radionuclide studies. In fact, though, the institutions were quite different, one of the consequences of this difference was that none of the patients in one hospital were available for comparative purposes.

---

[1] Predictive value generally means either the probability that a patient with an abnormal liver scan actually has liver disease, or, conversely, that a patient with a normal liver scan is actually free of liver disease.

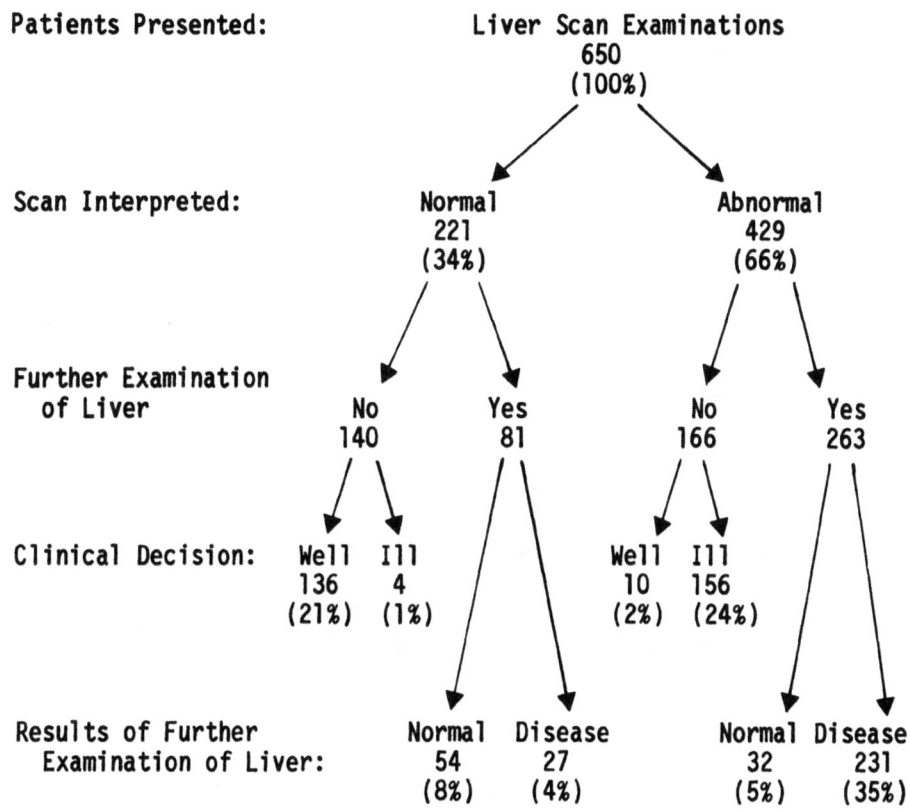

Figure 1. Clinical-Pathological Outcomes in 650 Sequential Liver Scans Performed in a Single Nuclear Medicine Unit. Of these, 61 percent of the abnormal scans and 35 percent of the normal scans had further histological liver examination. The prevalence of liver disease in the entire group (clinically ill or pathologically diseased) was estimated to be 64 percent.

Several facts emerge from a careful analysis of this study. First, the costs of the study were large, averaging about $450,000 for each hospital for a total of $2.2 million (Table 2) (5). Second, the total number of patients entered in each hospital was large, nearly 3,000, but the total number available for final analysis was small, only 136. This loss was due to a variety of factors, including incomplete follow-up, lack of histological data, lost copies of examinations, and so forth. Fortunately the sample was sufficient to make an analysis of the comparative accuracy of computerized tomography and radionuclide scanning. Finally, the cost per patient entered into the original study was about $765, but the cost per patient used for the analysis was $16,500.

Table 2 Comparison of Computed Tomography and Radionuclide Brain Scanning in the Diagnosis of Cerebral Tumors

Hospital	Total Cost	Total No. Patients	Total Patients Available for Analysis
A	$ 417,000	599	0
B	461,000	574	25
C	373,000	525	15
D	463,000	634	67
E	523,000	597	29
Total	$2,237,000	2,929	136

CRITERION-FREE MEASURES OF ACCURACY

If measures of accuracy are not criterion free, confusion may result. In practically all instances lax or strict criteria can be used to interpret diagnostic data from a wide variety of sources. Most diagnostic tests are not perfect. If they were, they would easily segregate normal populations from diseased populations. In fact, there is considerable overlap and room for type 1 (false negative) and type 2 (false positive) errors. A decision must therefore be made as to where to set the upper (lower) limits of normal or the lower (upper) limits of abnormal. Setting this value depends upon the percentages of false positive and false negative outcomes one is willing to accept. In the imaging modalities, the biased interpretation of individual readers produces a floating criterion. The best current method for deriving a criterion-free measure for imaging purposes is the receiver operating characteristic (ROC) curve or a plot of the true-positive ratio against the false-positive ratio (6,7). This method results in a continuum of inversely related sensitivities and specificities for a particular procedure. These curves can be very useful in the analysis of a host of problems, including the relative accuracy of two diagnostic tests, the utility of taking diagnostic tests together (2), and the construction of disjunctive analyses using multiple variables (8).

The ROC curve has been the principal quantitative instrument used in comparing two or more imaging modalities. As a result, indices have had to be developed which allow statistical comparison when the several tests have been applied to the same group or different group of patients (i.e. paired or unpaired samples) (14).

PHYSICIAN BEHAVIOR AND HEALTH OUTCOME

Cephalopelvimetry

Just as a new technology does not necessarily result in improved accuracy, so improved accuracy may not result in an improvement of health outcomes. In fact, relatively few controlled studies have been conducted in which such cause and effect relationships can be determined. Several years ago a study by Crichton (9) involved a prospective analysis of the use of cephalopelvimetry for the diagnosis of cephalopelvic disproportion and consequent improvements in morbidity and mortality in the perinatal period. In this protocol all patients referred to the radiology department for cephalopelvimetry were entered into the study on a random allocation basis. Approximately one half of the patients had x-ray examination and the other half did not. The test apparently had an influence on physician behavior in that 43 percent of patients who had pelvimetry underwent Caesarean section, while the corresponding value for the control group was 32 percent. The combined neonatal mortality and morbidity was 16 percent in the pelvimetry group and 25 percent in the control group. These differences are marginally significant.

Screening for Renovascular Disease

A number of recent studies have shown a less clear-cut relationship between certain diagnostic tests and health outcome. A number of years ago, we examined the impact of screening for renovascular hypertension on the frequency of subsequent morbid events, especially strokes and heart attacks (10,11). We found that several factors determined whether or not this screening procedure was likely to have an impact on outcome. Compliance was of particular importance; if compliance was high, little was gained by screening patients for renovascular hypertension versus treating them with hypertensive medication irrespective of cause. If compliance was low, then screening made a good deal of difference; surgical treatment had a greater impact than it did otherwise.

Radionuclide Brain Scan

In another study, George and Wagner (12) tried to evaluate the impact of the introduction of brain scanning and other neurodiagnostic procedures on the time course of brain tumors for the decade 1962-1972. During this time period, radionuclide brain scanning increased by a factor of 10; an analogous increase was seen in the number of cerebral angiograms performed over the same period. In 1962 brain scanning was an emerging technology; by 1972, it was a well-established technology. The sensitivity of the scan did not, however, change perceptively over the interval, although quite an impact occurred in terms of disease discovery. Before 1962 the duration of symptoms in patients with brain tumors was about four years. After these neurodiagnostic procedures were used, the duration of symptoms to the time of disease discovery was reduced to less than one year. Despite this, survival curves for patients with brain tumors were not significantly different from the beginning of that era to its end. The survival curves after operation were in fact virtually superimposable; and if one assumes that the time to operation was decreased over the period of ten years, then the survival of patients might actually have been shortened. In terms of survival, the value of a positive brain scan is not great. Alternatively, other issues must be considered in this case; perhaps the most obvious is the importance of prognostic information which is made available as a result of a normal test in a patient without a brain tumor. Most of the patients scanned fell into this category.

COST EFFECTIVENESS CALCULATIONS

Screening for Renovascular Disease

It is often easier to make a cost-effective calculation than it is to interpret one, although, at times the interpretation of cost-effectiveness calculations is straightforward. This is particularly true when two procedures of equal accuracy are compared. The cost per case found or the cost per year of life extended can then be compared in a straightforward manner. However, when an absolute judgment as to the value of cost-effectiveness ratio must be made, criteria for making judgements may or may not be available. Occasionally the complete analysis can be of some value. In screening patients for renovascular hypertension, we were able to calculate the cost per patient discovered as a function of the percentage of renovascular hypertensive patients identified, as well as the total cost of screening 100 patients as a function of the percentage of renovascular hypertensive patients identified (11). In both instances, one point appears to provide an optimal return for invested costs. In the first instance, the curve is parabolic and concave upward. There is a rather broad minimum, and a point at which about 90 percent of patients discovered is the extreme before the curve turns up again. This suggests that this point (which also maximizes the information content) optimizes the relationship between the fraction of patients discovered or identified and the cost per patient. With reference to the renogram as a screening procedure, the total costs also seem to change significantly at this same point, which represents an operating point taken before the total costs rise very steeply.

CT of the Head

The interpretation of cost-effectiveness calculations can be more problematic. As a theoretical exercise, I have attempted to evaluate the cost-effectiveness of computed tomography for neurological disorders. The data base is derived from a study of Abrams and McNeil (13) in which they analyzed the number of neurodiagnostic studies and neurological evaluations at two Boston hospitals before and after the introduction of CT of the head. If the accuracy data obtained from the study of Swets, et al. (6) are combined with these data, it is possible to tabulate the fraction of patients with disease identified, the percentage of patients found to have disease among those tested, the total costs of diagnosis, the cost per patient found, and the marginal cost (Table 3). As expected, the fraction of patients with disease who were identified rose from 75 percent to 86 percent. At the same time, the fraction of patients tested who had disease decreased from 66 percent to 36 percent; thus, physician behavior seemed to be influenced by the introduction of the test because of its perceived high degree of accuracy and noninvasive quality. Total diagnostic costs increased from $532,000 to $867,000, average costs increased from $565 to $805, and the marginal cost was $2,600 per patient discovered.

Table 3 Impact of Computed Tomography on Neuroradiological Costs and Case Finding at Two Boston Teaching Hospitals

	1974	1977
Fraction of patients with disease identified	75%	86%
Fraction of all patients tested who had disease	68%	36%
Total diagnostic costs*	$532,000	$867,000
Cost per patient found*	$ 565	$ 805

* In constant dollars relative to 1977 costs.

An appropriate question arising from these data concerns the meaning of the increase in the cost per patient discovered, as well as the increase in the number of patients examined by this method. Although the demonstration of a significant objective difference in health outcomes will be difficult, there undoubtedly has been a significant increase in the confidence of physicians whose patients have had this neurodiagnostic procedure and an increase in the peace of mind of those patients who have had a negative result. This analysis thus raises some critical questions. What is the value of physician confidence and patient peace of mind? Who should decide this worth policymakers, individual patients, or society as a whole?

References

1. McNeil, B.J. and S.J. Adelstein. Determining the value of diagnostic and screening tests. J. Nuc. Med. 17 (1976) 439.

2. McNeil, B.J., R. Sanders, P.O. Alderson, S.J. Hessel, H. Finberg, S.S. Siegelman, D.F. Adams, D.F., and H.L. Abrams. A prospective study of computed tomography, ultrasound, and gallium imaging in patients with fever. Radiology 139 (1981) 647.

3. Ransohoff, D.F. and A.R. Feinstein. Problems of spectrum and bias in evaluating the efficacy of diagnostic tests. N. Engl. J. Med. 299 (1978) 926.

4. Drum, D.E. and J.S. Christocopoulos. Hepatic scintigraphy in clinical decision-making. J. Nuc. Med. 13 (1972) 908.

5. McNeil, B.J. Pitfalls in and requirements for evaluations of diagnostic technologies. In Proceedings of the Conference on Medical Technology, ed. J. Wagner, pp. 33-39. DHEW Pub. No. (PHS) (1979) 79-3254.

6. Swets, J.A., R.M. Pickett, S.F. Whitehead, D.J. Getty, J.A. Schur, J.B. Swets, and B.A. Freeman. Assessment of diagnostic technologies. Science 205 (1979) 753.

7. Swets, J.A. ROC analyses applied to the evaluation of medical imaging techniques. Invest. Radiol. 14 (1979) 109.

8. McNeil, B.J., S.J. Hessel, W.T. Branch, L. Bjork, and S.J. Adelstein. Measures of clinical efficacy III. The value of the lung scan in the evaluation of young patients with pleuritic chest pain. J. Nuc. Med. 17 (1976) 163.

9. Crichton, D. The accuracy and value of cephalo-pelvimetry. J. Obs. Gyn. Brit. Comm. 69 (1962) 366.

10. McNeil, B.J., P.D. Varady, B.D. Burrows, B.D., and S.J. Adelstein. Measures of clinical efficacy: Cost-effectiveness calculations in the diagnosis and treatment of hypertensive renovascular disease. N. Engl. J. Med. 293 (1975) 216.

11. McNeil, B.J. and S.J. Adelstein. Measures of clinical efficacy: The value of case finding in hypertensive renovascular disease. N. Engl. J. Med. 293 (1975) 216.

12. George, R.O. and H.N. Wagner, Jr. Ten years of brain tumor scanning at Johns Hopkins: 1962-1972. In Noninvasive Brain Imaging, eds., H.J. DeBlanc and J.A. Sorenson, pp. 3-16. (1975) New York: Society of Nuclear Medicine.

13. Abrams, H.L. and B.J. McNeil. Medical implications of computed tomography. N. Engl. J. Med. 298 (1978) 255.

14. McNeil, B.J. and J.A. Hanley. Statistical approaches to the analysis of receiver operating characteristic (ROC) curves. Med. Decis. Making 4 (1984) 137.

The material in this lecture note is taken from: Adelstein, S.J. Pitfalls and biases in evaluating diagnostic technologies. In Critical Issues in Medical Technology, eds. (1982).B.J. McNeil and E. Cravalho Boston: Auburn House.

PERSPECTIVE OF DIFFUSION OF IMAGING TECHNOLOGIES

Roger Gariod
CEA-IRDI-LETI-CENG 85 X - 38041 Grenoble Cedex

1. INTRODUCTION

The perspectives for the diffusion of Medical Imaging are synthesized by numerous market forecasts, meaning that each partner should play its expected role.
The main partners are:

- private and public research laboratories;
- industry;
- medical world: research hospitals, clinics, private medicine;
- health management services (state and hospital) risk evaluation
- and cost.

Moreover, the economic situation is not favourable to the heavy equipment budget involved in Medical Imaging.

2 ECONOMIC DATA IN MEDICAL IMAGING

Medical Imaging depends on the following techniques:
Ultrasound, Conventional Radiology, Digital Radiology, X-Ray C.T., NMR, Nuclear Medicine. Networks, transmission, central image pr cessing systems and digital storage should be included in Medical Imaging.

Thermic tomography, biomagnetism, and high frequency imaging studies are now beginning and in the future their evaluation will perhaps offer interesting imaging methods.

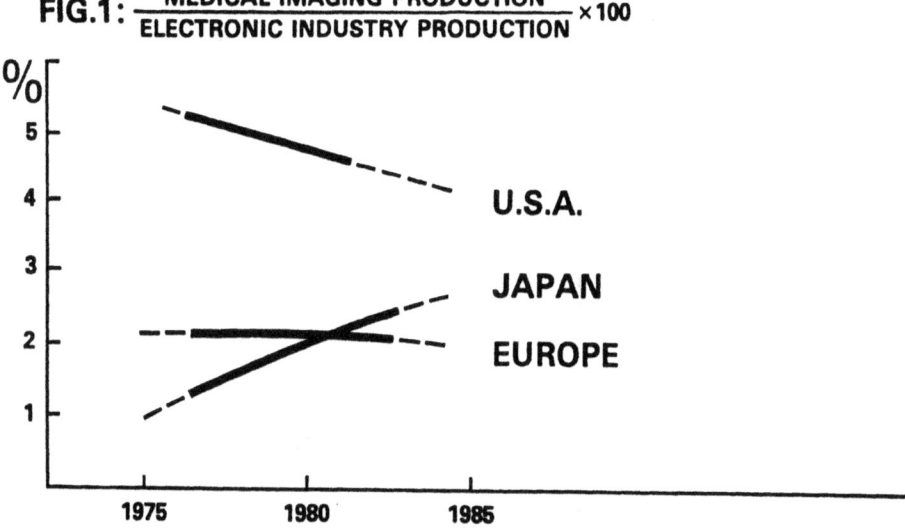

FIG.1: MEDICAL IMAGING PRODUCTION / ELECTRONIC INDUSTRY PRODUCTION ×100

In 1983 the Medical Imaging world turnover was around 4000 M $ and was only a small part (1) of the industrial electronic market (Fig.1). Benefitting from the recent rapid development of metrology, digital techniques, microcomputers and computers, Medical Imaging is ever evolving, as far as the detection and image construction techniques are concerned.

3 MEDICAL IMAGING AND HEALTH COSTS

Health service management, ruled by technocratic imperative, has the tendency to restrict the Medical Imaging diffusion, due to several factors:

- medical risks;
- evaluation of the diagnostic capacity and comparison with other techniques of diagnosis;
- economic evaluation and comparison with the cost of the other techniques.

A global evaluation can only be carried out after long experimentation, taking into account such relevant factors as the effect of the duration of hospitalization. The slowness with which Medical Imaging is spreading is also due to the reluctance of the medical world to accept a medicine too dependent on advanced technology.

FIG.2: RELATIONSHIP BETWEEN : HEALTH SPENDING, MEDICAL IMAGING SPENDING AND NATIONAL PRODUCT

1980	HEALT SPENDING		MEDICAL IMAGING SPENDING		RATIO IMAG.SPEN / HEALT SP. ‰	RATIO HEALT SP. / NAT.PROD. %
	TOTAL B $	PER CAPITA 10^3 $	TOTAL B $	PER CAPITA $		
U.S.A.	220	1	1.15	5	5	9.4
JAPAN	69	0.62	0.45	4	6.5	6
FRANCE	40	0.8	0.15	3	3.75	7.5
EUROPE			0.8	2.5		

FIG.3: RELATIVE EXPENSES

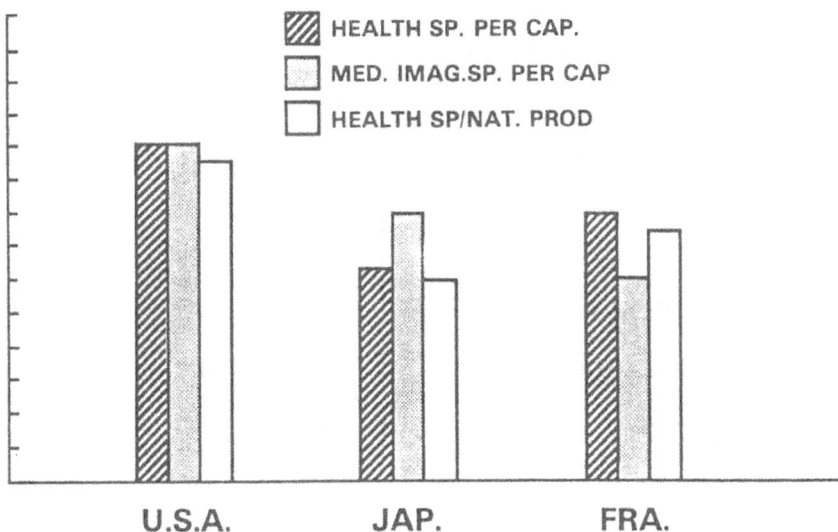

One can observe (Fig. 2 and 3) that there is no simple correlation between investments in advanced technologies and health costs. In conclusion, it seems that the relationship between the total cost and diagnostic efficiency is a good evaluation criterion. The diagnostic related group (DGR) was introduced in the United States since October 1983; it is highly codified and reviewed every four years.

Although health systems vary considerably from one country to another, it seems all the more reasonable in a period of economic difficulties that other countries adopt similar measures suited to their health systems.

4 FORECAST FOR DIFFUSION OF DIFFERENT TECHNIQUES

Fig. 4 shows the world market forecast (1983-93) of the expansion of Medical Imaging and the percentage of each technique.

FIG.4 : SUMMARY OF MARKET FIGURES AND SHARES OF THE DIFFERENT MEDICAL IMAGING TECHNIQUES

MILLION USD (CURRENT VALUE)	1983	1988[E]	1993[E]
MARKET FIGURE			
TOTAL	4000	6500	9500
CONVENTIONAL RADIOLOGY	1300	1200	900
DIGITAL RADIOLOGY	600	1600	3000
ULTRASOUND	750	1450	1950
NUCLEAR MEDICINE	250	350	450
X-RAY C.T.	1000	1100	1100
N.M.R.	100	800	2100
% SHARE OF THE MARKET			
TOTAL	100 %	100 %	100 %
CONVENTIONAL RADIOLOGY	33	19	9
DIGITAL RADIOLOGY	15	25	32
ULTRASOUND	19	22	20
NUCLEAR MEDICINE	6	5	5
X RAY C.T.	25	17	12
N.M.R.	2	12	22

(1) MEAN INFLATION : 5 TO 7 % IN THE U.S.A.

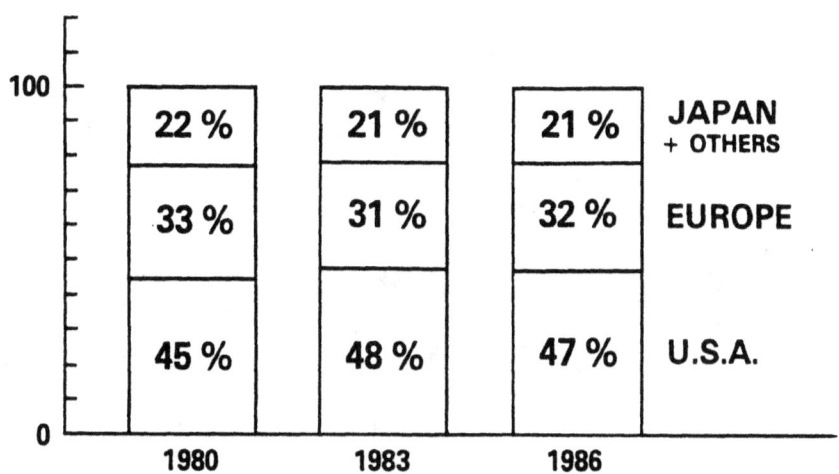

FIG.5: GEOGRAPHIC ZONE (% SHARE)

5 GEOGRAPHIC DIFFUSION

It seems probable that relative geographic diffusion (Fig.5) from 1986 onwards will be more favourable to other countries than the United States, in view of the decision taken in the United States to stabilize medical investments. It should be noted that in Europe Medical Imaging investment per capita is the lowest of the industrial countries (Fig.2).

6 ULTRASOUND

The Ultrasound market tendency and its different configurations are shown in Fig. 6 and 7.

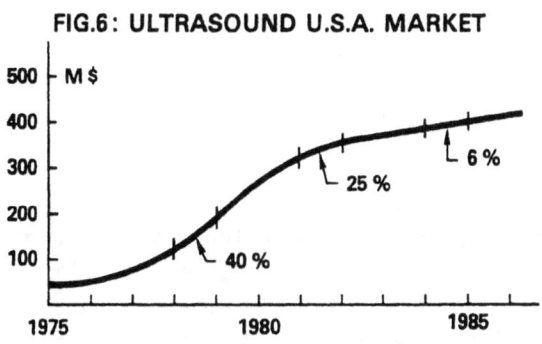

FIG.6: ULTRASOUND U.S.A. MARKET

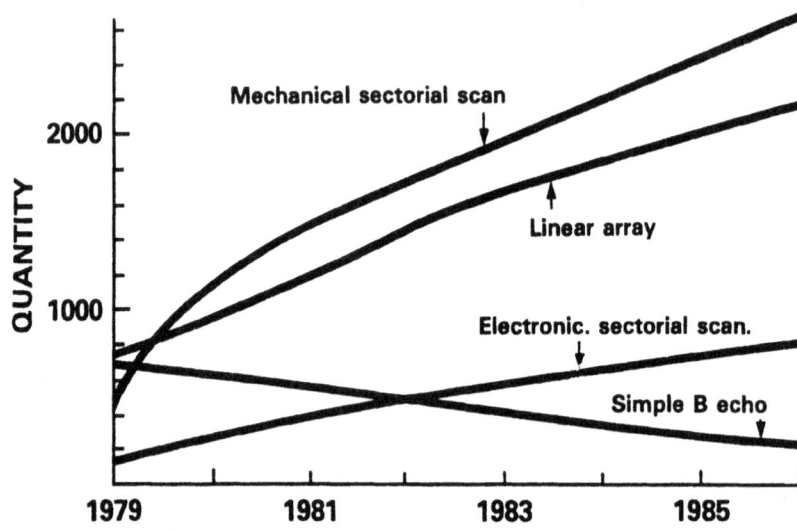

FIG.7: U.S.A. ULTRASOUND MARKET

Ultrasound, as is the case with all Imaging Techniques, has several basic aspects:

detection of the physical phenomena (probes) from a point to one dimension (1D) and to two dimensions (2D);

measurement techniques from analogue to digital;

image construction methods and techniques, from point by point to manual scanning, to mechanical scanning, to electronic scanning, to electronic focus, to echo tracking and to the synthesis method;

visualization;

from analogue vacuum to digital memory and video, to three-dimensional display.

The evolution of instrument design proceeds from the less to the more complex one. Such an evolution is worth examining over the whole field, but it would go beyond the scope of this paper.

The arrival on the market of high performance systems, which use an ever increasing part of digital processing has lead to the present trend in favour to these techniques. The expected decrease in future production costs of digital radiology will inevitably have a favourable effect on market prices for the latest equipment, evaluated today as being too expensive.

On the other hand, it should be noticed that a 3D visualization by ultrasound, at a given volume, will be limited by segmentation elimination capacities, because of the inaccurate quantitative meaning of each voxel. On this point the X-Ray C.T. has an advantage.

7 CONVENTIONAL RADIOLOGY AND DIGITAL RADIOLOGY

Market forecasts indicate a decrease in conventional radiology (Fig. 8) and an increase in digital radiology.

However, in 1983 the sales of digital equipment in the United States were considerably lower than in 1982. 600 systems in 1982, 400 systems in 1983, despite the fact that an increase by 25% per year from 1982 to 1986 had been foreseen.

The following reasons partly explain the optimistic forecast:

- all the digital techniques with their own large range of possibilities are attractive and the image processing, applied to angiography has been an immediate success;
- many other fields of radiological examinations have been favourably seen by medical consumers who were not very well informed.

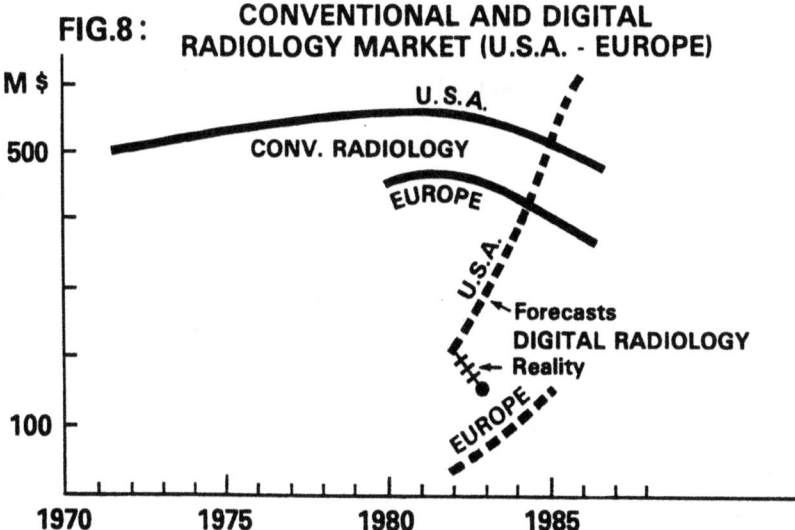

FIG.8: CONVENTIONAL AND DIGITAL RADIOLOGY MARKET (U.S.A. - EUROPE)

Long term forecast:

to extend the digital radiology techniques to a large field of examination, including digital radiography and digital radioscopy. The technical performance of these systems, above all X-Ray detection, must be improved.

Radiography (DRg)

The advantages offered by digital solutions such as thermoluminescent or optoluminescent stimulated screens, are not significantly superior to those offered by conventional radiographic film and presently, the increased costs cannot be justified until further progress will be made in speed, cost, digital storage.

Radioscopy (DRs)

Direct digital detectors try to replace the image intensifier tube. The linear array solution (1000 to 2000 cells) exists and gives sufficient spatial resolution. However, though it may solve a very small part of the digital radiography, it is inadequate for the digital radioscopy because the second dimension obtained by mechanical movement is too slow.

Many laboratories are studying new solutions such as bi-dimensional solid state direct converters and two-dimensional structure scintillator-detector.

Microelectronic techniques will be extensively used in order to reach a competitive cost and to solve, through repetition, the very difficult problem of reliability for a large number of elementary cells ($\sim 4 \times 10^4$ cells).

Other long term possibilities of the DR:

To gather two different applications of the conventional radiology and see that their intersection will lead to significant progress:
a) stereoscopic vision very often carried out, until now, without large success;
b) the longitudinal tomography has a real potential, even if the image is blurred.

Now we can reach the two previous goals, using real 3D reconstruction and 3D display of a volume. It should seem that some movement of a 2D X-Ray detector, adapted to the mechanical possibilities of the radiologic gantry, permits, with some algorithms corresponding to the movement, the obtaining of a real 3D reconstruction, with the same resolution as in the three-dimensions.

The three-dimensional visualization system will be necessary for a correct handling of the fourth dimension, i.e., density. Computer simulated surgery, taking into account the density value, allows us to choose or eliminate selected parts of the body, in order to easily visualize it in 3D representation. This last one is probably a very promising future technique.

8 X-RAY C.T.

The world total for installed C.T. scanners in 1984 is 5600. Fig. 9 shows the shares in the different countries at the end of 1982 (3).
1983 U.S. market forecast (Fig. 10) predicts a minimum figure for scanners.

FIG.9 : C.T. SCANNER WORLD REPARTITION DECEMBER 31,1982

	NUMBER OF SCANNERS	SCANNERS PER MILLION POPULATION
JAPAN	2120	18.5
UNITED STATES	2318	10.7
UNIT. KINGD.	115	2.1
WEST GERM.	230	5.4
FRANCE	80	1.5
SWEDEN		
ITALY	90	1.6
NETHERLANDS	80	5.7
CANADA	72	3.1

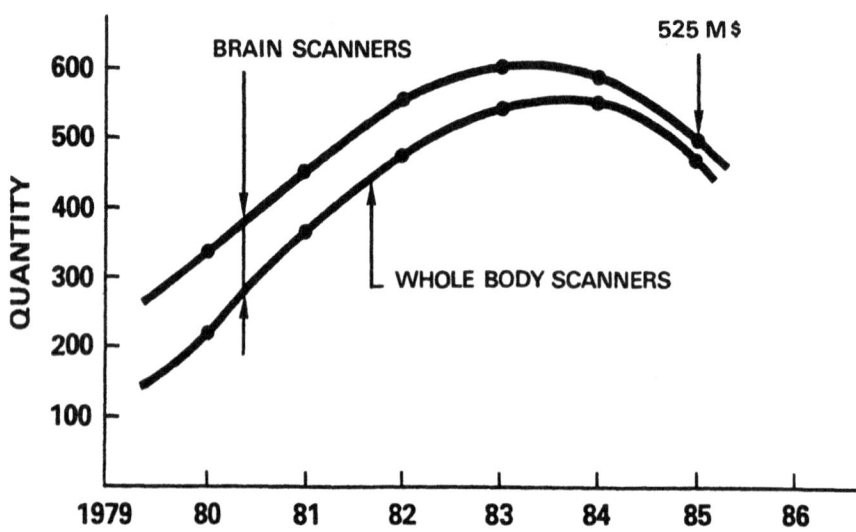

FIG.10: U.S. SCANNER MARKET FORECASTS

However, some experts now believe that the fast decrease in the X-Ray CT. market will occur later than 1985. The two main reasons are the "situation of expectancy" of Digital Radiology and NMR Imaging. The C.T. scanner is benefitting from premature consumer stimulation for these two very promising but immature techniques. There are other influencing factors on the long term market prospects of the C.T. scanners, that can be also discussed.

Favourable Factors for an Increased C.T. Market

Making diagnosis by C.T. is very simple and it facilitates its large scale diffusion, even in small hospitals, at the advantage of the C.T. market. This is favourable to the market extension in small hospitals.

C.T. prices can be reduced from ca. 1 M $ to ca.0.6 M $, 0.3 M $ expected.

It seems that in Japan, a reserve market in small hospitals exists.

FIG.11: BEDS PER HOSPITAL CLASS JAPAN 31 DECEMBER 1981

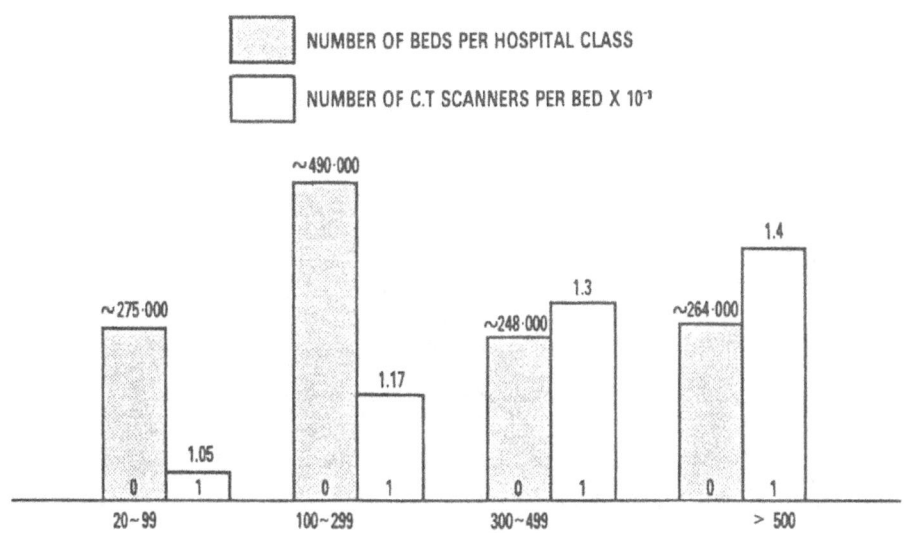

C.T. Scanners Feasible Technological Development

The detector could be developed with a multi-slice configuration, in order to improve the actual 3D performance. The low cost of future linear detectors can also significantly decrease the total C.T. cost.

Unfavourable Factors for the Long Term Market

Digital radiology, which could be adapted to a real 3D reconstruction image.

NMR imaging, which is promising but not yet fully established experimentally.

9 NMR IMAGING

The market potential of NMR is increasing all the time, but it should be noticed that the "take off" did not take place as early as it was initially expected. The U.S. market forecasts for 1982 are indicated in Fig. 12. In fact 39 experimental systems were installed in the U.S. in 1983. The most important factor is that every state and country is trying to control hospital demand.

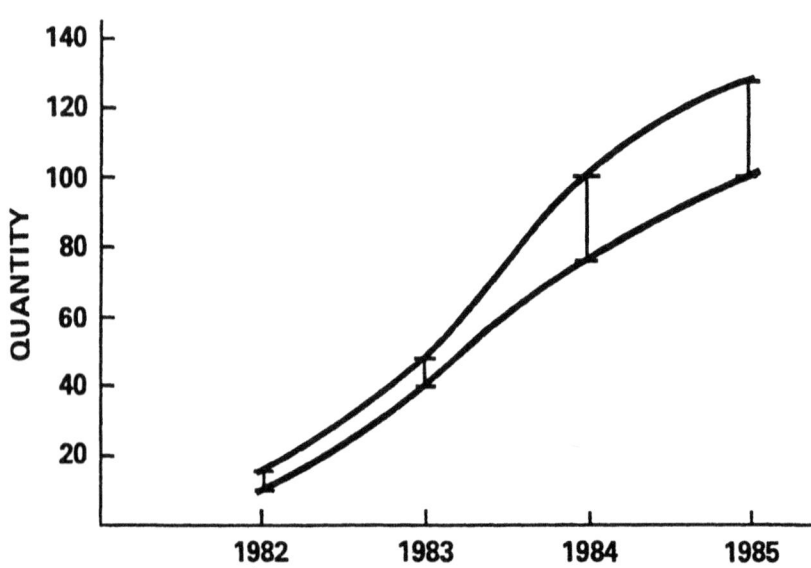

FIG.12: U.S. N.M.R. MARKET

The health management service has evaluated NMR in the following way:

- medical value of the diagnosis
- comparative cost of diagnosis (DRG: diagnosis related group/-tariff scale)

The diagnosis value of proton imaging compared to other diagnostic procedures (Fig.13) has encouraged the medical profession to adopt this technique.

The delivery of a "Certificate of Needs" by the health services initially limited the demand of NMR and this certificate enabled the accurate evaluation of the cost per examination in real hospital conditions. For example, the demonstration program with medical and financial evaluation organized by New York State involved approximately 10 hospitals (6).

These tests should, in the long term, enable each hospital to base its choice on the criteria of real cost/diagnosis efficiency, defined by DRG tariff scale.

Fig. 13 - EXAMPLES OF AVERAGE RESULTS OF DIAGNOSIS BY THE NMR

Place of the experimentation	Results
Huntington medical Research - Pasadena	2.000 neurological examinations NMR more accurat than tomo density in diagnosing that there is no cerebral lesion
MASSACHUSSETS General Hospital BOSTON CLEVELAND Clinic foundation University Hospital Cleveland (Technicare)	221 patients with cerebral lesions 39 healthy subjects NMR = 86 % of lesions detected Other imaging techniques = 72 %
SAN FRANCISCO University medical center SAN FRANCISCO General Hospital Letterman Army Hospital Veteran' administration medical center (Diasonics)	199 patients NMR Confirms diagnosis in 91 % of cases

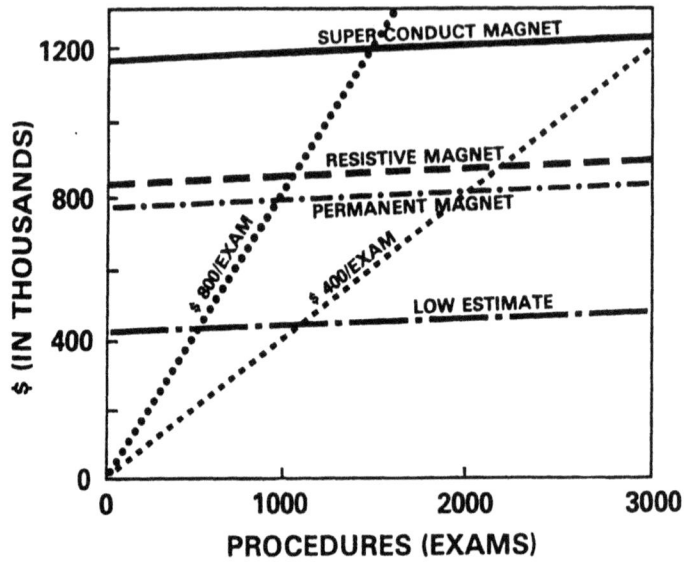

FIG.14: NMR BREAK-EVEN ANALYSIS (ANNUAL BASIS)

Numerous other evaluations and recommendations are being made in order to assure a future for NMR in hospitals.

Examples: ACR (American College of Radiology) (4)
AHA (American Hospital Association) (5)

AHA proposed a break-even analysis of the examination and annual cost of the different kinds of magnet (Supra, Resistif, Permanent) (Fig. 14).

Technical Origins of the Customer Hesitancy

The confusion created for the user by the "magnet field war", with optimum ranging from 0.15 to T, should be noted. This confusion very probably delays any decision-making.

We can be sure that the 3 classes of magnets already known, will continue to be used, but the analysis of the optimal use for each of them is far from being finished.

Probable Developments of NMR Techniques

Scientific progress will certainly disturb the present magnet distribution of field utilization. For example: low field 0.15 - 0.5 T will be used for applications, until now reserved for high fields (>1.5 T).

1st example: indirect imaging of C^{13} by imaging of coupled protons (7)

2nd example: water fat separation (8)

Technological and industrial progress may perhaps enable the range of each magnet type to be widened, thus increasing the overlap of their range. For example:

- an increased production of supra magnets optimized towards 0.2 T would allow a compromise (security/field homogenity/diagnostic quality) which could be unfavourable to resistive magnets.

- "bitter" coils promise higher fields (3KG) than "Helmotz coils" with an improved B_o/power ratio.

New magnetic material (Fe Nd Br) would enable the permanent magnet solution to reach more than 3 KG (B_o) for weights ∿ 15 tons. By the use of realistic weights, minimum consumption and maintenance, the permanent magnets will be better adapted, at least for mobile systems.

However, only the present test evaluation will perhaps enable a clarification of the correct total cost/diagnostic efficiency value to be made.

It will perhaps be possible to evaluate the total cost. But who will be able to estimate the percentage in dollars of loss or gain in diagnosing pathologies?

10 NUCLEAR MEDICINE

The U.S. nuclear medicine equipment market seems to be stabilized at ∿ 700 gamma cameras per year and roughly the same number in the other countries (Fig. 15)

Competition to nuclear medicine for conventional examination has come mainly from C.T. scanners. The development of single photon tomography, using principally rotating cameras, has not played a significant role, because of physical limitations and insufficient depth in spatial resolution.

Bedside cardiology examinations will require further development of the mobile cameras, well adapted to nuclear medicine specificity.

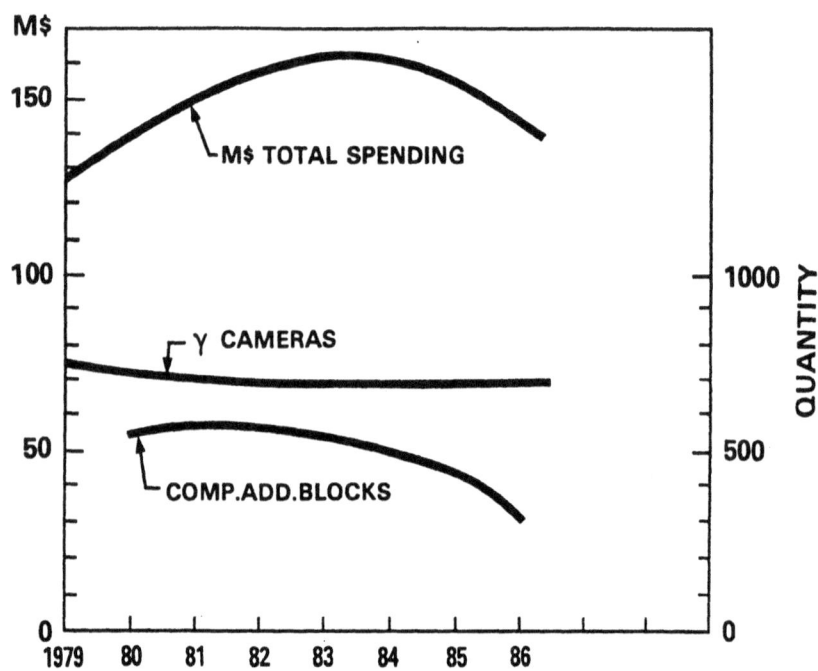

FIG.15: U.S. NUCLEAR MEDICINE MARKET

It is forecast that the complementary computer block market probably will strongly decline because of the increased number of computing parts included in the camera circuits.

Favourable Factors to Nuclear Medicine for Keeping a Good Position

High possibility of finding new radioisotopic utilizations as for example hepatolie (vesicle pathology), gold isotope Au-195 (cardiac examination), ioded Amphetamine (brain blow).
Application of labelled monoclonal antibodies, a direct tumor specific imaging technique, by gamma camera. Even if it is now applied to 2 or 3 specific cases, principally colon tumors, it may be widened to many others.

The monoclonal antibodies technique wil be developed for further applications and the market forecast for research and in vitro studies goes from 58 M $ in 1982 to 1000 M $ in 1990. Probably Medical Imaging will benefit from this support.

Positron Emission Tomography (PET)

Approximately 50 medical research centers in the world use PET equipments.

The scientific interest for fundamental medical research, chiefly for brain metabolism studies, has been confirmed. However, even in major hospitals, the high cost of PET equipment (cyclotron, radiochemistry, PET camera $\sim$ 5 M USD) limits PET installation.

The early discovery of NMR capacities in spectrometry (P^{31}, C^{13}) have had an effect on PET projects. It would seem that practical NMR applications are being delayed in favour of other projects.

The world market forecasts should vary considerably, ranging from 100 to 300 in the next 10 years.

Favourable Factors for Future PET Development

As in classical Nuclear Medicine, some generators of radio-nuclide positron emitter may more likely open the way to clinical than to research applications. For example: Ga^{68}, R_b^{82} "long life" positron emitters (Ga ÷ 68 mn), (R_b ÷ 1,25 mn).

An intense chemical research has to be carried out to improve compatibility with labelled molecules.

CONCLUSION

The economical influence on medical imaging equipment development works in two directions:
  selection criteria for the different techniques
  feedback from the total spending.

Figure 16 shows the approximate indication of the Imaging Techiques and their relative forecasts.

Now after a general economical overview of the Imaging Techniques, I will mention some factors, the future effect of which on the market trend has not been taken into account yet. These factors are related to different aspects of Medical Imaging:
- PAC Systems
- 3D Visualization
- Monoclonal Antibodies
- New Imaging Techniques (Thermic Imaging)

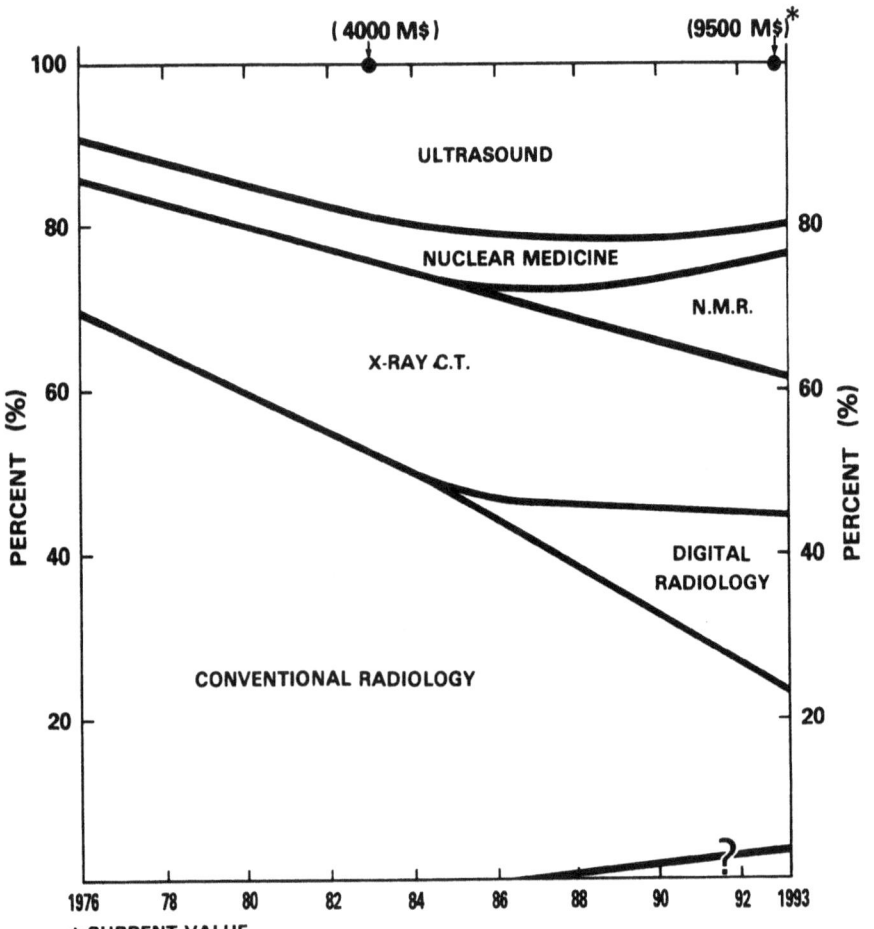

FIG.16: RELATIVE MEDICAL IMAGING WORLD EVOLUTION
* CURRENT VALUE

PAC Systems

Market forcasts (Ref 9) for PAC and related systems (Fig.17) indicate that PAC will probably involve several different industries. It would seem that medical imaging industries may be interested in image processing systems of PAC. The telecomunication industries, on the other hand, adapted to other needs, should be concerned with other aspects of PAC.

3D Visualization

Following the initial effort of some laboratories, this technique is actually very promising. The good knowledge of the algorithm and the feasibility of the real time computing will benefit from the microelectronic improvements in cost and performance.

It seems that the good adaptation of the different techniques to 3D visualization is of increasing interest in the following order:
1) X-Ray tomography 3D reconstruction (CT scanners multislices) or digital radioscopy with 2D detectors and 3D reconstruction.
2) NMR multislice (ρ, T_1, T_2 and spectrometric imaging)
3) Nuclear Medicine
   PET (multi-narrowslices)
   Single Photon Tomography with sufficient events per voxel
4) Ultrasound

Monoclonal Antibodies

Though Nuclear Medicine Imaging is advancing in the use of labelled monoclonal antibodies, on the other hand, NMR is very likely an actual competitor. In fact, labelling can be used to make either the classical proton imaging (ρ, T_1, T_2) or the spectroscopic imaging.

It is evident that all progress concerning the extension to the new specific organ tumors will be of benefit to both Imaging Modalities: N.M. and NMR.

New Imaging Techniques

I will focus only on those techniques able to carry out the body temperature imaging, which have also a great medical interest. In fact, Hyperthermia, selecting and increasing chemiotherapy, radiotherapy and pharmacotherapy effects, needs an accurate measurement of temperature in volume. The following new

FIG.17: MARKET ESTIMATES FOR PAC AND RELATED SYSTEMS
(millions of 1983 dollars)

	1983	1984	1985	1986	1987	1988	1989	1990
PAC systems	$8	$20	$35	$50	$70	$100	$145	$210
Prototype PACS (components)	25	40	50	60	70	70	70	60
Image processing systems	20	40	60	80	95	110	125	140
Image Transmission systems	15	25	40	60	80	105	135	170
Total	$68	$125	$185	$250	$315	$385	$475	$580

Numbers in parentheses are annual percent growth

techniques are able to do it:

- NMR T_1 Constant Measurement in volume can be used by means of its temperature relationship.
- Thermic Emission Tomography. Industries and laboratories try to obtain directly the body temperature profile, using the body emitted microwaves. This thermic tomography needs a healthy body computed model.
- High frequency Tomography. It is proposed by several research teams. Using gigaherz microwaves, the absorption and/or scattering measurements permit the computing of $\frac{\varepsilon}{\mu}$ coefficient on each elementary volume of the body.

Perhaps these new Imaging Methodologies will be the next generation of Medical Imaging.

REFERENCES

1 Sources : - Current Industrial report
   - Electronic Industries Association of Japan
   - Z.V.E.I.
   - F.I.E.E.

2 Sources : Biomedical Business International

3 Sources : O. Hasuike : Nikkei Medical 12(4) : 208 1983
   Ryu Niki M.D. Health Conference - France,
   Lille Sept. 14-16, 1983

4 American College of Radiology - Health planning criteria considerations for medical NMR

5 American Hospital Association
   AHA Hospital Technology Series Vol. 2 n°8 - NMR guideline report

6 - Cornell Medical Center
   - Columbia Presbiterian Medical Center
   - Mount Sinai Medical Center
   - New York University Medical Center
   - Montefiore Medical Center
   - Downstate Medical Center
   - Long Island Jewish Hillside Medical Center
   - Westchester Country Medical Center
   - New York Hospital
   - North Shore University Hospital
   - Memorial SLoan-Kettering Cancer Center.

7 ^{1}H observe C^{13} decouple spectroscopic measurements of Lactate and Glutamate in the rat brain in vivo.
   D.L. Rothman, K.L. Behar, H.P. Hetherington, J.A. den Hollander M.R. Bendall and R.G. Shulman.
   Third annual meeting of the Society of Magn. Reson. in medicine - New York August 13-17, 1984 - Abstract.

8 Proton Spectroscopic Imaging at 0,35 T - W. Dixon and D. Faul Third annual meeting of the Society of Magn. Reson. In. Medicine - New York August 13-17, 1984 - Abstract/.

9 Source : Drew Consultant

SUBJECT INDEX

1-123 amines 685
A-mode 12, 266
A-mode display 292
absolute 215
absorption and attenuation 269
accelerator 258
accidental coincidences 803
accuracy in PET 802
accuracy of diagnostic tests 937
acoustic imaging systems 318
acoustic impedance 319
acquired valvular diseases 221
active therapeutic cures 670
adaptive sampling 421
algebraic reconstruction 73
algorithms 73
amino acids 753
amount of information 42
amphetamine 657
analysis 50
Angio-CT 220
angiocardiography 117
angiography 250
angular data 678
anisotropy 479
antennae 478
aperture 324
archiving 595, 604
array processor 425, 426, 596, 598, 599, 601
ART3 710
ART3H 710
artificial intelligence 428
assessment of imaging 937
attenuation correction 637, 859
Au-195 964
automated radio synthesis system 770
automatic recognition and tracking 429
automation 792
automation network 765
autoradiographic technique 846
axial coverage 860
axial resolution 286, 887, 920

B 320
back projecting 479
back projection operator 80
backprojection 694
backscatter images 335
BaF2 861
barium fuoride (BaF^2) 928, 905
beam hardening 211
BGO 860, 874
BGO detectors 802
bikplane ateriography 102
bio medical image enhancement 428

bioavailability 47, 843
biochemical current flow 456
biomagnetism 455, 948
biomedical image processing 427
biomedicine 423
biplane 111, 250
Bismuth Germanate (BGO) 212, 884, 928
bistable ultrasonic displays 358
bit slice 596
bitter coils 963
BK subtraction 615
bloch equation 491
blood flow 119, 660, 846
blood volume 656
blurred mask subtraction 158
B-Maraviglia 489
B-mode 11, 265
B-mode display 290, 293
body surface potential mapping 474, 480
bone densitometry studies 201
br-77 715
76 Br 752
brain activity 465
Brain Glucose Metabolism 731
brain uptake 661
brain-scanning 677
brightness temperature 449
buffer memories 424

Cadmium tungstate (Cd W) 212
caesium-iodide (CsI) 212
calibre 250
carbon-11 750
cardiac computed tomography 231
cardiac gated MRI 538
cardiac gating 558
cardio-c.t. 222
cardiological application of PET 813
cardiology 340
cardiovascular imaging 110
cardiovascular nuclear medicine 171
central processing unit 425
cerebral arterio-venous malformation 254
cerebral blood flow 830
chest radiography 101
cine angiography 102
Cine-C.T. 231
cinematic display 235
circuit deadtime 866
classifier 422
cleon brain scanner 677
cleon two-dimensional 674
clinical nuclear magnetic resonance imaging 511
closed system 52

coded aperture 587
collimator 715
collimator system 649
Color Doppler technique 345
colour maps 481
communications 423
communication satellites 429
comparative cost of diagnosis 960
compartment 48
compartment model 42
compartmental analysis 842
components of quality assurance 414
compression algorithms 389
compton scattering 704, 863
Compton tomography 704
computed tomography 365, 479, 527
computer aided tomographic radiometry 448
computer languages 425
computer reconstruction 358
computer tomography 257, 428, 429
computerized infrared systems 446
computerized radiometric systems 445
Consensus Development Conferences 5
continuous wave doppler systems 295
contraction pattern analysis 116
contrast agents 368
contrast agents for MRI 559
contrast media 474
conventional DSA (CDSA) 106
conventional radiology 948, 955
converging collimators 585
convolution 46
convolution/back projection 478
convolution integral 44
coronary arteries 161, 254
correction for scatter 805
correlative aspects of cardiovascular nuclear medicine and digital angiography 178
correlative aspects with nuclear medicine 184
correlative imaging 514
cosine and sine transforms 418
cost-benefit analysis 2
cost-effectiveness 937
Crossed Cerebellar Diaschisis 830
crosstalk 875, 928
C.T. cost 959
C.T. market 958
C.T. scanner 385
current dipole 462
cyclotron 721, 784

2-D 418
2-D digital filtering 427
2-D flow mapping 334
2-D Fourier inversion 82
2-D space frequency response 419
3-D digital interpolations 428

3-D display 393
3-D display system coding schemes 398
3-D reconstruction 957
3-D visualization 965
data banks 429
data buses 424
data compression 157, 158, 421, 428, 429
decibel 269
decimation 422
decision table 420
decomposition of complex objects 428
decompression 421
densitometry 219
density 215
density resolution 209, 214, 215
deoxy-glucose uptake 848
dermatology 378
design programs 425
detection efficiency 858
detector material 860
detector ring 681
detectors 587
detector sampling modes 887
diagnosis 960
diagnosis related groups/tariff scale 960
diaphanography 477
diaphragm 475
dielectric scanning 480
digital 595, 596, 597, 598, 599, 601, 604
digital angiography 153, 385
digital archiving 385
digital filter coefficients 419
digital image acquisition systems 427
digital image processing 428
digital optical disks 385
digital process systems 216
digital radiography 21, 97, 183, 197
digital radiology 948, 955
digital subtraction angiography (DSA) 103
digital transformation 418
digital video-image processing 116
digitized image 880
discrete signal averaging 505
display 250
display of internal structures 406
DOPA 751
Doppler 327
Doppler data 365
Doppler signals 266
Doppler technique 295, 340, 344
dose reduction 475
D-SPECT 671
DYNAMATIC 254 647
dynamic SPECT 646
dynamic cardiovascular imaging 110
dynamic focus 327
dynamic range 475

ecg-gated reconstructions 231
echocardiography 340
ECT 600, 601, 603
edge detectors 420
electric transducer 320
electrical impedance imaging 478
electrical impedance methods 474
electrocardiographic 480
electroencephelographic signals 480
electronic focussing 281
emission computed tomography 16
emission tomography 623
endoscopic 359
energy and timing resolution 933
enhancement 419
equilibrium radionuclide angiography 615
error control coding techniques 427, 429

18F 751
fan beam 208
fast fourier transform (FFT) 82, 418
fast microprocessors 426
fast walsh transform 418
fatty acids 757
features 422
FFT 418
filtered Layergram method 83
filtered back-projection 82
filtered back-projection algorithms 625
filtering kernel 678
finite impulse response 419
flow imaging 551, 558
flow studies 367
focused-ray geometry scanner 674
focussing 280
Fourier 421
Fourier methods 73
Fourier transform 156, 418, 490
Fourier zeugmatography 495
fraction recirculated 68
fractional ejection fraction 236
Fredholm integral equation 449
Free Induction Decay 490
frequency 271
Fresnel zone plate 587
fully three dimensional 73
functional 646
functional imaging 111, 118, 157, 171, 456
funtional renal imaging 188
FWT 418

Ga-AS devices 423
Gadolinium Orthosilicate (GSO) 928
gamma camera 708, 963
Gated blood pool imaging with SPECT 643
general purpose computers 424
geometrical transformations 422, 427

germanium semiconductor detectors 581
global ejection fraction 175
glucose utilization 816
gradient system 555
grey and white cerebral matter 657
grey scale tomographic images 296
GSO 860

3H-deoxy-glucose 847
Haar 421
Haar transform 418
Hadamard 421
Hadamard transform 418
hardware implementation 423
hardware processors 426
health costs 949
heart 475
heart phantom 711
helium-neon laser 476
Helmotz coils 963
hemodynamics 670
hg^{12} 864
high density digital tape 424
high frequency imaging 948
high resolution magnified images 538
high sensitivity 655
highly focusing collimators 677
histoprojection 79
holograms 403
HPLC 762
hyperthermia 439

I-131 715
identification of active sources in the human brain 464
image acquisition 427
image analysis 41, 847
image clutter 327
image contrast 215
image converters 297
image correction 698
image presentation 424
image processing methods and techniques 418
image quality 215
image reconstruction 73
image subtraction 154
image texture analysis 364
image trapping 476
images 250
images processing 847
imaging 474
imaging of bioelectrical sources 455
imaging technologies 937
IMP distribution 657
impedance of medium 268
implementation systems 423
individual photon counting 197

infinite impulse response 419
infrared 439
infrared radiation 476
infrared radiometry 427
infrared transmission imaging 477
in-plane resolution 920
input acquisition unit 426
integer coefficients 424
integrated digital circuits 423
integrated optics 424
intensity 268
interaction 406
interdetector scatter 875
internal medicine 357
interplane axial resolution uniformity 803
interpolation 421
interventional radiography 474
interventional radiology 477
intraoperative ultrasound (IU) 259
intravenous 117
Intravenous angiography (IVA) 101
intrinsic resolution 878
inverse scattering 478
inversion formula 73
in vivo NMR spectroscopy 800
in vivo spectroscopy 551
IOD-123 amphetamine 646
ioded Amphetamine 964
IR multisensor array structures 446
ischemic heart diseases 221
isopotentials 479,
iterative reconstruction 479, 678
iterative techniques 84, 86
itracavitary 359

Josephson effect 423

Kalman filtering 449
Karhunen-Loeve 421
Karhunen-Loeve transform 418
K-edge energy subtraction 107
kuhl 647

Laplace's equation 479
large perfusion abnormalities 686
lateral resolution 288
least square procedures 73
light 477
light and infrared transmission 474
light collection efficiency 858
limited angle sampling 699
line scanning 501
linear 258
Linear and angular sampling 634
linear array 212
linear phase 419
local space operators 419

logistic 784
luminous efficiency 858
lung tissue 475

magnetic material 963
magnetic resonance imaging 551
magnetic shielding 555
magnetic storage techniques 387
magnetopharmaceuticals (MPs) 559
magnetric resonance imaging 385
mammography 524
manually-performed syntheses 770
manufacturing automation 423
mathematic model 696
maximum likelihood approach 87
maximum rates 922
measurement 119, 215
mechanical automatic or mixed mechanical electronic scanning 301
mechanical sector scanners 324
mediastinal regions 475
medical and non medical imaging 417
medical cyclotrons 768
medical images 385
medical imaging 412, 948
medical imaging department 385
medical risks 949
medical ultrasonics 429
medical ultrasound 378
medical value 960
medimatic 647
mercury/gold 571
microprocessors 426
microwave computerized active tomography 447
microwave imaging 474, 478
microwave radiometry 427, 439
minimum distance 422
minimum word-length 421
mirror systems 404
M-mode 340
mobile cameras 963
mode scanning 320
moments 45, 842
monochromatic beam 98
monoclonal antibodies 965
Monte Carlo methods 590
morbidity 937
mortality 937
MOS technologies 423
motion artifacts 679
MRI 514
MRI surface coil imaging 522
Multi-Wire Proportional Chamber(MWPC) 197, 581, 847
multi-line detectors 216
multi-ring detector 682

multidimensional moments 66
multiplan angocardiography 111
multiple detectors 675
multiple slices 671
MWPC 199, 201
mycardium 160
myocardial 846
myocardial infarction 818
myocardial ischemia 341, 813
myocardial perfusion imaging 708
myocardium 816

N.A. Lassen 660
neurofibroma 657
neurotransmitter studies 732
new imaging techniques 965
n-isopropyl-p-Iodoamphetamine 661
nitrogen-13 750
NMR 948
NMR image 489
NMR imaging 500, 958, 959
NMR imaging methods 492
NMR spectroscopy 489
noise 880
noise amplification 679
noise suppression 157
non iterative regularized solutions 86
non-circular orbits 585
non-converging moments 52
non-linear filtering 420
non-linear smoother 420
nonlinearity 479
nonuniform resolution and scatter 802
normal incidence 272
nuclear cardiology 708
nuclear magnetic resonance 13, 489
nuclear magnetic resonance imaging 24
nuclear medical tomography 674
nuclear medicine 183, 428, 948
nuclear scanner 674
Nyquist frequency 632

1-123 OMB 687
object motion 508
office automation 423, 426
offset correction 635
optical disk technology 385
optical fibers 426, 429
optical processors 426
optical scanner 848
optical storage 387
optical technologies 424
optimal magnetic field strength 553
optimization theory 84
oxygen-15 750

PACS 604

PAC systems 965
parallel processing 334
paramagnetic contrast agents 559
parametric images 154
partial 215
partial volume effects 211, 799
particulate media 474
pattern recognition 41, 422, 428
perfluoroctylbromide emulsions 474
perfusion 160
PET 16, 514, 769, 792, 797, 829, 874, 913
PET radiochemistry 782
phantom 696
phantom study 655
phase analysis 172, 178
phase encoding 555
phase synchronous integration 158
phase synchronous subtraction 158
phased array 318
phased array transducer 363
phased transducer array 312
photo-stimulable phosphor crystals 476
photomultiplier 476
phototube- solid state readout 915
pipeline 423
pipeline hardware 82
planar imaging 501
PMTS with fused silicate windows 933
point scanning 502
point-spread 678
polyvinylidene fluoride 378
Positron emission tomograph (PET) 765, 837, 855, 882, 902, 928, 965
positron emitters 571
positron emitting nuclides 570
positron emitting radionuclides 797
positron emitting radiopharmaceuticals 721
positron range 863, 903
positrons tomography 750
potential sensitivity 921
prediction 421
predictive outcome 937
primitive cardiomyopathies 221
processing programs 425
projection-reconstruction 492
projections 73
projection theorems 80
prototypes 422
pulmonary diseases 704
pulsed doppler 378
pulsed doppler systems 296
pulsed doppler transducer materials 362
pvf 2 362, 335

quality assurance 412, 595
quality control 601, 623
quality of life 937

quantum efficiency 858

rabidium/krypton 571
radar-sonar systems 423
radiation dose 210
radioactive microsphere 846
radio frequency signal 298
radiography (DRg) 957
radioimmunotherapy 714
radioisotope production 783
radionuclide angiography 171
radionuclide imaging 13
radionuclide production 722
radio-opaqueliposomes 475
radiopharmaceuticals 569, 750, 792
radiopharmacy 569
radioscopy (DRs) 957
radiotracers 769
Radon operator 75
Radon transform 73, 80
random coincidences 903
randoms rejection 922
raster scanned equalisation radiography 475
receiver operating characteristic (ROC) curve 942
receptor 758
recognition and tracking of moving objects 428
reconstruction 250
reconstruction algorithm 866
recording the moments 53
redundancy reduction 421
reference points 422
reflection 275
reflectivity 450
refraction 273
regional brain protein synthesis 734
regional ejection fractions 175
regional receptors 687
remote sensing 422, 423, 426
renal blood flow 613
renal function 611
representation 396
reproducibility 802
residence time 68
resolution 285, 802, 928
Rf coils 556
Rf energy deposition 554
rheumatology 378
ring 587
robotics 423
robust parameters 43
roentgen television computer techniques 110
rotating camera 623, 963
rotating gamma camera 676, 682
rotating images 404
rotating wheel (6) collimators 475

rotation 422
rotational artifacts 675
RV ejection fraction (EF) 615

safety 784
sampling motion 866
satellite communication systems 426
scaling the counting rate 57
scanning electron beam 231
scanning motion 258
scanning slot 475
scatter correction 588
scatter rejection 920
scattered radiation 208, 211
scattering 275
scintillation crystals 913
scintillation-photodiode crystals 231
screen-film 476
selective 117
selectively for brain 671
sense conductor 908
sensitive point 501
sensitivity 803, 903, 920, 937
septa 878
seven pinhole tomography 708
shaded surfaces 400
Shepp-Logan-Hanning filters 632
shielding aperture 920
short sampling time 663
signal amplification technique 883
signal to noise 879
silicon avalanche photodiodes 864
silicon photodiodes 864
simulation programs 425
Simultaneous Iterative Reconstruction Technique (SIRT) 710
Simultaneous Multiple Angle Reconstruction Technique (SMART) 710
single photon imaging 575
single photon tomography 674, 682
single-photon emission computer tomography (SPECT) 694
single-photon emitter radionuclide computed tomography 674
singular value decomposition (SVD) 418
skin blood flow 378
slant transform 418
slice projection theorem 81
5 slices of the rCcbf 653
small low-gain phototubes 864
smoothing 419
software implementation 423, 425
solid angle coverage 860
solid phase labelling 573
solid state detectors 212, 914
solid state photodetectors 864
sorting 395

source localization 462
spatial resolution 209, 215, 650, 678, 694
specialized processors 424
specificity 937
SPECT 16 , 514, 575, 598, 625, 646, 674, 699, 714
SPECT single/multiple slice systems 585
spillover 930
spin-warp 497
spiperone 752
SQUID 458
stable isotopes 730
standard collimator 651
statistical decision 422
stereo pairs 403
steroids 757
stochastic transport 44
stroke 656
structural methods 422
sub-patterns 422
sub-routines 425
substitution labelling 570
sugars 756
surface coil imaging 551
surface coil techniques 538
surface display algorithms 245
SVD 418
syntactical 422
synthesis 48
synthesizing radiotracers 765

T564 648
T1-201 SPECT studies of heart 699
tagging 570
tail 63
target cost 730
technetium lipophilic radiotracers 687
technetium-99m 572
techniques 358
telehistology 358
telematics 423, 426
telemedicine 429
telethermography 439
temporal filter 154
temporal resolution 903
temporal segmentation 120
textures 320
thermic tomography 948
thorax 478, 480
three dimensional 250
three dimensional Radon reconstruction 678
three dimensional imaging 503
three-dimensional emission distribution 710
three-dimensional visualization 956
Time Depth Compensation (TDC) 291
time gain compensation (TGC) 291
time motion 294

time-of-flight 79, 865, 902, 921
time-of-flight positron emission tomography 902
tissue characterisation 350, 364
tissue dissolution 245
tissue tracer concentration 799
tissues 320
TM-mode 266
tomographic image 625, 684
tomographic reconstruction 440, 675, 858
tomography-rotating gamma cameras 583
tomomatic 32 647
tomamatic 64 647
tomomatic 564 646, 648
tomomatic T564 652
tracee 53
tracer 53
tracer models 798
transducer 362
transducer arrays 329
transducer materials 361
transducers 277
transfer time 68, 843
transform 418
transform kernel 418
transient ischemia 815
transit time 68, 843
transmission 358
transmission computed tomography 13
transmission of biomedical images 429
transmission raster scanning 478
transmission unit 426
transmittance 449
transmural myocardial ischemia 342
true 3-D images 406
truncated moments 62
tumor 656
two-component chemical shift imaging 551, 559
two-dimensional 340
two-dimensional B-mode display 293

ultra short life generators 571
ultrasonic tissue characterization 340
ultrasound 13, 340, 522, 948, 953
ultrasound imaging 10, 263, 357, 361
ultrasound tissue characterisation 358
ultrasound tomographic images 264
uniform T 564 650
uniformity 635
uptake rate of 99mTc DMSA 611
use of transforms 421
UV transparent glass 933

value of information 42
variable word-length encoding 421
varifocal 404

vascular 250
vector maps 480
videodensitometry 113, 114
videometry 113, 115
VLSI 423
voludensitometry 88
volume effect 215
volume images 245

Walsh 421
Walsh transform 418
weight 49, 843
whole-body imaging 208
with short data sampling times or with long data sampling times 663

Xe-133 648
Xenon-133 646
Xenon-133 CBF 647
x-radiography 429, 474
x-ray 250, 251
x-ray CT 218, 948, 956
x-ray computed tomography 207
x-ray source 98, 198
x-ray tomography 704

y-ray techniques 429

PARTICIPANTS

S. James Adelstein
Harvard Medical School
Office of the Dean Building A
25 Shattuck Street
Boston, MA, 02115
U.S.A.

Patricia Agnew
Occupational Therapy
University of Queensland
St. Lucia 4067
Queensland
Australia

Luciano Alcidi
Istituto di Medicina Nucleare
e Fisica Medica
Università di Firenze
Viale Morgagni, 85
50134 Firenze
Italy

Robert Allemand
Laboratoire d'Electronique
et de l'Informatique
85 X, Avenue des Martyrs
38041 Grenoble Cedex
France

John Humprey Amuasi
Istituto di Medicina Nucleare
e Fisica Medica
Università di Firenze
Viale Morgagni, 85
50134 Firenze
Italy

Alberto Ancarani
SEPA S.p.A.
C.so G. Cesare, 294
10156 Torino
Italy

Turgay Baskaya
G.A.T.A.
Department of Nuclear Medicine
Etlik - Ankara
Turkey

Ronaldo Bellazzini
Dipartimento di Fisica
Università di Pisa
P.zza Torricelli, 2
56100 Pisa
Italy

Antonio Benassi
Consiglio Nazionale delle Ricerche
Istituto di Fisiologia Clinica
Via P. Savi, 8
56100 Pisa
Italy

Sergio Berti
Consiglio Nazionale delle Ricerche
Istituto di Fisiologia Clinica
Via P. Savi, 8
56100 Pisa
Italy

Luisa Biazzi
Istituto di Radiologia
Università di Pavia
Via Forlanini
27100 Pavia
Italy

Antonio Rui Borges
Departamento de Electronica
e Telecomunicaçoes
Universiade de Aveiro
3800 Aveiro
Portugal

Douglas P. Boyd
IMATRON ASSOCIATES
454 Carlton Court
South San Francisco, CA, 94080
U.S.A.

Arturo Brunetti
Istituto di Radiologia
Università di Napoli
Via Spansini
80100 Napoli
Italy

Paolo Camici
Consiglio Nazionale delle Ricerche
Istituto di Fisiologia Clinica
Via P. Savi, 8
56100 Pisa
Italy

Antonio Capone
911 Smith Street
Providence, RI, 62908
U.S.A.

Vito Cappellini
Consiglio Nazionale delle Ricerche
Istituto di Ricerca
sulle Onde Elettromagnetiche
Via Panciatichi, 64
50127 Firenze
Italy

Vittorio Chiarini
COMECER
Via Emilia Ponente, 390
48014 Castel Bolognese (RA)
Italy

Giovanna Chimini
Centro di Medicina Nucleare
Via G. Monti, 107
16151 Genova
Italy

Carlo Corsi
R.S.E. - Selenia
Via Tiburtina, Km 12,4
00131 Roma
Italy

Peter H. Cox
The Dr. Daniel De Hoed Cancer Center and
Rotterdam Radio-Therapeutic Institute
Groene Hilledijk, 301
3075 Ea Rotterdam
Holland

Michael Crabtree
CTI Computer Technology and Imaging, Inc.
215 Center Park Road
Knoxville, TN, 37922
U.S.A.

Christian Crouzel
Service Hospitaliér Fréderic Joliot
Département de Biologie
Commissariat à l'Energie Atomique
Hospital d'Orsay
91406 Orsay
France

Harold Davidson
Department of the Army
Office of the Deputy Chief
of the Staff for Research
Development and Acquisition
Washington, D.C., 20310
U.S.A.

Peter C. deLuca
PHOTON DIAGNOSTIC Inc.
45 West Street
Medfield, MA, 02052
U.S.A.

Stephen Derenzo
Lawrence Berkeley Laboratory
Bldg 55 Room 146
1 Cyclotron Road
Berkeley, CA, 94720
U.S.A.

Lucio Di Guglielmo
Istituto di Radiologia
Università di Pavia
Via Forlanini
27100 Pavia
Italy

Mario Di Lullo
NATO Scientific Affairs Division
B--1110 Brussels
Belgium

Alessandro Distante
Consiglio Nazionale delle Ricerche
Istituto di Fisiologia Clinica
Via P. Savi, 8
56100 Pisa
Italy

Luigi Donato
Consiglio Nazionale delle Ricerche
Istituto di Fisiologia Clinica
Via P. Savi, 8
56100 Pisa
Italy

Susan Edwards
Department of Clinical Physics
and Bioengineering
Guy's Hospital
St. Thomas Street
London, SE1 9RT
U.K.

Bernard Eid
KODAK-PATHE'
26 Avenue du Petit Parc
94300 Vincennes
France

Barbara Fedeli
Istituto di Radiologia
Università di Pisa
Via Roma 67
56100 Pisa
Italy

Ezio M. Ferdeghini
Consiglio Nazionale delle Ricerche
Istituto di Fisiologia Clinica
Via P. Savi, 8
56100 Pisa
Italy

Armando Ferraioli
SOXIL S.p.A.
Via G. Miranda, 25
80131 Napoli
Italy

Francesco Fusco
EURO-BIT S.p.A.
Via G. Armellini, 33
00100 Roma
Italy

Elena Gaggelli
Dipartimento di Chimica
Università di Siena
Pian dei Mantellini, 44
53100 Siena
Italy

Philippe Garderet
Laboratoire d'Electronique
et de Technologie de l'Informatique
85 X Avenue des Martyrs
38041 Grenoble Cedex
France

Roger Gariod
Laboratoire d' Electronique
et de Technologie de l'Informatique
85 X Avenue des Martyrs
38041 Grenoble Cedex
France

Amilcare Gentili
Division of Nuclear Medicine
University of Miami
Miami, FL, 33101
U.S.A.

Joseph N. Gitlin
U.S. Department of Health
Education & Welfare
Bureau of Radiological Health
1901 Chapman Avenue
Rockville, MD, 20857
U.S.A.

David Guilfoyle
Department of Physics
University of Nottingham
Nottingham, NG7 2RD
U.K.

Sadettin Günsoy
Department of Electrical
and Electronic Engineering
Middle East Technical University
Gaziantep
Turkey

Riccardo Guzzardi
Consiglio Nazionale delle Ricerche
Istituto di Fisiologia Clinica
Via P. Savi, 8
56100 Pisa
Italy

Dan J. Hawkes
Department of Medical Physics
St. George's Hospital
Blackshaw Road
London, SW17 OQT
U.K.

Paul H. Heintzen
Klinikum der
Christian-Albrechts-Universität-Kiel
Schwanenweg, 20
D-2300 Kiel
GFR

Karl Heinz Höhne
Universität-Krankenhaus-Eppendorf
Martinistr., 52
2000 Hamburg

Ziya Ider
Department of Electrical Engineering
Middle East Technical University
Inönü Bulvari
Ankara
Turkey

Tatsuo Ido
Cyclotron Radioisotope Center
Tohoku University
Aza Aoba, Amaraki
Sendai-Miyagi
Japan

Terry Jones
MCR Cyclotron Unit
Hammersmith Hospital
Ducane Road
London, W12 0HS
U.K.

Daniel Kaplan
THOMSON-CGR
Departement Etudes et Developpement
Imagerie Nouvelle
48, Rue Camille Desmoulins
92130, Issy Les Moulineaux
France

Arnold Kettschau
Federal Institute
for Materials Testing
Königin Luise Str. 74
1000 Berlin 33
GFR

Karin Knesaurek
Department of Medical Physics
Ruder Boskovic Institute
Bukovacka 8
8,41000 Zagreb
Jugoslavia

Robert Kruger
Department of Radiology
University of Utah
Salt Lake City, UT, 84132
U.S.A.

Gian Luigi Lenzi
Dipartimento di Scienze Neurologiche
Università "La Sapienza"
Viale dell'Università, 30
00185 Roma
Italy

Harry P.L. Levels
Optische Industrie De Oude Delft
P.O. BOX 72
2600 MD Delft
Holland

Robert R. Luypaert
AZ - VUB
Laarbecklaan, 101
B-1090 Brussels
Belgium

M. Antonietta Macrì
Dipartimento di Scienze Neurologiche
Università "La Sapienza"
Viale dell'Università, 30
00185 Roma
Italy

Thomas Malone
Channon Building
Room 132
9000 Rockville
Bethesda, MA, 20205
U.S.A.

Cesare Mangianti
TECHNICARE INTERNATIONAL
Viale Luca Gaurico, 209-211
00143 Roma
Italy

Peter Mansfield
Department of Physics
University of Nottingham
University Parc
Nottingham, NG7 2RD
U.K.

Bruno Maraviglia
Istituto di Fisica
Università di Roma
Piazzale Aldo Moro
00185 Roma
Italy

Paolo Marzullo
Consiglio Nazionale delle Ricerche
Istituto di Fisiologia Clinica
Via P. Savi, 8
56100 Pisa
Italy

Leonardo Masotti
Istituto di Elettronica
Università di Firenze
Facoltà di Ingegneria
Via di Santa Marta, 3
50139 Firenze
Italy

Roberto Minacapilli
C.G.E..
Via V. Emanuele Orlando, 83
00100 Roma
Italy

Renzo Moretti
Servizio di Fisica Sanitaria
Spedali Civili Brescia
P.le dell'Ospedale, 1
23100 Brescia
Italy

Pierluigi Mozzo
Servizio di Fisica Sanitaria
Policlinico Borgo Roma
Via Menegone
37100 Verona
Italy

Danilo Neglia
Consiglio Nazionale delle Ricerche
Istituto di Fisiologia Clinica
Via P. Savi, 8
56100 Pisa
Italy

S. Pors Nielsen
Department of Clinical Physiology
and Nuclear Medicine
Centralsygehsuet
DK-3400 Hillerod
Denmark

Raffaele Novario
Servizio di Fisica Sanitaria
Ospedale Regionale di Varese
Viale Borri, 57
21100 Varese
Italy

John R. Olsson
MEDIMATIC A/S
Gersonsvej, 7
DK-2900 Hellerup
Denmark

Atilla Ozmen
Institute of Science and Technology
Gazy University
Ankara
Turkey

Lino Palla
Consiglio Nazionale delle Ricerche
Istituto di Fisiologia Clinica
Via P. Savi, 8
56100 Pisa
Italy

Carlo Paoli
IBM - Italia
Via Santa Maria, 67
56100 Pisa
Italy

Oberdan Parodi
Consiglio Nazionale delle Ricerche
Istituto di Fisiologia Clinica
Via P. Savi, 8
56100 Pisa
Italy

Leon C. Partain
Division of Nuclear Medicine
Department of Radiology
Vanderbilt University
Nashville, TN, 37232
U.S.A.

Peter A. Payne
Department of Instrumentation
and Analytical Science
U.M.I.S.T.
P.O. BOX 88
Manchester, M60 1QD
U.K.

Alessandro Pepino
Dipartimento di Elettronica Biomedica
Università di Napoli
Via Claudia
80100 Napoli
Italy

Marco Peresson
Consiglio Nazionale delle Ricerche
Istituto di Elettronica
dello Stato Solido
Via Cineto Romano, 42
00156 Roma
Italy

Steffen Petersen
NOVO DIAGNOSTIC SYSTEMS
Novo Allé
DK-2880 Bagsvaerd
Denmark

Giuseppe Pozzi
ELSCINT S.r.l.
Via Negrelli, 55
20035 Lissone (MI)
Italy

Richard C. Reba
Division of Nuclear Medicine
George Washington University Hospital
901 Twenty-Third Street, N.W.
Washington, D.C., 20037
U.S.A.

Aldo Rescigno
Section of Neurological Surgery - 131 FMB
Yale University
School of Medicine
333 Cedar Street
New Haven, CT, 06510
U.S.A.

Anthony Ricci
Division of Nuclear Medicine
Department of Radiological Sciences
UCLA Medical School
405 Hilgard Avenue
Los Angeles, CA, 90024
U.S.A.

Alfredo Rinaudo
SEPA S.p.A.
C.so G. Cesare, 294
10100 Torino
Italy

Gianluca Romani
Consiglio Nazionale delle Ricerche
Istituto di Elettronica
dello Stato Solido
Via Cineto Romano, 42
00156 Roma
Italy

Per Rommer
MEDIMATIC A/S
Gersonsvej, 7
DK-Hellerup
Denmark

Jerome A.G. Russell
Brookhaven National Laboratory
Chemistry Department
Associates Universities, Inc.
Upton, N.Y., 11973
U.S.A.

Jean Salomon
ELSCINT
40 Rue Jéan Jaurés
93170 Bagnolet
France

Piero Salvadori
Consiglio Nazionale delle Ricerche
Istituto di Fisiologia Clinica
Via P. Savi, 8
56100 Pisa
Italy

Derek Shaw
INTERNATIONAL GENERAL ELECTRIC
Company of New York Ltd.
260 Bath Road
Slough
U.K.

Hugh. F. Stoddart
PHOTON DIAGNOSTIC Inc.
45 West Street
Medfield, MA, 02252
U.S.A.

Karl Thomaseth
LADSEB CNR
Corso Stati Uniti, 4
35100 Padova
Italy

Andrew Todd Pokropek
University College Hospital
Gower Street
London, W01B 6XD
U.K.

Maria Rita Torquati
Dipartimento di Fisica
Università di Pisa
P.zza Torricelli, 2
56100 Pisa
Italy

Alberto Torresin
Servizio di Fisica Sanitaria
Ospedale Maggiore
Policlinico di Milano
Via Pace, 9
20122 Milano
Italy

Guido Torrioli
Consiglio Nazionale delle Ricerche
Istituto di Elettronica
dello Stato Solido
Via Cineto Romano, 42
00156 Roma
Italy

Gerry van Oortmarssen
SIEMENS GAMMASONICS B.V.
1430 AB-Vithorn
Holland

Joris Vanregemorter
Vrije Universiteit Brussel
Academic Hospital
Department of Nuclear Medicine
Laarbeeklaan, 101
1090 Brussels
Belgium

Max Viergever
Department of Mathematics
and Informatics
Technische Hoogeschool Delft
P.O. Box 356
2600 AJ Delft
Holland

Andrea Villa
Istituto di Radiologia
Università di Pavia
Via Forlanini
27100 Pavia
Italy

Mosè Visconti
Servizio di Fisica Sanitaria
Ospedale Regionale di Varese
Viale Borri, 57
21100 Varese
Italy

Michael Waller
Queen Elisabeth College
Department of Physics
University of London
Campdem Hill Road, W.B.
London
U.K.

Joseph D. Weissman
TECHNICARE CORPORATION
P.O. BOX 5130
Cleveland, OH, 44101
U.S.A

Peter N.T. Wells
Bristol & Weston Health District
Bristol General Hospital
Department of Medical Physics
Guinea Street
Bristol, BSI 6SY
U.K.

Alfred P. Wolf
Brookhaven National Laboratory
Chemistry Department
Associated Universities, Inc.
Upton, N.Y. 11873
U.S.A.

Colour Section

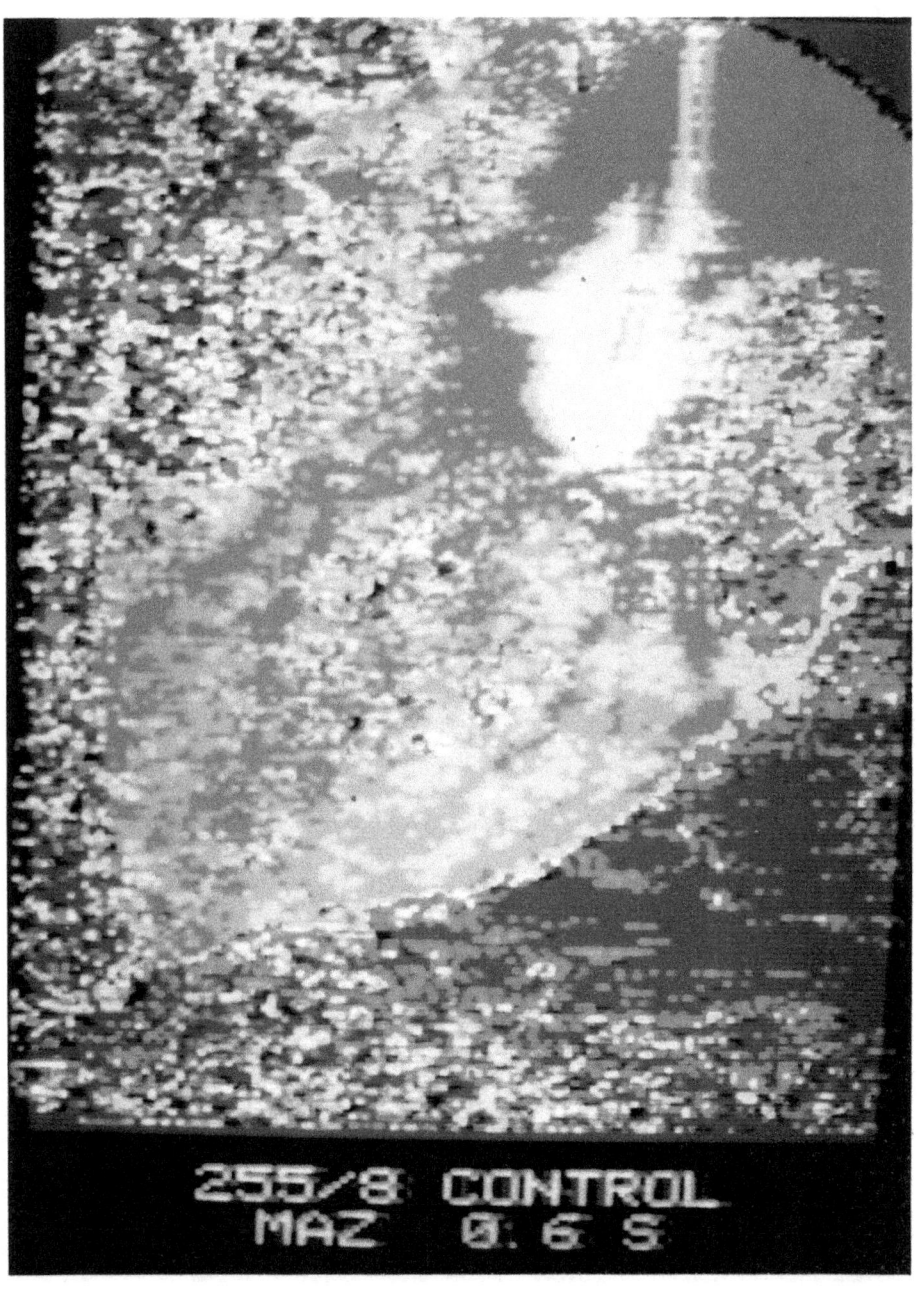

For text see page 148

4

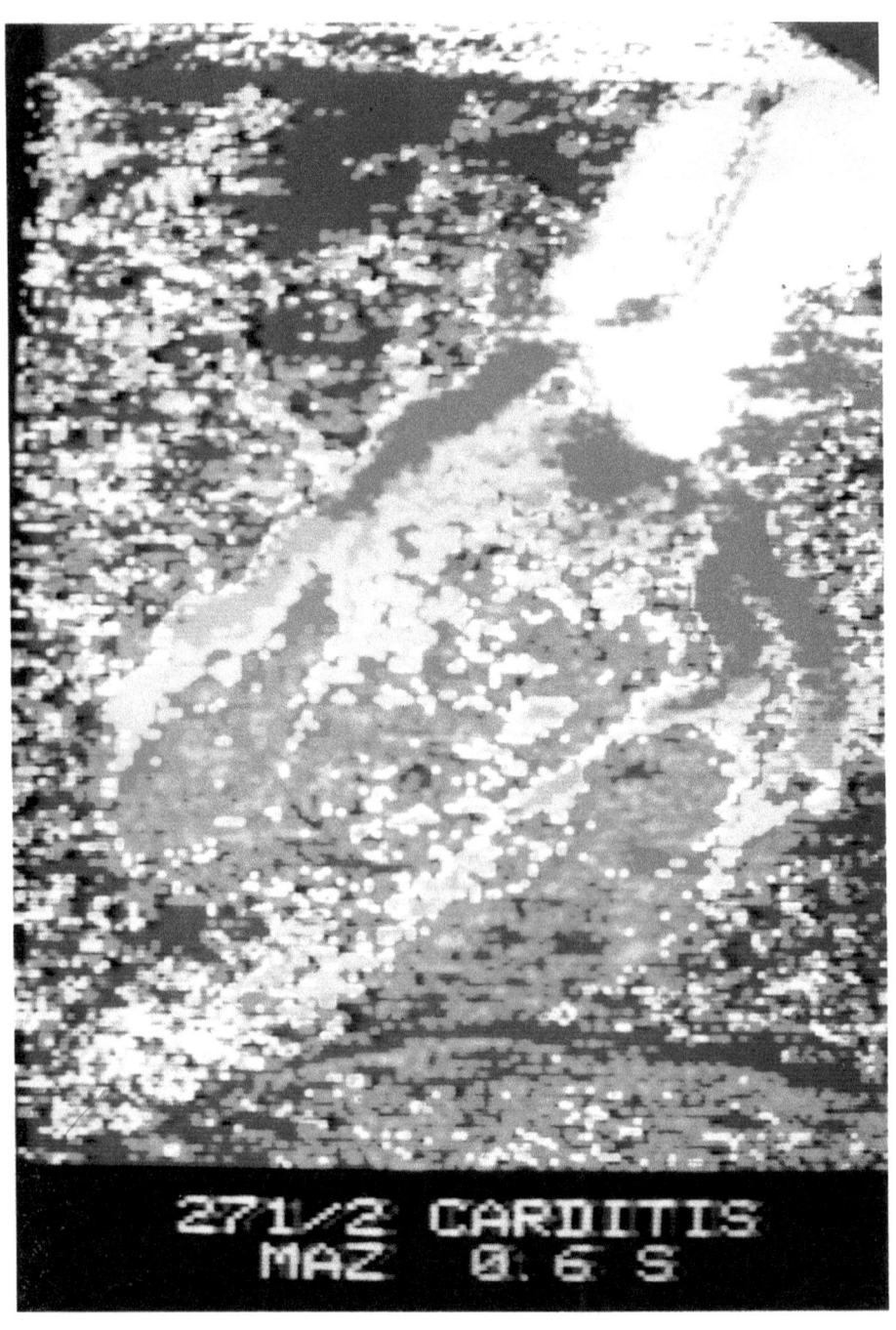

For text see page 149

5

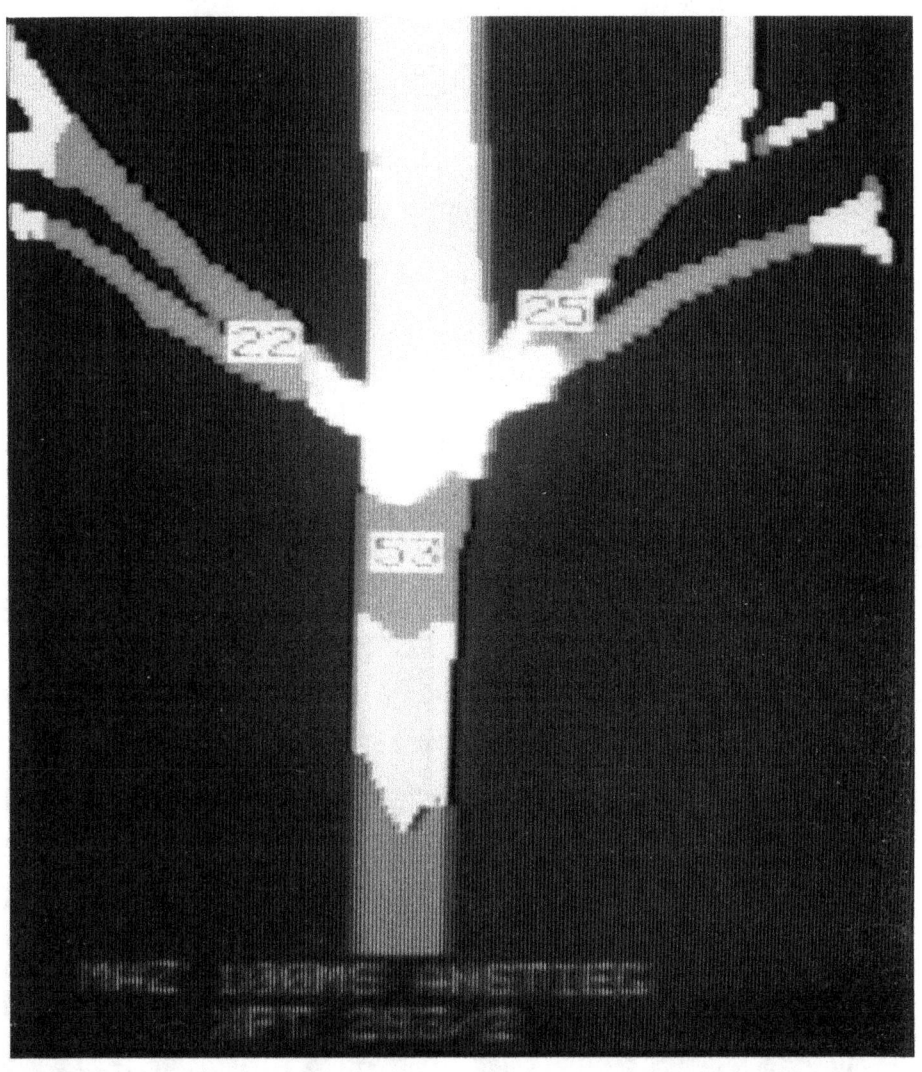

For text see page 150

6

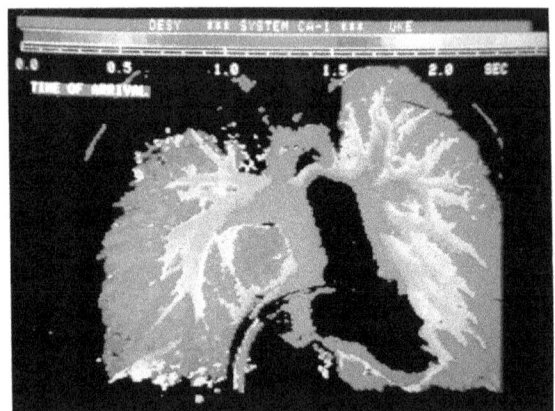

For text see page 166

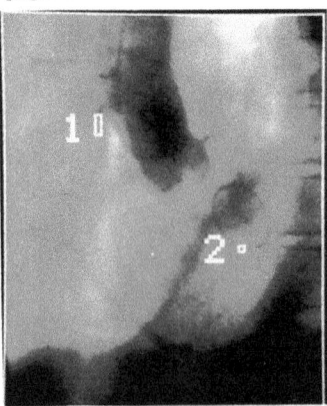

For text see page 166

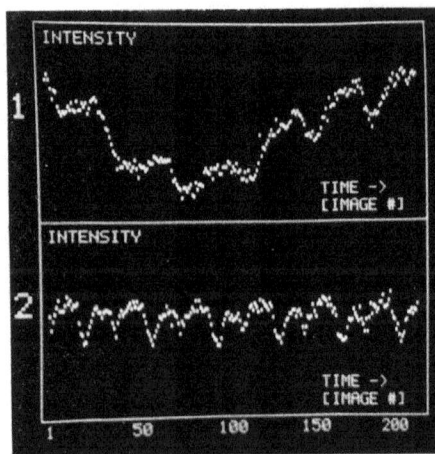

For text see page 167

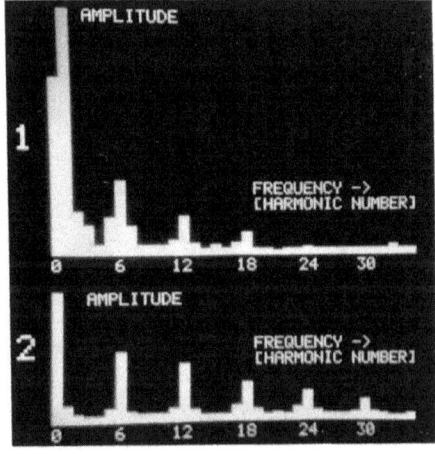

For text see page 167

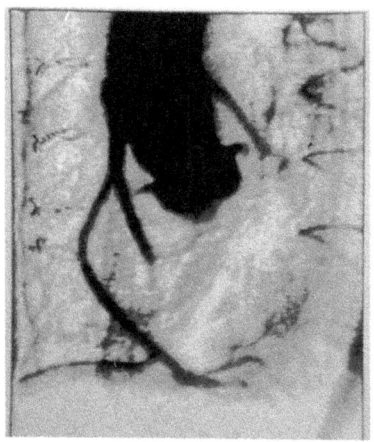

For text see page 168

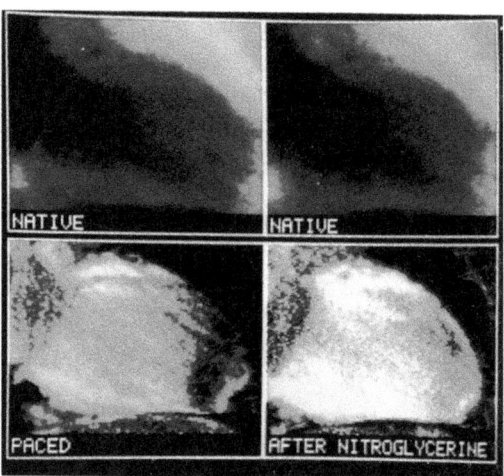

For text see page 168

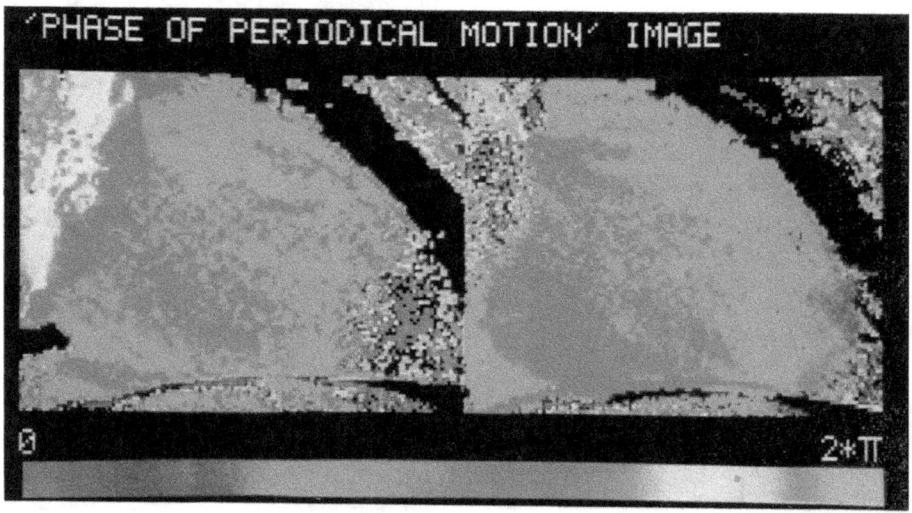

For text see page 169

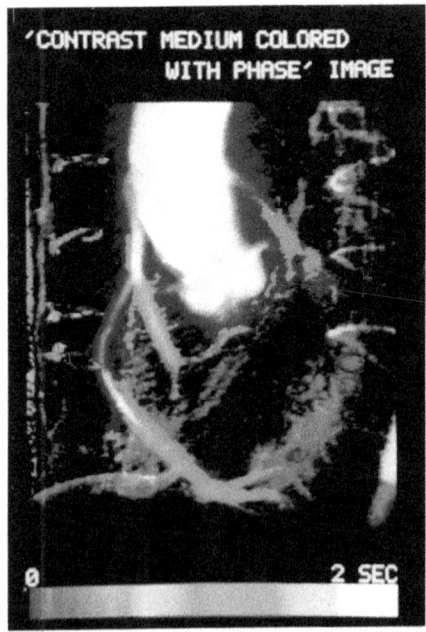

For text see page 169

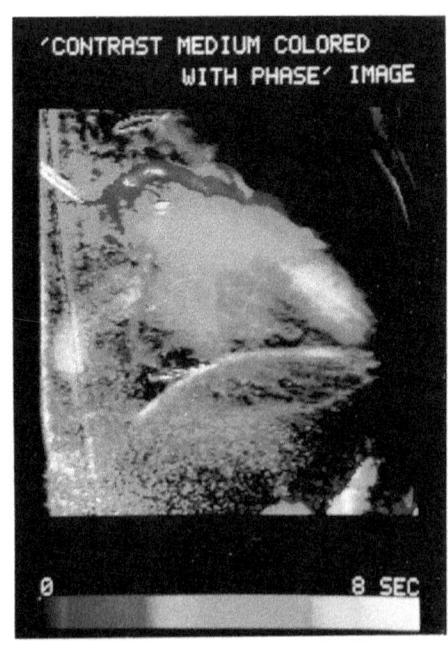

For text see page 169

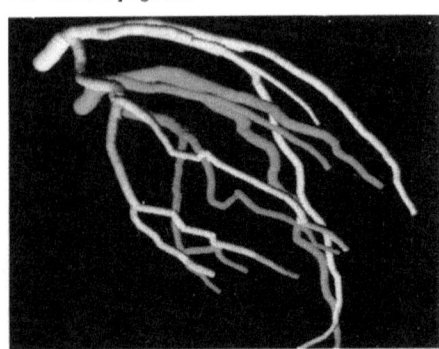

For text see page 254

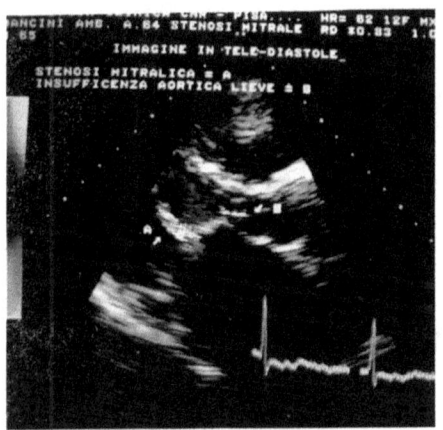

For text see page 346

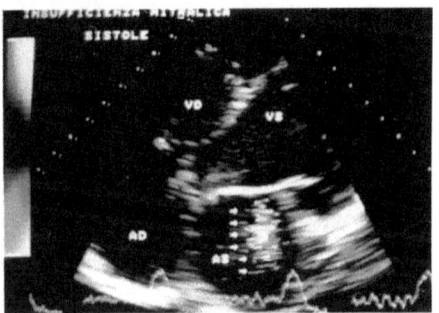

For text see page 347

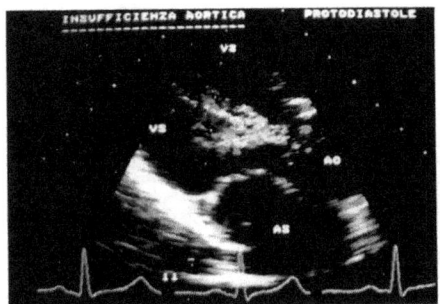

For text see page 347

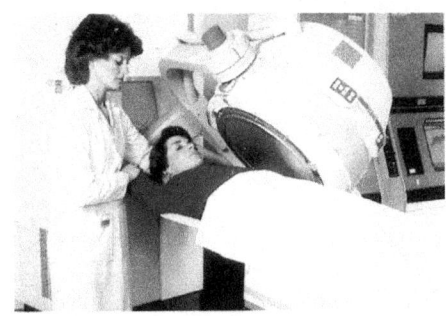

For text see page 627

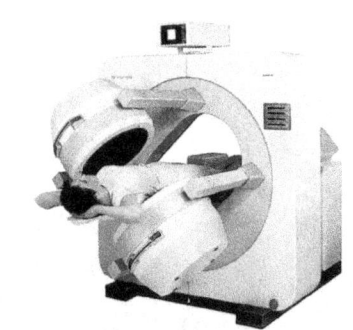

For text see page 627

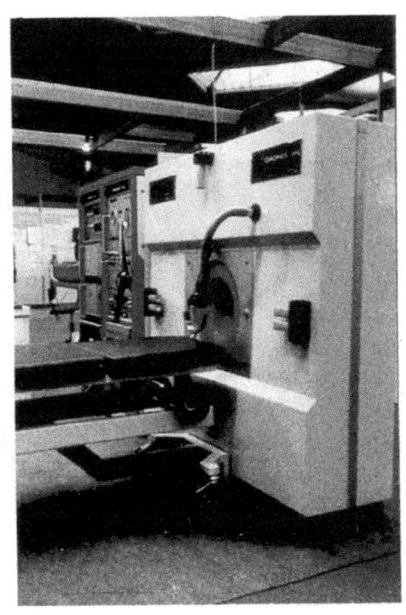

For text see page 648

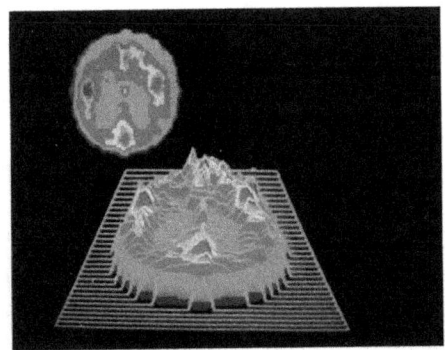

For text see page 652

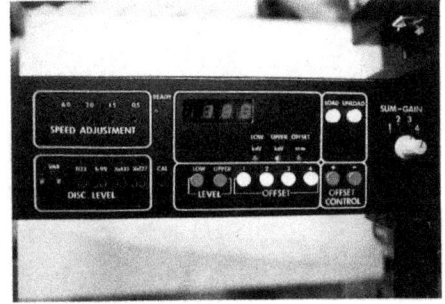

For text see page 655

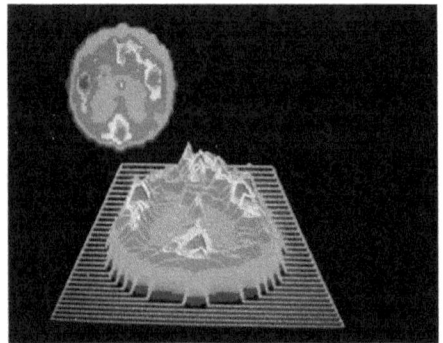

For text see page 655

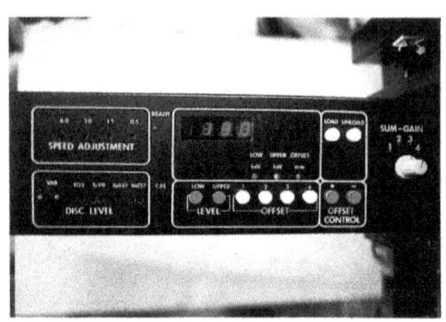

For text see page 656

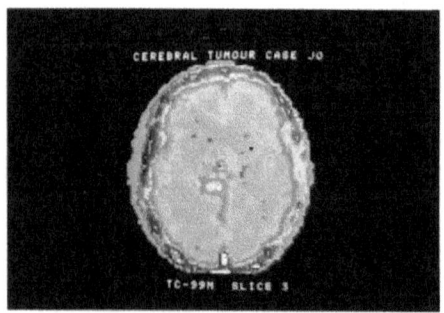

For text see page 656

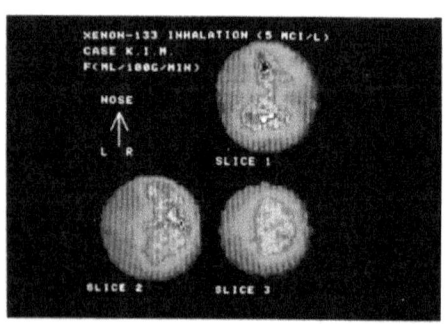

For text see page 657

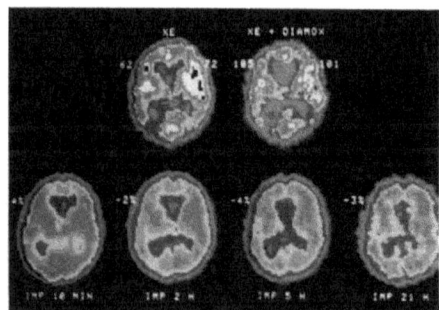

For text see page 657

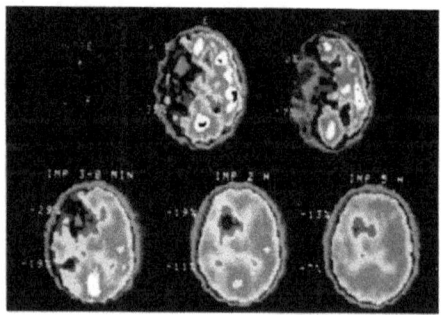

For text see page 662

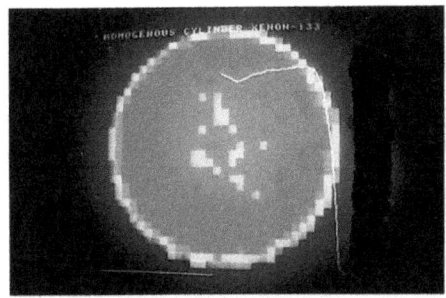

For text see page 666

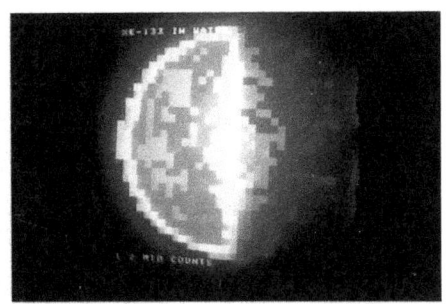

For text see page 666

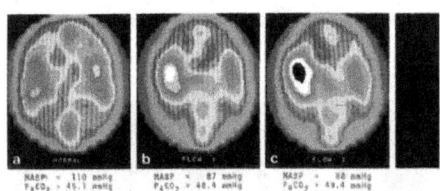

For text see page 669

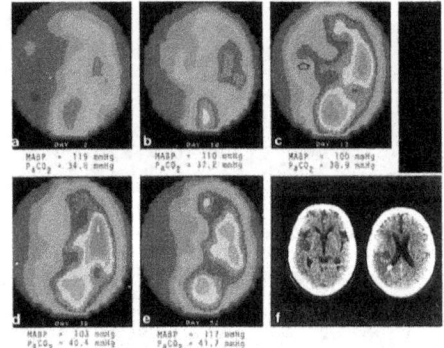

For text see page 669

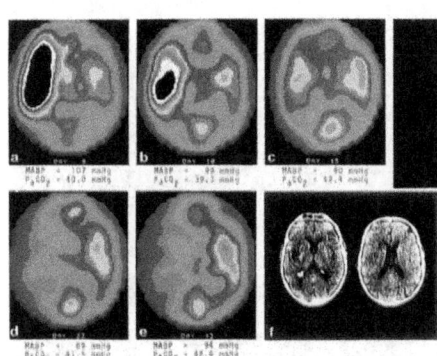

For text see page 670

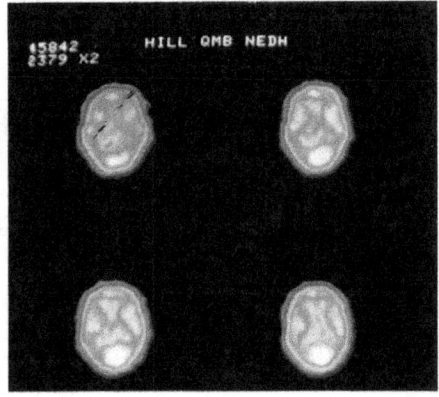

For text see page 688

12

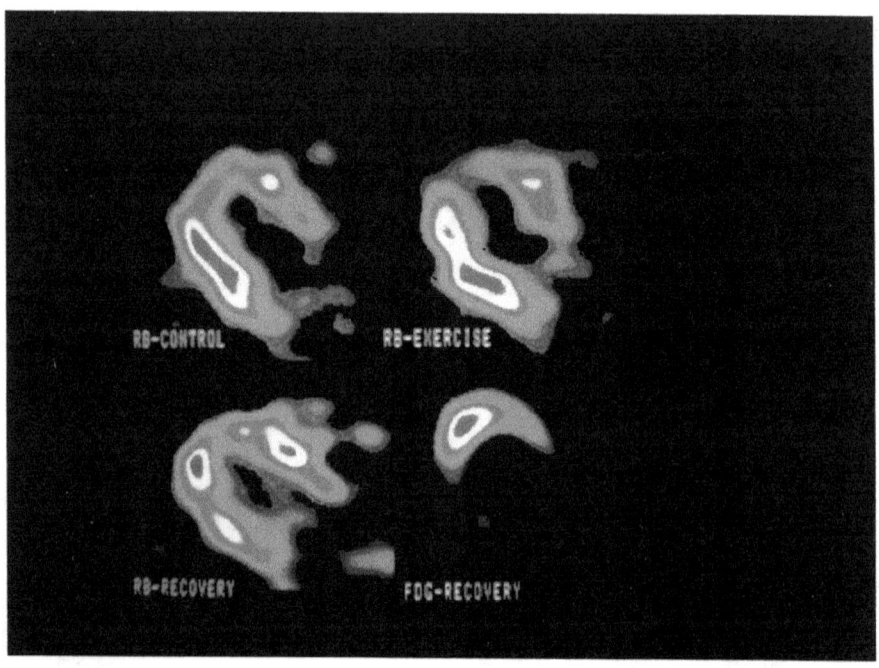

For text see page 823

For text see page 824

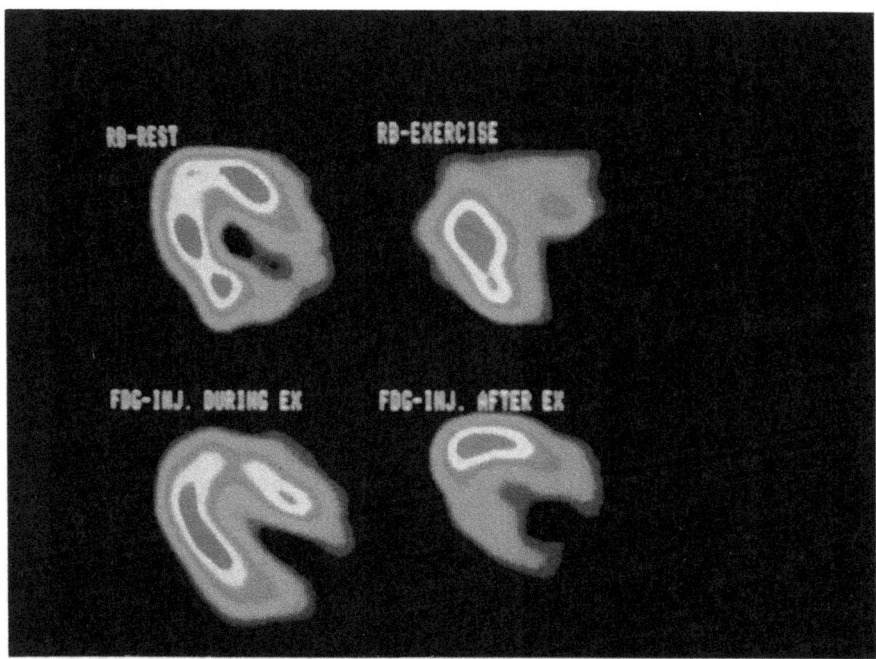

For text see page 825

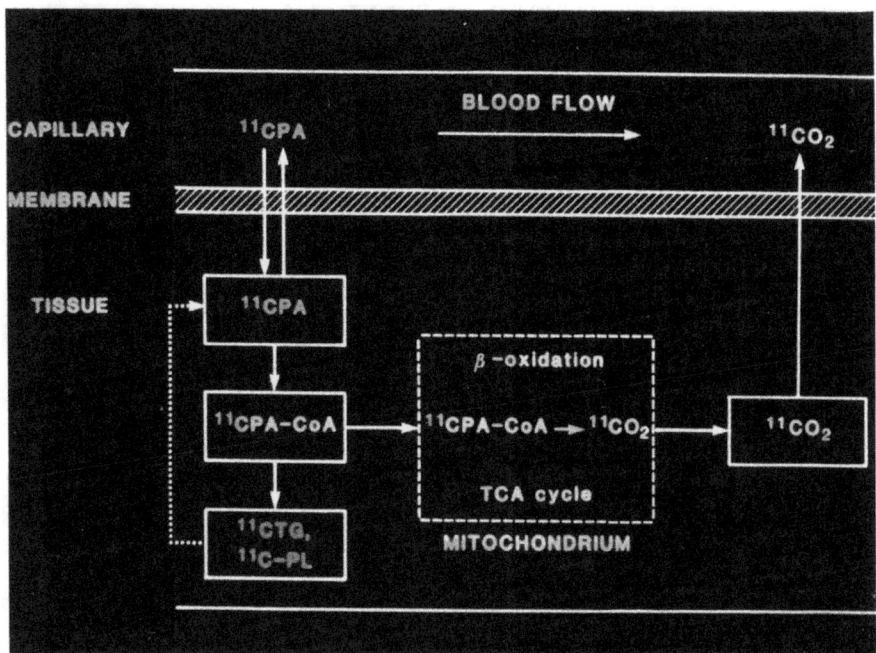

For text see page 826

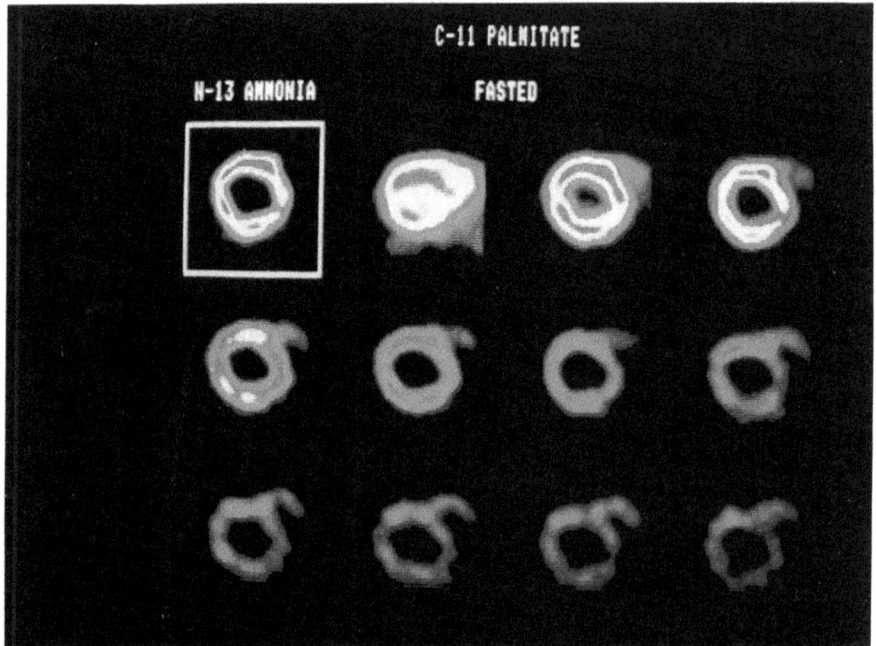

For text see page 827

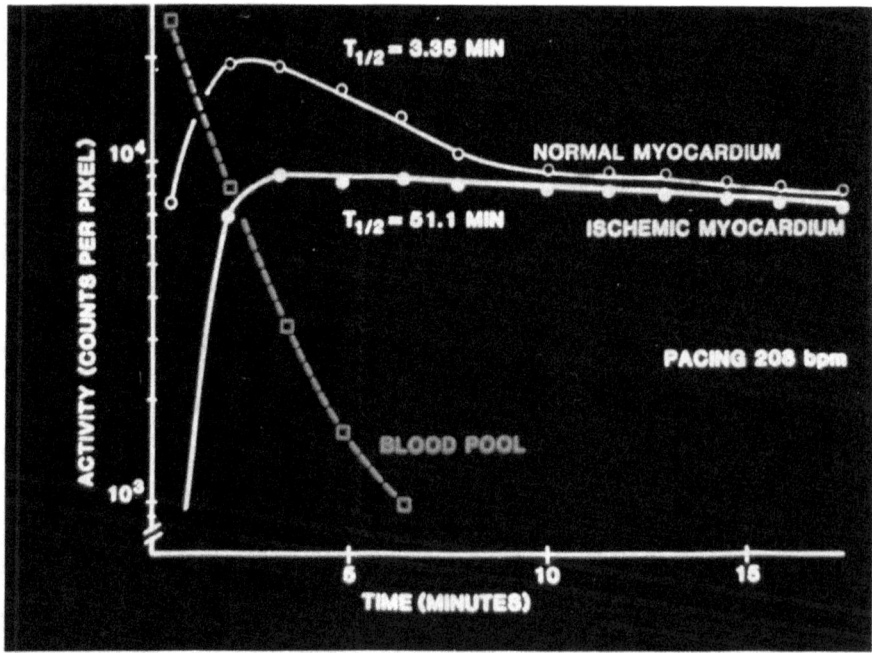

For text see page 828

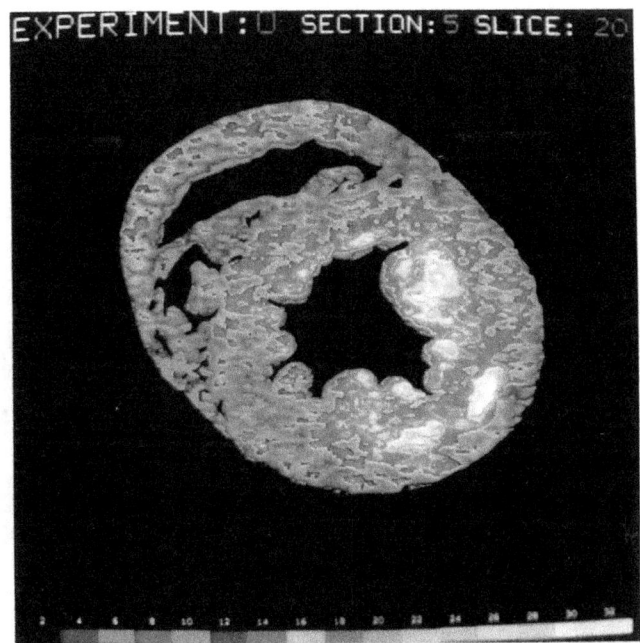

For text see page 848

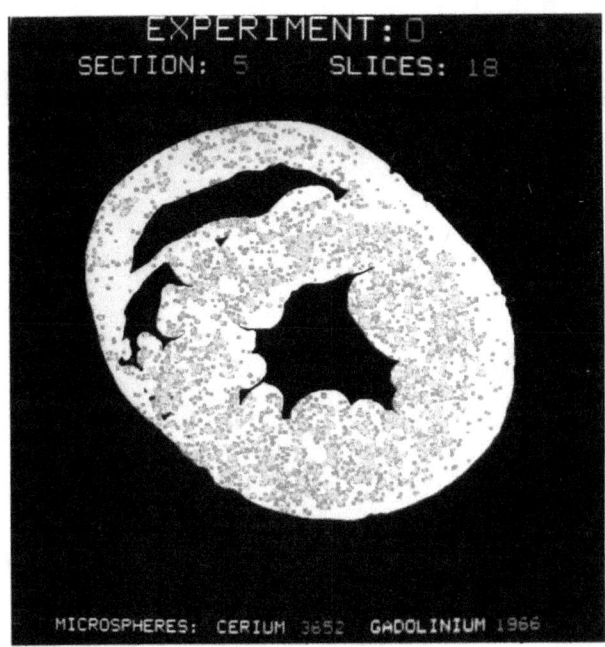

For text see page 849

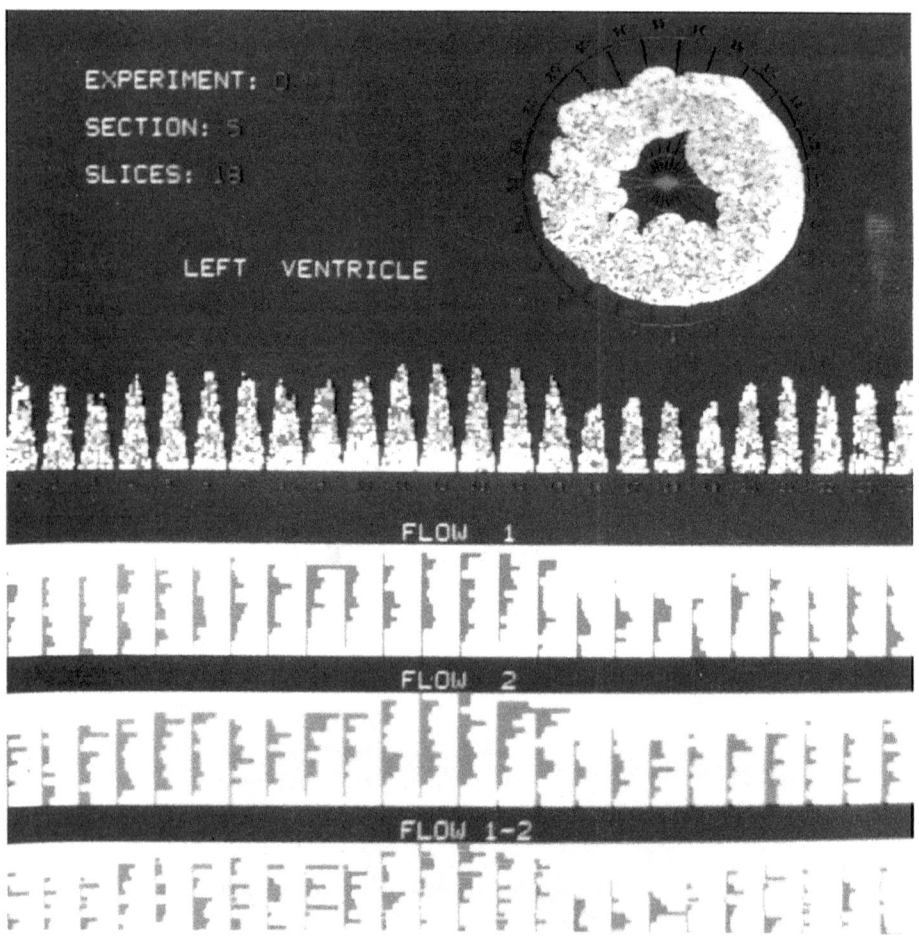

For text see page 850

GPSR Compliance

The European Union's (EU) General Product Safety Regulation (GPSR) is a set of rules that requires consumer products to be safe and our obligations to ensure this.

If you have any concerns about our products, you can contact us on

ProductSafety@springernature.com

In case Publisher is established outside the EU, the EU authorized representative is:

Springer Nature Customer Service Center GmbH
Europaplatz 3
69115 Heidelberg, Germany

www.ingramcontent.com/pod-product-compliance
Lightning Source LLC
LaVergne TN
LVHW021949060625
813236LV00001B/2